# PSYCHIATRIC-MENTAL HEALTH NURSING

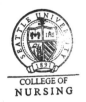

COLLEGE OF
NURSING

**JEFFREY S. JONES, DNP, PMHCNS, BC, LNC,** is a board certified psychiatric clinical nurse specialist, board certified sex therapist, legal nurse consultant, and entrepreneur. He is president and owner of Pinnacle Mental Health Associates, Inc., in Mansfield, Ohio. He received his doctorate from Case Western Reserve University in Cleveland, Ohio, and is currently fulltime visiting faculty at The University of Akron in Akron, Ohio. He was a contributing author on the role of the CNS in private practice in *Foundations of Clinical Nurse Specialist Practice* (Springer, 2009). He has served on the Richland County Mental Health Board, the Ohio Board of Nursing Standards and Practice Committee, and as a content expert on psychiatric nursing for the American Nurses Credentialing Center. Dr. Jones has provided service to the mentally ill in hospital settings, out-patient clinics, prisons, and in private practice.

**JOYCE J. FITZPATRICK, PhD, MBA, RN, FAAN,** is the Elizabeth Brooks Ford Professor of Nursing, Frances Payne Bolton School of Nursing at Case Western Reserve University in Cleveland, Ohio, where she was Dean from 1982 through 1997. She has received numerous honors and awards including the *American Journal of Nursing* Book of the Year Award 18 times. Dr. Fitzpatrick is widely published in nursing and health care literature, and is senior editor for Springer's revived Nursing Leadership and Management Series. Her most recent Springer books are *The Doctor of Nursing Practice and Clinical Nurse Leader: Essentials of Program Development and Implementation for Clinical Practice* and *Giving Through Teaching: How Nurse Educators Are Changing the World.*

**VICKIE L. ROGERS, DNP, RN,** is an Assistant Professor at the University of Southern Mississippi where she teaches in the undergraduate and graduate nursing programs. She received a Doctor of Nursing Practice from Case Western Reserve University, Cleveland, Ohio, and a MS and BS in Nursing from the University of Southern Mississippi. Dr. Rogers has previously held faculty appointments at various schools of nursing in Mississippi and Connecticut. Additionally, Dr. Rogers has international teaching experience in the Caribbean. She is a contributing author of a chapter in the book, *Giving Through Teaching: How Nurse Educators Are Changing the World.* She has worked in psychiatric clinical nurse specialist and management roles in the past. Research interests include the use of the Internet as a format to provide individual therapy to young adults. Dr. Rogers has presented her work internationally, and has published on this topic.

# PSYCHIATRIC-MENTAL HEALTH NURSING

## An Interpersonal Approach

**Jeffrey S. Jones,** DNP, PMHCNS, BC, LNC
**Joyce J. Fitzpatrick,** PhD, MBA, RN, FAAN
**Vickie L. Rogers,** DNP, RN

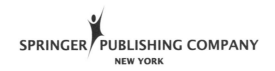

SPRINGER PUBLISHING COMPANY
NEW YORK

Springer Publishing Company, LLC
11 West 42nd Street
New York, NY 10036
www.springerpub.com

*Acquisitions Editor:* Allan Graubard
*Composition:* Newgen Imaging

ISBN: 978-0-8261-0563-9
E-book ISBN: 978-0-8261-0564-6
Student's Guide: 978-0-8261-7084-2 (Available at springerpub.com/Jones)
Drug Monographs: Available at springerpub.com/JonesDrugMonographs
Instructor's Companion: 978-0-8261-7083-5 (Available by contacting textbook@springerpub.com)

12 13 14 15/ 5 4 3 2

**Library of Congress Cataloging-in-Publication Data**
Jones, Jeffrey S. (Jeffrey Schwab)
  Psychiatric-mental health nursing : an interpersonal approach to professional practice / Jeffrey S. Jones, Joyce J. Fitzpatrick, Vickie L. Rogers.
      p. ; cm.
  Includes bibliographical references and index.
  ISBN 978-0-8261-0563-9 — ISBN 978-0-8261-0564-6 (e-book)
  I. Fitzpatrick, Joyce J., 1944- II. Rogers, Vickie L. III. Title.
  [DNLM: 1. Psychiatric Nursing. 2. Mental Disorders—nursing. 3. Nurse-Patient Relations. WY 160]
  LC classification not assigned
  616.89'0231—dc23                                                                 2012005583

Special discounts on bulk quantities of our books are available to corporations, professional associations, pharmaceutical companies, health care organizations, and other qualifying groups.

If you are interested in a custom book, including chapters from more than one of our titles, we can provide that service as well.

**For details, please contact:**
Special Sales Department, Springer Publishing Company, LLC
11 West 42nd Street, 15th Floor, New York, NY 10036–8002s
Phone: 877–687-7476 or 212–431-4370; Fax: 212–941-7842
Email: sales@springerpub.com

Printed in the United States of America by Bradford & Bigelow.

This book is dedicated to
Hildegard Peplau and Joyce Travelbee.

Their models in structuring the practice of psychiatric nursing
from an interpersonal/relationship-based perspective are
timeless, relevant, and invaluable.
We are pleased to honor their legacy with this text
so that new generations of nurses can be inspired
and guided by their pioneering work.

**Carolyn A. Baird, DNP, MBA, RN-BC, CARN-AP, ICCDPD**
Waynesburg University
Waynesburg, PA

**Audrey Marie Beauvais, DNP, MBA, RN-BC**
Sacred Heart University
Fairfield, CT

**Katherine R. Casale, MS, RN**
Bridgeport Hospital School of Nursing
Bridgeport, CT

**Angela S. Chesser, PhD, RN, PMHCNS-BC**
The Ohio State University Medical Center
Columbus, OH

**E. J. Ernst, DNP, MBA, APRN, FNP-BC, CEN**
California State University Dominguez Hills
Carson, California

**Joyce J. Fitzpatrick, PhD, MBA, RN, FAAN**
Case Western Reserve University
Cleveland, OH

**Loraine Fleming, MA, APRN, PMHNP-BC**
Hawaii Pacific University
Honolulu, HI

**Patricia Ann Galon, PhD, PMHCNS-BC**
The University of Akron
Akron, OH

**Marianne Goldyn, MSN, PMHCNS-BC**
Community Support Services, Inc.
Akron, OH

**Vicki P. Hines-Martin, PhD, CNS, RN, FAAN**
University of Louisville
Louisville, KY

**Áine Horgan, RPN, BNS, MSc**
University College Cork
Cork, Ireland

**Emily K. Johnson, DNP, PMHNP-BC, RN**
Mayo Clinic
Rochester, MN

**Jeffrey S. Jones, DNP, PMHCNS-BC, LNC**
Pinnacle Mental Health Associates, Inc.
Mansfield, OH

**Betty Jane Kohal, DNP, PMHCNS-BC**
Cumberland University
Lebanon, TN

**Melanie S. Lint, MSN, PMHCNS-BC**
New Horizons Youth & Family Center
Lancaster, OH

**Patricia Smythe Matos, DNP, RN**
Mount Sinai Medical Center
New York, NY

# CONTRIBUTORS

**Declan McCarthy, MA HDip (Integ. Psychother.), RPN**
South Lee Mental Health Services
Cork, Ireland

**Geraldine McCarthy, RGN, RNT, MEd, MSN, PhD**
University College Cork
Cork, Ireland

**Kimberly S. McClane, RN, MBA, PhD**
International University of Nursing
St. Kitts, West Indies

**Lori A. Neushotz, DNP, PMHCNS-BC, NPP, CASAC**
Private practice
New York, NY

**James O'Mahony, MSc, PgDip Cog Psych, BSc, RPN**
North Lee Mental Health Services
Cork, Ireland

**Patti Hart O'Regan, DNP, ARNP, ANP-C, PMHNP-BC, LMHC**
Village Health, LLC
Port Richey, FL

**Kathleen L. Patusky, MA, PhD, RN, CNS**
University of Medicine and Dentistry of New Jersey
School of Nursing
Newark, NJ

**Patrice Ellen Rancour, MS, RN, PMHCNS-BC,**
The Ohio Sate University Medical Center
Columbus, OH

**Vickie L. Rogers, DNP, RN**
University of Southern Mississippi
Hattiesburg, MS

**Shirley A. Smoyak, PhD, MPhil, MS**
Rutgers University
New Brunswick, NJ

**John F. Sweeney, PhD, MSc DipANS, RNID, RPN, RNT, CNT T.Nur**
University College Cork
Cork, Ireland

**Amanda Alisa Townsend DNP, APRN, FNP-C**
Gulf Coast Mental Health Center
Gulfport, MS

**Kathleen Tusaie, PhD, PMHCNS-BC**
The University of Akron
Akron, OH

**Mark P. Tyrrell, RGN, RPN, RNT, BNS, Med**
University College Cork
Cork, Ireland

# Psychiatric-Mental Health Nursing

*Psychiatric-Mental Health Nursing: An Interpersonal Approach* uniquely focuses on interpersonal relationships as the foundation for therapeutic practice in psychiatric nursing. The book satisfies the most current competencies.

**Student Materials** include a handy per-chapter review guide with a glossary, summaries of Learning Objectives and Need to Know sections from each chapter, 2 to 6 hyperlinks to online videos or commercial films illustrating content, and care planning practice exercises.

**Faculty Materials** include the same features PLUS additional films and videos (with brief descriptions), answers and rationales to NCLEX questions, and responses for the How Would You Respond? case scenarios.

# Chapter Feature Boxes:

### CHAPTER CONTENTS

Historical Perspectives

Epidemiology

Diagnostic Criteria

Etiology

Treatment Options

Applying the Nursing Process from an Interpersonal Perspective

### EXPECTED LEARNING OUTCOMES

**After completing this chapter, the student will be able to:**

1. Define anxiety
2. Identify the disorders classified as anxiety disorders
3. Describe the historical perspectives and epidemiology associated with anxiety disorders
4. Discuss current scientific theories related to the etiology of anxiety disorders, including relevant psychodynamic and neurobiological influences
5. Distinguish among the diagnostic criteria for anxiety disorders as outlined in the *Diagnostic and Statistical Manual of Mental Disorders, 4th edition, Text revision (DSM-IV-TR)*

**EXPECTED LEARNING Outcomes** lists what the reader will be able to do after completing a chapter.

**DIAGNOSTIC CRITERIA** lists the key symptoms of a disorder for consideration when making a diagnosis. Features DSM-IV and NANDA-I guidelines.

---

**BOX 12-1: DIAGNOSTIC CRITERIA**

MAJOR DEPRESSIVE DISORDER

In addition to the depressed mood or loss of interest or pleasure in usual activities, at least four of the following must be present:

- Significant weight loss without dieting or weight gain or markedly decreased or increased appetite
- Hypersomnia or insomnia
- Psychomotor agitation or slowness
- Fatigue or energy loss
- Feelings of worthlessness or guilt
- Difficulty concentrating or indecisiveness
- Recurrent thoughts of death, either with or without suicide ideation
- Symptoms cause significant distress or impair social, occupational, educational, or other functioning
- Symptoms are not caused by a substance or a general medical condition.

DYSTHYMIC DISORDER

In addition to the individual's chronic depressive symptoms, the individual has never been with

## PLAN OF CARE 13-1:
### THE PATIENT WITH AN ANXIETY DISORDER (WITH PANIC) AND OBSESSIVE COMPULSIVE DISORDER

NURSING DIAGNOSIS: Anxiety (*severe*); related to exposure to traumatic event; manifested by perceived threats and recurrent panic attacks. Ineffective coping; related to anxiety of perceived need to check and re-check things; manifested by participation in repeated ritualistic behavior to reduce anxiety.

Patient will demonstrate participation in fewer ritualistic behaviors with an improved level of independent function.

| INTERVENTION | RATIONALE |
|---|---|
| Assess the level of the patient's anxiety; stay with the patient and provide for safety and security | Determining the level of the patient's anxiety provides a baseline from which to intervene |
| Maintain a calm, reassuring approach; keep verbal exchanges short and direct | Maintaining a calm, reassuring approach prevents adding to the patient's anxiety Keeping exchanges short and direct redu~ |

**PLAN OF CARE** offers interventions for a specific nursing diagnosis and includes the rationales for the interventions.

## HOW WOULD YOU RESPOND? 12-1:
### A PATIENT WITH DEPRESSION AND SUICIDAL THOUGHTS

Carol is a 24-year-old female being admitted to the acute care psychiatric unit. She has been diagnosed with Bipolar I disorder. Carol has no medical conditions or illnesses. During the nursing assessment, Carol states she was treated for Bipolar I disorder when she was 18 but did not require hospitalization. Carol was prescribed lithium but stopped taking it about a year ago. She reports that she recently moved to the city to teach secondary school, has a limited support system, and lives alone. Approximately three weeks ago, she experienced a burst of energy and wasn't able to sleep for several days.

She states she then started feeling sad, worthless, hopeless, lonely, and guilt about leaving her parent's home. Carol has a blunted affect, unkempt, and her clothes are dirty. She frequently bursts into tears during her intake. Carol has lost 11 pounds over the past two weeks, has no appetite, and difficulty sleeping. She has missed several days of work this past week due to her not having the "energy to get out of bed." Carol admits to recurrent thoughts of hanging herself but is afraid if she commits suicide she will "go to hell." You are assigned to provide care to Carol.

### CRITICAL THINKING QUESTIONS
*1. How would you describe what Carol is experiencing?*

**HOW WOULD YOU RESPOND?** presents case scenarios followed by critical thinking questions.

## THERAPEUTIC INTERACTION 13-1:
### INTERVENTIONS FOR OCD

Ms. Cox is admitted to an inpatient psychiatric unit for obsessive thoughts that her hands are dirty and compulsive hand washing. The compulsive hand washing has resulted in skin breakdown and impaired social and professional functioning.

| | |
|---|---|
| The nurse enters the patient's room and finds Ms. Cox sitting on her hands on her bed, rocking back and forth. The nurse gains permission to come in and sit down across from the patient. The nurse maintains a calm, pleasant demeanor and speaks in a slow, simple manner. | Showing respect strengthens the bond between the nurse and the patient and is a predictor of a successful intervention. Moving slowly and staying calm minimizes the potential for an increase in anxiety. |
| **Nurse:** "Ms. Cox, you appear anxious. I would like to show you a way to help you relax." | Provides reassurance that you are there to empower the patient to learn a way to decrease her anxiety level. |
| **Ms. Cox:** "Please, I need some help here. I'm trying not to obsess about my hands but I can't stop." | |

**Therapeutic Interaction** provides an exemplar therapeutic dialogue between nurse and patient with rationales for the nurse's interaction methods.

**(Continued)**

**Patient and Family Education** offers tips and guidelines to help the patient and family manage a disorder.

**Consumer Perspective** gives a first-hand account of what it's like to live with a particular disorder.

**Evidence-Based Practice** offers a relevant study, with study summary and outcome, applications to practice, and questions to ponder.

**Drug Summary** lists the common drugs used in the treatment of a disorder and their implications for nursing care. Expanded drug monographs are available for reference.

**DRUG SUMMARY 13-1:**
**AGENTS USED FOR ANXIETY DISORDERS\***

| DRUGS | IMPLICATIONS FOR NURSING CARE |
|---|---|
| **BENZODIAZAPINES** | |
| aprazolam (Xanax)<br>clonazepam (Klonopin)<br>diazepam (Valium)<br>lorazepam (Ativan) | • Institute safety precautions to prevent injury secondary to sedative effects of the drug; warn the patient of these effects including decreased response time, slowed reflexes<br><br>• Encourage the patient to change positions slowly to minimize the effect of orthostatic hypotension<br><br>• Teach the patient that the full effects of the drug may not be noted for several weeks. Work with the patient to use other methods such as guided imagery and progressive relaxation to assist in relieving anxiety until drug reaches its therapeutic effectiveness<br><br>• Counsel the patient that one or more agents may need to be tried to determine the most effective drug |

**SUMMARY POINTS**

• Anxiety disorders include panic disorder, obsessive-compulsive disorder (OCD), posttraumatic stress disorder (PTSD), generalized anxiety disorder (GAD), acute stress disorder, and phobias. Anxiety disorders were not officially recognized as a psychiatric illness until 1980. They are the most common and most costly psychiatric illness in the United States.

• The exact cause of anxiety disorders is not known. Psychodynamic, behavioral, and learning theories are prominent. Additionally, biological influences, including brain structures, neurotransmitters, and

monoamine oxidase inhibitors (MAOIs); beta blocker propranolol; and anticonvulsants such as lamotrigine or topiramate.

• Individual psychotherapy involves a combination of supportive and insight-oriented therapy which is helpful for patients with PTSD. Eye movement desensitization and reprocessing (EMDR) is a new type of psychotherapy gaining popularity for treating PTSD. Cognitive behavioral therapy is considered the first line treatment strategy for patients with depression and anxiety disorders. Flooding or implosion therapy is a type of exposure therapy in which the

**Summary Points** gives key takeaways from each chapter.

**NCLEX-Prep** questions at the end of each chapter evaluate the reader's comprehension and help predict performance on related questions in an NCLEX exam.

**NCLEX-PREP**

1. A patient with PTSD is exhibiting hypervigilance. Which statement would the nurse interpret as indicating this?
   a. "I'm having trouble sleeping at night."
   b. "I've been really irritable and angry."
   c. "I always have to watch my back."
   d. "I just can't seem to relax."

2. A group of nursing students is reviewing information about anxiety disorders. The students demonstrate a need for additional study when they identify which of the following as a compulsion?
   a. Hearing voices that tell a person he is the king
   b. Repeat...

   c. Acute stress disorder
   d. Specific phobia

4. A patient with panic disorder is prescribed venlafaxine. The nurse identifies this agent as which of the following?
   a. Selective serotonin reuptake inhibitor (SSRI)
   b. Serotonin/norepinephrine reuptake inhibitor (SNRI)
   c. Benzodiazepine
   d. Atypical antipsychotic

5. A nursing instructor is preparing a class on anxiety disorders and the biological influences associated with this group of illnes...

---

• Boxes in each chapter elucidate and elaborate on chapter content.
• Cumulative NCLEX review, NANDA-I guidelines, and full glossary at the end of the book.

# CONTENTS

There is an old saying: "What goes around comes around." This textbook returns to life the promise of Hildegard Peplau's pioneering work. When Peplau wrote *Interpersonal Relations in Nursing* in 1952, she was clear that the relationship between the nurse and the patient was the core of all nursing practice. In that book she demonstrated the key elements of that practice. Herein were also the roots of all specialty practice in psychiatric-mental health nursing. Some years after she published her work, I once asked Peplau if she had ever considered revising and publishing a new edition. Her answer was direct and to the point. She said that if and when there was something new to be added she might consider it but nothing had appeared on the horizon to contradict the material presented in the book. She went on to say that if the concepts and ideas presented in the book had merit, they would still be relevant even after 50 years. And she was right, of course; they still have merit. In this textbook, the editors and contributors have eloquently and persuasively rendered much of the wisdom found in the 1952 book. They also use the complementary work of Joyce Travelbee who, in the same time period, pursued very similar ideas to those of Peplau.

I have been a nurse for more than 50 years. I have witnessed the shifting sands of my profession as it follows fads and trends. For us in psychiatric nursing, we have typically followed the trends in psychiatry. So, in the late 1960s when what was thought to be the "magic bullet" for the treatment of serious mental illness was discovered with the advent of thorazine and the subsequent explosion of interest in and demand for psychotropic drugs, nursing followed. Then, when the "decade of the brain" was announced in the 1990s, nursing followed. Now, when current research informing best practices suggests that "talk therapies" are equal to and often have better outcomes than biophysical regimens, nursing is rediscovering its power, precisely in the practice of the relationships that help and heal.

This textbook is a major step in that direction. The editors and contributors are to be congratulated for their clear effort to bring some degree of correction to the singular emphasis on pharmacotherapy found in many advanced practice work roles as well as in general psychiatric care. While it is clear that pharmacotherapy has a role to play in treatment, it is equally clear that the use of relationships as therapy has an equal if not more important

# FOREWORD

role to play. It is this point that this text makes in compelling fashion.

However, a word of caution to the reader is in order on this point. One should not try too hard to impose phases on the nurse-patient relationship as Peplau described. The stages may merge and overlap and often may take place over a short interval of time, or they may take place over an extended period, in which case they are usually more easily discernable. What was most important was that the nurse and the patient began as strangers and would be engaged for a time-limited period, and that the limits inherent in their engagement should be understood by both the nurse and the patient.

There are several other features of this text that commend it to the student and to the nurse seeking a review or refresher. First, the authors have done an excellent job in noting historical context. Understanding where and how these ideas and practices have had their origins allows the reader to appreciate the growth and development of information. Information when tested in practice/experience leads to knowledge. Hopefully, it also encourages the idea that there is more to know as well as to appreciate in the developmental nature of information.

Second, the authors have made extensive use of the current research literature and have well used the nursing research literature. The embedded web links will allow the reader to easily explore the treasure trove to be found inside the wonderful world of the internet.

In short, I would wish that this text, your experience, the teachers who will guide that experience, and the excellent role models that you will undoubtedly meet in your experience will give you an appreciation for the rewards of practicing in this field. If not that, I am certain that the knowledge gained from these experiences will be a central part of your practice in all other areas of nursing. I am often asked what is the one thing I would say about my many years of experience. My reply is always the same, "I have never been bored, not even for a minute!"

May you too never be bored and may you have fun with the challenges!

*Grayce M. Sills, PhD, RN, FAAN*
Emeritus Professor
College of Nursing
Ohio State University

This textbook is the result of our belief in the need to reaffirm and strengthen interpersonal relationships as the core component of psychiatric-mental health nursing practice. Throughout the book we have used the interpersonal theories of Hildegard Peplau and Joyce Travelbee so that the student can develop an understanding of the nature of the nurse-client relationship in the care of persons with psychiatric illnesses. Prevailing curricular guidelines were used in the text's construction; thus, the book is divided into six key areas of foci.

**SECTION I: THE PRACTICE OF PSYCHIATRIC-MENTAL HEALTH NURSING** lays the groundwork for understanding the history and nature of this specialty area. The theories of Peplau and Travelbee are introduced in the early chapters. Additional chapters in this section focus on therapeutic use of self and boundary management in nursing practice. **SECTION II: HEALTH PROMOTION AND ILLNESS PREVENTION** continues to build the fundamental skill sets by presentation of topics such as critical thinking, clinical decision making, and counseling interventions. Crisis intervention and the case management role are also discussed. System and group dynamics

are emphasized as key to understanding various mental health treatment modalities. This section also provides an overview of theories of mental health disorders, information about known risk factors for select illnesses, and related nursing interventions.

**SECTION III: ACUTE AND CHRONIC ILLNESS** provides detailed discussion of the most common psychiatric disorders utilizing the *Diagnostic and Statistical Manual of Mental Disorders, 4th Edition, Text Revision (DSM-IV)* to describe criteria and enrich understanding. This section also includes important content related to mental health care of the medically ill person. Key to this section and unique to this book is the integration and application of the Peplau/Travelbee theories to the four step Assessment, Planning/Diagnosing, Implementation, and Evaluation (APIE) nursing process. The North American Nursing Diagnosis Association (NANDA 2009–2011) approved diagnoses are utilized in examples for care planning practice. Case study questions augment the chapter's content with reflective questions both in the text and in the student and instructor companions. **SECTION IV: GROWTH AND DEVELOPMENT AND MENTAL HEALTH CONCERNS ACROSS**

**THE LIFE SPAN** covers essential nursing concerns related to care for children, adolescents, the elderly, and victims of abuse. **SECTION V: MENTAL HEALTH CARE SETTINGS** details psychiatric nursing across the continuum of care with special content on vulnerable populations and alternate settings and roles for the psychiatric-mental health nurse. **SECTION VI: CULTURAL, ETHICAL, LEGAL, AND PROFESSIONAL ASPECTS OF MENTAL HEALTH CARE** covers integral aspects to providing competent care from a culturally sensitive perspective. Essential ethical and legal components are delineated for safe practice. Prevailing curricular guidelines for psychiatric-mental health nursing education are discussed.

The text contains features such as NCLEX preparation questions, clinical scenarios with "how would you respond?" questions, and consumer perspectives describing what it is like to live with a specific illness. Also included are evidence-based practice summaries from the psychiatric-mental health nursing literature and related research literature. Two student companions are available: the Student's Guide is available at springerpub.com/ Jones and drug monographs are available at springerpub. com/JonesDrugMonographs. The Student Guide contains carefully selected hyperlinks that complement and augment the chapters' themes, supplemental case study questions and answers, and review of key terms. The Instructor's Companion (available via textbook@ springerpub.com) expands upon the Student Guide and also contains PowerPoint highlights of each chapter and recommended films to further illustrate major diagnostic concepts.

This book will assist the beginning professional nurse in the development of knowledge of the interpersonal relationship, the importance of self-reflection and discovery, and in acquiring the skill to use these processes to assist patients in their journey toward mental health. The role of the professional psychiatric nurse and the power to heal an individual's suffering from mental illness from an interpersonal relationship perspective remains timeless and relevant. This textbook intentionally guides curricula toward interpersonal relationships in nursing as being the key fundamental practice skill set in psychiatric-mental health nursing, and thus serves as a testimony to the original architects of relationship-based care.

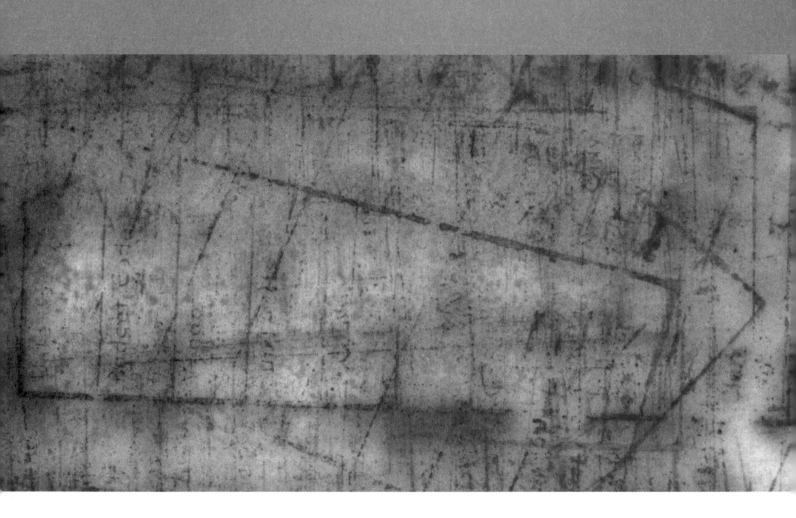

## CHAPTER CONTENTS

## CHAPTER 1
# MENTAL HEALTH TRENDS AND THE HISTORICAL ROLE OF THE PSYCHIATRIC-MENTAL HEALTH NURSE

Joyce J. Fitzpatrick

Jeffrey S. Jones

## EXPECTED LEARNING OUTCOMES

**After completing this chapter, the student will be able to:**

1. Identify key events that helped to shape the current view of psychiatric-mental health care.

2. Describe the early role of the psychiatric nurse.

3. Identify the changes in the field of mental health that correlate with the evolution of psychiatric-mental health nursing.

4. Define interpersonal relationships as being the foundation for clinical practice.

5. Delineate between the roles and functions of basic and advanced practice in psychiatric-mental health nursing.

## KEY TERMS

Deinstitutionalization

Interpersonal models

Milieu management

Process groups

Psychopharmacology

Psycho-educational groups

Somatic

Therapeutic communication

Professional nursing originated from the work of a visionary leader, Florence Nightingale, who identified a need to organize the profession into a respectable discipline with its own body of knowledge and practice skill sets. As professional nursing evolved, so too did the practice of psychiatric-mental health nursing. This evolution paralleled the development in the field of mental health care. Subsequently, mental health care and psychiatric-mental health nursing practice have evolved from a poorly understood and poorly organized area of concern to a highly specialized area of health care.

This chapter provides an overview of the key historical events associated with the evolution of mental health care and their influences on psychiatric-mental health nursing. It also describes the current status of psychiatric-mental health nursing, focusing on the scope of practice for the two levels of psychiatric-mental health nursing practice: basic and advanced. This chapter emphasizes the interpersonal models of practice as the standard of care across the full range of settings and client groups. Relationships, interactions, and environment are important components of these models. This focus was selected to enhance this crucial element of nursing practice, the nurse-patient relationship, and, in particular, to establish interpersonal relations as the cornerstone of psychiatric-mental health nursing practice to assist patients in meeting their needs.

## HISTORICAL OVERVIEW OF MENTAL HEALTH AND MENTAL ILLNESS CARE

History reveals that mental illness has been around since the beginning of time. However, it was not until the late eighteenth century when the view of mental illness became that of a disease requiring treatment and humane care. Overall, the views of mental health and mental illness closely reflect the sociocultural climate of the time.

### The Earliest Years

Mental illness is a complex experience, with different values and meanings worldwide. While some cultures considered mental illness in a negative light, attributing it to possession by spirits or demons, other cultures considered mental illness somewhat differently, even as an exceptional state; one that would prepare that person to become a healer as, for example, in shamanism. However classified or viewed, the complexity of mental illness has prompted treatment, from ridding the person of spirits or demons to enabling the person to explore the possibility that he or she is a potential healer. For the former, magical therapies such as charms, spells, sacrifices, and exorcisms were used. For the latter, various initiation rituals were used.

In the West, however, the prevailing view of mental illness involved possession. A person who exhibited an odd or different kind of behavior without identifiable physical injury or illness was seen as possessed, specifically by an evil spirit or demon and the patient's behavior was the result of this state of possession. In response, treatments such as magical therapies were commonplace. Physical treatments such as bleeding, blistering, and surgically cutting into the skull to release the spirit also were done. If the patient was not disruptive, he or she could remain in the community. However, if the patient's behavior was violent or severe, the patient often was ostracized and driven from the community.

During the Middle Ages and the Renaissance period, the view of mental illness as demonic possession continued. Witch hunts and exorcisms were common. In addition, the strong religious influences at that time led to the belief that mental illness was a punishment for wrong doings. Persons with mental illness were inhumanely treated, being placed in dungeons or jails and beaten.

### The Eighteenth and Nineteenth Centuries

The early to middle eighteenth century laid the groundwork for future developments in the latter half of this century and the next, especially in the United States. Society was beginning to recognize the need for humane treatment, which led to a gradual reshaping of the view of mental illness. Treatment, rather than punishment, exorcisms, and magical therapies, was becoming the focus. During this time, public and private asylums, buildings specially constructed to house persons with mental illness, were developed. Individuals with mental illness were removed from their homes and placed in these institutions.

This need for treatment prompted the development of institutions where care could be provided. For example, in 1751, Benjamin Franklin established Pennsylvania Hospital in Philadelphia. This was the first institution in the United States to provide treatment and care for individuals with mental illness. As the late eighteenth century approached, medicine began to view psychiatry as a separate branch. At the time, mental illness embraced only such medical interventions as bloodletting, immobilization, and specialized devices such as the tranquilizer chair both in the United States and abroad. These practices continued until the very late eighteenth and early nineteenth centuries. Through the work of Dr. Benjamin Rush in the United States, the focus of treatment began to shift to supportive, sympathetic care in an environment that was quiet, clean, and pleasant. Although humane, this care was primarily custodial in nature. Moreover, individual states were required to undertake financial responsibility for the care of people with mental illnesses, the first example of government-supported mental health care.

A key player in the evolution of mental health and mental illness care during the nineteenth century was Dorothea Dix. A retired school teacher, Dix was asked to teach a Sunday school class for young women who were incarcerated. During her classes, she witnessed the deplorable conditions at the facility. In addition, she observed the inhumane treatment of the women with mental illness. As a result, she began a crusade to improve the conditions. She worked tirelessly for care reform, advocating for the needs of the mentally ill through the establishment of state hospitals throughout the United States (Mental Health America, 2009). Unfortunately, these state institutions became overcrowded, providing only minimal custodial care. Although she was a nurse, her impact on the evolution of mental health and mental illness may be overlooked because her work was primarily humanitarian.

> *Dorothea Dix was instrumental in advocating for the mentally ill. She is credited with the development of state mental hospitals in the United States.*

## The Twentieth Century

The twentieth century ushered in a new era about mental health and illness. Scientific thought was coming to the forefront. In the beginning of the 1900s, two schools of thought about mental illness were prevalent in the United States and Europe. One school viewed mental illness as a result of environmental and social deprivation that could be treated by measures such as kindness, lack of restraints, and mental hygiene. The other viewed mental illness as a result of a biologic cause treatable with physical measures such as bloodletting and devices. This gap in thinking—deprivation on one end of the spectrum and biologic causes on the other end—led to the development of several different theories attempting to explain the cause of mental illness.

One such theory was the psychoanalytic theory developed by Sigmund Freud. His theory focused on a person's unconscious motivations for behaviors, which then influenced a person's personality development. Freud, a neuropathologist, examined a person's feelings and emotions about his or her past childhood and adolescent experiences as a means for explaining the person's behavior. According to Freud, an individual develops through a series of five stages: oral, anal, phallic/oedipal, latency, and genital. He considered the first three of these five stages (oral, anal, and phallic) to be the most important. If the person experiences a disruption in any of these stages, experiences difficulty in moving from one stage to the next, remains in one stage, or goes back to a previous stage, then that individual will develop a mental illness. Freud's views became the mainstay of mental health and mental illness care for several decades.

The development of **PSYCHOPHARMACOLOGY**, the use of drugs to treat mental illness and its symptoms, also revolutionized treatment for mental illness. The control of symptoms through the use of drugs allowed many individuals to be discharged from institutions and return to the community where they could live and function. Subsequently, the numbers of persons requiring hospitalization dramatically decreased. Moreover, psychopharmacology provided a lead-in to the future for deinstitutionalization and for addressing the underlying biologic basis for mental illness.

Research into the causes or factors associated with mental illness exploded during the 1990s, which became known as the "the decade of the brain." Information about neurotransmitters and their role in influencing mental illnesses grew. New medications were developed from a greater understanding of how medications could regulate neurotransmitter reuptake. This era led to a major shift away from therapy as the main psychiatric treatment to one involving medical-somatic options as first line intervention.

### Governmental Involvement and Legislation

Governmental involvement in mental health care took on an expanded role during the twentieth century. In the United States at the time of World War II, individuals were rejected for military service due to psychological problems. Additionally, those returning from combat often were diagnosed with emotional or psychological problems secondary to the effects of the war. The view that anyone could develop a mental illness was beginning to take root. As a result, the National Mental Health Act was passed in 1946. This act provided governmental funding for programs related to research, mental health professional training, and expansion of facilities including state mental health facilities, clinics, and treatment centers. It also called for the establishment of a National Advisory Mental Health Council and a National Institute of Mental Health (NIMH), which was formally established in 1949. NIMH focused its activities on research and training in mental health and illness.

In 1955, the Mental Health Study Act was passed, which called for a thorough analysis of mental health issues in the nation. This resulted in a Joint Commission on Mental Illness and Health which prepared a major report titled "Action for Mental Health." The report established a need for expanded research and training for personnel, an increase in the number of full-time clinics as well as supplemental services, and enhanced access to emergency care and treatment. In addition, the report recommended that consumers should be involved in planning and implementing the delivery systems and that funding would be shared by all levels of government.

The impact of psychopharmacology coupled with the social and political climate of the 1960s led to the passage of the Mental Retardation Facilities and Community Mental Health Centers Act. This act was designed to expand the resources available for community-based mental health services. It called for the construction of mental health facilities throughout communities to meet the needs of all those experiencing mental health problems. The result was to ease the transition from institutionalized care to that of the community. The ultimate goal was to provide comprehensive humane treatment rather than custodial care. This legislation was part of President John F. Kennedy's New Frontier program and led to the **DEINSTITUTIONALIZATION** (the movement of patients in mental health institutions back into the community) of many who had been in state-run and other mental health facilities that had provided long-term mental health care and treatment.

At this time, the NIMH expanded its service role and assumed responsibility for monitoring the community mental health centers programs (National Institutes of Health [NIH], 2010). Unfortunately, the number of community mental health centers grew slowly and often were understaffed. Care was fragmented and inadequate. Thus, the demands resulting from deinstitutionalization became overwhelming.

> *In the late 1960s, care of the mentally ill began to shift to community clinics.*

The overwhelming demands faced by the community mental health centers continued. In addition, society was changing. Population shifts, a growing aging population, changes in family structures, and increased numbers of women in the workforce further complicated the system. In 1980, the Mental Health Systems Act was passed in response to the report findings of the President's Commission on Mental Health. This act was designed to establish research and training priorities and address the rights of patients and community mental health centers. However, the election of a new president led to dramatic changes in focus. In 1981, the Omnibus Budget Reconciliation Act (OBRA) was passed, which provided a set amount of funding for each state. Each state would then determine how to use these funds. Unfortunately, mental health care was not a priority for the majority of states and, subsequently, mental health care suffered. Individuals with chronic mental illness often were placed in nursing homes or other types of facilities. In an attempt to address the issues associated with OBRA, Congress passed the Omnibus Budget Reconciliation Act of 1987, which was to provide a means for ensuring that the chronically mentally ill would receive appropriate placement for care. However, the political climate of concern for an ever-widening federal budget deficit led to a significant decrease in funding for mental health care.

In 1992, NIMH joined the National Institutes of Health (NIH) as one of the institutes that continues today to fund research on mental health and illness. NIMH also serves as a national leadership organization for mental health issues (NIH, 2010).

As a result of the changes in society and the political climate of the times, mental health care suffered once again. In response, Surgeon General David Satcher issued The Surgeon General's Report on Mental Health in 1999. This was the first national report that focused on mental health. The report included recommendations for broad courses of action to improve the quality of mental health in the nation as follows: continuing the research on mental health and illness to build the science base; overcoming the stigma of mental illness; improving public awareness of effective treatment; ensuring the supply of mental health services and providers; ensuring delivery of state-of-the-art treatments; tailoring treatment to age, gender, race and culture; facilitating entry into treatment; and reducing financial barriers to treatment (Satcher, 1999). Subsequently, mental health care was brought to the forefront.

## Current Perspectives

Following publication of the Surgeon General's Report in 1999, another key report focusing on children's mental health was published. The Report of the Surgeon General's Conference on Children's Mental Health: A National Action Agenda called for:

- Improved recognition/assessment of children's mental health needs and promotion of public awareness of children's mental health issues.

- Continued development, dissemination, and implementation of scientifically proven prevention and treatment services.
- Reduction and/or elimination of disparities in access to mental health services and increased access and coordination of quality mental health services (U.S. Public Health Service, 2000).

This report further emphasized the need for improved mental health care.

Continued problems in the mental health system prompted the launch of the President's New Freedom Commission on Mental Health in 2001. Its goal was to promote increased access to educational and employment opportunities for people with mental health problems. This Commission was specifically targeted with reducing the stigma associated with mental illness, lifting the financial and access barriers to treatment, and addressing the system fragmentation. The report, *Achieving the Promise: Transforming Mental Health Care in America*, was issued in 2003 with several recommendations for service delivery. It identified the need for changing the current system to one that is more consumer- and family-driven and that underscored the need for mental illnesses to receive the same attention as other medical illnesses. Many of these changes are in the process of being implemented on the national and state levels (President's New Freedom Commission on Mental Health, 2003).

Mental health, which first appeared as a major priority area in the Healthy People 2000 objectives, continued to be a priority for Health People 2020. In December of 2010, the Healthy People 2020 objectives were released. As in 2010, mental health and mental disorders are a priority concern. The Healthy People 2020 objectives for mental health and mental disorders are highlighted in **Box 1-1**.

---

### BOX 1-1: HEALTHY PEOPLE 2020 OBJECTIVES

#### MENTAL HEALTH AND MENTAL DISORDERS

1. Reduce the suicide rate.
2. Reduce the rate of suicide attempts by adolescents.
3. Reduce the proportion of adolescents who engage in disordered eating behaviors in an attempt to control their weight.
4. Reduce the proportion of persons who experience major depressive episode.
    4.1. Adolescents aged 12 to 17 years.
    4.2. Adults aged 18 years and older.
5. Increase the proportion of primary care facilities that provide mental health treatment onsite or by paid referral.
6. Increase the proportion of children with mental health problems who receive treatment.
7. Increase the proportion of juvenile residential facilities that screen admissions for mental health problems.
8. Increase the proportion of persons with serious mental illness who are employed.
9. Increase the proportion of adults with mental health disorders who receive treatment.
    9.1. Adults aged 18 years and older with serious mental illness.
    9.2. Adults aged 18 years and older with major depressive episode.
10. Increase the proportion of persons with co-occurring substance abuse and mental disorders who receive treatment for both disorders.
11. Increase depression screening by primary care providers.
    11.1. Increase the proportion of primary care physician office visits that screen adults aged 19 years and older for depression.
    11.2. Increase the proportion of primary care physician office vistits that screen youth aged 12 to 18 years for depression.
12. Increase the proportion of homeless adults with mental health problems who receive mental health services.

*From the U. S. Department of Health and Human Services. (2010). Healthy People 2020 Objectives. Available at: http://www. healthypeople.gov/2020/topicsobjectives2020/overview.aspx?topicid=28*

## EVOLUTION OF PSYCHIATRIC-MENTAL HEALTH NURSING

The evolution of the nursing profession and the evolution of mental health care have striking similarities. **Figure 1-1** depicts a timeline of events, highlighting significant events in the evolution of mental health care in conjunction with significant events in the evolution of psychiatric-mental health nursing. As seen in the timeline, as mental health care evolved, so too did psychiatric-mental health nursing.

Nurses have always been available to care for the mentally ill. At first, this care occurred in sanitariums where the focus of care was custodial. From the 1890s to after World War II, nurses did things to and for patients, rather than with patients. Mental illness was poorly understood and the role of the nurse was focused on making the environment comfortable, safe, and amenable to healing. While there was a body of knowledge regarding practices that were unique to nursing, this was a new and developing field. Thus, many of the nursing activities were focused on carrying out of medical regimes.

## Early Emergence of the Profession

The early beginnings of psychiatric-mental health nursing can be traced back to Florence Nightingale, who first identified the need to view the patient holistically. Her focus was not mental illness; she was an advocate for patient self-care, believing that when a patient developed independence, he or she would be better able to face illness with lessened anxiety.

Specialization for psychiatric-mental health nursing arose along the same time that humane treatment for mental illness was coming to the forefront. Linda Richards, the first nurse trained in the United States, opened a training school for psychiatric-mental health nurses (PMHNs) in 1882. Although the training primarily consisted of meeting the patient's physical needs, Richards strongly emphasized the need to assess a patient's physical and emotional needs both. Thus, she is credited as being the first American psychiatric nurse.

Approximately 40 years later, the first nursing program for psychiatric-mental health nursing was established by

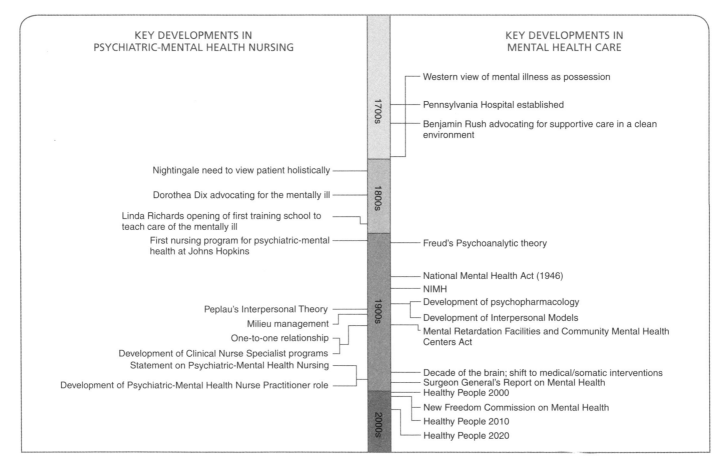

**Figure 1–1** *Evolution of mental health care and psychiatric-mental health nursing.* Events listed at the right identify key developments associated with mental health care. Events listed at the left identify key developments associated with psychiatric-mental health nursing. Note how significant events in mental health care parallel those in psychiatric-mental health nursing.

Effie Taylor at Johns Hopkins Phipps Clinic. Taylor, like Nightingale, emphasized the need to view the patient as an integrated whole. She also believed that general nursing and mental health nursing were interdependent. This was the first time that a course for psychiatric-mental health nursing was included in a curriculum.

## Continued Evolution

During the first half of the twentieth century, the mental health field continued to evolve through the discovery of new therapies and theories. With the introduction of these new therapies, PMHNs were required to adapt the principles of medical-surgical nursing care to the care of psychiatric patients. In 1920, the first textbook of psychiatric-mental health nursing was written by Harriet Bailey. This book primarily focused on procedure-related care by nurses.

Continued involvement with the use of therapies resulted in a struggle for PMHNs to define their role. However, the social climate of the time promoted a view of women as subservient to men. This view also carried over into the realm of nursing.

Near the middle of the twentieth century, INTERPERSONAL MODELS (those that focus on the interaction of the person with others) by leaders such as Harry Stack Sullivan and others began to emerge. Sullivan believed that personality was an observable reflection of an individual's interaction with other individuals. Thus, a person's personality, be it healthy or ill, was a direct result of the relationship between that person and others. Sullivan also identified two key needs: the need for satisfactions (biologic needs) and the need for security (state of well-being and belonging). Any block to satisfactions or security results in anxiety (Sullivan, 1953).

Again, the emergence of interpersonal models paralleled a shift in nursing practice as interpersonal models of nursing practice were being developed. Interpersonal systems became prominent in mental health around 1945 and then in nursing practice in 1952. Both the field of mental health and the field of nursing flourished during this time period with an abundance of theorists contributing to their respective disciplines.

Nursing as a profession began to refine itself with the emergence of theorists such as Hildegard Peplau (1952) who defined nursing as "*a significant, therapeutic, interpersonal process. It functions cooperatively with other human processes that make health possible for individuals and communities. Nursing is an educative instrument, a maturing force that aims to promote forward movement of personality in the direction of creative, constructive, productive, personal, and community living*" (p. 16). Nurse educators thus began to emphasize the importance of interpersonal relations and integrated relevant content in the curricula. Peplau further clarified the PMHN's role as that of counselor, differentiating PMHNs working as general staff nurses from those who were expert practitioners with advanced degrees. According to Peplau, "psychiatric nursing emphasizes the role of counselor or psychotherapist...From my viewpoint, a psychiatric nurse is a specialist and at this time specialist status can be achieved by two routes—experience and education" (Peplau, 1962, p. 51). (For a more in-depth discussion of Peplau, see Chapter 2.)

As a result, nurses were being educated in modes of THERAPEUTIC COMMUNICATION (patient focused interactive process involving verbal and nonverbal behaviors), which were seen as integral parts of the patient's recovery. It was not uncommon for nurses to carry a case load of patients and to spend significant portions of their shift having one-to-one, planned, structured conversations. These conversations were then recorded in the nursing record and their content was processed by the psychiatrist and other health professionals in their evaluation of progress in treatment. (For a more in-depth discussion of therapeutic communication, see Chapter 3.)

MILIEU MANAGEMENT, which developed after 1950, was adopted by psychiatric care facilities. Milieu management refers to the provision and assurance of a therapeutic environment that promotes a healing experience for the patient. This treatment approach is reflected in everything from the physical attributes of the mental health unit such as wall color and choice and arrangement of furniture, to source and levels of lighting. Nurses became the managers of the milieu, responsible for recognizing that they themselves were part of the milieu and thus had to conduct themselves in a manner conducive to supporting a therapeutic environment. This required an ever-conscious focus on dress, body language, tone, and style of verbal interaction, as well as vigilant awareness of surroundings and environment. For example, it would not be unusual for a nurse who was mindful of milieu management therapy to sense that the unit was tense and volatile and to respond by slowly and subtly adjusting the level of light or noise to produce a more relaxed environment. As much thought was spent about how to manage the unit as on how to manage any individual patient.

Nurses also conducted groups. Sometimes these were with a psychiatrist or other psychiatric staff member. Nurses led PSYCHO-EDUCATIONAL GROUPS (groups designed at imparting specific information about a select topic such as medication) and co-facilitated PROCESS GROUPS (more traditional form of psychotherapy where deep feelings, reactions, and thoughts are explored and processed in a structured way). Regardless of the treatment modality, the energy expended by the nurse in the delivery of psychiatric care revolved around the development and maintenance of a therapeutic relationship and the promotion of a therapeutic environment.

From 1954 onward, the discovery and use of antipsychotic medications such as chlorpromazine (Thorazine) revolutionized the understanding of and care for the severely mentally ill. It signaled a change of course for both nursing and mental health care. Medication administration and monitoring were added to the nurse-patient experience. Because of the effectiveness of newer longer acting medications (such as haloperidol [Haldol] and fluphenazine [Prolixin]), the 1960s were a time of care transition from hospital setting to community setting. However, the one-to-one nurse-patient relationship still remained important in nursing (Doona, 1979).

During the 1960s, the Division of Psychiatric and Mental Health Nursing Practice of the American Nurses Association (ANA) published the Statement on Psychiatric Nursing Practice. This was the first document to address the PMHN's holistic view of the patient. It emphasized involvement in a wide range of activities addressing health promotion and health restoration. Since its initial publication, the document has been updated three times, expanding and clarifying the roles and functions of the PMHN to reflect the status of the current society.

By the 1990s, research and understanding of brain chemistry exploded so rapidly that it became known as the "decade of the brain." Again, this signaled a shift in both mental health care and nursing practice because medical **SOMATIC** (referring to the body) interventions became the primary focus of treatment.

Inpatient stays became shorter and funding for mental health treatment began to diminish both at the inpatient and community levels. The role of the psychiatrist changed from the provider of therapy and medication to that of diagnostic and pharmacological expert as schools of medicine no longer offered therapy as part of physician training. Therapy was also now seen as the domain of the PhD-prepared psychologist and other independent providers such as social workers and advanced practice psychiatric nurses. With less time, less money, and less integrated service lines, the generalist psychiatric nurse's role shifted to more of case manager of care. Duties were now more focused on admission and discharge proceedings, medication administration and monitoring, community linkage, and crisis management. These changes are still evident today.

## CONTEMPORARY PSYCHIATRIC-MENTAL HEALTH NURSING PRACTICE

Psychiatric-mental health nursing is "a specialized area of nursing practice committed to promoting mental health through the assessment, diagnosis, and treatment of human responses to mental health problems and psychiatric disorders" (ANA, 2007, p. 14). A major component of this specialized practice is the therapeutic use of self in conjunction with theoretical and research-based foundations from the various scientific disciplines. Psychiatric-mental health nursing occurs across a continuum of care encompassing a wide variety of settings (**Box 1-2**).

### Scope and Standards of Practice

Initially developed in 1973, and most recently revised in 2007, the Scope and Standards of Practice delineate the specific responsibilities for psychiatric-mental health nursing. The Standards are divided into two areas: Standards of Practice and Standards of Professional Performance. The Standards of Practice address six major areas: assessment, diagnosis, outcomes identification, planning, implementation, and evaluation. The Standards of Professional Performance address nine areas including quality of practice, education, professional practice evaluation, collegiality, collaboration, ethics, research, resource utilization, and

---

**BOX 1-2: SETTINGS FOR PSYCHIATRIC-MENTAL HEALTH NURSING PRACTICE**

- Crisis intervention services
- Emergency psychiatric services
- Acute inpatient care
- Intermediate and long-term care
- Partial hospitalization programs
- Intensive outpatient treatment programs
- Residential services
- Community-based care: home, work sites, clinics, health maintenance organizations, shelters, schools, and colleges
- Assertive community treatment (ACT) programs
- Primary care
- Integrative programs
- Telehealth
- Self-employment
- Forensic mental health: correctional facilities
- Disaster response

leadership. Each area includes specific criteria for use in measuring achievement of the standard.

## Phenomena of Concern

The psychiatric-mental health practice division of the ANA has developed a list of 13 specific areas or "phenomena of concern." The phenomena provide the focus of patient care for PMHNs. These areas reflect the holistic view of the patient including the needs of the patient, family, group, and community. Therefore, when providing care to patients, PMHNs focus on the following:

- Health promotion (optimal mental and physical health and well-being) and prevention of mental illness
- Impaired ability to function
- Alterations in thought, perception and communication
- Potentially dangerous behaviors and mental states
- Emotional stress
- Management of symptoms, side effects or toxicities related to treatment
- Treatment barriers
- Changes in self-concept, body image, and life process; issues related to development and end-of-life
- Physical symptoms associated with changes in psychological status
- Psychological symptoms associated with changes in physiologic status
- Effects of interpersonal, organizational, sociocultural, spiritual, or environmental aspects
- Issues related to recovery
- Societal factors (ANA, 2007)

## Levels of Psychiatric-Mental Health Nursing Practice

Two levels of psychiatric-mental health nursing currently are recognized: basic and advanced. The levels are distinguished by the educational preparation, complexity of practice, and specific nursing functions (ANA, 2007). The American Nurses Credentialing Center (ANCC) certifies both basic and advanced practice psychiatric nurses through an examination and credential review process.

Basic level PMHNs are registered nurses who have graduated from an accredited nursing education program and are licensed to practice in their state. In addition, basic level PMHNs possess specialized knowledge and skills to care for patients with mental health issues and psychiatric problems. They apply the nursing process through the use of the therapeutic nurse-patient relationship, therapeutic interventions, and professional attributes such as

self-awareness, empathy, and the therapeutic use of self (ANA, 2007). The ANCC recognizes the baccalaureate degree in nursing as the preferred level of educational preparation.

Advanced practice PMHNs are educated at the master's or doctorate level of education in the specialty and have achieved certification in this specialty by the ANCC. Advanced practice focuses on the "application of competences, knowledge, and experience to individuals, families, or groups with complex psychiatric-mental health problems" (ANA, 2007, p. 19). Mental health promotion, collaboration, and referral are key components of the advanced practice PMHN.

When graduate programs in psychiatric-mental health nursing were first introduced, the focus was on preparing educators to teach in basic nursing programs. Faculty members also were prepared to integrate psychiatric-mental health concepts throughout the undergraduate nursing curricula. Components such as communication skills, process recordings, and understanding of the emotional dimensions of physical illness were integrated into all nursing courses. The first psychiatric advanced practice role was the psychiatric clinical nurse specialist implemented by Hildegard Peplau. During the mid-1960s, more clinical nurse specialist (CNS) programs were introduced, emphasizing the preparation of specialists for both psychiatric-mental health nursing direct care roles, and for teaching, consultation, and liaison with other nurses in clinical practice. The core focus of CNS practice today emphasizes three spheres of influence: organizational and systems; nursing practice; and client (patient). The CNS seeks to improve patient outcomes by influencing nursing practice via research and mentorship, influencing organizational systems via consultation, or through direct care to individuals or communities (Fulton, Lyon, & Goudreau, 2010). Most psychiatric CNSs have training in individual psychotherapy, group psychotherapy, organizational consultation and liaison work, and research. More recently, some psychiatric CNSs have opted to add prescriptive authority to their set of services.

In the early 1960s the Nurse Practictioner (NP) role was introduced in rural areas of the United States. By the late 1990s, the psychiatric-mental health NP role was introduced. Traditionally, this role has been seen as a provider of common physician services such as direct patient care for complex diagnosis and management of medical illnesses with medication prescription. More recently, the development is the blending of the CNS and NP roles for preparation of advanced practice nurses (APNs) in psychiatric-mental health nursing. The challenge to educators, however, is how to combine the two roles while

> *Psychiatric nursing is practiced at two educational levels: generalist practice (ADN, Diploma, BSN) and advanced practice (MSN, DNP, PhD). Advanced practice nurses are clinical nurse specialists (CNS) and nurse practitioners (NP).*

preserving the uniqueness of each (Jones, 2010). The American Psychiatric Nurses Association (APNA) and the International Society of Psychiatric Nurses (ISPN),

two professional psychiatric-mental health nursing organizations, are in the process of reviewing the standards for credentialing for future psychiatric-mental health nursing practice at both basic and advanced levels.

## Roles and Functions of the PMHN

Both basic and advanced practice PMHNs are guided by the Scope and Standards of Practice developed by the ANA. However, specific standards and criteria used for measurement are expanded for the advanced practice PMHN. **Table 1-1** highlights the key functions for each level of practice.

| TABLE 1-1: FUNCTIONS OF PMHNs | |
|---|---|
| **BASIC LEVEL** | **ADVANCED PRACTICE LEVEL (CNS / NP)** |
| Establishment of the therapeutic nurse-patient relationship<br>Use of the nursing process<br>Participation as a key member of the interdisciplinary team<br>Health promotion and health maintenance activities<br>Intake screening, evaluation, and triage<br>Case management<br>Milieu management<br>Administration of psychobiological treatments and monitoring and evaluation of response and effects<br>Crisis intervention and stabilization<br>Psychiatric rehabilitation | *In addition to basic level functions:*<br>Collaboration<br>Referral<br>Primary psychiatric-mental health care delivery<br>Comprehensive psychiatric and mental health evaluation (assessment and medical diagnosis)<br>Prescription of psychopharmacological agents (if allowed by state)<br>Integrative therapy interventions<br>Psychotherapy<br>Complex case management (individual- or population-based)<br>Consultation/liaison<br>Clinical supervision<br>Program development and management |

### SUMMARY POINTS

- Early views of mental illness in the West focused on demonic possession with treatment consisting of charms, spells, witch hunts, and exorcisms. As the late eighteenth century approached, medical interventions such as bloodletting, immobilization, and specialized devices were used to treat mental illness. These practices were eventually stopped as the focus changed to supportive, sympathetic care in a quiet, clean environment.

- Dorothea Dix was instrumental in the care of the mentally ill in the United States, advocating for their needs through the establishment of state hospitals.

*(cont.)*

- During the twentieth century, Freud's psychoanalytic theory and the development of psychopharmacology played key roles in the treatment of mental illness. The passage of the National Mental Health Act in 1946 provided funding for research, mental health professional training, and facility expansion programs, and established the National Advisory Mental Health Council and a National Institute of Mental Health (NIMH). Mental health was beginning to gain focus as an important area of health.

- In the 1960s, deinstitutionalization occurred. However, community mental health centers were not equipped to deal with the large numbers of persons who were deinstitutionalized. Care became fragmented and inadequate.

- In 1999, the Surgeon General issued the first national report that focused on mental health that called for improving the quality of mental health in the nation. In 2001, the President's New Freedom Commission on Mental Health was created and led to recommendations for changing the current system to one that is more consumer- and family-driven and emphasizing the need for mental illnesses to receive the same focus of attention as medical illness.

- Although not a psychiatric-mental health nurse, Florence Nightingale first identified the need to view the patient holistically, advocating for self-care. Linda Richards, credited as being the first American psychiatric nurse, emphasized the need to assess a patient's physical and emotional needs.

Forty years later, the first psychiatric-mental health nursing program was established.

- With the evolution of the mental health field, psychiatric-mental health nurses were required to adapt the principles of medical-surgical nursing care to that of psychiatric patients. The emergence of interpersonal models in the fields of psychiatry and nursing led to a refinement in the nurse's role. Hildegard Peplau emphasized the importance of interpersonal relations and the need to integrate this relevant content into the curricula.

- Publication of the ANA's Statement on Psychiatric Nursing Practice was the first document to address the psychiatric-mental health nurse's holistic view of the patient and emphasized involvement in a wide range of activities addressing health promotion and health restoration.

- The "decade of the brain" shifted the focus of care to medical somatic interventions.

- Two levels of psychiatric-mental health nursing are recognized: basic and advanced. Basic level psychiatric-mental health nurses apply the nursing process through the use of the therapeutic nurse-patient relationship, therapeutic interventions, and professional attributes such as self-awareness, empathy, and the therapeutic use of self. Advanced practice psychiatric-mental health nurses have a master's or doctoral degree and have received certification by the ANCC. Mental health promotion, collaboration, and referral are key components of advanced practice.

### NCLEX-PREP*

1. A nursing instructor is preparing a class discussion about the development of mental health care over time. Which of the following would the instructor include as occurring first?

   a. Development of psychoanalytic theory
   b. Establishment of the National Institute of Mental Health
   c. Use of medical treatments such as bloodletting and immobilization
   d. Emphasis on supportive, sympathetic care in a clean, quiet environment

2. A group of nursing students are reviewing information related to the development of psychiatric-mental nursing. The students demonstrate understanding of the information when they identify which person as emphasizing the use of the interpersonal process?

   a. Florence Nightingale
   b. Linda Richards
   c. Dorothea Dix
   d. Hildegard Peplau

3. A psychiatric-mental health nurse (PMHN) is preparing a presentation for a group of student nurses about psychiatric-mental health nursing. Which statement would the nurse include in the presentation about this specialty?

   a. A PMHN needs to obtain a graduate level degree for practice.
   b. Advanced practice PMHNs can engage in psychotherapy.
   c. Basic level PMHNs mainly focus on the patient's ability to function.
   d. PMHNs primarily work in acute in-patient settings.

4. When describing the results of integrating interpersonal models in psychiatric-mental health nursing, which of the following would be least appropriate to include?

   a. Therapeutic communication
   b. Milieu management
   c. Psychopharmacology
   d. Process groups

5. Deinstitutionalization occurred as a result of which of the following?

   a. Mental Retardation Facilities and Community Mental Health Centers Act
   b. National Mental Health Act
   c. Omnibus Budget Reconciliation Act (OBRA)
   d. The Surgeon General's Report on Mental Health

*Answers to these questions appear on page 639.

## REFERENCES

American Nurses Association, American Psychiatric Nurses Association, International Society of Psychiatric-Mental Health Nurses. (2007). Psychiatric-Mental Health Nursing: Scope and Standards of Practice. Silver Springs, MD: American Nurses Association Publishing Program.

Doona, M.E. (1979). *Travelbee's Intervention in Psychiatric Nursing.* (2nd ed.) Philadelphia: F.A. Davis.

Fulton, J.A., Lyon, B.L., & Goudreau, K.A. (2010). *Foundations of Clinical Nurse Specialist Practice.* New York: Springer Publishing.

Jones, J.S. (2010). Credentialing and Psychiatric Clinical Nurse Specialist Practice—Current Issues, *Clinical Nurse Specialist: The Journal for Advanced Nursing Practice,* 24(1), 38–40.

Mental Health America (2009). Mental Health America Recognizes Contributions of Dorothea Dix as Part of National Women's History Month, 100th Anniversary. Available at: http://www.nmha.org/index.cfm?objectid=C8DDFD65–1372-4D20-C82C20F3FCC1FE7A. Accessed 10/22/2010.

National Institutes of Health. (2010). National Institute of Mental Health. Retrieved August 1, 2010 from http://www.nih.gov/about/almanac/organization/NIMH.htm

Peplau, H. (1952). *Interpersonal relations in nursing.* New York: G.P. Putnam.

Peplau, H. (1962). "Interpersonal Techniques: The crux of psychiatric nursing," *American Journal of Nursing,* 62(6): 50–54.

President's New Freedom Commission. (2003). Final report to the President. Retrieved from http://www.mentalhealthcommission.gov/ August 1, 2010.

Satcher, D. (1999). Mental health: A report of the Surgeon General. Retrieved from http://www.surgeongeneral.gov/library/mental-health/home.html, August 1, 2010.

Sullivan, H.S. (1953). *The interpersonal theory of psychiatry*. New York: W.W. Norton.

U.S. Department of Health and Human Services (2009). Proposed HP2020 Objectives. Available at: http://www.healthypeople.gov/hp2020/Objectives/TopicArea.aspx?id=34&TopicArea= Mental+Health+and+Mental+Disorders; Retrieved October 20, 2010.

U.S. Department of Health and Human Services (2010). Healthy People 2020 Objectives. Available at: http://www.healthypeople.gov/2020/topicsobjectives2020/overview.aspx?topicid=28 Retrieved January 16, 2011.

U.S. Public Health Service (2000). Report of the Surgeon General's Conference on Children's Mental Health: A national action agenda. Retrieved from http://www.surgeongeneral.gov/topics/cmh/childreport.html#sum Retrieved October 20, 2010.

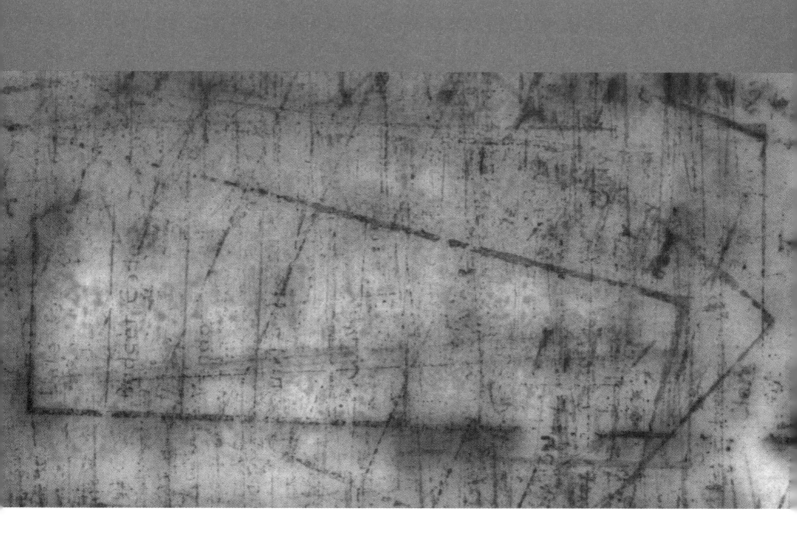

## CHAPTER CONTENTS

Hildegard E. Peplau

Joyce Travelbee

## EXPECTED LEARNING OUTCOMES

**After completing this chapter, the student will be able to:**

1. Define interpersonal relationships.

2. Identify the two predominant interpersonal models in psychiatric nursing.

3. Discuss the stages of the interpersonal process as described by Hildegard Peplau.

4. Explain the six roles that nurses may assume during Peplau's interpersonal process.

5. Correlate Peplau's stages of the interpersonal process with the steps of the nursing process.

# CHAPTER 2
# INTERPERSONAL RELATIONSHIPS: THE CORNERSTONE OF PSYCHIATRIC NURSING

Jeffrey S. Jones

Joyce J. Fitzpatrick

6. Identify the three key concepts associated with Joyce Travelbee's Human to Human Relationship Theory.

7. Discuss the five phases of Travelbee's model.

8. Describe the importance of these theories in the professional practice of psychiatric mental health nursing.

9. Apply Peplau's and Travelbee's theories to patient care delivery in the clinical setting.

10. Incorporate the models of interpersonal relationships in professional psychiatric nursing practice.

## KEY TERMS

Emerging identities

Empathy

Empathetic linkages

Exploitation phase

Hope

Human being

Identification phase

Interpersonal relationship

Orientation phase

Original encounter

Rapport

Resolution phase

Suffering

Sympathy

An INTERPERSONAL RELATIONSHIP, often referred to as an IPR, is the connection that exists between two or more individuals. Observation, assessment, communication, and evaluation skills serve as the foundation for an interpersonal relationship. Development of any interpersonal relationship requires the individual to have a basic understanding of self and what that individual brings to the relationship. The second most important skill is that of communication, including both nonverbal and verbal communication.

The relationship that nurses have with their patients is considered the cornerstone of all other components of nursing. Regardless of the patient's health status—ranging from well individuals living in the community to patients who are critically or terminally ill—establishing a nurse-patient relationship is one of the nurse's primary goals. It is this relationship that is reflected and integrated into the plan of care for any patient of any age, culture, or socioeconomic background.

The interpersonal relationship in nursing is often considered to be the one-to-one relationship between the nurse and patient. However, the nurse also needs to develop interpersonal relationships with the patient's family and key individuals in the patient's environment.

Interpersonal relationships form the basis of nursing interventions for psychiatric-mental health nursing. To do this, nurses must learn how to build the relationship and develop the skills for enhancing the interaction between the nurse, patient, family, and other important individuals in the patient's life.

This chapter provides an introduction to interpersonal relationships which serves as the foundation for the rest of the book. Several interpersonal models have been developed in nursing. Two prominent nursing theories that specifically address the interpersonal relationship as the core concept are described. These are the theories of Hildegard Peplau and Joyce Travelbee.

> *Interpersonal relationships are the connections between two or more people. Skillful management of interpersonal relationships is essential to psychiatric-mental health nursing.*

## HILDEGARD E. PEPLAU

Hildegard E. Peplau is considered the founder of psychiatric-mental health nursing theory and professional practice. She has been referred to as the "mother" of psychiatric nursing and, in an authorized biography by Callaway (2002), as the psychiatric nurse of the century. She is well known within the national and global nursing communities, not only for her contributions to psychiatric nursing but also for her activism throughout nursing. During her professional career, she served as President of the American Nurses Association (ANA) and subsequently as the ANA Executive Director. She also served as a Board member of the International Council of Nurses (ICN). In 1997, she received the highest award from this organization, the Christine Reimann Prize.

Peplau was always a staunch supporter of professional education for nurses and of specialization for post-basic preparation. She was responsible for developing the first master's degree clinical nurse specialist psychiatric-mental health nursing program at Rutgers University School of Nursing in New Jersey.

> *Peplau is considered the founder of psychiatric-mental health nursing.*

## Biographical Background

Hildegarde Peplau was born September 1, 1909, in Reading, Pennsylvania; she died in 1999 at the age of 89 (**Figure 2-1**). She was the second in a family of five children. Her parents had immigrated to the United States from Poland before any of the children were born. Throughout her school years, Peplau excelled; she decided on a career in nursing to advance her education and to provide a means for making her own way in the world. She graduated from the Pottstown Hospital School of Nursing in 1931 and from Bennington College in 1942 with a Bachelor of Arts degree with a major in interpersonal psychology.

While studying at Bennington, Peplau was exposed to the work of Harry Stack Sullivan. Sullivan's theory described personality as behavior in relation to others. He identified a person's need for satisfaction and security with the development of anxiety if these needs are not met. Sullivan's work greatly influenced Peplau who also emphasized basic needs and anxiety.

Peplau served in the Army Nurse Corps as a first lieutenant in World War II. Following her service, she received a master's degree from Columbia University in 1947 and a doctorate in education in 1953.

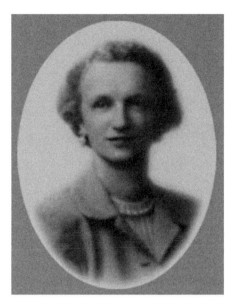

Figure 2-1. *Hildegard E. Peplau.*

Peplau was a dedicated nurse and scholar and quickly rose to the top of her profession. She directed the graduate program in psychiatric nursing at Columbia Teachers College from 1948 to 1953. It was during this time that she wrote the seminal text: *Interpersonal Relationships in Nursing: A Conceptual Frame of Reference for Psychodynamic Nursing.* Although the book was completed in 1948, it was not published until 1952 (Peplau, 1952). Her book was considered most unusual in nursing because it was one of the first nursing books written by a nurse without a physician as co-author. In fact, the three-year delay in publication was because the book was considered too revolutionary for a nurse to publish (O'Toole & Welt, 1989).

## Peplau's Theory of Interpersonal Relationships

Peplau viewed nursing as an interpersonal process between two or more persons directed toward a therapeutic goal. Therapeutic goal attainment is achieved by the nurse's deliberate actions that occur along a sequence of phases.

The environment also plays a key role in human development (Peplau, 1992). The environment included factors such as culture, adult presence, economic status, and prenatal environment, as well as the interactions between the patient and others, i.e., family, parents, or nurse.

Anxiety is another key component of Peplau's theory. (See Chapter 13 for a more in-depth discussion of anxiety.) Drawing on the work by Sullivan and his interpersonal theory, she identified different levels of anxiety and their effect on an individual. Peplau emphasized the need

for nurses to recognize anxiety and intervene accordingly to improve the individual's state.

Peplau believed that the interpersonal competencies of nurses are essential to assisting patients to regain health and well-being. These interpersonal competencies are based on the nurse's ability to understand his or her own behavior. Peplau stressed the need for nurses to be able to feel within themselves the feelings that others are communicating verbally or nonverbally. Most commonly, these feelings are anxiety or panic. Nurses then integrate this understanding and self-awareness to assist others in indentifying their problems. (See Chapter 3 for more information on developing self-awareness.)

> *According to Peplau, nurses integrate an understanding of their own behaviors and self-awareness to assist patients in identifying problems and in working toward achieving health and well-being.*

## Phases of the Interpersonal Process

Initially, Peplau described four phases in the interpersonal process: the orientation phase, identification phase, exploitation phase, and resolution phase (Peplau, 1952, 1991). Later, these four stages were condensed into three stages: orientation phase, working phase, and termination phase (Peplau, 1988, 1997). The four-stage model is described in **Figure 2-2**.

### Orientation

The first phase of Peplau's interpersonal process is the ORIENTATION PHASE. This phase includes the initial contact the nurse has with the patient. During this phase, the patient seeks assistance. The nurse identifies him- or herself and the purpose and nature of the relationship. It is in this orientation phase that the nurse also communicates the temporal dimension of the relationship to the patient; that is, he or she informs the patient about the timeframe available for the therapeutic interaction.

Peplau emphasizes that the patient is the focus of the communication. Personal information about the nurse is not needed. The patient conveys his or her needs, asks questions, and shares information. The nurse observes the patient and makes assessments of the patient's status and needs during this phase of the relationship. Acting as a participant observer, the nurse

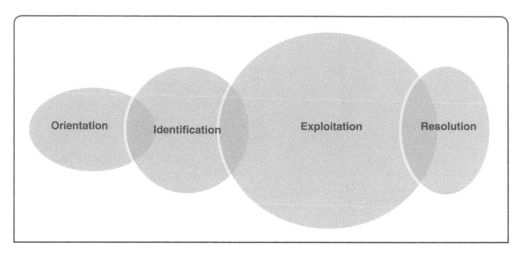

**Figure 2-2.** *Peplau's Model of Interpersonal Relationships.* Peplau initially identified four phases of the interpersonal process as orientation, identification, exploitation, and resolution. Note that the exploitation phase is the largest because the majority of work occurs at this time. In follow-up research, Peplau combined the phases of identification and exploitation, calling it the "working phase." (From Jones, 2010.)

uses his or her knowledge about influencing factors and takes into account the patient's previous experiences, values, beliefs, culture, and expectations. The nurse also is cognizant of his or her own previous personal experiences, values, beliefs, culture, preconceived ideas, and expectations, assesses his or her own self, and determines how these may influence the nurse-patient relationship. This knowledge of self is an important factor in the relationship.

At the beginning of the orientation phase, the nurse and patient meet as strangers, but as the relationship is developed, the problem is identified. The nurse explains routines, roles, and expectations to elicit the full participation of the patient. Subsequently, the patient begins to develop a sense of belonging and the ability to deal with the present difficulties. The patient and the nurse are ready to move to the next phase of the relationship.

## Identification

In the **IDENTIFICATION PHASE**, the patient recognizes his or her health care needs for which the nurse can provide assistance. The patient views the nurse as a skilled provider of care capable of helping the patient meet these needs and accepts the nurse's help. The nurse, in turn, senses that the patient has identified the needs and has cast him or her in the role of care provider. Additionally, the nurse identifies personal knowledge, attributes, and skills that he or she can bring to the relationship when providing nursing care. Together, the patient and nurse develop mutual goals and begin working together to address the patient's needs. Expression and exploration of the patient's feelings are key during this time.

## Exploitation

During the **EXPLOITATION PHASE**, the bulk of the work in the nurse-patient relationship is accomplished with the patient taking full advantage of the nursing services offered. This phase encompasses all of the therapeutic activities that are initiated to reach the identified goal. Throughout this phase the nurse and patient must continue to clarify expectations and goals and to define the work to be done based on identification of patient needs. **Evidence-Based Practice 2-1** highlights a research study that applies Peplau's theory to women with depression.

Open communication is essential during this time and requires a trusting relationship between nurse and patient. Without this trust, the work essential to meeting the therapeutic goals cannot be completed.

The relationship between the nurse and patient during this phase is intense as the patient begins to take responsibility for his or her own health goals. This shift in responsibility from the nurse to the patient characterizes this phase. However, this transition to greater responsibility may be the most difficult point in the nurse-patient relationship. The exploitation phase requires that the nurse begins to foster independence in the nurse-patient relationship and starts the process of "letting go" in preparation for the next phase. Health care providers, including nurses, sometimes have difficulty in relationships when their clients are not dependant upon them. This may indicate a boundary issue. (For more information on health boundary management in therapeutic relationships, see Chapter 4.) While the patient may initially be dependent upon the nurse, as the exploitation phase progresses the patient develops independence.

**EVIDENCE-BASED PRACTICE 2-1:
DEPRESSION AND PEPLAU'S THEORY**

STUDY

Peden, A. R. (1993). Recovering in depressed women: Research with Peplau's theory. *Nursing Science Quarterly, 6*(3): 140–146.

SUMMARY

Depression is a signficant problem among women. This study was guided by Peplau's theory of nursing. The author conducted in-depth interviews of seven women who at one time had been hospitalized for depression and were now recovering. The findings indicated that the process of recovering consisted of three phases: (1) a turning point and professional support; (2) determination, support of family and friends, and successes; and (3) self-esteem and maintaining balance. The participants described recovery as a dynamic process, with movement among phases.

APPLICATION TO PRACTICE

Nurses need to understand the dynamic nature of the recovery process and help individuals who have experienced depression move through the phases of recovery. This can be accomplished through the interpersonal process described by Peplau.

QUESTIONS TO PONDER

1. *How prevalent is the problem of depression among women?*
2. *What are the phases of the recovery process from the perspective of the women in this study and how do the women describe their experiences of recovery?*
3. *Describe the role that the professional nurse can play in the recovery process based on Peplau's theory.*

## Resolution

The **RESOLUTION PHASE** of the relationship occurs when the patient's needs have been met through the collaborative work of nurse and patient. The nurse's evaluation of the patient's readiness to move through termination of the relationship is crucial to resolution. During a successful termination, the patient moves away from the nurse and understands that he or she can manage independently. The patient assumes the power to meet his or her needs and set new goals. However, if the relationship is terminated prematurely, the patient may relapse and thus require a rebuilding of the therapeutic relationship.

> *The four phases of the interpersonal process as identified by Peplau are the orientation phase, identification phase, exploitation phase, and resolution phase. Later, she condensed these phases into three phases: orientation phase, working phase, and termination phase.*

## Roles

Peplau defined six primary roles that the nurse assumes throughout the interpersonal process to assist the patient in meeting his or her needs (Tomey, 1989). These roles, described in **Table 2-1**, may overlap and occur at any time during any phase of the nurse-patient relationship. She also identified other roles that the nurse may assume, such as consultant, tutor, mediator, administrator, researcher, and observer. However, she did not define these roles specifically but rather left them up to the reader to define (Peplau, 1952).

> *Nurses may find themselves in any or all of six roles (stranger, resource person, teacher, leader, surrogate, or counselor) when working with patients.*

## Application to Psychiatric-Mental Health Nursing Practice

The nurse must integrate the use of therapeutic communication and interviewing skills while helping the patient through the phases of the interpersonal relationship. Peplau (1997) describes the need for participant observation, which consists of the following three foci: the nurse, the patient, and the relationship. Thus, the nurse must be ever vigilant about him- or herself and others and the interaction between him- or herself and patient. The nurse must be cognizant of all of the messages, verbal and nonverbal, communicated to patients.

As a component of the observation required in the nurse patient interaction, Peplau describes **EMPATHETIC LINKAGES**, the ability to feel in oneself the emotions experienced by another person in the same situation. It is the nurse's role to reframe the observed feelings into verbal communications.

Peplau (1997) noted several challenges in the interpersonal relationships that develop between nurses and patients. These may include avoiding rather than dealing with the patient's anger or one's own anger, avoiding discussion of emotionally laden topics, and competing with the patient on some dimension. As these challenges test the competence of the nurse, it is important for the nurse to identify them and their effect on the nurse-patient relationship.

Peplau understood that patients want relationships with others, including therapeutic relationships with nurses. The connectedness developed through the interpersonal relationship helps decrease the anxiety that is a

| TABLE 2-1: ROLES OF THE NURSE | |
|---|---|
| **ROLE** | **DESCRIPTION AND CONSIDERATIONS** |
| Stranger | Usually during orientation phase<br>Need for a climate of courtesy and acceptance since the nurse and patient are strangers to each other; facilitation of identification phase<br>No prejudgment of patient |
| Resource person | Nurse as a valuable source of information<br>Nurse responsible for determining how best to answer questions: Are there larger issues that need to be addressed? How much information can the patient handle at this point in his or her illness? Is the patient ready to hear the response to be given? |
| Teacher | Occurrence along many points throughout the relationship<br>Decision as to what mode best fits situation: brief instructional moment with review of printed material; experiential meeting with demonstration<br>More likely advantageous during exploitation phase |
| Leader | Direction for understanding therapeutic goals<br>Accomplishment of therapeutic activities with cooperation and active participation |
| Surrogate | Clients seeing those who care for them as they would others who have cared for them in their lives, i.e., mother, father, sister, wife<br>Assistance to help patient develop awareness of mindset and understand differences from recalled person |
| Counselor | Emphasis on therapeutic communication strategies<br>Awareness of therapeutic use of self in patient encounters<br>Expected outcome of patient being able to integrate the illness into their lives rather than see it as a separate experience |

predominant emotion in many patients' experiences. The relationship further serves as a means to decrease the space between persons.

## Application to the Nursing Process

Peplau's four phases of the nurse-patient relationship closely parallel the steps of the nursing process. Both focus on the therapeutic relationship and occur sequentially, with each phase dependent upon the previous phase. Peplau's orientation phase is similar to the assessment phase. In each, the nurse and patient meet for the first time as strangers because of a need on the patient's part. Information is collected and problems are identified. During planning and Peplau's identification phase, outcomes and goals are established and actions are set forth to meet these goals. Her exploitation phase, which correlates to implementation, provides the opportunity to put the plan into motion, using the necessary interventions and therapeutic activities to meet the established goals. The patient is an active participant in his or her care with the nurse facilitating and promoting increasing patient independence. Lastly, Peplau's resolution phase, like evaluation, occurs with the achievement of the patient's goals and the patient's ability to resume his or her own care independently. Chapter 5 decribes the nursing process in greater detail.

## Use of Peplau's Theory in Practice

Consider the following scenario. As a student nurse, you will have a chance to interact with patients on a mental health unit. This may be your first time caring for someone with a psychiatric disorder. In this situation, a female patient is diagnosed with panic disorder (recurrent, unexpected periods of intense discomfort accompanied by physical signs and symptoms such as palpitations, sweating, shaking and shortness of breath) with agoraphobia (anxiety about being in places or situations from which escape may be difficult or embarrassing or in which help may not be available). When you walk into the room to meet the patient for the first time, what should you expect? What will someone with panic disorder look like, act like? What should the patient expect? Should you smile or be serious? Should your body posture be relaxed or stiff? Should you introduce yourself with a handshake or let them make the first move? All of these questions are important ones to consider as you prepare to engage with your first patient.

When you meet the patient, you are a stranger. In this first phase, "orientation," the goal is to engage the patient in such a way that you and the patient begin to identify

with each other. If the patient can perceive you as trustworthy, knowledgeable, and helpful, then you will have progressed into the identification phase.

In the identification, you and the patient will begin discussions focusing on what her health situation is, what problems she is having, and how she can benefit from mutual goal setting. You and the patient decide to focus on her awareness of triggers for the panic attacks. Moving into the phase of exploitation provides you with the opportunity to function in the roles of counselor, teacher, and resource person. You may have helpful printed material about panic disorder and ways patients can learn to become aware of triggers for the condition and begin to manage the anxiety with self-relaxation techniques. You may meet several times with this patient to review the material, teaching her these techniques, offering suggestions to reduce her exposure to the triggers, and providing support through active listening. These actions are focused on achieving the mutual goal. As your time on the unit as a student comes to an end, you now need to disengage from and terminate the relationship. You meet with the patient and review her accomplishments so far and the gains that she has made in treatment. Your actions foster independence in the patient. Subsequently, you have now experienced resolution to the relationship.

## JOYCE TRAVELBEE

Joyce Travelbee viewed nursing as an interpersonal process that assists individuals, families, or communities to prevent or cope with illness and suffering with the goal of finding meaning in these experiences (Travelbee, 1971). Her Human to Human Relationship Theory focuses on caring and the therapeutic use of self.

## Biographical Background

Joyce Travelbee was born in 1926 and received a diploma in nursing from Charity Hospital School of Nursing in New Orleans in 1946 (**Figure 2-3**). She then obtained a baccalaureate degree in nursing (BSN) from Louisiana State University in 1956 and a master's degree in nursing (MSN) from Yale University in 1959. She had just begun a doctoral program in Florida at the time of her death in 1973. Travelbee began her nursing career in education, teaching psychiatric nursing in New Orleans in 1952. She also taught psychiatric nursing at schools of nursing and universities in New York and Mississippi (Marriner Tomey & Alligood, 2006).

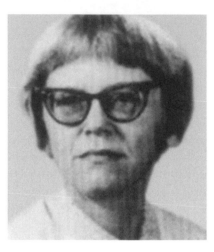

**Figure 2-3.** *Joyce Travelbee*

## Travelbee's Human to Human Relationship Theory

Travelbee's Human to Human Relationship Theory developed from a convergence of three significant influences. The first influence was her experiences in practice. She felt that what she witnessed was a lack of compassion on the part of her colleagues and that the time was right for professional nursing to undergo a "humanistic revolution" (Marriner Tomey, 2006).

A second influence was that of Ida Jean Orlando, another nurse theorist. Orlando was one of Travelbee's instructors at Yale University and was in the process of further developing and teaching her Nursing Process Theory (1958–1961). Orlando's work focused on medical-surgical patients, not psychiatric-mental health patients. However, she emphasized the need for nurses to view the patient as a whole, not just a disease entity.

The writings of Victor Frankl, a philosopher, were a third influence on Travelbee. Frankl was a survivor of Nazi concentration camps and developed the theory of Logotherapy based on observations of others and his experience of suffering (Marriner Tomey, 2006). Logotherapy is founded upon the belief that it is the striving to find a meaning in one's life that is the primary, most powerful motivating and driving force in humans. Frankl, an existentialist, felt that all life, even the most desperate of situations, had meaning and it was these situations that gave a person a reason to live.

### Major Concepts

In her theory, Travelbee identified three main concepts: **HUMAN BEING**, **SUFFERING**, and **HOPE** (Travelbee, 1971).

She defined a human being as "a unique irreplaceable individual, a one-time being in this world, like yet unlike any person who has ever lived or ever will live" (Travelbee, 1971). This individual is continuously evolving, changing, and becoming. Human being referred to any person. The nurse and the patient both would be considered human beings.

Suffering is defined *"a feeling of displeasure which ranges from simple transitory mental, physical, or spiritual discomfort to extreme anguish, and to those phases beyond anguish, namely, the malignant phase of despairful not caring, and the terminal phase of apathetic indifference"* (p. 62).

One of the main functions of nursing is to relieve suffering, be it physical or emotional suffering. Physical pain and suffering is often easy to assess and address for a variety of reasons. Consider the example of a wound. A nurse can often see the wound and have a clinical frame of reference about its severity and the probable level of pain associated with it. The patient also may be able to report the level of pain on a scale that correlates to the nurse's concept of pain given the injury. The nurse then has a variety of protocols available, such as analgesics, repositioning, and massage to alleviate the patient's suffering.

Conversely, emotional pain and suffering is more difficult to assess, understand, and treat because of its inherent subjective nature. The nurse often has to rely on the patient's statements to assess the level of suffering.

Travelbee described suffering using four levels, which can be depicted as a continuum (**Figure 2-4**). The first level is simple transitory mental, physical, or spiritual discomfort. All human beings have experienced this discomfort. For example, something goes wrong in your life, you have an argument with a friend, you get a lower grade on an exam than you expected, or your seasonal allergies flare up due to a high pollen count. As the name implies, the suffering is short-lived. While unpleasant and uncomfortable, it is usually self-resolving. The person can usually return to a previous state of equilibrium.

Sometimes a more serious stressor impacts a person's life, such as a serious physical injury (broken leg or slipped disc), or an emotional trauma (loss of a pet or the ending of a romantic relationship). These are examples of events possibly triggering extreme anguish. Most individuals have also experienced this level of suffering. Although potentially self-resolving, this phase may lead to the next level of suffering if intervention does not occur.

If extreme anguish is left unattended, despairful not caring may emerge. As the term despair implies, this phase is characterized by the patient who has suffered extreme anguish without intervention or relief of symptoms for such a long period of time that they are now experiencing

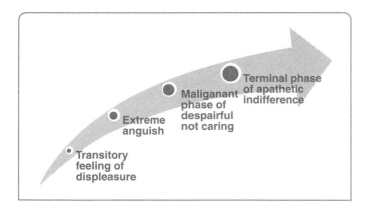

Figure 2-4. *Continuum of suffering.* (Conceptualized by J. Jones, based on Travelbee's definitions.)

angry feelings of pending hopelessness. Loss of a spouse, loss of a child, or other catastrophic event may trigger this level of suffering.

The prolonged unrelenting suffering of anguish can lead to despair as well. If left without intervention, the person progresses to the terminal phase of apathetic indifference. This level is characterized by the person experiencing utter hopelessness. Nurses and other health care professionals describe patients as having lost their will to live (Travelbee, 1971). In psychiatric mental health nursing, despairful not caring is considered an interpersonal emergency that requires immediate intervention to prevent the development of apathetic indifference.

Hope, according to Travelbee, is "*a mental state characterized by the desire to gain an end or accomplish a goal combined with some degree of expectation that what is desired or sought is attainable. Hope is related to dependence on others, choice within, trust and perseverance, and courage, and is future oriented*" (p. 77). One of the most powerful interventions a nurse can provide to a patient is the instillation of hope.

> *Human being, suffering, and hope are the three main concepts of Travelbee's Human to Human Relationship Theory.*

## Phases and the Nurse-Patient Relationship

Travelbee defined the nurse-patient relationship as a human-to-human relationship. The human-to-human relationship in nursing is the means through which the purpose of nursing is accomplished. She stressed that interpersonal relationships are primarily an experience between the nurse (a human being) and recipient of the care (another human being). The major characteristic of these experiences is that the nursing needs of the individual (or family) are met. Travelbee (1971) felt that "*the human-to-human relationship is established when the nurse and the recipient of care have progressed through four interlocking phases. The phases are the original encounter, emerging identities, empathy, and sympathy*" (p. 119). Progression through these phases culminates in a fifth phase, rapport (**Figure 2-5**).

- **ORIGINAL ENCOUNTER** is the first phase of the nurse-patient relationship. It is characterized by first impressions by the nurse of the ill person and by the ill person of the nurse. Both the nurse and the ill person perceive each other in stereotypical or traditional roles.
- **EMERGING IDENTITIES** phase is characterized by the nurse and the ill person perceiving each other as unique individuals. The bond of a relationship is beginning to form.
- **EMPATHY** phase is characterized by the ability to share in the other person's experience. It is "an intellectual process and, to a lesser extent, emotion comprehension of another person..." (Travelbee, 1964, p. 68). The result of the empathic process is the ability to predict the behavior of the individual and to "perceive accurately his thinking and feeling" (Travelbee, 1964, p. 68). Empathy is necessary to develop sympathy.
- **SYMPATHY** goes beyond empathy and occurs when the nurse desires to alleviate the cause of the patient's illness or suffering. This phase requires a combination of the disciplined intellectual approach combined with the therapeutic use of self. The nurse creates a helpful nursing action as a result of reaching a phase of sympathy.
- **RAPPORT** is characterized by nursing actions that alleviate an ill person's distress. The nurse and ill person are relating as human being to human being. Rapport includes a "concern for others and an active interest in them, a belief in the worth, dignity, uniqueness, and irreplaceability of each individual human being, and an accepting, nonjudgmental approach" (Travelbee, 1963, p. 71). The ill person exhibits both trust and confidence in the nurse.

> *The five phases of the Travelbee's nurse-patient relationship are original encounter, emerging identities, empathy, sympathy, and rapport.*

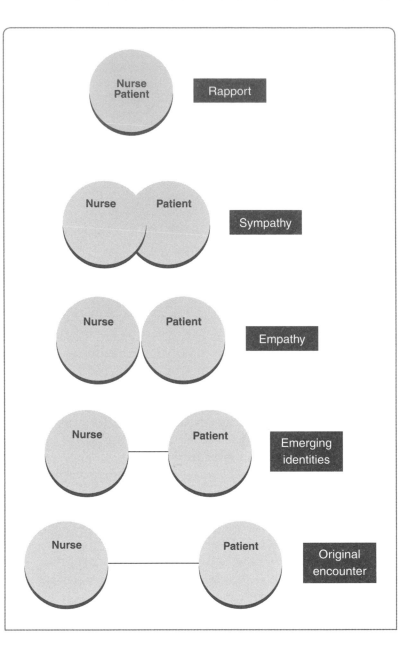

**Figure 2-5.** *Phases of Travelbee's nurse-patient relationship.* (Adapted from Hobble & Lansinger, *Nursing Theorists and Their Work*, Ann Marriner-Tomey, 2nd Ed, 1989.)

## Application to Psychiatric-Mental Health Nursing Practice

Travelbee's theory has been applied most easily and readily when working with patients who are suffering from depressive disorders. It also has been used by hospice nurses when caring for terminally ill patients.

### Application to the Nursing Process

Travelbee's theory can be integrated within the nursing process. The assessment phase of the nursing process would correlate to Travelbee's first and second phases, the original encounter and emerging identities. During the original encounter/emerging identities, the nurse forms a first impression of the patient and the patient, in turn, forms a first impression of the nurse. The nurse and the patient are just beginning to get a mutual sense of what the problems are as the nurse collects information about the patient and the problems at hand (assessment). The empathy phase most closely correlates to the diagnosis/planning in the nursing process. The nurse has now experienced an emotional sense of the patient's situation and has begun to consider interventions based on this perspective. The next phase of Travelbee's model, sympathy, involves the nurse now actively wanting to alleviate the patient's suffering and correlates to the implementation phase of the nursing process in that the actions designed in the plan of care during empathy are now implemented. During rapport, the nurse and the patient enjoy a close human-to-human relationship where the nurse has opportunities, along with the patient, to evaluate the effectiveness of the interventions; this phase reflects the evaluation aspect of the nursing process. The patient now demonstrates trust and confidence in the nurse and the actions being implemented.

## Use of Travelbee's Theory in Practice

Consider the following scenario that is typical in psychiatric care delivery. It deals with the issue of depression and suicide. You are working on the afternoon shift as a nurse at the local mental health unit. You have been informed that a new admission has just been triaged from the emergency department and has been cleared for admission to the unit. You are assigned this person as part of your caseload. You prepare the room as the patient is brought to the unit by the emergency department staff.

Applying Travelbee's model you know that the *original encounter* will occur the moment you greet the patient. You may have some preliminary information about the patient (54-year-old Caucasian female diagnosed with depression who is suicidal) and she may have some preliminary information about nurses (are generally nice and caring).

The patient arrives on the unit and you and the patient are now alone in the room as you begin your admission assessment. You are now entering the emerging identities phase. You are getting to know the patient as a human being and she is getting to know you as a human being. You hear her story and the circumstances leading to her admission and you may begin to feel something emotionally toward the patient. She, too, is mentally forming an impression of you, for example, based on how you are asking the questions, the tone of your voice, your body posture, and your attitude. She is deciding if you are trustworthy, caring, and competent.

You skillfully navigate the sensitive issues around suicidality, which allows the patient to feel comfortable enough to disclose information. Details of the emotional pain leading to her suicide attempt have touched you and you recognize that you have now entered the *empathy phase* of the relationship. You may actually experience a brief sense of your own mood shifting as you navigate this phase.

You return to the nursing station to document your assessment and begin the plan of care. As you put the information together and start your work, you may next experience *sympathy*. Developing a plan of care with goals of safety, restoration of internal control, reduction of depressive symptoms, and instillation of hope indicates that you desire to provide nursing interventions that alleviate the cause of the patient's illness and reduce her suffering. It may also occur to you that this patient was probably experiencing at least prolonged extreme anguish or likely despairful not caring, as viewed by Travelbee's continuum of suffering.

As the days pass, you and the patient meet regularly during your shift. You have meaningful conversations that allow her to express her feelings and explore solutions to the circumstances that led to her admission. She uses her time with you productively and you have been able to relate to each other, human being to human being. Subsequently, you have now established *rapport*. This is where the bulk of the work and healing is done in the nurse-patient relationship.

---

### ☯ SUMMARY POINTS

- Interpersonal relationships form the basis of nursing interventions for psychiatric-mental health nursing. Observation, assessment, communication, and evaluation skills serve as the foundation.

- Development of an interpersonal relationship requires an individual to have a basic understanding of him- or herself and what he or she brings to the relationship.

- Hildegarde Peplau is considered the founder of psychiatric-mental health nurse theory and professional practice, often referred to as the "mother of psychiatric nursing."

*(cont.)*

## SUMMARY POINTS (*CONT.*)

- Her Theory of Interpersonal Relationships views nursing as an interpersonal process between two or more persons directed toward goal achievement. Nurses need interpersonal competencies (based on the nurse's ability to understand his or her own behavior) to assist patients to regain health and well-being.

- Peplau identified four phases in the interpersonal process: orientation, identification, exploitation, and resolution. Later, these four stages were condensed into three: orientation, working, and termination phases. Her phases closely parallel those of the nursing process.

- Peplau identified six primary roles assumed by the nurse in the interpersonal process.

These include stranger, resource person, teacher, leader, surrogate, and counselor.

- Joyce Travelbee viewed nursing as an interpersonal process assisting individuals, families, or communities to prevent or cope with illness and suffering in an attempt to find meaning in these experiences. She identified three main concepts: human being, suffering, and hope. She described suffering using four levels: simple transitory discomfort; extreme anguish; despairful not caring; apathetic indifference.

- According to Travelbee, the nurse-patient relationship consisted of five phases: original encounter, emerging identities, empathy, sympathy, and rapport.

## NCLEX-PREP*

1. A nurse who will be providing care to a psychiatric-mental health patient is in the orientation phase of the relationship. The nurse would most likely assume which role?

   a. Counselor
   b. Teacher
   c. Stranger
   d. Surrogate

2. A group of nursing students are reviewing information about Peplau's phases of the nurse-patient relationship and how they apply to the nursing process. The students demonstrate understanding of the

information when they identify which of Peplau's phases as correlating to the implementation step of the nursing process?

   a. Orientation
   b. Identification
   c. Exploitation
   d. Resolution

3. Travelbee identifies three major concepts for her theory. Which concept provides the nurse with the most powerful intervention?

   a. Hope
   b. Suffering
   c. Human being
   d. Empathy

(*cont.*)

### NCLEX-PREP* (CONT.)

4. A nurse is integrating Travelbee's theory of the nurse-patient relationship into the care being provided to a patient. Which of the following is demonstrated when the nurse implements actions to alleviate the ill person's distress?

   a. Emerging identities
   b. Empathy
   c. Sympathy
   d. Rapport

5. During the orientation phase of the nurse-patient relationship, the nurse focuses communication on which of the following?

   a. Reason for the patient seeking help
   b. The patient as a whole
   c. Expected routines
   d. Time frame for interaction

6. A group of nursing students is reviewing information about the interpersonal theorists, Peplau and Travelbee. The students demonstrate understanding of the information when they identify which person as a key influence on Peplau?

   a. Harry Sullivan
   b. Victor Frankl
   c. Ida Orlando
   d. Sigmund Freud

*Answers to these questions appear on page 639.

## REFERENCES

Beeber, L.S., Canuso, R., & Emory, S. (2004). Instrumental inputs: Moving the interpersonal theory of nursing into practice. *Advances in Nursing Science, 27*(4): 275–286.

Callaway, B. J. (2002). *Hildegard Peplau: Psychiatric nurse of the century.* New York: Springer Publishing Co.

Marriner Tomey, A. & Alligood, M. R. (2006). *Nursing theorists and their work,* (6th ed.) St. Louis: Mosby.

Orlando, I. J. (1961). The dynamic nurse-patient relationship: Function, process and principles. New York: G. P. Putman. Sons. [Reprinted 1990, New York: National League for Nursing.]

O'Toole, A.W., & Welt, S.R. (1989). *Interpersonal theory in nursing practice: Selected works of Hildegarde E. Peplau.* New York: Springer Publishing Co.

Peplau, H. (1952). *Interpersonal relations in nursing.* New York: G.P. Putnam.

Peplau, H.E. Interpersonal techniques: The crux of psychiatric nursing. *American Journal of Nursing, 62*(6): 50–54.

Peplau, H.E. (1991). *Interpersonal relations in nursing.* New York: G.P. Putnam.

Peplau, H.E. (1992). A theoretical framework for application in nursing practice. *Nursing Science Quarterly, 5*(1): 13–18.

Peplau, H.E. (1997). Peplau's theory of interpersonal relations. *Nursing Science Quarterly, 10*(4): 162–167.

Reed, P.G, (2006) The force of nursing theory guided-practice. *Nursing Science Quarterly, 19*(3):225.

Travelbee, J. (1963). What do we mean by rapport? *American Journal of Nursing, 63*(2): 70–72.

Travelbee, J. (1964). What's wrong with sympathy? *American Journal of Nursing, 64*(1); 71.

Travelbee, J. (1971). *Interpersonal aspects of nursing.* (2nd ed.). Philadelphia: F.A. Davis.

Vandemark, L.M. (2006). Awareness of self and expanding consciousness: Using nursing theories to prepare nurse therapists. *Mental Health Nursing, 27*(6): 605–615.

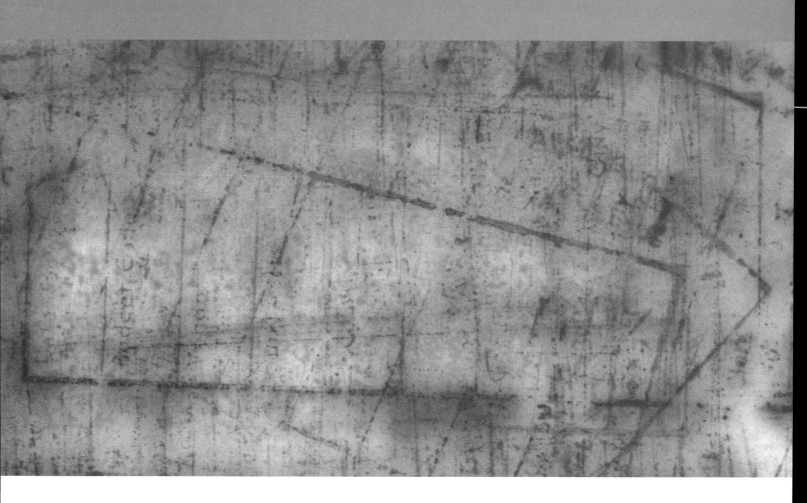

## CHAPTER CONTENTS

The Concept of Self

Theoretical Foundations for Self and the
Therapeutic Use of Self

Development of the Therapeutic Use of Self

Therapeutic Use of Self and the
Interpersonal Process

Therapeutic Communication

## EXPECTED LEARNING OUTCOMES

**After completing this chapter, the student will be able to:**

1. Define the term self.
2. Define therapeutic use of self.
3. Identify key concepts associated with the therapeutic use of self.
4. Describe ways to develop greater self-awareness.
5. Define therapeutic communication.
6. Discuss the key concepts of therapeutic communication.

## CHAPTER 3

# THERAPEUTIC USE OF SELF AND THERAPEUTIC COMMUNICATION: FROM SELF-DISCOVERY TO INTERPERSONAL SKILL INTEGRATION

John F. Sweeney

Declan McCarthy

7. Explain the significance of therapeutic communication to establish and maintain therapeutic nurse-patient relationships.

8. Identify techniques of therapeutic communication.

9. Describe barriers to effective therapeutic communication.

## KEY TERMS

Active listening

Attitudes

Beliefs

Communication

Empathy

Process recording

Self

Self-awareness

Self-disclosure

Self-reflection

Therapeutic

Therapeutic communication

Therapeutic use of self

Values

*No man can come to know himself except as an outcome of disclosing himself to another person* (Jourard, 1971). Thus, one's self is not just a single abstract idea, but rather the whole of the person including his or her experiences with others. When working with any patient, but especially a psychiatric-mental health patient, nurses integrate the nurse-patient relationship with the nursing process. This integration is complex and dynamic and requires that the psychiatric-mental health nurse develop a specialized skill set—THERAPEUTIC USE OF SELF. The therapeutic use of self is complex and involves a process of self-awareness through one's own growth and development as well as one's interactions with others. While the concepts of self and therapeutic use of self are usually referred to in psychiatric-mental health nursing practice, the beginning psychiatric-mental health nurse is encouraged to recognize the importance of these skills and practice using them when dealing with all patients or family members, regardless of diagnosis.

This chapter explains therapeutic use of self including its theoretical foundations and how nurses use this skill during the nurse-patient relationship, especially when working with psychiatric-mental health patients. The chapter also addresses therapeutic communication as a key component of the therapeutic use of self, describing effective techniques and potential barriers to effective communication.

## THE CONCEPT OF SELF

Beginning psychiatric-mental health nurses need to understand the concept of SELF to provide quality patient care. Self is defined as the entire person of an individual; an individual's typical character and an individual's temporary behavior; and as the union of elements (body, emotions, thoughts, and sensations) that constitute the individuality and identity of a person (Merriam-Webster, 2011). An awareness of a sense of the self is core to a human being's personal identity (Gallop & O'Brien, 2003). From an early age, individuals become aware of physical, psychological, social, and cultural similarities with others. Insights into these similarities and dissimilarities emerge as individuals begin to understand the unique, interactive, and shared experiences of him- or herself and others that occur across one's lifespan. The sense of self develops from early childhood experiences and continues as the individual transitions from family, school, social, and work life toward old age. Self-reflections are triggered by the developmental and incidental encounters with others as the individual moves along in life. Whether joyful, neutral, or painful, the processes of feedback from others,

self discovery, learning, experience, travel, and memory forge insights into the complexity of life as an individual and shared reality. This experience of the self represents a lifelong journey of discovery of personal identity.

> *The concept of self refers to a person's entirety that develops throughout the lifespan as an individual experiences similarities and differences with others and gains insight into his or her identity.*

Consider the intricacy of the universe then reflect upon your own complexity. They are both more intriguing and fascinating. Work through the exercise outlined in **Box 3-1** to examine your "self."

Based on the exercise, the point is that the self is a complex entity that is interconnected to others through interpersonal, intrapersonal, and external relationships and through environmental forces. Additionally, the more one magnifies something, the more one sees. Thus, individuals realize that they know very little about the deep self.

Yet the true authentic self can often remain elusive. To acknowledge and accept this means one must confront the limits to current awareness of self, an issue of reflective practice that is paramount to psychiatric-mental health nurses (Prestwood, 2009). The important part of the psychiatric-mental health nurse is the "person." Knowing one's personal self helps one to engage more fully with others. To a certain extent, it is impossible to think of the self without considering a mutual relationship with others in one's environment. The way reality is constructed depends as much on a person's response to feedback from significant others, as on perception through a process of inter-subjective sharing of beliefs, cognitions, and feelings (Gallimore, Goldenberg, & Weisner, 1993; Vatne & Hoem, 2008). As psychiatric-mental health nurses, the use of self in the nurse-patient relationship is the crux of professional engagement (Lego, 1999). This is the paramount therapeutic use of the self.

## THEORETICAL FOUNDATIONS FOR SELF AND THE THERAPEUTIC USE OF SELF

Several theorists and researchers have provided information about self, the therapeutic use of self, the nurse-patient

> **BOX 3-1: COMPLEXITY OF SELF AND UNIVERSE**
>
> 1. Consider the universe in which we live. Write down all the types of celestial bodies and planets that you know. Write a sentence or two to reflect the multitude of orbits and their conjunction with each other
> 2. Consider your own "self." Think about what keeps you alive and helps you to grow – physically, emotionally, socially, and spiritually. Draw a spider diagram with your "self" in the center and add those supports that help you to grow and develop.
> 3. What do you think are the connections between your "self" and the universe? (There are no right and wrong answers here.)
> 4. *Practical Activity:* Plant a seed or a seedling and care for it. Keep a diary of what is needed to stimulate its growth.
> 5. When you are working with a person, what do you think are the cognitive, emotional, and spiritual ingredients necessary for a psychiatric-mental health nurse?
>
> From this exercise you will have possibly gathered that when a human being's self is separated from the universe, growth is impaired. The more one splits the self, the more disintegrated, fragmented, and complicated everything and everyone becomes. Remember that the self represents an integration of multiple elements. For more exercises on complexity, see *The Möbius Strip* (Pickover, 2006).
>
> *From Pickover, C. (2006). The Möbius Strip: Dr. August Möbius's Marvelous Band in Mathematics, Games, Literature, Art, Technology, and Cosmology: Thunder's Mouth Press. Cited in Mathforum, 2009.*

relationship, and the importance of integrating these concepts for the psychiatric-mental health nurse. The information provided expounds on from Chapter 2.

## Carl Rogers

Carl Rogers, although not a nurse, is one theorist who addressed the concept of self. Rogers is known as the founder of person-centered counseling. He contends that when listening to another, a number of major conditions are imperative in supporting development in the other. Namely, these core conditions are:

- Congruence (the mind being in tune with the body)
- Empathy (being able to put yourself in the other persons shoes emotionally)
- Unconditional positive regard (not judging anyone and having a positive and supportive attitude to them) (Rogers, 1951)

According to Rogers, these elements, when present in the therapeutic relationship, would lead patient's to develop these conditions in themselves. Contemporary psychiatric-mental health nursing understandings, skills, and treatment approaches have been influenced by his philosophies.

> *Carl Rogers, the founder of person-centered counseling, identified three core conditions needed to support development of the other person: congruence, empathy, and unconditional positive regard.*

## Other Theorists

It is one thing to become more aware of one's own self, it is altogether another to be able to assist others to explore the dimensions of their own sense of self, reality, and connection to the world. The term "*therapeutic use of self*" primarily came from the work of three theorists writing about the one-to-one nurse-patient relationship, namely Hildegard Peplau, June Mellow, and Ida Jean Orlando (Lego, 1999). Lego synthesized the work of these early theorists to provide a seminal definition of the concept *therapeutic use of self* as:

*…the relationship between a psychiatric nurse and his/her patient, formed for the purpose of brief counselling, crisis*

*intervention, and/or individual psychotherapy. The empha- sis is on the interpersonal relationship between the nurse and the patient, with all its vicissitudes, as opposed to physi- cal care of the patient.* (1999, p. 4)

Peplau's theory (see Chapter 2 for more informa- tion) developed over a 40-year period and was enhanced by research focused on barriers to interpersonal closeness and her reflections on clinical observations (Coatsworth- Puspoky, Forchuk, & Ward-Griffin, 2006; Lego 1999). Drawing on Peplau's theory, Karen Lee Fontaine defined the therapeutic use of self as "using one's personhood to provide psychiatric nursing care" (Fontaine, 2009, p.168). Fontaine notes that a distinction has to be drawn between the therapeutic use of self in a one-to-one nurse-patient relationship and its use within a specialized milieu that focuses on the shaping of group behaviors within a thera- peutic community.

In addition to Peplau, other nursing theorists such as Joyce Travelbee (1971), Annie Altschul (1972), and Phil Barker (1998, 2001b) have described the nurse-patient relationship. Still others have suggested that psychiatric- mental health nurses define the development of a thera- peutic relationship with their patients as a foundational aspect of nursing care (O'Brien, 2001).

In the twenty-first century, the term "patient" began to be replaced with terms such as "client," "service user" or "survivor of psychiatric-mental health services" as a result of a gradual paradigm shift from a biomedical to a social psychiatric viewpoint that placed greater empha- sis on increased patient autonomy. Prior to this shift in viewpoint, the more medical model approach resulted in patients being disempowered. With this greater emphasis on patient autonomy, patient involvement and collabora- tive care planning were taking place.

Terminology related to psychiatry and psychiat- ric illness also is changing due to the shift in attitudes and patient involvement. The terms mental health and recovery (a view that encompasses the whole person) are coming to the forefront. For example, in Ireland, new in-patient units are being renamed as mental health and recovery units instead of psychiatric units. Such a change initiates a gentler and more embracing sense of a unique personal recovery journey, thus transforming a pure bio- medical model of care into one focusing on dialogue and a shift in patient-therapist power relations. In the United States, recovery, too, is a major focus. The Executive Summary of the President's New Freedom Commission on Mental Health cited a need for transforming mental health service delivery with recovery as the goal of this transformation (President's New Freedom Commission,

2003). In addition, The Substance Abuse and Mental Health Services Administration (SAMHSA) in their National Consensus Statement described "mental health recovery as a journey of healing and transformation enabling a person with a mental health problem to live a meaningful life in a community of his or her choice while striving to achieve his or her potential" (SAMHSA, 2006). Thus the term, "recovery" is now used more frequently.

Recovery is a process that includes a person's lifestyle, work, and aspirations. It is about the person's quality of life, not about the illness. SAMHSA has identified ten fundamental components of recovery:
- Self-direction
- Individualized and person-centered (based on unique strengths and resiliencies, needs, preferences, experi- ences, and cultural background)
- Empowerment (authority to choose from a range of options and to participate in all decisions)
- Holistic (mind, body, spirit, and community; all aspects of life)
- Non-linear (continual growth, occasional setbacks, and learning from experience)
- Strengths-based
- Peer support
- Respect
- Responsibility
- Hope (SAMHSA, 2006)

Psychiatric-mental health nurses are in a strong position to support patients as they reintegrate into society. Nurses have the knowledge and skills to enable people to help themselves toward the goal of normal living as productive members of communities. Further collaboration between the professional and the patient is an important component of the treatment plan. This is evident in Phil Barker's Tidal Model approach (Barker, 1998; Barker, 2001b).

Barker's Tidal Model (2001a) provides a meaningful way of empowering both the nurse and patient to work ther- apeutically toward recovery (Buchanan-Barker & Barker, 2006; Buchanan-Barker & Barker, 2008). Barker's Tidal Model is the first mental health recovery model developed conjointly by psychiatric-mental health nurses and people who have used mental health services. It is also the first recovery-focused model of psychiatric-mental health nurs- ing recognized internationally as a significant middle-range theory of nursing (i.e., theory that is more concrete and less abstract in scope). This model has been used as the basis for interdisciplinary mental health care; it focuses on begin- ning the recovery journey when the person is at his or her lowest ebb. Barker advocates that the psychiatric-mental health nurse affirms the person's view of the experience of mental ill health, helping him or her to retain emotional and physical safety while exploring the types of supports necessary for re-establishing connections within life.

## DEVELOPMENT OF THE THERAPEUTIC USE OF SELF

Self has been defined earlier in this chapter. The term THER-APEUTIC means of or relating to the treatment of disease or disorders by remedial agents or methods (a therapeutic rather than a diagnostic specialty; Merriam-Webster, 2011). While the term therapeutic use of self is not defined in the dictionary, it is a concept widely accepted by professionals working in the psychiatric-mental health field. The therapeutic use of self integrates theory, experiential knowledge, and self awareness to assist patients in exploring their impact with others to promote behavioral changes in the patient (American Nurses Association [ANA], American Psychiatric Nurses Association [APNA], and International Society of Psychiatric-Mental Health Nurses [ISPN], 2007).

Joyce Travelbee (1971) described the therapeutic use of self as the ability of nurses to be self aware and consciously use themselves (their reactions and verbal and nonverbal interactions) to establish a sense of relatedness with patients and to structure therapeutic nursing interventions. This skill is critical. Without it, the nurse-patient relationship could easily drift into being no more than a pleasant social interaction.

The therapeutic use of self keeps the psychiatric-mental health nurse focused on the patient's needs by requiring the nurse to reflect on and monitor his or her own reactions to the verbal and nonverbal interactions between them. A psychiatric-mental health nurse's reactions to and interactions with a given patient can help or hinder the nurse's ability to accurately assess the patient's needs and plan therapeutic interventions. For this reason, the therapeutic use of self requires the psychiatric-mental health nurse to develop self-awareness and engage in both self-reflection and reflection about his or her clinical work with other experienced psychiatric nurses.

> *Therapeutic use of self is a key element of the therapeutic nurse-patient relationship. The psychiatric-mental health nurse develops it through self-awareness and self-reflection.*

## Self-Awareness

SELF-AWARENESS refers to the process of developing an understanding of one's own values, beliefs, thoughts, feelings, reactions, motivations, biases, strengths, and limitations, and recognizing their effect on others. It is an introspective process that requires an in-depth examination of attributes alone and in conjunction with others. Input from others is key to preventing an unrealistic, biased perception. Also important here are values, beliefs, and attitudes.

VALUES are abstract positive or negative concepts that represent ideal conduct and goals. They help to establish a sense of what is right and wrong, providing a "code of conduct." This is different from real conduct, that is, how the person actually behaves.

Values are developed from one's experiences with family, friends, culture, and the environment throughout one's lifespan. Values do not develop spontaneously, however. Individuals need to discover what their values are through a process of values clarification. This process reflects how an individual actually comes to have the values that he or she does. It is not what the values should be or which values should be followed. With values clarification the individual looks at all the possible values and then identifies those that seem right for that individual (choosing). Then the individual looks at the chosen values and, being satisfied with the choices, publicly affirms those choices (prizing). Lastly, the individual integrates and demonstrates the values in his or her behavior consistently and repeatedly (acting). These values ultimately determine the person's behavior.

BELIEFS are ideas that an individual holds to be true. They often arise from the person's values. However, a belief is different from a value in that a belief is not acted on. For example, a person may hold specific beliefs but he or she may not act on the beliefs. Beliefs can be rational (based on objective evidence), irrational (idea held despite contradictory evidence), blind (idea held without any objective evidence such as faith), and stereotypical (idea describing an oversimplified or undifferentiated concept that is socially shared).

ATTITUDES refer to general feelings or that which provides a frame of reference for an individual. Attitudes generally reflect a person's values and provide a person with a means for organizing how to view the world. Thus, attitudes provide meaning in an individual's life. **Box 3-2** provides three exercises that can help promote the development of self-awareness.

## Self-Reflection

One way a psychiatric-mental health nurse can evaluate whether his or her interpersonal nurse-patient relationship

**BOX 3-2: EXERCISES FOR DEVELOPING SELF-AWARENESS**

### ACTIVITY 1:

1. Bring to class a portion of clay that can be molded or sculpted. Also bring old clothes or a plastic apron to protect your clothing
2. Then, in a quiet part of the room, sculpt a symbol or a shape representing psychiatric-mental health nursing. Allow the thoughts and the feelings to integrate with your hands as you mold the clay.
3. In group discussion, briefly give feedback on the symbolic representation of psychiatric-mental health nursing that you have created and what thinking influenced you in creating this sculpture.
4. Then break into groups of three and provide objective feedback to each other about the objects after observing the others' work.

This activity can help incorporate an essential artistic component into the work and everyday skills of a psychiatric nurse.

### ACTIVITY 2:

1. Split into pairs. Discuss your different perceptions of things, e.g., an apple, a mountain, or a mouse. What does it mean to you personally? Choose anything you like.
2. Describe your perception to your partner in a few minutes. Practice the active listening skills you have picked up or read about.
3. Include the different colors and things involving your image, such as its surroundings.
4. Then reverse roles and listen to how your partner describes the same thing, person, or place.
5. Note and identify how each person has different thoughts and images about the same things.

### ACTIVITY 3:

1. Working in pairs with a peer, write your personal response to the following questions. Then exchange papers with your peer and explore each other's answers.
   a. If you were to be an animal, which species would you be?
   b. Which characteristics of this creature appeal to you most?
   c. What does this choice say about the way you see yourself at present?
2. Now with the same partner, write your personal response to the following questions. Then exchange papers with your peer and explore each other's answers.
   a. What attracted you to a career as a nurse?
   b. What experience and qualities from your life do you bring to your studies?
   c. What qualities do you think you will need to become a good nurse?

is therapeutic and focused on meeting patient needs in a professional versus social way is to ask: "Whose needs are being met in this interaction?" Unconsciously, a nurse's earlier experiences of communicating with others or with patients encountered in the past could subtly influence the nurse's way of relating to a patient in the present. Mannerisms, body language, speech, or behavior could trigger unconscious responses of attraction, anxiety, or dislike in the nurse based on earlier encounters with persons who remind the nurse of this patient. One way of bringing these reactions to conscious awareness is through reflection on one's self.

SELF-REFLECTION refers to a process of becoming conscious of largely tacit or intuitive knowledge, motives, and attitudes that underlie a professional interpersonal interaction. Questions that psychiatric-mental health nurses might use for self-reflection and to better understand how their own reactions and needs might be impacting their clinical decision making with patients include:

1. What in my past or current life circumstances helps or hinders my ability to respond therapeutically to this patient?
2. Of whom does this patient remind me?
3. What am I thinking about while the patient talks?
4. How does this patient make me feel?
5. Why did I react to the patient in this particular manner?
6. Who talked the most in this patient interaction?
7. Why am I seeking out or avoiding this patient?
8. How did my reactions to this patient help or hinder meeting his or her needs?

Answers to these questions can help psychiatric-mental health nurses understand how personal needs and reactions impact their therapeutic nurse-patient relationships.

> *Self-awareness develops by examining one's values, attitudes, and beliefs. Self-reflection focuses on examining whose needs are being met.*

## THERAPEUTIC USE OF SELF AND THE INTERPERSONAL PROCESS

Although development of greater awareness into hidden motives or unconscious reactions by the psychiatric-mental health nurse is important to professional development, insight alone will not assist in skill development. Structuring a meaningful therapeutic interaction is addressed in terms of the process and the therapeutic listening and response skills needed by the nurse. The therapeutic use of self and the interpersonal process has been the subject of much investigation. Several studies have addressed this topic and the effects on the nurse and on the patient. The therapeutic use of self has been shown to require conscious effort, competency, role support, commitment, and sensitivity on the part of the nurse and to be a positive force for growth of the nurse and patient.

### Importance of the Therapeutic Use of Self

Recall that the interpersonal relationship begins with the initial or first encounter with the patient. Researchers have evaluated methods used to open up initial conversations

between psychiatric-mental health nurses and their patients. One study by McAllister et.al. (2004) examined conversation starters between psychiatric-mental health nurses and their patients in Australia. From the study, McAllister and colleagues proposed a means of structuring first encounters with patients through the use of effective conversation starters (McAllister, Matarasso, Dixon, & Shepperd, 2004). The researchers argued that use of tentative opening invitations to restructure an interview into a mental status evaluation through conversation required sensitivity as to pacing, answering, and the posing of questions. It is suggested that psychiatric-mental health nurses should exercise "wise authority" to enable vulnerable people to make informed decisions as they balance the demands of citizenship (that is, the demands and responsibilities of being a member of a wider society), with those of the patient role as they negotiate their recovery. This involves giving information and sometimes justifiable opinions based on experience. However, patients may have cognitive challenges due to underlying organic or functional issues. This then presents a fine line in relation to human rights and freedom of choice, especially where their or society's health is at stake. The sharing of information and the open, frank discussion that is given honestly induces personal growth for both patient and staff. This development is healthy and progressive and is the basis for many if not all therapeutic relationships. It is the cornerstone for change in the way the nurse relates to the patient in terms of therapeutic intervention.

> *Therapy is seen as a journey with twists and turns in a landscape, which is largely unknown territory, wherein many conversations are possible. The aim of this approach is for a respectful, non-blaming approach, in which the client is central as the expert in his/her own life.* (McAllister et al., 2004, p. 578)

A phenomenological study (a study designed to describe the lived experience) by Moyle (2003) recounts two aspects of an effective therapeutic relationship valued by patients during treatment for depression. These are "being with the patient" and "the need for comfort," in contrast with two alternative approaches perceived as non-therapeutic—"focusing on the physical" and "lack of comfort" (Moyle, 2003). These alternative approaches were experienced as avoidance of emotional engagement through the nurse's business and emotional coolness within the context of maintaining professional boundaries. While subscribing to a positive view of the therapeutic use of self as nurturing, caring, insight developing, and behavior challenging, Moyle suggests that over-involvement can be detrimental.

To establish a meaningful interpersonal relationship, the nurse needs role competence (skills for practice), role support (effective supervision), and a commitment to engage therapeutically (Lauder, Reynolds, Reilly, & Angus, 2000). In other words, claims of it being someone else's job, there is not enough time, no one supports or coaches me, or values my efforts, will inhibit the nurse from engaging or taking professional accountability for the quality of the therapeutic relationship that he or she has with a patient.

The therapeutic use of self can be burdensome. For some, the notion of the emotional burden of nursing suggests that the therapeutic use of self as a nursing intervention may be problematic (Smith, 1988, 1989; Smith & Gray, 2001a; Smith & Gray, 2001b; Smith & Lorentzon, 2005). The therapeutic use of self can be burdensome if the nurse does not receive adequate support and clinical supervision. For example, a psychiatric-mental health nurse may often experience an emotional burden from his or her sharing one's presence with a person rather than by retreating into task activity or psychological distancing of the self; that is, not getting involved with the person's issues at times of personal painful distress (Finfgeld-Connett, 2006). Also, establishment and maintenance of an effective interpersonal relationship require skilled personal disclosure by the nurse where appropriate, in which the therapeutic use of self is akin to Smith's understanding of the emotional labor of mental health nursing (Smith 1989; Smith & Gray, 2001a; Smith & Lorentzon, 2005). Mitchell and Smith (2003, p. 109) suggest that "the concept of emotional labor provides a means of describing and understanding the often invisible work employed, among others, by those in the caring professions. It involves using emotions and the appearance of emotions to provide security and confidence in others." Trying to meet the needs of patients in distress over a prolonged period can take its toll on the psychiatric-mental health nurse. In short, the emotional labor of psychiatric-mental health nursing requires resources of resilience, perseverance, compassion, and access to clinical support.

Clinical supervision provides an objective view crucial to therapeutic relationships. Without adequate support and clinical supervision, the nurse may experience role strain and uncertainty about what he or she is likely to encounter in the clinical setting and may feel overwhelmed. One way in which such role strain may be manifested is by physical and emotional distancing from the person through activities such as being too busy, engaging in tasks, or avoiding accompanying the person through the painful episodes of distress. Using the four stages of Peplau's interpersonal theory, Forchuk investigated the

behavior of nurse and patient during the outcomes of each stage. The results showed that psychiatric-mental health nurses were competent and did to assist patients therapeutically to traverse the four stages of the nurse-patient relationship as described by Peplau (1952) (Forchuk, 1991a, 1991b; Forchuk, 1992, 1994; Forchuk et al., 1989; Forchuk & Brown, 1989).

Another study by Welch (2005) demonstrated that psychiatric-mental health nurses experienced "trust," "sharing of power," "mutuality," "self-revelation," "congruence" and "authenticity" as their true self at pivotal moments of a therapeutic relationship (**Evidence-Based Practice 3-1**). The psychiatric-mental health nurses interviewed gained a sense of mastery of the essential art of interpersonal nursing (Welch, 2005). There is evidence that mental health service users can articulate what they seek and value from psychiatric-mental health nurses in the context of a therapeutic relationship.

Patients have expressed a desire for the nurse to be able to "relate to me," "know me as a person" and to "get to the solution" (Shattell, Starr, & Thomas, 2007). To be effective, patients wanted a nurse to treat them compassionately with respect, sensitivity, caring, and support. They wanted to be listened to and provided with companionship and to have confidence in the nurse's skills to interact effectively with them. Specifically, it meant providing emotional support; having appropriate knowledge, training, and experience; and having a capacity to challenge verbal and nonverbal cues honestly and congruently (Shattell, Starr, & Thomas, 2007). To relate in a human-to-human manner, to know a person intimately, and to apply therapeutic use of self, requires the psychiatric-mental health nurse to assess the professional boundaries between patient and nurse.

Despite shorter admissions, an individual's journey through a period of mental distress toward recovery can be lengthy. This requires that the nurse be skilled with focused compassion and a willingness to challenge and support a person through a period of mutually disconcerting exploration. These existential challenges affect one's ways of knowing how to relate to others and events and turn them into new ways of relating to self, others, and the world (Shattell, Starr, & Thomas, 2007).

Self-awareness is a necessary component of therapeutic use of self. A self-awareness program for undergraduate nursing students was devised to assist in the development of therapeutic relationships with their patients (Kwaitek, McKenzie, & Loads, 2005). The course was developed drawing on the work of Patricia Benner and Judith Wrubel (1989) on the primacy of caring in professional nursing and on Dawn Freshwater's (1999) work on

**EVIDENCE-BASED PRACTICE 3-1:**
**SIGNIFICANT MOMENTS IN THERAPEUTIC RELATIONSHIPS**

### STUDY

Welch, M. (2005). Pivotal moments in the therapeutic relationship. *International Journal of Mental Health Nursing, 14*(3): 161–165.

### SUMMARY

The purpose of this study was to explore and describe significant factors for a therapeutic relationship. A series of one-on-one interviews were conducted with six experienced psychiatric-mental health nurses who were asked to think about therapeutic relationships that they have had with patients and describe times within those relationships when everything seemed to change and the quality of the relationship improved. The nurses identified several factors that were associated with the change in the relationship, including empathy, uniqueness, meaning and purpose, and appropriate self-disclosure.

### APPLICATION TO PRACTICE

Many psychiatric-mental health nurses have had difficulty explaining exactly what the therapeutic relationship is, even though the majority agreed that it is the foundation of psychiatric-mental health nursing. Psychiatric-mental health nurses could employ the factors associated with the changes in the relationship identified by this study as key characteristics of the relationship. These terms are readily describable and familiar to most individuals. Psychiatric-mental health nurses can also integrate knowledge of these factors when engaging in the interpersonal process with patients to promote a quality, effective relationship.

### QUESTIONS TO PONDER

1. *Think back to a time when you had a pivotal moment with a patient. What made this time therapeutic?*
2. *Have you ever experienced a time when a pivotal moment was not therapeutic? If so, what happened and why?*

psychotherapeutic application of emotional intelligence of the psychiatric-mental health nurse described in the following. It used exploration of clinical vignettes to focus on four key themes—"knowing self," "knowing others," "unknowing," and "presencing." Through exploration of these dimensions of the self particularly related to what was unknown about self or others, participants gained insights into their personal attitudes and conscious and unconscious ways of human relating. The development

of capacity to reflect on the self and the personal impact on others form part of what is referred to as "emotional intelligence" (Freshwater & Stickley, 2004). This realization is key to understanding one's unconscious ways of responding to others that are complementary to, yet distinct from, intentional, interpersonal interactions. The notion of "doing for" a person and the conscious experience of "being with" a person at times of mental anguish or distress need to be cultivated in the nurse to facilitate a therapeutic healing process. Recognition of the nurse's own unconscious need for approval, respect, and love through the caring process constitutes a necessary, if at times painful, journey of self-discovery, without which the nurse will be unable to relate empathetically to others (Freshwater & Stickley, 2004).

This sense of unknowing is explored in the deliberate creation, valuing, and usage of inter- and intrapersonal space in the therapeutic relationship (Stickley & Freshwater, 2006). It is cultivated through experiential learning using art, creative therapies, role modeling and clinical supervision as an alternative to propositional knowledge. Failure to acknowledge interpersonal space by being busy with tasks creates the risk that the nurse may compound alienation, prejudice, and the replacement of meaningful dialogue. What is termed "phatic" conversation or social chit chat, though of benefit in the early stages of a professional relationship, may be over used to the expense of authentic, shared interaction (Bloor & Fonkert, 1982).

Dealing with a patient's distress could become unidimensional unless considered from the patient's perspective of a therapeutic nurse-patient relationship. Early attempts by psychoanalysts to delve into the chaotic existence of a patient tended to rely on the techniques and expertise of the therapist to shape the reframing of mental distress (Shattell, Starr, & Thomas, 2007). This gave way to the later human-to-human theories developed by psychiatric nurses such as Hildegard Peplau and Joyce Travelbee. Both advocated for greater power equity in the therapist-patient relationship. A warm, secure, trusting, and companionable relationship is the type sought by contemporary service recipients in a mental health setting (Shattell et al. 2007). Specific characteristics in the nurse valued by patients included a capacity to relate to the patient as a person rather than as patient, the instillation of hope, and the building of authentic rapport. While the art of effective listening, mutual understanding, touch and self-disclosure were prized, these could be undermined if a nurse withheld the commitment to time, presence, and genuine effort to understand the person's needs and perspectives (Shattell et al. 2007). This then leads to the question: What could be the indicators of an effective therapeutic relationship? A number of writers (Dziopa & Ahern, 2009; Stockmann, 2005) have identified the qualities or constituents of such a relationship. These are identified in **Table 3-1**.

It is one thing to identify the constituents of the therapeutic relationship but altogether another to attempt to define the role of the psychiatric-mental health nurse and the needs and preferences of the patient for such an encounter. **Table 3-2** links the stages of Peplau's (1952,

1997) interpersonal process with contemporary views of patients and the interventions identified through clinical studies. It provides exemplars drawn from the wide body of research that has engaged with and explored the application of Peplau's theory in the everyday practice of the psychiatric-mental health nurse over the past 50 years since it was first formulated. In general, contemporary views of patients reveal that they want and feel the need to be in control of their own recovery. They feel positive when being listened to and when given a choice of treatments if appropriate.

> *Different skills need to be applied by the psychiatric-mental health nurse as he or she accompanies the patient through the therapeutic journey across the four stages of Peplau's interpersonal therapeutic relationship.*

## Positive Components of the Self

Therapeutic interaction is facilitated by certain components. The most important component the nurse brings to any interpersonal relationship is self. This is body and mind and unique life experience. Patients view the relationship as the cornerstone of in-patient care (Forchuk & Reynolds, 2001). Three factors are thought to contribute to the development of the professional relationship: (a) caring characteristics of the nurse; (b) how the relationships were conducted; and (c) implementation of the goals during the therapeutic meetings.

**EMPATHY** is often another core principle highlighted in relationship literature. Empathy is not simply active listening but more a recognition of the person hearing what the other is saying while being able to occupy a shared space. Empathy can be defined as putting yourself in the other person's shoes, or seeing the world through the other person's eyes.

When trying to access what a person is feeling, it is important not to complicate things. Rather, it should be kept simple. Six emotional expressions have been recognized at the core—feeling shock, anger, sadness, awe, elation, and disgust (Ekman, Friesen, & Ancoli, 1980). Other words—such as confused, bothered, and agitated—camouflage the core emotions. It is important to remember that feelings are never right or wrong. They exist and are the

**TABLE 3-1: CONSTITUENTS AND QUALITIES OF A THERAPEUTIC RELATIONSHIP**

| EXEMPLIFYING CONSTRUCTS[a] | DEMONSTRATED QUALITIES IN NURSE[b] |
|---|---|
| Conveying understanding and empathy | Empathy |
| Accepting individuality | Openness |
| Providing support | Hope, forgiveness |
| Being there/available | Presence, unconditional positive regard |
| Being genuine | Congruence |
| Promoting equality | Empowerment, self-esteem building |
| Demonstrating respect | Respect, trust |
| Maintaining clear boundaries | Patient centered goals and objectives setting, value clarification |
| Demonstrating self awareness | Self-disclosure, self-awareness |

From [a]*Dziopa, F., & Ahern, K. (2009). Three different ways mental health nurses develop quality therapeutic relationships. Issues in Mental Health Nursing, 30(1):14–22;* [b]*Stockmann, C. (2005). A literature review of the progress of the psychiatric nurse-patient relationship as described by Peplau. Issues in Mental Health Nursing, 26(9):911–919.*

raw materials that nurses engage with when involved with patients therapeutically. No judgments should be afforded to them. A psychiatric-mental health nurse might find it impossible to have had the type of experience that gives rise to the emotional responses in the patient. As a result, the nurse may feel personally inadequate. However, listening attentively and empathetically can enable the person to recognize that, although out of the realm of the nurse's personal experience, the nurse is genuine in the attempt to engage and comprehend the person's emotional turmoil.

> *For a therapeutic relationship, the psychiatric-mental health nurse must develop empathy, the ability to put him- or herself in the patient's shoes or see the world through the patient's eyes.*

All engagement with others, especially in the domain of feelings, carries a certain risk of misunderstanding. This is an element of being human and sometimes mistakes are made. However, these times afford opportunities for reflection and learning for the nurse and patient. How did I misinterpret this person's intentions, body language, or expressed emotion? Many people encountered in clinical practice will experience uncertainty around a major transition in their life or health. There is a human temptation to try to fix or rescue a person in distress as part of therapeutic communication. However, giving reassurance prior to grappling with the underlying emotional pain or distress can lead to frustration in the person, who may feel misunderstood or patronized, both of which could serve as blocks to recovery of the healthy self.

## THERAPEUTIC COMMUNICATION

**COMMUNICATION** refers to the transmission of information or a message from a sender to a receiver. The sender initiates the interaction and encodes the message, which is conveyed through channels. These channels can be auditory (spoken), visual (sights, observations, and perceptions), and kinesthetic (via touch). The receiver then translates and interprets the message and makes the appropriate response. The receiver demonstrates that the message has been received through feedback. This feedback returns to the sender, thus making communication a reciprocal process. **THERAPEUTIC COMMUNICATION** refers to the interaction between a nurse and patient that is focused on the patient, based on the patient's needs, and geared to promoting the patient's health and well-being and positive outcomes. The patient shares personal information about him- or herself and the nurse shares information about his or her role as a professional. Therapeutic communication is the basis for the nurse-patient relationship. It is different from social communication, which focuses on the individuals sharing information often similar in type and quantity to meet mutual needs and achieve mutual benefits.

Communication typically is in the form of verbal and nonverbal communication. Verbal communication, as the term implies, refers to information that is spoken. It also includes the written word. Nonverbal communication refers to information that is sent without words. **Box 3-3** highlights major elements of nonverbal communication.

## TABLE 3-2: A COMPARISON OF PEPLAU'S INTERPERSONAL PROCESS WITH CONTEMPORARY VIEWS

| INTERPERSONAL PROCESS | CONTEMPORARY VIEWS | |
| --- | --- | --- |
| PHASES OF THE INTERPERSONAL PROCESS (Peplau 1952, 1991, 1997) | CLIENT PREFERENCE (Shattell, Starrs & Thomas, 2007; Moyle, 2003; Langley & Klopper, 2005; Coatsworth-Puspoky, Forchuk & Ward-Griffin, 2006) | NURSING INTERVENTIONS (Dziopa & Ahern, 2009; Stockmann, 2005; Welch, 2005) |
| Orientation | "To relate to me"; "being with the patient" and "the need for comfort"; "trust"; "a glimmer of hope" | Listening attentively with openness – trying to understand<br>Conveying understanding and respect<br>Authenticity – congruence, consistency<br>Building self-esteem<br>Relating non-judgmentally<br>Using touch appropriately<br>Showing warmth – holding and caring<br>Developing trust—instilling hope<br>Acknowledging reality of client's experience<br>Presence – being available, accessible<br>Pacing development |
| Identification | "To know me as a person"; "not focussing on the physical" | Seeing beyond the diagnosis<br>Providing emotional care and support<br>Containing focus on strengths, reality<br>Timing, pace, consistency of input<br>Promoting equality and mutuality<br>Using self-disclosure<br>Encouraging self-exploration<br>Setting and maintaining boundaries |
| Exploitation | "a working relationship" "focus"; "exploring"; "problem solving" | Exploring person behind defensive strategies – rejection, splitting, transference, sabotage<br>Sharing of power – defining responsibility, choices, decision-making responsibility<br>Enlisting support – working alliance<br>Empowering – allowing mistakes<br>Setting person-centered goals |
| Resolution | "To help me get to a solution"; "carrying on"; "constancy and commitment"; "saying goodbye" | Validation of experience<br>Questioning, speaking plainly, confronting and challenging assumptions<br>Giving information and self-revelation<br>Monitoring progress, eliciting feedback<br>Applying insights learned experientially<br>Using creative solutions to augment verbal and nonverbal strategies<br>Using clinical supervision to stay on track |

*Communication involves a sender, message, receiver, and feedback. With therapeutic communication, the patient is the focus of the interaction.*

The key to successful therapeutic communication is to ensure that the verbal message is congruent to the nonverbal message. In other words, body language, posture, and tone of voice must correspond to and match the words being spoken. Otherwise, conflicts in the message occur. For example, a nurse tells a patient that all morning to talk about the patient's problem, but as the nurse and patient begin to talk, the nurse continuously looks at the wall clock. The patient will most likely receive the message

> ### BOX 3-3: ELEMENTS OF NONVERBAL COMMUNICATION
>
> - Body language
>   - Facial expressions
>   - Gestures
>   - Posture
>   - Reflexes
>   - Body motions/gait
>   - Eye contact
> - Sounds
>   - Voice tone, inflection, rate
>   - Groaning, laughing, crying, grunting
> - Touch
> - Space/proximity (comfort zone)
> - Appearance
>   - Clothing
>   - Makeup, jewelry
>   - Grooming, hygiene

that the nurse is in a hurry and uninterested in spending time with the patient.

## Therapeutic Communication Techniques

Numerous verbal communication techniques can be used with patients. These include: silence, giving recognition, offering general leads, sequencing events in time, encouraging descriptions and/or comparisons, restating, reflecting, exploring, clarifying, validating, and voicing doubt to name a few. If, for example, patients appear angry or are shouting or visibly upset, then offer time and support. Create a therapeutic environment and space for patients to express themselves and be heard. Perhaps the most important communication technique is active listening.

### Active Listening

ACTIVE LISTENING refers to a concentrated effort on the part of the nurse to pay close attention to what the patient is saying, both verbally and nonverbally. The nurse focuses on the words being spoken and the meaning of the message being sent. The nurse demonstrates acceptance of the patient, thereby resulting in the establishment of trust. Trust facilitates open, honest expression by the patient. **Therapeutic Interaction 3-1** provides an example of therapeutic communication with the nurse using active listening.

A number of indicators for active listening have been identified as key hallmarks of non-competitive, purposeful, and active attending to another person with congruence between body language and spoken words in the nurse (Stickley & Freshwater, 2006). Further, there must be a synergy between spoken and nonverbal cues, illustrated in the following.

To enable active listening and attending to the patient, Egan (2003) developed a model for positioning oneself. This model is a valuable tool for framing the therapeutic part of ourselves (physical) in relation to others. The model is based on the acronym SOLER:

S = Sit squarely with the nurse facing the patient

O = Open posture with legs and arms uncrossed

L = Lean slightly forward to convey interest and involvement in the interaction

E = Eye contact to demonstrate interest and willingness to listen

R = Relax

In addition to applying the model just described, psychiatric-mental health nurses use open-ended questions to allow the patient to guide the direction of the interaction. An example of an open question would be: "*Good morning. After all that happened yesterday, tell me how you are feeling about your session today?*" This allows the patient to describe in greater detail more about him- or herself and ideally permits more of a cathartic nature to the rapport. This also makes a connection about how the person is relating the current emotional state to the recent experience. Open-ended questions are more effective than closed-ended questions, which typically require a yes or no response from the patient. An example of a closed-ended question would be: "*Did your session go well today?*" This allows the patient to affirm that it either went well or badly. It does not allow the patient to express what he or she is feeling and can interfere with further discussion, possibly even blocking additional interaction.

There are many verbal and nonverbal cues that a nurse must pay attention to because they can help or hinder the therapeutic relationship. Some helpful ones are listed in **Table 3-3.**

> *Active listening is an important therapeutic communication technique that requires the nurse to focus closely on the patient's message and evaluate the congruency between the verbal and nonverbal messages.*

Words, although important in communication, do not alone provide the message. Words mean different things

**THERAPEUTIC INTERACTION 3-1:**
**INTERACTION BETWEEN A NURSE AND A PATIENT WITH PARANOID SCHIZOPHRENIA**

K. is a young adult female who has been diagnosed with paranoid schizophrenia. She is admitted to the acute care unit of the psychiatric facility. She has been resistant to taking her medications at times because she "feels" the staff is trying to control her thoughts by poisoning her.

| | |
|---|---|
| **RN:** "Hello K., My name is C. I am your nurse and will be helping you with your care." | Establishment of who you are and your role |
| **Patient**: "I don't know you. How will you help me?" | Seeking clarification |
| **RN:** "We will spend time talking about how you are feeling. I will be giving you your medications." | Providing clarification; identifying his or her role through explanation |
| **Patient:** "I don't think I will be taking any medications from you today." | Guarded and suspicious of the RN |
| **RN:** "Are you saying you are afraid of taking the medications?" | Validating and clarifying the underlying feelings behind the patient's statement |
| **Patient:** "Yes. I think you may poison me so you can control my behavior." | Voicing fear |
| **RN:** "That must be a scary feeling to be so afraid." | Voicing empathy |
| **Patient:** "Yes. So you understand what I am saying?" | Starting to feel a connection with the nurse |
| **RN:** "I understand that you feel scared. It is important for you to take your medication. I will let you watch me take the pills out of the package so you can feel safer about taking them." | Validating that the nurse heard the patient and working to develop trust with patient |
| **Patient:** "I think I can trust you so, yes, I will take my medication as long as you let me watch you open the package." | Patient feels safer now and agrees to be compliant with medication regime |

to different people. Each person is unique and individual when it comes to thoughts and images. Consider the concept of time. Individuals spend time, give it, and keep it. For example, patients feel time is valuable and request time. Sometimes they verbalize they do not get enough of one-to-one time. Protected one-to-one therapeutic time is highly important for a successful engagement and therapeutic relationship.

| TABLE 3-3: VERBAL AND NONVERBAL CUES TO PROMOTE ACTIVE LISTENING | |
| --- | --- |
| **NONVERBAL CUES** | **VERBAL CUES** |
| Eye contact<br>Smiles<br>Nodding<br>Close proximity<br>Not rushing off<br>Appropriate use of touch<br>A mirrored position<br>Open gestures and body position | Using non-judging language<br>Not being quick to problem solve<br>Inviting interaction<br>Using open-ended questions<br>Valuing the other person<br>Being honest<br>Congruence with nonverbal actions<br>Calm, even tone of voice<br>Eliciting feedback by being reflexive<br>Allowing silence for review and reflection |

All these words are similar in their description of what one does with time. Through active listening, exploring, and checking one's understanding of the words and metaphors used in conversation, additional insight into the perception one has of the self becomes clearer. Posture, gait, and how individuals hold themselves can reflect congruence to how individuals feel. Thus being attentive to the words and the meanings associated with the words are important. **Box 3-4** provides an activity to help foster active listening.

Paying attention to one's own posture, tone of voice, type of questions and responses can appear artificial and stilted to the nurse. Sometimes usual or routine communication becomes more difficult because the nurse is constantly thinking about which therapeutic techniques he or she should be using. Thus, psychiatric-mental health nurses can use self-reflection and seek out clinical supervision with other experienced registered nurses and faculty to explore actions, motives, and intention, thereby fostering more effective therapeutic listening skills. Exploring such generally unnoticed aspects of the self may cause nurses to feel uncomfortable and uneasy. However, this exploration will help the nurse develop greater awareness of the self and, thus, more effective communication skills (Stickley & Freshwater, 2006). Acquiring the art of effective listening provides a key foundation to the nurse's therapeutic use of self to assist patients to work through their mental distress on the road to recovery.

One means for evaluating and analyzing a therapeutic interaction and for promoting self-reflection is through a **PROCESS RECORDING**. A process recording involves the written report of an interaction. The interaction between the patient and nurse is recorded verbatim to the extent possible and includes both verbal and nonverbal communication of both parties. The content of the interaction is analyzed for meaning and pattern of interaction. The process recording also helps to identify positive and negative communication strategies used.

## Silence

Silence is another important therapeutic communication technique. It is not the mere absence of words. Rather, it is a purposeful, deliberate tool used to allow the patient time to become comfortable, gather his or her own thoughts, and respond when he or she is ready. Silence promotes patient autonomy and control over the situation such that the patient can proceed at his or her own pace to share relevant information. The patient can explore and organize his or her thoughts, think something through, or identify issues that may be of greater concern. Silence also allows the psychiatric-mental health nurse time to interpret the patient's nonverbal messages and provide time for the nurse to think about his or her response. Maintaining silence in the therapeutic relationship may be difficult because of the nurse's own anxiety level or feeling that he or she is just sitting there and doing nothing for the patient. Psychiatric-mental health nurses need to be vigilant in monitoring their own anxiety levels during silence to prevent inappropriate interruptions. Sometimes, instead of verbally breaking silences, eye contact and a facial expression of acceptance and acknowledgment is as effective.

## Self-Disclosure

Self-disclosure is an effective communication technique if it is used appropriately and for therapeutic purposes only. **SELF-DISCLOSURE** refers to the nurse revealing genuine feelings or personal information about him- or herself. A psychiatric-mental health nurse uses self-disclosure only if it will help:

- Educate the patient about him- or herself to better deal with the issues at hand.
- Build rapport, so that the patient feels free to share information more freely
- Encourage reality testing, thereby helping to support the patient's feelings in response to the current situation.

The belief surrounding self-disclosure is that the nurse's sharing of information or feelings will promote the patient to do the same. Additionally, it may help strengthen the trust and rapport of the relationship. However, when using self-disclosure, the psychiatric-mental health nurse needs to ensure that the information or feelings to be shared is

---

**BOX 3-4: ACTIVE LISTENING THROUGH IMAGERY**

Language is not the only route to discovering the self. Other media, such as paint, clay, or music open up different channels. For example, dance opens up a different level of awareness around the body. The key is active listening. Use the activity below to promote active listening skills.

- Break into groups of three
- Have one person act as the listener, one person as the describer, and the other as the dreamer
  - The describer tells the others of a type of animal portrays him- or herself and the situation; e.g., a horse in a field or a lion in the jungle. The describer tells a little bit about why they see themselves as that particular animal.
  - The listener uses open questions and applies the SOLER model described earlier in the chapter to facilitate the describer.
  - The dreamer closes his or her eyes and plays with imagery in relation to colors, concepts, and anything that comes up. This information can be fed back and a discussion held to see if and where the images fit.
- Explore and play with what happened. Compare the information presented by the describer, listener, and dreamer and determine if the information is congruent.

---

appropriate and relevant. In addition, he or she must keep it brief and to the point, ensuring that the disclosure is focused on the patient's needs and for the patient's benefit. Once the disclosure occurs, the psychiatric-mental health nurse then deflects the communication to focus back to the patient. For example, a nurse may state that he or she knows the feeling being experienced by the patient. Then the nurse would ask the patient to say how he or she deals with it. The nurse would then go on to help the patient explore better ways of improving his or her coping mechanisms.

> *Self-disclosure can be an effective therapeutic communication technique if it is used to benefit the patient.*

## Barriers to Effective Therapeutic Communication

What are the barriers to effective communication? There are several. Think about the simple things that stop individuals from being emotionally present to another human being. Minds tend to wander off or concentration lapses. Perhaps individuals are more comfortable with themselves than with someone else, and shy away, especially when dealing with difficult issues. Communication and active listening are much different than hearing alone. Actually,

listening to what someone says and understanding it takes place at an advanced level of relating. One should also think about what is *not* being said, what the nurse or patient avoids, or what the underlying theme or meaning in the conversation is.

Physical barriers can negate meaningful engagement and dialogue. Noise, furniture, temperature and lighting extremes, or equipment can interfere with therapeutic communication. In addition, sometimes the fast-paced, emotional, and chaotic pace of in-patient facilities are contrary to peaceful grounded chatting between people. Task-orientated work may distract the nurse and take away from a meaningful engagement.

> *Physical surroundings such as noise or furniture, as well as communication techniques such as giving advice, using clichés/stereotypical or judgmental comments, or providing false reassurance can act as barriers to effective therapeutic communication.*

Moreover, certain communication techniques can create barriers to effective therapeutic communication. Clichés, false reassurance, advice, closed-ended questions,

## TABLE 3-4: A SELECTED TECHNIQUES ACTING AS BARRIERS TO THERAPEUTIC COMMUNICATION

| TECHNIQUE | DESCRIPTION | EXAMPLE(S) |
|---|---|---|
| Cliché/stereotypical comments | Discounts the patient's feelings making them feel trite or insignificant | "Everything will be okay."<br>"You have nothing to worry about."<br>"Hang in there. Tomorrow is another day." |
| False reassurance | Focuses on the positive outcomes even when the chances for such are not realistic | "Everybody feels depressed now and then. Don't worry about it." |
| Advice | Imposes nurse's view on patient implying that nurse is better than the patient | "I think you really should stop drinking."<br>"Walking every day will definitely help you get your mind off of things." |
| Closed-ended questions | Requires a "yes" or "no" answer without any opportunity to provide additional information | "Are you feeling sad today?"<br>"Do you understand everything I told you about your medications?" |
| Judgmental comments | Imposes the nurse's view on the patient | "You are acting like a child."<br>"You should be sorry for the pain you caused your family" |
| Belittling | Discounts the patient's feelings; infers that patient's concerns/issues are not as significant as the patient feels they are | "Perk up, at least you didn't die this time." |
| Challenging comments | Disputes the patient's beliefs through the use of logic or arguments | "If you are the king of the world, where's your crown?" |
| Defending comments | Discounts the patient's concerns or feelings indicating the patient has no right to these concerns or feelings by arguing, justifying nurse's position | "Everybody here is doing the best they can to help you." |

and stereotypical, judgmental, belittling, challenging, or defending comments or statements can be detrimental to the therapeutic interaction. **Table 3-4** highlights several of these negative techniques.

## Therapeutic Communication Within Challenging Nursing Situations

Maintaining a distant, cool, yet professional therapeutic relationship, overconcentration on physical care, or being too busy completing tasks can erode the sense of interpersonal, mutual trust between nurse and client. Certain settings or patients also can challenge the psychiatric-mental health nurse to develop a close therapeutic interpersonal rapport. These include working with clients who find it hard to trust, those who may lack insight, or those who are out of touch with reality. The range of issues with which patients will present may vary enormously from anxiety to addiction to aggression and psychosis. Regardless of the issue, a sincere and

respectful demeanor and attitude by the nurse is necessary to foster engagement by the patient in the relationship. For example if a patient is experiencing severe depression or a psychotic episode and does not have the concentration span or willingness for meaningful engagement, the nurse should convey acceptance and empathy and indicate that he or she will support the person by being close until the patient feels able to open up in conversation. Similarly, if a patient is expressing frustration in the form of challenging behavior, the nurse should review the timing of interactions with his or her clinical supervisor and carry out a risk assessment as to when and if an intervention should begin. Using a care pathway that follows a four-phase engagement process involving a structured set of goals and types of interactions and skills for each stage can clarify expectations for a patient and the psychiatric-mental health nurse. This can assist a patient to attain a therapeutic alliance leading to a meaningful interpersonal relationship (Rayner, 2005).

## SUMMARY POINTS

• An awareness of the sense of self is crucial to a human being's personal identity. As an individual grows and develops, he or she develops an awareness of the similarities and differences that are unique or shared with others, leading to the development of self.

• Carl Rogers is considered the founder of person-centered counseling and identified three core conditions that must be present in the therapeutic relationship: congruence, empathy, and unconditional positive regard.

• Therapeutic use of self involves the integration of theory, experience, and self-awareness to promote behavioral changes in patients as they explore their impact with others. Psychiatric-mental health nurses need to engage in self-awareness and self-reflection to develop therapeutic use of self.

• Three factors are thought to contribute to the development of the therapeutic relationship: caring characteristics of the nurse; how the relationships were conducted; and implementation of the goals during the process. Empathy is an essential principle associated with the therapeutic relationship.

• Therapeutic communication refers to the interaction between a nurse and patient that is focused on the patient, the patient's needs, and aimed at promoting positive outcomes for the patient.

• The verbal message must be congruent to the nonverbal message to ensure successful therapeutic communication.

• Therapeutic communication techniques include active listening, silence, giving recognition, offering general leads, sequencing events in time, encouraging descriptions and/or comparisons, restating, clarifying, reflecting, exploring, validating, and voicing doubt.

• Self-disclosure is appropriate if it will help educate the patient, build rapport, or encourage reality testing. It must be focused on the patient's needs.

• Techniques that can impede therapeutic communication include cliché/stereotypical comments, false reassurance, advice, closed-ended questions, and judgmental, belittling, challenging, or defending statements.

## NCLEX-PREP*

1. When describing the concept of self, which of the following would be most appropriate to include?
    a. Discovery of personal identity throughout life
    b. A typically positive process of feedback
    c. The similarities shared with others in the environment
    d. An interaction among two or more individuals

2. A group of nursing students in a psychiatric-mental health rotation are reviewing information about various theorists associated with self, therapeutic use of self, and the therapeutic relationship. The students demonstrate understanding of the materal when they identify which theorist as having identified three core conditions for a therapeutic relationship?
    a. Hildegard Peplau
    b. Phil Barker
    c. Carl Rogers
    d. Joyce Travelbee

*(cont.)*

### NCLEX-PREP* (CONT.)

3. A psychiatric-mental health nurse is engaged in a therapeutic dialogue with a patient. The patient states, "I've been feeling so down lately." Which of the following would the nurse identify as being congruent with the patient's statement?

   a. Wide facial grin
   b. Low tone of voice
   c. Fidgeting
   d. Erect posture

4. When engaging in therapeutic communication for the initial encounter with the patient, which of the following would be most appropriate for the nurse to use?

   a. Silence
   b. "What would you like to discuss?"

   c. "Are you having any problems with anxiety?"
   d. "Why do you think you came here today?"

5. A patient states, "I get so anxious sometimes. I just don't know what to do." The nurse responds by saying, "You should try to do some exercise when you start to feel this way. I know it helps me when I get anxious." The nurse is using which of the following?

   a. Clarifying
   b. False reassurance
   c. Validating
   d. Giving advice

*Answers to these questions appear on page 639.

## REFERENCES

Altschul, A. (1972). *Nurse-patient interaction: A study of interactive patterns on an acute psychiatric ward.* Edinburgh: Churchill Livingstone.

American Nurses Association, American Psychiatric Nurses Association, International Society of Psychiatric-Mental Health Nurses. (2007). Psychiatric-Mental Health Nursing: Scope and Standards of Practice. Silver Springs, MD: American Nurses Association Publishing Program.

Barker, P. (1998). The future of the theory of interpersonal relations? A personal reflection on Peplau's legacy. *Journal of Psychiatric Mental Health Nursing,* 5(3):213–220.

Barker, P. (2001a). The Tidal Model: developing a person-centered approach to psychiatric and mental health nursing. *Perspective Psychiatric Care,* 37(3):79–87.

Barker, P. (2001b). The Tidal Model: Developing an empowering, person centred approach to recovery within psychiatric and mental health nursing. *Journal of Psychiatric and Mental Health Nursing,* 8:233–240.

Benner, P., & Wrubel, J., (1989). *The primacy of caring: stress and coping in health and illness.* Menlo Park, California: Addison-Wesley.

Bloor, M., & Fonkert, J. (1982). Reality construction, reality exploration and treatment in two therapeutic communities. *Social Health Illness,* 4(2):126–140.

Buchanan-Barker, P., & Barker, P. (2006). The ten commitments: A value base for mental health recovery. *Journal of Psychosocial Nursing Mental Health Service,* 44(9): 29–33.

Buchanan-Barker, P., & Barker, P. (2008). The Tidal Commitments: extending the value base of mental health recovery. *Journal of Psychiatric Mental Health Nursing,* 15(2):93–100.

Coatsworth-Puspoky, R., Forchuk, C., & Ward-Griffin, C. (2006). Nurse-client processes in mental health: Recipients' perspectives. *Journal of Psychiatric Mental Health Nursing,* 13(3): 347–355.

Dziopa, F., & Ahern, K. (2009). Three different ways mental health nurses develop quality therapeutic relationships. *Issues in Mental Health Nursing,* 30(1):14–22.

Egan, G. (2003). *The skilled helper : a problem-management and opportunity-development approach to helping.* Pacific Grove, CA: Brooks/Cole Pub. Co.

Ekman, P., Friesen, W., & Ancoli, S. (1980). Facial signs of emotional experience. *Journal of Personality and Social Psychology,* 39, 1125–1134.

Finfgeld-Connett, D. (2006). Meta-synthesis of presence in nursing. *Journal of Advanced Nursing,* 55(6):708–714.

Fontaine, K. L. (2009). *Mental Health Nursing.* 6th ed. New Jersey: Pearson Prentice Hall.

Forchuk, C. 1991a. A comparison of the works of Peplau and Orlando. *Archives of Psychiatric Nursing,* 5(1):38–45.

Forchuk, C. (1991b). Peplau's theory: Concepts and their relations. *Nursing Science Quarterly,* 4(2):54–60.

Forchuk, C. (1992). The orientation phase of the nurse-client relationship: How long does it take? *Perspective of Psychiatric Care,* 28(4):7–10.

Forchuk, C. (1994). The orientation phase of the nurse-client relationship: Testing Peplau's theory. *Journal of Advanced Nursing, 20*(3):532–537.

Forchuk, C., Beaton, S., Crawford, L., Ide, L.,Voorberg, L., & Bethune, J. (1989). Incorporating Peplau's theory and case management. *Journal of Psychosocial Nursing Mental Health Services, 27*(2):35–38.

Forchuk, C., & Brown, B. (1989). Establishing a nurse-client relationship. *Journal of Psychosocial Nursing Mental Health Services, 27*(2):30–34.

Forchuk, C., & Reynolds, W. (2001). Clients' reflections on relationships with nurses: comparisons from Canada and Scotland. *Journal of Psychiatric Mental Health Nursing, 8*(1):45–51.

Freshwater, D. (1999). Polarity and unity in caring: the healing power of symptoms. *Complementary Therapies in Nursing Midwifery, 5*(5):136–139.

Freshwater, D., & Stickley, T. (2004). The heart of the art: Emotional intelligence in nurse education. *Nursing Inquiry, 11*(2):91–98.

Gallimore, R., Goldenberg, C., & Weisner, T. (1993). The social construction and subjective reality of activity settings: Implications for community psychology. *American Journal of Community Psychology, 21*(4):537–559.

Gallop, R., & O'Brien, L. (2003). Re-establishing psychodynamic theory as foundational knowledge for psychiatric/mental health nursing. *Issues in Mental Health Nursing, 24*(2):213–227.

Jourard, S. 1971. *The Transparent Self.* Princeton, NJ: Van Nostrand.

Kwaitek, E., McKenzie, K., and Loads, D. 2005. Self-awareness and reflection: exploring the "therapeutic use of self." *Learning Disability Practice 8*(3):27–31.

Langley, G., & Klopper, H. (2005). Trust as a foundation for the therapeutic intervention for patients with borderline personality disorder. *Journal of Psychiatric Mental Health Nursing, 12*(1):23–32.

Lauder, W., Reynolds, B., Reilly, A., & Angus, N. (2000). The development and testing of the Mental Health Problems Perception Questionnaire. *Journal of Psychiatric and Mental Health Nursing 7*:221–226.

Lego, S. (1999). The one-to-one nurse-patient relationship. *Perspectives in Psychiatric Care, 35*(4):4–23.

Mathforum (2009) [Internet] Available from:<http:mathforum. org/sum95/math_and/moebius.html/#todo>[Accessed 21, January 2009]

McAllister, M., Matarasso, B., Dixon, B., & Shepperd, C. (2004). Conversation starters: re-examining and reconstructing first encounters within the therapeutic relationship. *Journal of Psychiatric Mental Health Nursing, 11*(5), 575–582.

Merriam Webster. (2011) [Internet]. Retrieved online January 3, 2011, from http://www.merriam-webster.com/dictionary/self

Merriam Webster. (2011) [Internet]. Retrieved online January 3, 2011, from http://www.merriam-webster.com/dictionary/therapeutic

Mitchell, D. and Smith, P. (2003). Learning from the past: Emotional labor and learning disability nursing. *Journal of Learning Disabilities, 7*(2), 109–117.

Moyle, W. (2003). Nurse-patient relationship: A dichotomy of expectations. *Internation Journal of Mental Health Nursing, 12*(2), 103–109.

O'Brien, A.(2001). The therapeutic relationship: Historical development and contemporary significance. *Journal of Psychiatric Mental Health Nursing, 8*(2):129–137.

Orlando, I. (1961). *The Dynamic Nurse-Patient Relationship: Function, Process, and Principles.* New York: G.P. Putnam.

President's New Freedom Commission. (2003). Final report to the President. Retrieved from http://www.mentalhealth commission.gov/ )

Peplau, H.(1997). Peplau's theory of interpersonal relations. *Nursing Science Quarterly, 10*(4):162–167.

Peplau, H.(1952). *Interpersonal relations in nursing.* New York City, New York: G.P. Putnam & Sons.

Peplau, H.(1991). *Interpersonal relations in nursing: A conceptual framework of reference for psychodynamic nursing.* New York: Springer Publishing Co. Inc.

Pickover, C.(2006). *The Mobius Strip: Dr. August Mobius's Marvelous Band in Mathematics, Games, Literature, Art, Technology, and Cosmology.* Thunder's Mouth Press.

Prestwood, C. (2009). The person with an eating disorder. In *The art and science of metal health nursing: A textbook of principles and practice*, edited by I. Norman and R. Ryrie. Maidenhead, UK: McGraw-Hill.

Rayner, L. (2005). Language, therapeutic relationships and individualized care: addressing these issuesin mental health care pathways. *Journal of Psychiatric and Mental Health Nursing 12*(4):481–487.

Rogers, C. (1951). *Client-centered therapy.* London: Constable & Co.

Shattell, M., Starr, S., & Thomas., S. (2007). "Take my hand, help me out": Mental health service recipients' experience of the therapeutic relationship. *International Journal of Mental Health Nursing, 16*:274–284.

Smith, P. (1988). Recruit and retain. The emotional labour of nursing. *Nursing Times 84*(44):50-51.

Smith, P. (1989). Nurses' emotional labor. *Nursing Times, 85* (47): 49–51.

Smith, P., & Gray, B., (2001a). Emotional labour of nursing revisited: Caring and learning 2000. *Nurse Education in Practice, 1*(1):42–49.

Smith, P., & Gray, B. (2001b). Reassessing the concept of emotional labour in student nurse education: Role of link lecturers and mentors in a time of change. *Nurse Education Today, 21*(3):230–237.

Smith, P., & Lorentzon, M. (2005). Is emotional labour ethical? *Nursing Ethics, 12*(6): 638–642.

Stickley, T., & Freshwater, D. (2006). The art of listening in the therapeutic relationship. *Mental Health Practice, 9*(5):13–18.

Stockmann, C. (2005). A literature review of the progress of the psychiatric nurse-patient relationship as described by Peplau. *Issues in Mental Health Nursing, 26*(9):911–919.

Substance Abuse and Mental Health Services Administration (2006). National Consensus Statement on Mental Health Recovery. Retrieved from: http://store.samhsa.gov/shin/content//SMA05–4129/SMA05–4129.pdf

Travelbee, J. (1971). The nature of nursing. In *Interpersonal aspects of nursing*, edited by J. Travelbee. Philadelphia, PA: F.A. Davis.

Vatne, S., & Hoem, E. (2008). Acknowledging communication: a milieu-therapeutic approach in mental health care. *Journal of Advanced Nursing, 61*(6):690–698.

Welch, M. (2005). Pivotal moments in the therapeutic relationship. *International Journal of Mental Health Nursing, 14*(3):161–165.

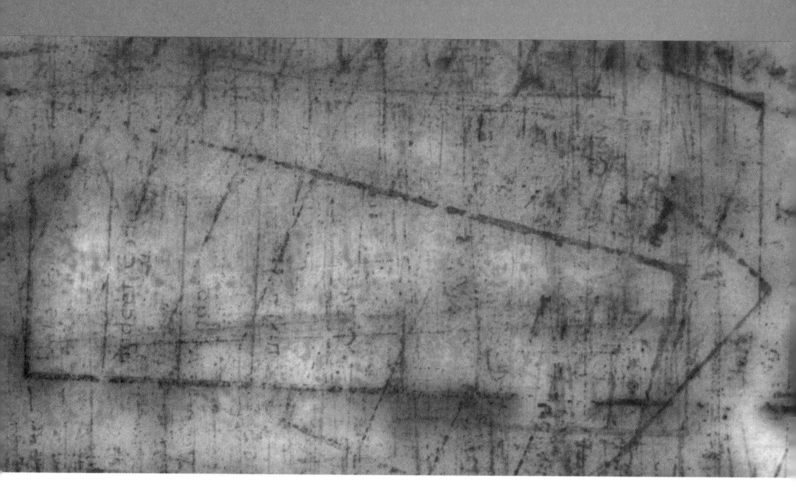

## CHAPTER CONTENTS

# CHAPTER 4
# BOUNDARY MANAGEMENT

Jeffrey S. Jones

## EXPECTED LEARNING OUTCOMES

**After completing this chapter, the student will be able to:**

1. Define boundaries.
2. Identify tangible boundaries that can be established in an interpersonal relationship.
3. Explain the intangible boundaries important in interpersonal relationships.
4. Differentiate between a boundary crossing and a boundary violation.
5. Identify risk factors for establishing unhealthy boundaries.
6. Apply the concepts of boundary management when engaging in an interpersonal relationship.

## KEY TERMS

Boundaries

Boundary crossing

Boundary violation

Counter transference

Transference

In the therapeutic relationship, a nurse must be careful not to be over involved or under involved. The nurse, as a professional, must gain the trust and respect of the patient by presenting him- or herself as genuine and empathic while maintaining therapeutic **BOUNDARIES**, the professional spaces between the nurse's power and the patient's vulnerability (National Council of State Boards of Nursing [NCSBN], 1996). All nurses, especially novice nurses and those new to psychiatric-mental health nursing, need to continually think about their practice in terms of boundaries and relationships as this area is important to the professional practice of psychiatric-mental health nursing. This chapter describes professional boundaries and discusses the importance of boundary management as an integral part of the interpersonal process between the nurse and the patient.

## BOUNDARIES

The term "boundary" typically refers to the physical and psychological space that a person denotes as his or her own. An individual's boundaries provide a separation for that person from another's physical and psychological personal space. Thus, a person's boundaries are unique to that person and reflect his or her own self.

Boundaries may be physical or psychological. Privacy, physical proximity, touching, and sexual behavior are examples of physical boundaries. Feelings, choices, interests, and spirituality are examples of psychological boundaries. Each person delineates the limits of his or her own physical and psychological boundaries that are important. What may be a boundary for one person may or may not be a boundary for another individual.

Boundaries also can be classified as rigid, flexible, or enmeshed. A person with rigid boundaries is unwilling to consider alternative views or ways of doing things. The person refuses to accept new ideas or experiences and often remains distant, possibly withdrawing from others. A person with flexible boundaries is able to relinquish his or her boundaries when necessary. The person is open to allowing others who are viewed as safe to enter their space. A person with enmeshed boundaries experiences a blending or overlapping with another person's boundaries. Thus, it is difficult to determine where that person's boundaries begin and end. Often the boundaries are blurred so that there is no clear delineation of boundaries for each person. Often, individuals with enmeshed boundaries cannot identify feelings or beliefs as his or her own or different from the other person.

> *Boundaries may be physical or psychological, and can be classified as rigid, flexible, or enmeshed.*

## Establishment of Professional Boundaries

The first step in understanding professional boundaries between nurses and patients is to remember that there is an imbalance of power in the nurse-patient relationship. Patients, by nature of their illness, are dependent upon nurses for some aspects of their care. In psychiatric-mental health nursing, the patient also is vulnerable due to the mental illness. This vulnerability is highly evident for patients who are psychotic, have problems with communication, or who have been involuntarily committed. In contrast, nurses are in a position of power based on their knowledge, experience, and status.

The nurse-patient relationship must remain professional because of this imbalance of power. The patient expects that a nurse will respect his or her dignity. Throughout the interpersonal relationship, the nurse must abstain from obtaining personal gain at the patient's expense. The nurse also refrains from inappropriate involvement in the patient's personal relationships.

The American Nurses Association (ANA) Code of Ethics for Nurses (Section 2.4) describes the nurse-patient relationship, addressing boundaries in this relationship: *When acting in one's role as a professional, the nurse recognizes and maintains boundaries that establish appropriate limits to the relationship. In all encounters nurses are responsible for maintaining professional boundaries* (ANA, 2001).

Failure to maintain professional boundaries can result in a disciplinable offense by a state board of nursing or regulating body. Most states have language regarding the need to maintain professional boundaries in the nurse-patient relationship. In the United States, the National Council of State Boards of Nursing (NCSBN) has taken a strong position about failing to maintain professional boundaries and issued the following to facilitate disciplinary action at the local level:

*Professional boundaries are the spaces between the nurse's power and the patient's vulnerability. The power of the nurse comes from the professional position and the access to private knowledge about the patient. Establishing boundaries allows the nurse to control this power differential and allows a safe connection to meet the patient's needs* (NCSBN, 1996, p. 3).

## Boundaries Within the Nurse-Patient Relationship

Applying Peplau's or Travelbee's theories about the nurse-patient relationship, boundaries are initially established during the orientation or original encounter phase and then maintained throughout the other phases. At any time during the relationship, new boundaries may be established or current boundaries may need to be adapted depending upon the situation. However, regardless of the phase of the relationship, professional objectivity is essential to maintain boundaries. Without it, trust, the foundation of the interpersonal relationship, is destroyed. When boundaries are considered and attended to in a way of enhancing interpersonal relations, the process promotes health for the patient and growth for the nurse (Peplau, 1991).

> *Boundaries are initially established during the orientation or original encounter phase.*

Recall that during Peplau's first phase, orientation, and Travelbee's original encounter, the nurse and patient are new to each other. Opinions may be formed about each other in the first few moments of meeting. This is the ideal time to begin establishing healthy boundaries within the relationship. The patient needs to know who the nurse is, why he or she is there, what the nurse can offer the patient, and what the patient can expect in return. Mutually agreed upon goals can be introduced and discussed; these goals will be reviewed throughout the interpersonal relationship.

During the second phase, identification, the nurse identifies what he or she can now bring to the relationship to help the patient achieve the therapeutic goals. This phase allows the nurse to examine further opportunity for boundaries within the relationship. Potential issues of transference and counter-transference, if not apparent during the orientation phase, may emerge. TRANSFERENCE is a psychodynamic term used to describe the patient's emotional response to the health care provider. In this case, the patient may feel and/or think that the nurse reminds him or her of a relative or a past romantic interest

because there is some emotional or physical similarity to someone else in the patient's life. The feelings generated may be either positive or negative. Likewise, the nurse may find that he or she is responding to the patient's transference by developing COUNTER-TRANSFERENCE. Counter-transference occurs when the health care professional develops a positive or negative emotional response to the patient's transference. For example, a nurse is assigned to care for an elderly woman who has been admitted with depression. This client is very seclusive but seems to gravitate toward the nurse. She perks up when the nurse is around and when she does comes out of her room she asks for the nurse at the desk. The nurse later discovers that the patient has a daughter about the same age as the nurse. It is possible that the patient is responding to the nurse based on feelings about her daughter. The nurse, on the other hand, notices she is becoming irritated and uncomfortable when around this patient. The more she seeks out the nurse, the more the nurse avoids the patient. Not only does the patient's physical appearance remind the nurse of her recently deceased grandmother, the grandmother also suffered from bouts of depression toward the end of her life. The nurse may not have fully completed processing her grandmother's death. This patient's attraction to the nurse may be triggering personal feelings and thus interfering with the establishment of a therapeutic relationship. Being able to manage transference and counter-transference is very important in boundary management to maintain a professional interpersonal relationship and to deliver appropriate nursing care.

In the third phase, exploitation, the bulk of the work in the nurse-patient relationship is accomplished. Consider this example. A nurse is working with a young woman who has found herself chronically depressed and disillusioned about her ability to have long, sustained, healthy relationships with men. Within the interpersonal relationship, information was discovered that the young woman's father abused alcohol and was physically and psychologically abusive to the mother. The young woman has stated that she never wanted to marry or be with a man like her father, yet she has continued to develop relationships with men who are very similar to her father. The nurse senses that the patient wants to develop insight and understanding of her own behavior. Subsequently, using skillful conversation, the nurse guides the patient toward awareness in recognizing that the young woman is simply following paths of least resistance, and entering into relationships that feel most comfortable to her. During moments of insight from the work in this phase, the nurse and the patient may feel a strong connection to each other. If not managed appropriately, boundaries could be violated.

The patient may feel grateful that the nurse has helped her solve a particularly troubling dilemma. The nurse, in turn, feels a sense of deep reward in having skillfully done so. As a result, the relationship is vulnerable and at risk for becoming personal rather than remaining professional. During this time, the nurse must manage transference and counter-transference with the ever-present reminder that the power of the nurse comes from the professional position with access to private knowledge about the patient. The maintenance of boundaries allows the nurse to control this powerful differential and allows a safe interpersonal relationship to develop to meet the patient's needs.

During resolution, the last phase, the nurse and patient review the work done and the goals accomplished. If no further goals are set and the identified needs have been met, then the relationship is terminated. Boundaries are maintained based on the understanding that the professional relationship will end. Resolution can be problematic for nurses who have obtained personal gain from a successful experience in the exploitation phase. They desire to continue and to prolong that feeling, and thus delay terminating the relationship even though the goals have been met and the therapeutic work is complete. Careful attention to whose needs are truly being met will help the nurse make the best decision during this phase of the relationship.

Maintaining boundaries during the last phase is best addressed by focusing on conversations that summarize what was accomplished in the relationship and the reinforcement of goals. In addition, other aspects of terminating the relationship can be difficult, particularly if the patient is so thankful that he or she wants to give gifts, exchange personal phone numbers, or initiate other strategies to prolong the ending of the relationship. The idea is for the nurse to manage the therapeutic relationship and maintain boundaries that keep the relationship within the Zone of Helpfulness (**Figure 4-1**) until resolution (NCSBN, 2006).

> *Managing transference and counter-transference are essential to boundary management.*

## BOUNDARY ISSUES

Issues related to boundaries of therapeutic relationships may occur at any time in the course of treatment. However, they are best dealt with at the outset of the therapeutic encounters. It may be helpful to think of boundaries as rules or expected behaviors that regulate healthy conduct in meetings between patients and nurses. Establishing boundaries takes on added significance in mental health work because symptoms experienced with some patients put them at risk. It is the responsibility of the nurse to set clear boundaries, both tangible and intangible, for the therapeutic relationship. **Box 4-1** lists some examples of tangible and intangible boundaries.

In the therapeutic relationship, tangible boundaries typically are established and negotiated at the beginning

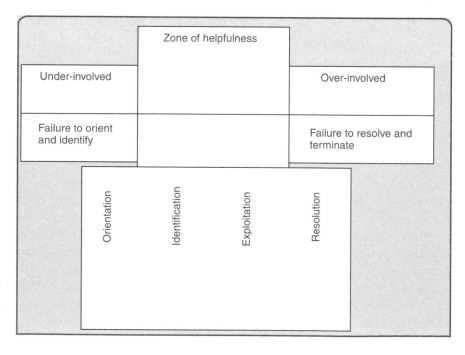

**Figure 4-1** *Zone of helpfulness* as seen alongside Peplau's phases of the nurse/patient relationship. Adapted from NCSBN Professional Boundaries—A Continuum of Professional Behavior (1996).

of the relationship. Intangible boundaries also must be addressed because these are as important in the nurse-patient relationship as tangible boundaries are. For example, sexually explicit or vulgar language violates boundaries and should never be used. In addition, the nurse and patient need to mutually negotiate and agree upon whether to use first or full names. This decision typically reflects the customs where the treatment takes place. Self-disclosure, a very powerful tool, must be done appropriately and only when its purpose is to model, educate, foster a therapeutic alliance, or validate a patient's reality. Self-disclosure is never to be used to meet the nurse's needs. Misuse or overuse of self-disclosure could lead to over involvement and a weakening of the professional relationship.

> *The nurse dresses appropriately, addresses patients by their proper names, and uses self-disclosure appropriately to maintain intangible boundaries.*

## Boundary Testing

Sometimes boundaries in the relationship will be tested by a patient. Some examples of boundary-testing behaviors include: (a) attempting to initiate a social relationship; (b) attempting role reversal where the patient offers care to the nurse; (c) soliciting personal information about the nurse; and (d) violating the personal space of the nurse. The nurse is responsible for maintaining the structure of the therapeutic relationship by reinforcing the boundaries.

Not all therapeutic relationships run smoothly. Patients are dynamic human beings that experience a wide range of emotions and feelings such as fear, sadness, or frustration. Being the recipient of health care can leave one feeling helpless and vulnerable. Additionally, the stressors of dealing with an illness, physical or emotional, can lead to challenges in the therapeutic relationship. **Therapeutic Interaction 4-1** provides an example of how to maintain boundaries when a patient tests them.

One of the biggest challenges to boundaries occurs when patients attempt to convert therapeutic relationships into social ones, thereby testing the boundaries of therapeutic encounters. At times in the therapeutic relationship, social exchanges are appropriate, for example, during recreation times. In these instances, the nurse may use the interaction to acquire information about the patient's behaviors, his or her perception of self, and his or her ability to sustain a social relationship. An activity, such as playing pool, can be a therapeutic strategy to develop trust and rapport, thereby assisting in the progression through the identification phase of the relationship.

Testing behavior will challenge the nurse to remain focused and goal oriented. Careful, self-assessment in such situations will enable the nurse to use what the patient is saying and doing to intervene therapeutically. When the relationship proceeds therapeutically and is successful, the patient and nurse will arrive at outcomes such as independence, spontaneity, mutual trust, self-awareness, honesty, responsibility, and acceptance of reality that allows

---

### BOX 4-1: BOUNDARIES: EXAMPLES OF TANGIBLE AND INTANGIBLE BOUNDARIES

**TANGIBLE BOUNDARIES:**

- Time, place, frequency, and duration of meetings
- Guidelines that prohibit the exchange of gifts
- Guidelines regarding physical contact between the patient and the nurse
- Understanding that sexual contact is never permitted

**INTANGIBLE BOUNDARIES:**

- Setting kind yet firm limits with patients if boundary violations are attempted by the client
- Dressing professionally (suggestive, flamboyant, or seductive clothing may send mixed messages and is unacceptable)
- Using language that conveys caring and respect
- Using self-disclosure very discriminately

**THERAPEUTIC INTERACTION 4-1:
TESTING BOUNDARIES**

Mr. K. has been admitted with severe depression. You have been assigned as his primary nurse. During your visits with him, he reveals that his wife recently left him and he is very scared about moving on in life without her. He is very uncomfortable being alone. During your visits, he tries to sit as close to you as possible and has asked you to sit by him on the bed. He offers you a hug after your visits. The interaction that follows illustrates a therapeutic response to maintain boundaries.

| | |
|---|---|
| **Nurse:** (standing in the doorway smiling) "Hello, Mr. K. I have some time to talk now. Is this a good time for you?" | Introduces self and established purpose |
| **Mr. K.:** "Yes, I've been looking forward to this. Here, sit down by me." (Mr. K. pats the bed) | Attempts to interact with nurse on a personal level and tests boundaries |
| **Nurse:** "Thank you, Mr. K., but it's more appropriate if I sit in the chair rather than beside you on the bed." | Sets the limits of the boundaries: Positions a chair to be facing him about 5 ft away. Sits comfortably with hands folded on lap. Maintains eye contact and smiles |
| **Mr. K.:** "Why? Don't you care for me?" (looking puzzled) | Doesn't understand the response |
| **Nurse:** "Yes, as a patient, not as a personal friend." | Provides clarification (serious but relaxed expression) (conversation ensues for about 20 minutes....) |
| **Mr. K.:** "Thanks for the talk; I always find them helpful." (stands to walk toward nurse) | Showing appreciation for interaction |
| **Nurse:** "Glad to hear you are feeling better. I will plan to talk with you tomorrow." (stands to move chair back) | Validates client's emotion |
| **Mr. K.:** "Can I have a hug?" (smiles and stretches arms out) | Testing boundaries |
| **Nurse:** "No, but a handshake is fine." (smiles and shakes his hand before leaving the room) | Re-establishing boundaries |

The nurse maintains both appropriate physical and emotional boundaries in this scenario. Mr. K. has clearly begun to view the nurse in a more personal capacity. The nurse, sensing this, uses the therapeutic conversation, body posture, and physical space to reinforce the boundaries of the professional relationship. If the nurse had sat on the bed, received a hug, or allowed herself to be pulled into conversation of a personal nature, Mr. K.'s view of the relationship would have been reinforced. If the nurse had left the room when Mr. K. invited her to sit by him on the bed rather than continuing the conversation, the nurse would have sent a confusing message to the patient and would not have been able to clarify the role.

both to achieve resolution. Adhering to the guidelines for professional boundaries will aid in maintaining and stabilizing the boundaries of the therapeutic interpersonal relationship.

> *Patients commonly test boundaries by attempting to change a therapeutic relationship into a social one.*

## Boundary Crossing Versus Boundary Violation

Professional nurses need to differentiate a boundary crossing from a boundary violation. This difference can be conceptually confusing to both student nurses and practicing nurses. Both may be engaging in boundary crossings that do not necessarily lead to boundary violations (Jones, Fitzpatrick, & Drake, 2008). At times, the distinction between the two may not be very clear (**Evidence-Based Practice 4-1**).

### Boundary Crossing

A **BOUNDARY CROSSING** refers to a transient, brief excursion across a professional boundary. The action may be inadvertent, unconscious, or even purposeful (if done to meet a specific therapeutic need), (NCSBN, 1996). Boundary crossings can result in a return to established boundaries. However, repeated boundary crossings should be avoided. Additionally, if they occur with increased frequency or severity, the boundary crossing can become a boundary violation. In every instance, the nurse needs to evaluate the boundary crossing for potential patient consequences and implications.

An example of a boundary crossing would be a patient who shares with a nurse that the patient's mother has passed away, and begins sobbing profusely. In the nurse's effort to comfort and console the patient, the nurse embraces the patient and offers a hug. Typically, physical contact, beyond a handshake, between a nurse and a psychiatric-mental health patient is not a routine part of the relationship. Thus, this action could be considered a boundary crossing. In this situation, physical contact between two people carries with it different messages. Therefore, the nurse needs to examine thoroughly the underlying message that the action may convey before attempting it. For example, the patient may misinterpret

the embrace. Also, the nurse needs to question him- or herself as to whose needs are being met by the action. Overall, the nurse must conclude that the benefits outweigh the risks.

> *Boundary crossings between nurses and patients can be reversible and in some instances therapeutic.*

### Boundary Violation

A **BOUNDARY VIOLATION** results when there is confusion between the needs of the nurse and those of the patient (NCSBN, 1996). Boundary violations allow the nurse to meet his or her own needs rather than the patient's needs. Thus, the foundation of the nurse-patient relationship, to meet the patient's needs, is violated.

Commonly, such violations involve issues such as excessive personal disclosure by the nurse to the patient, keeping secrets with the patient, or possibly role reversal between the nurse and the patient. Boundary violations can cause distress for the patient, for example, ambivalence, mistrust, increased guilt, or increased shame. However, the patient may not recognize or feel the distress until harmful consequences occur.

> *Boundary violations are never helpful and can lead to harm for the patient and possible criminal charges for the nurse. Detachment from a patient to the point of neglect is also a boundary violation.*

An extreme form of boundary violation is sexual misconduct. Professional sexual misconduct includes any behavior that is considered seductive, demeaning, harassing, or reasonably interpreted as sexual by the patient. Professional sexual misconduct is an extremely serious violation of the nurse's professional responsibility to the patient and breaches trust (NCSBN, 1996). Some state boards of nursing or nursing regulating bodies also may consider this a criminal offense with further action by the state prosecutor's office. Even if a patient consents and/or initiates the sexual conduct, a sexual relationship would still be considered sexual

---

**EVIDENCE-BASED PRACTICE 4-1: .**
**BOUNDARY CROSSING OR BOUNDARY VIOLATION?**

STUDY

Glass, L.L. (2003). The gray areas of boundary crossings and violations. *American Journal of Psychotherapy*, *57*(4), 429–444.

SUMMARY

Glass (2003) attempted to define the parameters associated with boundary crossings and boundary violations to clarify current ambiguities. According to the author, "It is crucial to demarcate the differences between boundary violations and boundary crossings as clearly as possible, to describe the 'gray areas' of each, and to recognize the heterogeneity of boundary violations and boundary crossings." The author used this example of a boundary crossing—not charging a long established patient a no-show fee when he or she misses an appointment even though it is the policy. In this instance, a boundary violation would be waiving an office fee in exchange for some handy work around the office or the practitioner's own home. Glass emphasized the need for early training in this area as crucial for mental health professionals to discern the difference between boundary crossings and violations and practice of boundary navigation.

APPLICATION TO PRACTICE

A firm understanding of the terms *boundary crossing* and *boundary violation* are essential to psychiatric-mental health nursing practice because of the nature of the nurse-patient relationship. At times, the line between a boundary crossing and boundary violation may not be clear-cut, leaving the psychiatric-mental health nurse to second-guess him- or herself after the event has occurred. However, armed with the knowledge of the differences and the ability to integrate this knowledge within the nurse-patient relationship, the nurse can ensure that the needs of the patient and not the nurse are being met.

QUESTIONS TO PONDER

1. *Are there certain situations where it would be appropriate, maybe even helpful, to cross a boundary in a nurse-patient relationship?*
2. *If you are about to do something and have trouble determining if it's a boundary crossing or a boundary violation, what should you do?*
3. *What should you do if you feel you have violated a boundary in the nurse client relationship?*

---

misconduct for the nurse because such an action places the nurse's needs first (NCSBN, 1996). Other evidences of potential boundary violations are presented in **Box 4-2**. Detachment to the point of neglect also has been suggested as a boundary violation (Peternelj-Taylor, 2002).

## RISK FACTORS FOR UNHEALTHY NURSE-PATIENT BOUNDARIES

Nurses often find themselves working in a fast-paced environment with little time for reflective analysis of relationship dynamics. This can lead to impulsive and

## BOX 4-2: POTENTIAL BOUNDARY VIOLATIONS

IN ADDITION TO SEXUAL MISCONDUCT, OTHER SITUATIONS THAT MAY BE POTENTIAL BOUNDARY VIOLATIONS INCLUDE:

- Lack of objectivity in the delivery of care
- Personal emotional attachment
- Excessive self-disclosure by the nurse
- Secret keeping with the patient
- Nurse viewing him- or herself as the only one who understands the patient and meet the patient's needs
- Inappropriate amounts of time spent with a single patient (such as visiting the patient when off-duty, switching assignments to be with the patient)
- Failure to explain actions and aspects of care, selective reporting or "double messages"
- Flirtatious communication with the patient
- Overprotectiveness of the patient (siding with patient at all times)
- Failure to recognize feelings related to sexual attraction to the patient
- Neglect (underinvolved)

spontaneous responses to patients rather than thoughtful and planned interactions. There is no short cut to healthy boundary management. Even seasoned psychiatric nurses report that the intellectual energy required to manage boundaries during the course of a shift can be emotionally exhausting (Welch, 2005). Nurses need to be alert for some early warning signs that may indicate the need to step away and take some additional time to process information about the nurse-patient relationship. These signs may include:

- *Feeling frustrated with the job:* Drifting away from a relationship-based mode of practice often leaves the nurse, regardless of setting, feeling frustrated and unfulfilled in the role. The nurse then seeks to recapture the feelings he or she had that were sources of inspiration early in his or her education and professional practice. The nurse should examine his or her own needs and not attempt to meet those needs through the nurse-patient relationship. Relationships with patients based on transference are never healthy groundwork for relationship building.
- *Not connecting with peers:* Having difficulty developing a sense of collegiality within a peer group can lead to feelings of isolation. The nurse needs to explore the reasons for the difficulty in connecting. Unfortunately some nurses choose to seek solace in patient care and thus operate in a vacuum, emotionally disconnected from their colleagues. The boundary work with patients benefits from careful personal reflection as well as thoughtful peer feedback.

*Warning signs of boundary problems include:*

- *Not monitoring transference and counter-transference*
- *Over/inappropriate use of self-disclosure*
- *Feeling as though the relationship with a patient is "special"*
- *Getting personal needs met (e.g., admiration, physical compliments) through a relationship with patients*
- *Becoming distant and secretive from peers*

- *Finding one's self focusing on one patient disproportionately:* Looking forward to going into work just to see a particular patient, becoming embroiled in a patient's personal issues, overuse of self-disclosure and thinking that the relationship is somehow special are all important warning signs of boundaries that require attention and management.

## STRATEGIES FOR MAINTAINING BOUNDARIES

Boundary management in the psychiatric-mental health interpersonal relationship is crucial to the effectiveness of the relationship. As in any interpersonal relationship, nurses need to adhere to the standards of practice and ethical code for conduct. In addition, nurses need to be aware of potential areas in which boundaries may be crossed or violated. Regardless of the situation, the patient's needs and safety are paramount. Nurses also need to develop a keen sense of self-awareness, being cognizant of his or her own personal feelings and behavior. Ultimately, psychiatric-mental health nurses must act in the patient's best interests.

When dealing with patients, be sure to establish clear boundaries early on in the relationship. If warning signs do appear, address them with the patient as soon as they occur, making sure to stress the importance of maintaining the boundaries to achieve the mutually agreed upon goals. If self-disclosure is used, be sure that the information shared directly relates to the patient's goals. Clarify roles and boundaries as often as necessary because patients may not always interpret words and actions in the same manner as what the nurse was attempting to communicate.

Additional help can be obtained from peers and clinical supervisors. Peer support and review of practice are helpful in identifying potential issues related to boundaries. Feedback from peers as well as clinical supervisors or mentors about situations can help the nurse process his or her feelings and actions about patient. This interaction also can help promote growth collegially with peers in the same arena. Any potential issues regarding boundaries with patients should be addressed with the nurse's immediate supervisor, e.g., the nurse manager.

Throughout the interpersonal relationship, nurses need to continually ask themselves the following question: "Whose needs are being met by this action, the nurse's or the patient's?" In addition, it is helpful to quickly evaluate any issues that possibly may be related to transference or counter-transference. Identification of these issues allows the nurse to take corrective measures to ensure that professional boundaries are maintained. **How Would You Respond? 4-1** highlights a case study involving boundary management.

---

**HOW WOULD YOU RESPOND? 4-1**
**BOUNDARY MANAGEMENT**

Abby Rhodes is a registered nurse working at a community mental health center. She obtained her Bachelor of Science degree in nursing from a local university a year ago and is planning to sit for her certification as a psychiatric-mental health nurse generalist as soon as she accrues enough hours in the specialty area. Her role as a community mental health psychiatric nurse is a combination of case management, brief supportive counseling interventions, psychoeducation, and medication monitoring for the patients on her caseload. She has found that the favorite part of her job is the time she spends talking with patients. Most of the patients also see a therapist for therapy and a psychiatrist or psychiatric advanced practice nurse for medication management. Some of her patients share the content of their therapy sessions with her. One patient in particular has discussed some cognitive behavioral strategies (CBT) that his therapist wants

him to start trying to help relieve his anxiety. This patient complains to Abby that these strategies "aren't working," and asks "Can't the doctor just up my Xanax?" Abby assess the patient's level of distress and determines that he is anxious, fidgety, and tense. She tells the patient that "CBT is too slow of a process for someone with your level of anxiety." She decides to approach the patient's doctor to try to get the Xanax increased. The doctor is initially hesitant as the overall treatment plan was to use Xanax for short-term stabilization only and then begin a titration off of the medication. Abby finds herself wanting to advocate for the patient's distress and keeps assuring the doctor that she will monitor the patient's use closely but really thinks he needs it for now. The doctor agrees to increase the Xanax and Abby returns to her office to inform the patient of the news. The patient seems relieved and Abby is happy that she has made the patient

*(cont.)*

## HOW WOULD YOU RESPOND? 4-1 (*CONT.*)
## BOUNDARY MANAGEMENT

feel better. The following day the therapist learns of the situation and comes to talk with Abby about the matter. He is frustrated that he wasn't involved in the decision-making process for this patient and feels that some important therapy was "undone" with the patient getting more Xanax rather than learning to manage his anxiety with other techniques. The therapist then also discusses the case with the psychiatrist who in turn comes back to Abby and says "I don't know why I let you talk me into that. I should have followed my instincts." Abby now feels upset and confused. After all, all she wanted to do was help her patient feel better. The nursing department at the agency where Abby works offers monthly peer group supervision with a psychiatric Clinical Nurse Specialist.

### CRITICAL THINKING QUESTIONS

1. *How did Abby fail to manage the boundaries?*

2. *Whose needs were being met?*

3. *How could Abby have maintained the boundaries?*

### APPLYING THE CONCEPTS

Several elements of this scenario speak to poor boundary management. First, and most importantly, is Abby's rescuing behavior. Rather than finding out which CBT techniques the patient was instructed to use and which ones were or were not working, she immediately follows through on his request for medication changes. Was she responding to her own anxiety? Peplau has noted that most clinicians are uncomfortable with anxiety and are unable to tolerate it. Therefore, they try to restore comfort to both the patient and themselves (Field, 1979). It would have been more productive for Abby to have explored the anxiety with her patient and used the time to talk about it rather than trying to get the medication changed. Peplau suggested that the nurse should first check his or her own anxiety so that the patient does not empathize with it (O'Toole & Welt, 1989). Abby also could have discussed the situation with the therapist first before deciding on the medication change strategy. Her persistence in advocating for this patient, even when the doctor initially resisted, was also an important clue to possible boundary problems. She seems to have confused her nursing role as patient advocate by considering herself as the only one who could save this patient in the present situation. She not only exhibited rescuing behavior but also took part in splitting the staff by not supporting the therapist or the doctor. Lastly, as a BSN-prepared nurse, her knowledge of CBT is limited. As psychotherapy is the domain of advanced practice, she should have deferred commentary about this therapy with the patient. Finally, Abby should avail herself to the monthly peer group supervision with a psychiatric Clinical Nurse Specialist where she can process what happened and understand how things went wrong.

## SUMMARY POINTS

- Boundary management is an integral part of the interpersonal process between the nurse and the patient. There is an imbalance of power in the nurse-patient relationship. Patients are vulnerable and dependent on nurses for their care; nurses are in a position of power based on their knowledge and status.

- The nurse establishes professional boundaries at the beginning of the nurse-patient relationship. Transference and counter-transference can occur during any phase of the relationship but may emerge during the identification phase and can interfere with boundary management.

- Tangible boundaries include: time, place, frequency, and duration of meetings; guidelines that prohibit the exchange of gifts; guidelines regarding physical contact between the patient and the nurse; and understanding that sexual contact is never permitted. Intangible boundaries include: setting kind yet firm limits; dressing professionally; using caring, respectful language; and using self-disclosure very discriminately.

- Patients test boundaries at any time during the interpersonal relationship. One common example is when patients attempt to convert a therapeutic relationship into a social one. Nurses need to remain focused and goal oriented.

- Boundary crossing refers to a brief impingement across a professional boundary. A boundary violation allows a nurse to meet personal needs rather than the patient's needs. Examples of boundary violations include: excessive personal disclosure by the nurse; keeping secrets with patients; role reversals; and sexual misconduct, an extreme form of boundary violation.

- Nurses need to be aware of possible risk factors contributing to unhealthy nurse-patient boundaries such as frustration with the job, isolation from peers, and disproportionate focus on one patient.

- Peer support and clinical supervision are helpful in identifying potential boundary issues and can provide feedback to help nurses process feelings about specific patient situations.

## NCLEX-PREP*

1. When describing physical boundaries to a group of nursing students, which of the following would the instructor use as an example of this type of boundary?
   a. Feelings
   b. Choices
   c. Touching
   d. Spirituality

2. During an interpersonal relationship, a patient identifies that a nurse reminds him of his grandmother and begins to respond to the nurse as he would his grandmother. The nurse recognizes this as which of the following?
   a. Boundary testing
   b. Transference
   c. Boundary crossing
   d. Counter-transference

3. A nurse is establishing boundaries with a patient who is coming to a community mental health center for treatment. Which

**≡ NCLEX-PREP\* (CONT.)**

of the following would be least appropriate to do during the orientation phase?

   a. Give the patient some information about the nurse's personal life.

   b. Explain to the patient the reason for the nurse being there.

   c. Describe what it is that the nurse can provide for the patient.

   d. Discuss the time, place, and frequency for the meetings.

4. A group of nursing students are reviewing information on boundaries, boundary crossings, and boundary violations. The students demonstrate understanding of the information when they state which of the following?

   a. "Most times, a boundary crossing will lead to a boundary violation."

   b. "Boundary violations can be therapeutic in some instances."

   c. "Boundaries are unnecessary if the patient and nurse view each other as equals."

   d. "Boundary crossings can result in a return to established boundaries."

5. While interacting with a patient, the patient says, "How about we meet later after you are done with work and go grab a cup of coffee and talk?" Which response by the nurse would be most appropriate?

   a. "That sounds like fun but I'm busy after work."

   b. "Remember, I'm here as a professional to help you."

   c. "Don't be silly. I can't meet you after work."

   d. "Okay, but this needs to be our secret."

\*Answers to these questions appear on page 639.

## REFERENCES

American Nurses Association, *Code of Ethics for Nurses (2001)*. Available at: www.ana.org Retrieved May 15, 2010.

Dziopa, F., & Ahern, K. What makes a quality therapeutic relationship in psychiatric/mental health nursing: A review of research literature. *The Internet Journal of Advanced Nursing Practice*, 10(1). Available at: http://www.ispub.com/journal/the_internet_journal_of_advanced_nursing_practice. Accessed 10/4/2010.

Field, W.E., Jr. (1979). *The psychotherapy of Hildegard Peplau*. TX: PSF Productions.

Glass, L.L. (2003). The gray areas of boundary crossings and violations. *American Journal of Psychotherapy, 57*(4), 429–444.

Holder, K.V., and Schenthal, S.J. (2007). Watch your step: Nursing and professional boundaries. *Nursing Management, 38*(2): 24–29, February.

Jones, J., Fitzpatrick, J.J., & Drake, V. (2008). Frequency of post-licensure Registered Nurse boundary violations with patients in the State of Ohio: A comparison based on type of pre-licensure Registered Nurse education. *Archives of Psychiatric Nursing, 22*(6), 356–363.

National Council of State Boards of Nursing. (1996). *Professional boundaries; A nurse's guide to the importance of appropriate professional boundaries* [Brochure].

O'Toole, A.W., and Welt, S.R. (1989). *Interpersonal theory in nursing practice: Selected works of Hildegard E. Peplau*. NY: Springer Publishing.

Peplau, H.E. (1991). *Interpersonal relations in nursing: A conceptual frame of reference for psychodynamic nursing* (Rev. ed.). NY: Springer Publishing.

Peternelj-Taylor, C. (2002). Professional boundaries: A matter of therapeutic integrity. *Journal of Psychosocial Nursing & Mental Health Services, 40*(4), 22.

Peternelj-Taylor, C.A., & Yonge, O. (2003). Exploring boundaries in the nurse-patient relationship: Professional roles and responsibilities. *Perspectives in Psychiatric Care, 39*(2): 55–62, April-June.

Welch, M. (2005). Pivotal moments in the therapeutic relationship. *International Journal of Mental Health Nursing, 14,* 161–165.

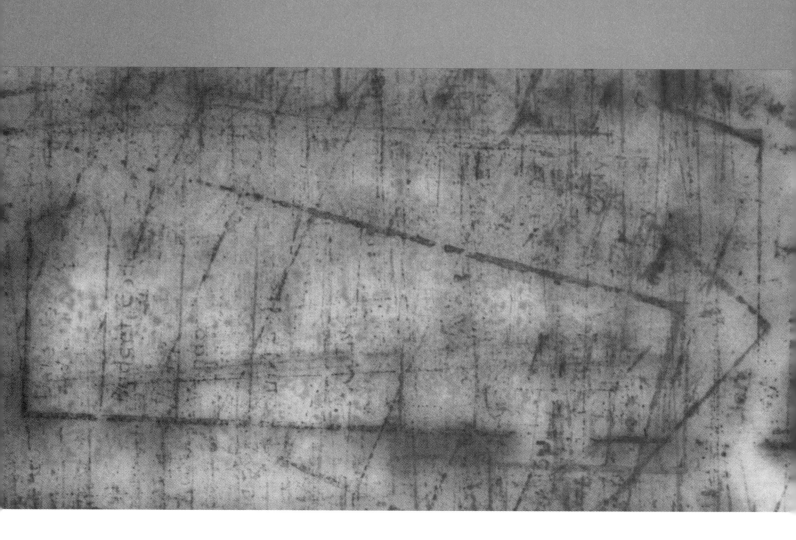

## CHAPTER CONTENTS

## CHAPTER 5
# CRITICAL THINKING, CLINICAL DECISION MAKING, AND THE INTERPERSONAL RELATIONSHIP

Angie S. Chesser

## EXPECTED LEARNING OUTCOMES

**After completing this chapter, the student will be able to:**

1. Identify the basic concepts involved in critical thinking.
2. Correlate critical thinking with clinical decision making.
3. Describe the framework for critical thinking.
4. Describe how the nursing process is related to critical thinking and clinical decision making.
5. Correlate the stages of the nursing process with Peplau's phases of the interpersonal relationship.

## KEY TERMS

Critical thinking

Critical Thinking Indicators™ (CTIS)

Dispositions

Nursing process

Psychoeducational intervention

Psychiatric-mental health nursing care is practiced in multiple settings across the health care continuum. Patients of all ages in need of psychiatric-mental health nursing care can be found in hospitals, community agencies, and residential settings. Across all these settings and age groups, psychiatric-mental health nurses integrate critical thinking skills for clinical decision making throughout the interpersonal relationship. Critical thinking and clinical decision making are crucial elements to ensure that the patient's needs are assessed, relevant problems are identified, and therapeutic nursing interventions are planned, implemented, and evaluated.

Clinical decision making based on critical thinking is similar across all clinical settings. One unique dimension of critical thinking in psychiatric mental health nursing is the importance of the interpersonal relationship as a major healing factor in delivering psychiatric nursing care. This chapter focuses on how psychiatric nurses integrate the concepts of critical thinking, clinical decision making, and the nursing process within the interpersonal relationship to address patient needs and delivery of nursing care. Throughout this textbook, a recurring special feature, "How Would You Respond?" is used to promote the development of critical thinking and clinical decision-making skills.

## CRITICAL THINKING AND CLINICAL DECISION MAKING

**CRITICAL THINKING** refers to a purposeful method of reasoning that is systematic, reflective, rational, and outcome-oriented. It is an important part of psychiatric-mental health nursing and the interpersonal relationship. Through the use of critical thinking, psychiatric-mental health nurses make clinical decisions that translate into an appropriate plan of care for the patient.

Critical thinking correlated with clinical decision making does not refer to thinking that is judgmental, negative, or dismissive about a given strategy, plan, or subject under consideration. Rather, it is a conscious, organized activity that requires development over time through consistent effort, practice, and experience. Critical thinking is dynamic, not static, and ever-evolving based on the circumstances of the individualized situation.

Numerous definitions have been developed about critical thinking and how it applies to nursing practice. Scheffer and Rubenfeld (2000), in a consensus statement, described critical thinking in nursing as

*…an essential component of professional accountability and quality nursing care. Critical thinkers in nursing exhibit these habits of mind: confidence, contextual perspective, creativity,*

*flexibility, inquisitiveness, intellectual integrity, intuition, open mindedness, perseverance and reflection. Critical thinkers in nursing practice the cognitive skills of analyzing, applying standards, discrimination, information seeking, logical reasoning, predicting, and transforming knowledge. (p. 357)*

This consensus statement indicates that critical thinking is a positive skill set used by nurses to plan patient care.

> *Critical thinking is a purposeful method of reasoning that is systematic, reflective, rational, organized, and outcome-oriented. Effort, practice, and experience are necessary to develop critical thinking.*

## Domains of Critical Thinking

Four specific domains have been identified as essential to critical thinking (Paul, 1993). These domains include:

- *Elements of Thought*—The basic building blocks of thinking, such as purpose (what one hopes to accomplish), question or problem at issue, points of view or frame of reference, empirical dimension (evidence, data, or information), concepts and ideas, assumptions, and implications and consequences.
- *Abilities*—The skills essential to higher-order thinking, such as evaluating the credibility, analyzing arguments, clarifying meanings, generating possible solutions, and developing criteria for evaluation.
- *Affective Dimensions*—The attitudes, dispositions, passions, and traits of mind essential to higher-order thinking in real settings, such as thinking independently, being fair-minded, developing insight, intellectual humility, intellectual courage, perseverance, and developing confidence in reasoning and intellectual curiosity.
- *Intellectual Standards*—The standards used to critique higher-order thinking, such as clarity, specificity, consistency, preciseness, significance, accuracy, and fairness (Paul, 1993).

## Elements Necessary for Critical Thinking

Critical thinking requires practice, effort, and experience. It involves the use of cognitive skills and working through **DISPOSITIONS**, the way a person approaches life and living (Facione, 2010). **Boxes 5-1 and 5-2** highlight the cognitive skills and dispositions important for critical thinking.

In addition to these cognitive skills and dispositions, evidence-based research has identified specific behaviors that demonstrate the knowledge, characteristics, and skills needed to promote critical thinking for clinical decision making. These behaviors are termed **CRITICAL THINKING INDICATORS**™ **(CTIS**™**)** (Alfaro-LeFevre, 2010). The two major categories of CTIs address knowledge and intellectual skills and competencies. Knowledge indicators involve:

• Clarifying nursing versus medical information, normal and abnormal function including factors that affect normal function, rationales for interventions, policies and procedures, standards, laws and practice acts that are applicable to the situation, ethical and legal principles, and available information resources

• Demonstrating focused nursing assessment skills and related technical skills, and clarifying personal values, beliefs and needs, including how one's self may differ from others' preferences and organizational mission and values.

Intellectual skills and competencies involve:

• Application of standards, principles, laws, and ethics

## BOX 5-1: COGNITIVE SKILLS ASSOCIATED WITH CRITICAL THINKING

### INTERPRETATION

• Comprehension and expression of the meaning or significance of wide-ranging experiences, situations, data, events, beliefs
• Ability to categorize, decode, and clarify the meaning and significance of the information

### ANALYSIS

• Identification of intended and inferred relationships
• Examination of ideas
• Detection and analysis of arguments

### EVALUATION

• Assessment of credibility
• Assessment of logical strength of actual or intended inferential relationships

### INFERENCE

• Ability to draw reasonable conclusions, conjectures, hypotheses
• Ability to arrive at consequences based on data evidence, beliefs, opinions, and descriptions
• Evidence queries, alternative conjectures, conclusion drawing

### EXPLANATION

• Presentation of coherent, logical, and rational reasoning
• Description of methods and results, justification of procedures, proposal and defense of one's explanations or points of view, and presentation of full, well-reasoned arguments for seeking the best understanding

### SELF-REGULATION

• Ability to self-consciously monitor one's cognitive activities, elements used in activities, and results obtained
• Self-examination and self-correction

*Adapted from Facione, R. W. (2010). Critical thinking: What it is and why it counts. Available at: http://www.insightassessment. com/pdf_files/what&why2006.pdf*

> **BOX 5-2: DISPOSITIONS ASSOCIATED WITH CRITICAL THINKING**
>
> - Independent thinking
> - Inquisitiveness toward a wide range of issues
> - Concern to be and remain well-informed
> - Self-confidence in own abilities
> - Open-mindedness, fair-mindedness
> - Flexibility for alternatives and other options
> - Honesty related to one's own biases, prejudices, and stereotypes
> - Intellectual courage: willingness to reconsider and revise views when change is necessary
> - Creativity or "thinking outside the box"
>
> *Adapted from Facione, R. W. (2010). Critical thinking: What it is and why it counts. Available at: http://www.insightassessment. com/pdf_files/what&why2006.pdf*

- Systematic and comprehensive assessment
- Detection of bias and determination of information credibility
- Identification of assumptions and inconsistencies
- Development of reasonable conclusions based on evidence
- Determination of individual outcomes with a focus on results
- Risk management; priority setting
- Effective communication
- Individualization of interventions.

Nurses also need to possess personal CTIs that support the critical thinking characteristics. These personal CTIs, reflect the nurse's behaviors, attitudes, and qualities that are associated with critical thinking.

> *The four domains of critical thinking are: elements of thought, abilities, affective dimensions, and intellectual standards. Critical thinking involves the use of cognitive skills and working through dispositions or the way a person approaches life and living.*

## Framework for Critical Thinking and Clinical Decision Making

The question is, "How is critical thinking related to clinical decision making in psychiatric-mental health nursing?" First, critical thinking is a skill set involving cognitive skills and dispositions. It is a framework which structures

psychiatric-mental health nurse's clinical decision making for psychiatric-mental health patients and their needs throughout the interpersonal relationship. One way that psychiatric-mental health nurses use critical thinking as a framework for clinical decision making is to answer a structured series of questions either through individual reflection or in consultation with other nurses. Facione (2010) developed the "IDEALS" approach to assist psychiatric-mental health nurses in making therapeutic clinical decisions. This framework includes "Six Questions for Effective Thinking and Problem Solving" (Box 5-3).

Reflecting upon and answering these questions can promote critical thinking involving cognitive skills and dispositions when a psychiatric-mental nurse is engaged in the interpersonal relationship and faces a clinical problem in delivering care. One example of psychiatric-mental health nurses using critical thinking skills to solve patient care problems may include situations that involve the need to alter a non-effective plan of care after a nurse-patient interaction. Another example may occur when the nurse requests clinical supervision to better understand how personal feelings may be influencing the nurse-patient relationship. A third example may be when a nurse participates in a case conference related to developing a more consistent approach to a patient's needs. Thus, when issues arise for a patient or within the interpersonal relationship,

> *The psychiatric-mental health nurse uses critical thinking skills to find the answer to the question about what to do or say to meet the patient's needs.*

> ### BOX 5-3: SIX QUESTIONS FOR EFFECTIVE THINKING AND PROBLEM SOLVING: "IDEALS"
>
> | | |
> |---|---|
> | **I**dentify the problem: | "What's the real question we're facing here?" |
> | **D**efine the context: | "What are the facts and circumstances that frame this problem?" |
> | **E**numerate choices: | "What are our most plausible three or four options?" |
> | **A**nalyze options: | "What is our best course of action, all things considered?" |
> | **L**ist reasons explicitly: | "Exactly why we are making this choice rather than another?" |
> | **S**elf-correct: | "Okay, let's look at it again. What did we miss?" |
>
> *From Facione, P. (2010) Critical Thinking: What It Is and Why It Counts. 2010 Update. Available at: http://www.insightassessment.com/pdf_files/what&why2006.pdf*

the psychiatric-mental health nurse's critical thinking skills can help find the answer to the question, "What should I say or do now to meet this patient's needs?"

## THE NURSING PROCESS

The **NURSING PROCESS** is a systematic method of problem solving that provides the nurse with a logical, organized framework from which to deliver nursing care. It is an ongoing, complex, cyclical process which requires the nurse to continually collect data, critically analyze it, and incorporate it into the patient's treatment plan (Fortinash, 2008). Thus, the nursing process integrates critical thinking skills and clinical decision making. According to the American Nurses Association and the American Psychiatric Nurses Association (2007):

> "the six Standards of Practice describe a competent level of psychiatric-mental health nursing care as demonstrated by the critical thinking model known as the nursing process…The nursing process encompasses all significant actions taken by registered nurses, and forms the foundation of the nurse's decision making."

The nursing process used in this text includes four key stages: assessment, planning/diagnosing, implementation, and evaluation (APIE). Nurses use the nursing process to deliver safe, effective therapeutic nursing care regardless of the setting. The challenge for psychiatric-mental health nurses is to integrate the specialized focus of their work with patients—the therapeutic use of self within the interpersonal relationship—with their nursing process skills. The integration of Peplau's four-phase interpersonal model with the four-step nursing process model challenges the nurse to use critical thinking skills to provide care for psychiatric-mental health patients.

Both the nursing process and the interpersonal relationship reflect a problem-solving approach to providing care. Their integration is important because it is the foundation for sound clinical decision-making in psychiatric-mental health nursing.

### The Nursing Process and the Interpersonal Relationship

Recall from Chapter 2 that Peplau identified four phases of the interpersonal relationship: orientation, identification, exploitation, and resolution. These phases closely parallel the stages of the nursing process. **Figure 5-1** depicts the correlations among critical thinking, clinical decision making, the interpersonal relationship, and the nursing process.

> *Both the nursing process and the interpersonal relationship reflect a problem-solving approach to providing care. Psychiatric-mental health nurses integrate the nursing process and interpersonal relationship for sound clinical decision making in psychiatric-mental health nursing.*

### Assessment
The first stage of the nursing process is assessment, which involves the collection of patient data through a patient history and physical assessment. For the psychiatric-mental

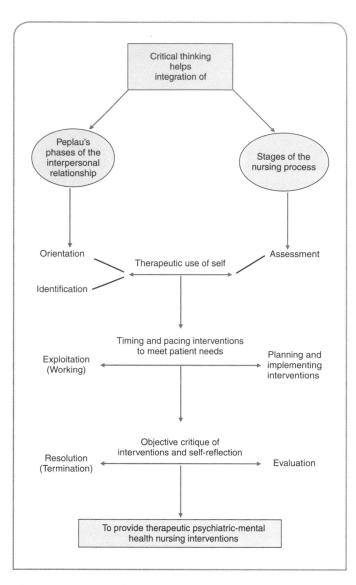

**Figure 5-1** *Interrelationship Among Critical Thinking, Clinical Decision Making, the Interpersonal Relationship, and the Nursing Process.*

health patient, a mental status examination and psychosocial assessment are essential components. The nurse obtains additional information from the patient's medical record as well as from his or her own knowledge of relevant and current literature. This data collection process is ongoing, with the nurse continuously updating and validating the information.

Peplau's orientation and identification phases correspond to the assessment phase of the nursing process. In some clinical situations, a psychiatric-mental health nurse will have information about the patient prior to meeting him or her. This information may come from a variety of sources. The nurse may have information from a nursing

report, another professional, records from other agencies, the patient's significant others, or a patient having filled out an assessment questionnaire prior to the meeting. At other times, a psychiatric-mental health nurse may need to respond to a patient's needs without any previous clinical history, such as in a crisis situation. The nurse uses observation skills to gather clinical information which can guide nursing interventions in the orientation and identification phases of such a relationship. A nurse might encounter a psychiatric patient in a hospital unit day room after an angry outburst in which the patient threatens to harm him- or herself. While the nurse may have only minimal background information on the patient, the nurse can gather data based on the patient's current emotional and behavioral status, which will guide the assessment and planning of care.

Information about a patient's prior clinical history is important because it can influence the orientation and identification phases when the nurse and patient interact. When reviewing a patient's clinical history, a psychiatric-mental health nurse needs to mobilize therapeutic use of self skills to analyze and monitor his or her own reactions to the information and how it might help or hinder the establishment of a therapeutic relationship. Information that a psychiatric-mental health nurse has prior to meeting the patient, whether it is historical in nature or immediately in the here and now, can trigger a range of reactions for the nurse. The psychiatric nurse needs to develop self-awareness about how either a stereotypically biased reaction (for example, questioning how any mother could attempt to harm her newborn) or a personal reaction (such as a nurse who works in substance abuse recovery reacting negatively to a patient's suicide attempt during a relapse) can impede the development of a therapeutic relationship before it even begins. **How Would You Respond?** 5-1 provides a practical example for the therapeutic use of self during the assessment stage and orientation phase.

The assessment stage begins when the patient and nurse meet, often for the first time. According to Peplau (1952), the orientation and identification phases begin when the nurse and patient meet together and begin to structure a relationship that can therapeutically address the patient's needs. Whether this is an encounter where the nurse meets the patient for the first time or the patient is known to the nurse from a previous therapeutic relationship and has now returned for further help, the assessment stage and the orientation and identification phases set the stage for how the nursing process and interpersonal relationship will unfold. Anxiety for both the nurse and patient is common during this time because each has

## HOW WOULD YOU RESPOND? 5-1: ASSESSMENT STAGE/ORIENTATION PHASE

You are completing a nursing assessment on a newly admitted patient on an in-patient psychiatric unit. Ms. Baker is a single 22 year old. For the past few weeks, she has become increasingly depressed, experiencing trouble eating, sleeping, and functioning at work. She reports increasing thoughts about killing herself "to end this pain" by driving her car into a bridge. She has no previous history of psychiatric problems or treatment. She identifies no recent events in her life that might relate to her current depression. When you ask the question relating to religious beliefs, the patient asks you, "Are you a Christian?"

### CRITICAL THINKING QUESTIONS

Based on the scenario described, which response would be most appropriate in demonstrating the therapeutic use of self when responding to the patient?

1. *Ignore the question.*

2. *Tell her, "My religious faith is not important now. What are your religious beliefs?"*

3. *State, "Yes, I am a Christian/No, I am not a Christian."*

4. *Clarify by asking, "Can you share with me how knowing if I am a Christian would be helpful to you?"*

### APPLYING THE CONCEPTS

The most therapeutic response would be Response 4. Because you are in the assessment stage and orientation phase of the interpersonal relationship with Ms. Baker, your focus is getting information from her to identify and meet her needs. Your goal is to understand more about how her need to know about your religious beliefs connects with the problems she is currently experiencing.

The other answers could lead to non-therapeutic results. Ignoring a patient's question can be seen by a patient as rude or as an area you are uncomfortable discussing. Response 1, therefore, does not foster or create a trusting relationship with the patient or a climate where any concern can be shared. Although it redirects the focus back to the patient, telling her that your religious faith is not important now and then asking what her religious beliefs are sounds somewhat punitive and dismissive, which would not further communication. Stating whether or not you are a Christiam directly answers the question but can lead to non-therapeutic results. In the assessment stage/orientation phase, the nurse is always operating with incomplete or unknown information. The nurse attempts to expand and clarify information. Because you have no way of knowing how or if this patient's religious beliefs are related to her depression, you cannot predict how the patient's reaction to your answer may impact your ability to identify and meet her needs. Does the patient think only a Christian nurse can understand her or does she believe a Christian nurse might condemn her for some past thoughts, beliefs, or behaviors? Asking the question directly may meet your need to be polite or finish up paperwork, but it would not be helpful in establishing a therapeutic nurse-patient relationship.

preconceptions about the other as well as uncertainty about how and if help can be provided.

The nurse collects bio-psychosocial clinical assessment data using the formats specific to the setting, for example, the hospital unit, emergency department, community agency, residential setting, or home health care setting. This clinical assessment occurs within the nurse-patient relationship. The psychiatric-mental health nurse works to build a trusting alliance with the patient so that the patient will share his or her perceptions about why this meeting is occurring and what his or her needs are. Using critical thinking skills, the nurse and patient identify the problem and define the context, thereby providing the basis for determining future strategies to address the problems.

Not all psychiatric-mental health patients voluntarily seek help or feel they need it. The psychiatric-mental health nurse begins to develop an interpersonal relationship with the patient by creating a climate of respect and inquiry regarding how the patient came to be in this psychiatric setting. If the patient is a stranger to the nurse and is voluntarily seeking help, the nurse and patient can begin to explore what assistance is available to help with his or her needs and how it will be provided. If the patient is not seeking help voluntarily, for example the admission was initiated by the patient's parents, ordered by the court, or the spouse threatened to leave if help was not sought, and believes he or she has no psychiatric needs, the nurse and patient can explore how this situation can be better understood while they are working together. If the patient is known to the nurse from previous treatment, the orientation and identification phases may be somewhat abbreviated but will still focus on how the patient's current needs led him or her to seek further help and how that help will be provided. The psychiatric-mental health nurse employs critical thinking and clinical decision making along with the therapeutic use of self to assist the patient in determining his or her needs.

During the assessment stage and orientation and identification phases, the nurse conveys a hopeful and optimistic attitude such that, through their work together, the patient's needs can be identified. Once identified, the nurse and patient can work together in meeting the patient's needs. This is especially important for patients already known to the nurse who are in need of assistance and treatment again. These patients may be experiencing feelings such as anger, shame, denial, or hopelessness about the need for help again. These feelings may lead them to assume that the nurse will also feel negatively about them and their prospects for the future. Through

the therapeutic use of self, the nurse identifies and deals with his or her own personal reactions to the patient's return for help such as frustration or inadequacy or failure in helping. In doing so, the nurse and the patient will be more likely to use the assessment stage and the orientation and identification phases of the relationship to focus on identifying the patient's present needs rather than focusing on what did not go well in the past. Thus, the therapeutic nurse-patient relationship can be re-established.

## Planning and Implementation

The next two stages of the nursing process are planning and implementation. These two stages correspond to Peplau's third phase of the interpersonal relationship, the exploitation phase. After completing the assessment stage and the orientation and identification phases, the nurse and the patient examine the needs and determine what it is that the patient ultimately wants to achieve (goals or outcomes). They now begin to work together to focus on strategies to assist the patient in meeting the identified needs and achieving the mutually determined goals or outcomes.

A wide range of nursing interventions can be proposed and provided to assist the patient in understanding and coping in healthier ways depending on what problematic issues brought him or her for psychiatric treatment. The nurse, in concert with the patient, uses critical thinking skills to determine the most plausible strategies, analyzing these strategies, and ultimately arriving as the best courses of action for the patient.

Through the interpersonal relationship established, nurses plan and implement nursing interventions focused on patient needs. Patients can explore how their thoughts, feelings, and behaviors relate to their needs and how dealing with these needs can impact their ability to live a more fulfilling life. During the planning and implementation stages and exploitation phase, patients can become partners in the treatment process by trying out new ways of thinking, feeling, behaving, and sharing what strategies are working for them in meeting their needs in new ways.

The implementation stage and exploitation phase can be difficult and painful for patients. It is not easy for anyone to change behavior, and it is often more difficult for those with mental illness as they must confront their own behavior and its negative consequences. Yet, it is also a time in which patients can experience help and increased self-confidence. Patients are asked to look at their thoughts, feelings, and behaviors in new ways and answer the question, "How is that working for you?" These new viewpoints may be anxiety producing for the patient but also provide them with insight and guidance in dealing with the problems now and potentially in the future. The interpersonal relationship provides a safe and affirming context for a patient to face problems, identify needs, and try out new skills. Psychiatric-mental health nurses use communication techniques and counseling skills to help guide patients to recognize how dealing with their problems in new ways can have beneficial results. **How Would You Respond?** 5-2 provides a practical example of appropriate communication to foster the interpersonal relationship.

*During the planning and implementation stages of the nursing process and the exploitation phase of the interpersonal relationship, the nurse works with the patient and uses critical thinking skills to determine the most plausible strategies, analyze these strategies, and ultimately arrive at the best courses of action for the patient.*

### HOW WOULD YOU RESPOND? 5-2: ASSESSMENT/IMPLEMENTATION/EXPLOITATION

You are in the nursing station when a psychiatric aide comes to tell you that your patient Joe is in the dayroom pacing and studying the ceiling in an anxious manner. When the aide approached the patient, he was counting the fire suppression devices in the ceiling. You know Joe was admitted two days ago. He is a graduate student who had a decline in his academic performance over the past few months. After a meeting with his dean, he retreated to his dorm room and began behaving strangely (putting all furniture against a wall, covering his window with bed sheets). The campus police brought him to the hospital for evaluation. Since admission, he has been anxious and suspicious. He feels the Dean is "listening in on his thoughts." He has refused medication, sleeps poorly, and has to be reminded about daily hygiene. You go to the dayroom and approach the patient. You share that you can see he is upset and ask him to come to a quieter area of the unit so he can tell you what is troubling him. He reluctantly agrees. The patient tells you he noticed these "things" in the ceiling in his room and when he came to the dayroom found more of them. Now he is counting them to see how many ways the dean has to listen in on his thoughts.

#### CRITICAL THINKING QUESTIONS

Based on the scenario described above, consider the following interventions. Which of these would be most appropriate for this patient and why?

1. *Remain quiet and just look at the patient in an interested manner to see if he will say more.*

2. *Tell the patient you have medication that will help the thoughts about the dean go away. Tell the patient you will go get him the medication.*

3. *Say, "Joe, feeling that the dean is listening in on your thoughts must be very frightening. What can you tell me about your relationship with the dean?"*

4. *Tell Joe, "Why would the dean have time to monitor your thoughts? These thoughts are delusions and that is why the doctor wants you to start taking the medication he prescribed. Those things in the ceiling are only required fire suppression devices."*

### APPLYING THE CONCEPTS

You are faced with a situation that requires you to intervene. The most therapeutic response to this patient would be Response 3. Whenever you are responding to a patient who is delusional, your first goal is to reduce the patient's anxiety by acknowledging that their thoughts are contributing to an uncomfortable emotional state. You then want to encourage the patient Response to link the delusional ideas to some reality-based event, if possible. (In this case, it would be the meeting with the dean regarding his academic performance.) You wish to convey a concerned interest in the patient's thoughts without agreeing with them or actively disputing them in any way. You want more information from the patient: Does he feel the dean plans to hurt him? Does he have plans to hurt the dean? What is his perception about his meeting with the dean? After you know more about how the patient thinks and feels about the situation, you can reassure the patient about his safety and explain what the "things" in the ceiling are. You might also inquire how the patient feels about trying some medication to help him relax and gain better control of these disturbing thoughts. You are working to form a therapeutic trusting alliance with this patient in order to understand and manage his delusional thoughts.

The other responses are not likely to lead to a therapeutic result. Continuing to remain quiet and just looking at the patient in hopes he will say more most likely will increase the patient's anxiety. The patient has just shared a frightening scenario with you (the belief that his thoughts are being monitored) and he may be anxious about your reaction. Patients who are suspicious and paranoid may believe others can or are trying to read their minds, so not reacting and just staring at the patient may reinforce the patient's fear. When patients with delusions become anxious within the context of an interaction, they may try to protect themselves by incorporating the other person into the delusion. This patient might begin to believe you are working with the dean to monitor his thoughts and begin to avoid contact with you.

Because you are uncertain as to why the patient has been refusing medication, beginning your interaction with him by telling him you will get medication is unlikely to be helpful. First, it does not acknowledge your understanding of how the patient is thinking and feeling, and it does not express an interest in how these thoughts and feelings are impacting the patient now. Second, leaving a patient alone right after he shares a frightening experience can be seen as uncaring. You would want to discuss medication with the patient after you had begun to develop a trusting alliance with him.

Finally, disputing the patient's beliefs as your initial response will raise his anxiety level and force him into a situation where he feels he must defend his delusions to you. Defending delusional beliefs only makes it more difficult for a patient to be able to examine the reality of his disturbing thoughts. Listening to patients who are delusional can be anxiety provoking for the nurse at times. The anxiety a patient is experiencing can be felt by the nurse, which can lead to the nurse wanting to "help" the patient feel better quickly. Challenging whether the dean has time to monitor the patient can feel dismissive and uncaring to the patient. Sharing the reality of the fire suppression devices and pressuring the patient about taking medication for his delusional (wrong) thoughts initially will block the development of a trusting therapeutic relationship.

Psychiatric-mental health nurses use an important strategy, **PSYCHOEDUCATIONAL INTERVENTIONS,** (interventions that include a significant educational component), to assist patients in understanding and dealing with their problems. Patients need information about diagnoses, medications, coping skills, and support to manage the impact their problems have on their ability to live a healthy and fulfilling life. Psychiatric-mental health nurses provide psychoeducational interventions using a variety of formats based upon patient needs. These formats may include one-on-one conversational settings, group settings, or the use of media via handouts, films, and computer sites and programs. The nurse uses critical thinking skills to decide which format(s) would work best for the specific patient.

> *Psychoeducaton is an excellent intervention that can consist of verbal one-on-one interaction, printed handouts, or other audio-visual materials.*

The planning and implementation stages and the exploitation phase rarely occur in a smooth fashion. The psychiatric-mental health nurse, through the therapeutic use of self, must recognize and manage the interplay of needs between the him- or herself and the patient to ensure that interventions planned and implemented are truly patient focused. Timing and pacing of interventions to correspond to what a patient is able to acknowledge and use is essential to psychiatric nursing clinical decision making. Planning and implementing nursing interventions that are poorly timed or paced usually result in negative patient reactions and problems within the nurse-patient relationship. For example, a patient struggling to accept that he or she has bipolar disorder should not be immediately assigned to attend a psychoeducational group focusing on managing bipolar disorder as a chronic disease. The timing and pacing of this planned intervention could backfire because it failed to meet the patient's immediate needs. The patient may not yet acknowledge what this diagnosis might mean for the future. If pushed to attend this group, the patient may feel less understood by the nurse and become disheartened or angry. It is unlikely that the patient could use any of the content provided. Within the nurse-patient relationship, the patient might react angrily or begin avoiding the nurse who is now perceived as not understanding his or her needs. Critical thinking about the timing and pacing of this intervention within the context of the nurse-patient relationship would have yielded a better result.

Often mismatches in timing and pacing of therapeutic interventions with patient needs relates back to monitoring the therapeutic use of self skills so crucial to psychiatric-mental health nursing. Through self-reflection or in consultation with other psychiatric nurses, the nurse might question how he or she was feeling about the patient's resistance to accepting the bipolar diagnosis and how this impacted the relationship. For example, was the nurse feeling angry, frustrated, or impatient? What kept the nurse from further exploring what was behind the patient's resistance? Was it something in his or her personal history or a supervisor pushing for the patient's discharge? Better understanding of how the nurse's reactions to the patient may have led to a poorly timed and paced intervention can assist the nurse in employing the therapeutic use of self, thereby avoiding similar ineffective nursing interventions in the future.

> *Interventions need to be appropriately timed and paced to be successful.*

## Evaluation

The final stage of the nursing process is evaluation and correlates to Peplau's final phase of interpersonal relationship, resolution. Evaluation and resolution are planned when patients are better able to manage their needs and cope with the problems that brought them for care. It is a time for both the nurse and the patient to reflect together on what has been accomplished by the patient since the nurse-patient relationship began. It also focuses on how the patient can take what has been learned and use it for future success in meeting his or her needs.

For both the nurse and patient, evaluation and resolution can be a time to celebrate successes and gains made by the patient because the outcomes and goals have been achieved. It can also be a time of loss and sadness. The termination of the relationship can reawaken feelings in both the nurse and patient about prior losses and separations. Patients may react to an upcoming termination by redeveloping needs and symptoms present during the assessment stage and orientation and identification phases. They may avoid contact with the nurse, trying not to think about or discuss their ending relationship. **How Would You Respond? 5-3** provides a practical example of a nurse and patient involved in evaluation and resolution.

The psychiatric-mental health nurse may also have reactions to a patient termination. The nurse may have difficulty in seeing a patient as ready to terminate or may avoid the painful aspects of a termination by rushing the process. Nurses can apply their therapeutic use of self skills to monitor their own reactions to a patient's termination and its impact on the patient. The nurse also needs to identify a patient's needs in the evaluation stage and resolution phase more clearly, thus therapeutically assisting the patient to manage thoughts, feelings, and behaviors regarding the upcoming termination of their relationship.

Finally, the evaluation stage and resolution phase provide the nurse an opportunity to determine what went well in the nurse-patient relationship and what might be an opportunity for improvement in the nurse's clinical decision-making skills. Nurses use this time to self-correct, asking themselves if they were able to integrate the stages of the therapeutic relationship to meet patient needs while assessing, planning, implementing, and evaluating nursing care. Did the nurse time and pace interventions to correspond to what a patient needed and could utilize at each stage of the relationship? How self aware was the nurse about the impact of his or her own reactions to the patient and the effect on the stages of their relationship? This self-reflection or reflection with other nurses can improve a nurse's critical thinking and clinical decision making skills in assessing, planning, and implementing psychiatric-mental health nursing care.

## HOW WOULD YOU RESPOND? 5-3: EVALUATION/RESOLUTION

You are working with Christina and are in the evaluation stage and resolution phase of the nurse-patient relationship. Christina had been hospitalized involuntarily after a manic episode led her to drive recklessly, crashing her car into a tree. She had not slept for days and she had run up huge credit card bills. She had also stopped taking her prescribed medications and began to drink heavily. Now, Christina is no longer manic and is taking her medications. She acknowledges she has bipolar disorder and will need on-going outpatient treatment and support.

As you are reviewing her discharge plan (appointments with psychiatrist, counselor, and support group) with her, Christina says to you, "I know I need on-going care. I feel we have a special relationship. It will be hard to talk about things with these people the way I feel I can talk to you. Can I have your number so if I recognize I am getting manic again, I can contact you for help? I promise not to call and bother you often, just when I need help." Your unit has a policy against continuing contact with discharged patients.

### CRITICAL THINKING QUESTIONS

*Based on the scenario described below, you need to respond to the patient. Which response would be most appropriate and why? Are boundaries being violated here?*

1. *"No, Christina, I cannot give you my number. It is against the rules. I could be fired."*

2. *"Christina, I too feel we worked well together. You worked hard to stabilize your mania here at the hospital. Needing to end our relationship so you can move forward to outpatient care isn't easy. Let's talk about how that feels to you and what you might want to share with your doctor and counselor about what you learned in the hospital."*

3. *"We have worked well together so in your case I will bend the rules. Only call me if you really feel manic and don't share my number with anyone else."*

4. *"Christina, you are capable of managing things without me now. I'm sure your new doctor and counselor will be helpful to you."*

## APPLYING THE CONCEPTS

The most helpful response to Christina would be Response 2. Patients being discharged frequently have anxiety about managing their problems outside the hospital with new doctors and counselors and seek ways to continue contact with you. While these requests can be flattering to your sense of professional competence, they do not meet the patient's needs. Unit policies about not maintaining contact with discharged patients are designed to assist patients in moving to the next level of out-patient care and assist nurses in maintaining professional boundaries with patients.

During the resolution phase, feelings about ending the nurse-patient relationship can surface for both parties. Christina's request alerts you to her distress about terminating her relationship with you and beginning a relationship with new caregivers as an out-patient. It is important to acknowledge your relationship and the feelings ending the relationship can evoke in the patient. It is also important to link how what she learned about herself and about managing her illness while in the hospital can be part of her relationship with out-patient providers. Discussing how she feels about ending her relationship with you keeps the focus on her transition to out-patient care and maintains your professional boundaries as her in-patient nurse. You can share with the patient the importance of her establishing a positive helpful relationship with her out-patient caregivers, just as she was able to do with you, after you better understand how ending your relationship feels to her now. Also, your focus on reviewing with her out-patient providers the things she learned in the hospital helps remind the patient what she has accomplished and takes with her at discharge. Anxiety about moving from the safety of an in-patient setting to being responsible for one's self as an out-patient is a common patient response. Acknowledging the patient's feelings and monitoring your own reactions can assist you to focus on the patient's need to make a transition to out-patient care in a therapeutic manner.

Choosing Response 1 would not be a therapeutic response to the patient's request. While it might relieve your anxiety about how to end your nurse-patient relationship, it will leave the patient feeling chastised and perhaps worried about you. This response is not focused on the patient's needs and will not assist her in making a therapeutic transition to out-patient care.

The third response is not therapeutic and is problematic for both the patient and for you. By acknowledging that your relationship has gone well but then offering to continue it when she is an out-patient sends confusing messages to the patient. It may be perceived by the patient that you, too, have doubts that she is ready for discharge or that the out-patient providers are not competent to help her.

Confirming a patient's anxiety about discharge is not focused on meeting the patient's needs. Ask yourself whose needs are being met by this response. Whenever a psychiatric nurse is tempted to ignore unit rules or policies with a patient, it is time to seek consultation from a more experienced supervisor or co-worker. Continuing a relationship with the patient in a manner that is against unit rules forces you to conduct it in secret. This separates you from any supervision of your work and undermines the work of the out-patient caregivers whom the patient should call if manic symptoms reoccur. Monitoring your therapeutic use of self within your nurse-patient relationship should help you either avoid such responses or if you make one, prompt you to seek consultation in order to take corrective action on behalf of the patient. Failure to do so can put the patient at risk for not having a successful transition to out-patient care and your job and nursing license at risk for not maintaining professional boundaries.

Response 4 would not be helpful to the patient. Christina has just expressed that she has doubts about terminating your relationship and being able to talk with her out-patient providers. Your response, while perhaps factually correct, sounds as if you either weren't listening to her or are being dismissive of her anxiety. When patients feel unheard, they frequently do not continue to express their concerns and withdraw from interacting with the nurse. Christina might then be left with unresolved feelings about ending your relationship and continued doubts about how to begin a new relationship with out-patient providers. This would put her at risk for non-compliance with out-patient care and possible readmission to the hospital.

## IMPLICATIONS FOR PSYCHIATRIC-MENTAL HEALTH NURSING

As a psychiatric-mental health nurse gains skill and experience integrating critical thinking skills, clinical decision making, the therapeutic relationship and the nursing process, it becomes clear that neither the nurse nor the patient moves through the stages or phases in a lock-step fashion. There is an ebb and flow between stages and phases. A patient may revisit issues in any stage or phase that the nurse thought were resolved in a previous one. For example, a patient in the resolution phase begins feeling suicidal again. To reassess patient needs, a nurse during the implementation stage or exploitation phase with a patient may need to revisit the assessment stage or orientation and identification phases after a patient develops new symptoms. It is important for the nurse to recognize this ebb and flow between stages and phases to time and pace interventions that best meet patients' needs. The patient's revisiting of needs and issues brought up in earlier stages and phases of the therapeutic relationship are to be expected. This revisiting of needs and issues, however, does not mean that a patient is not making progress. In fact, such situations can be an opportunity for a patient to solidify gains made earlier by thinking about them in new ways. For example, the patient in the resolution phase who feels suicidal again can be guided by the nurse to use skills learned in the exploitation phase to manage suicidality. If the patient can do this successfully, he or she may experience greater confidence in his or her ability to keep safe after discharge.

### SUMMARY POINTS

- Psychiatric-mental health nurses integrate critical thinking skills for clinical decision making throughout the interpersonal relationship to ensure that a patient's needs are assessed, relevant problems are identified, and therapeutic nursing interventions are planned, implemented and evaluated.

- Critical thinking is a purposeful, systematic, reflective, rational, outcome-oriented method of reasoning. It is a conscious, organized activity that requires development over time through consistent effort, practice, and experience.

- There are four domains essential for critical thinking: elements of thought, abilities, affective dimensions, and intellectual standards.

- Cognitive skills required for critical thinking include: interpretation, analysis, evaluation, inferences, explanation, and self-regulation. Important dispositions for critical thinking include: independent thinking; inquisitiveness; self-confidence; flexibility, honesty, and creativity; and intellectual courage.

- Psychiatric-mental health nurses can use the mnemonic, IDEALS (Identify the problem; Define the context; Enumerate choices; Analyze options; List reasons explicitly; Self-correct), to foster critical thinking and clinical decision making.

- The nursing process is a systematic method of problem solving that closely parallels Peplau's four phases of the interpersonal relationship. Both are an ongoing, cyclical process.

- The assessment stage of the nursing process correlates with Peplau's orientation and identification phases. The planning and implementation stages of the nursing process parallel Peplau's exploitation phase. Evaluation in the nursing process correlates with Peplau's resolution phase.

- The nursing process and interpersonal relationship reflect a problem-solving, critical thinking approach to providing care. Their integration is important because it is the foundation for sound clinical decision making in psychiatric-mental health nursing.

**NCLEX-PREP***

1. A nursing instructor is creating a teaching plan for a class about critical thinking. Which of the following would the instructor be least likely to include as a necessary cognitive skill?

   a. Analysis
   b. Creativity
   c. Inference
   d. Self-regulation

2. When engaging in critical thinking, the psychiatric-mental health nurse draws a reasonable conclusion after looking at the evidence and proposing alternatives. The nurse is using which cognitive skill?

   a. Evaluation
   b. Explanation
   c. Interpretation
   d. Inference

3. A nurse is in the resolution phase of the interpersonal relationship with a patient. The nurse would also be engaged in which step of the nursing process?

   a. Assessment
   b. Planning
   c. Implementation
   d. Evaluation

4. When integrating critical thinking, clinical decision making, the interpersonal relationship, and the nursing process, which of the following would be of primary importance?

   a. Nurse's self-awareness
   b. Setting for care
   c. Patient's needs
   d. Achievement of outcomes

5. When engaging in critical thinking, which of the following would the nurse ask first?

   a. "What would be the best course of action?"
   b. "What is the issue at hand?"
   c. "What could have been missed?"
   d. "What factors might be affecting the patient?"

*Answers to these questions appear on page 639.

## REFERENCES

Alfaro-Lefevre, R. (2009). *Critical thinking and clinical judgment: A practical approach (4th ed)*. St. Louis: Saunders Elsevier.

Alfaro-LeFevre, R. (2010). *Applying nursing process: A tool for critical thinking (7th ed)*. Philadelphia: Lippincott Williams and Wilkins.

American Nurses Association, American Psychiatric Nurses Association, & International Society of Psychiatric–Mental Health Nurses. (2007). *Scope and Standards of Psychiatric-Mental Health Nursing Practice*, Washington, D.C.: American Nurses Publishing.

Doona, M. E. (1979). *Travelbee's intervention in psychiatric nursing (2nd edition)*. Philadelphia: F. A. Davis.

Eckroth-Bucher, M. (2001). Philosophical basis and practice of self-awareness in osychiatric nursing. *Journal of Psychosocial Nursing, 39* (2), 33–39.

Facione, P. A. (2010). Critical Thinking: What it is and why it counts. 2010 Update. Available at: http://www.insightassessment.com/pdf_files/what&why2006.pdf. Retrieved 12/15.09.

Forchuck, C., Westwell, J., Martin, M. L., Bomber-Azzapardi, W., Kosterewa-Tolmon, D., & Hux, M. (2000). The developing nurse-client relationship: Nurses perspectives. *Journal of the American Psychiatric Nurses Association, 6* (1), 3–10.

Fortinash, K.M. and Holoday Worret, P.A. (2008). Psychiatric Mental Health Nursing (4th edition). St. Louis: Mosby Elsevier.

Fortinash, K. M., & Holoday Worret, P.A. (2003). *Psychiatric nursing care plans (4th edition)*. St. Louis: Mosby Elsevier.

Krause, J. B. (2000). Protecting the legacy: The nurse-patient relationship and the therapeutic alliance. *Archives of Psychiatric Nursing, 14(2)*, 49–50.

Lego, S. (1999). *The one to one nurse-patient relationship. Perspectives in Psychiatric Care, 35* (4), 336–338.

Paul, R. W. (1993). Critical thinking: How to prepare students for a rapidly changing world. Santa Rosa, CA: Foundation for Critical Thinking.

Peplau, H. (1952). *Interpersonal relations in nursing*. NY: G. Putnam & Sons.

Peternelj-Taylor, C. (2002) Professional boundaries: A matter of therapeuticiIntegrity. *Journal of Psychosocial Nursing, 40* (4), 22–29.

Scheffer, B. K., & Rubenfeld, M. G. (2000). A consensus statement on critical thinking in nursing. *Journal of Nursing Education, 39*, 352–359.

Scheffer, B. K., & Rubenfeld, M. G. (2006). Critical thinking tactics for nurses. Sudbury, MA: Jones and Bartlett.

Travelbee, J. (1971). *Interpersonal aspects of nursing (2nd edition)*. Philadelphia: F. A. Davis.

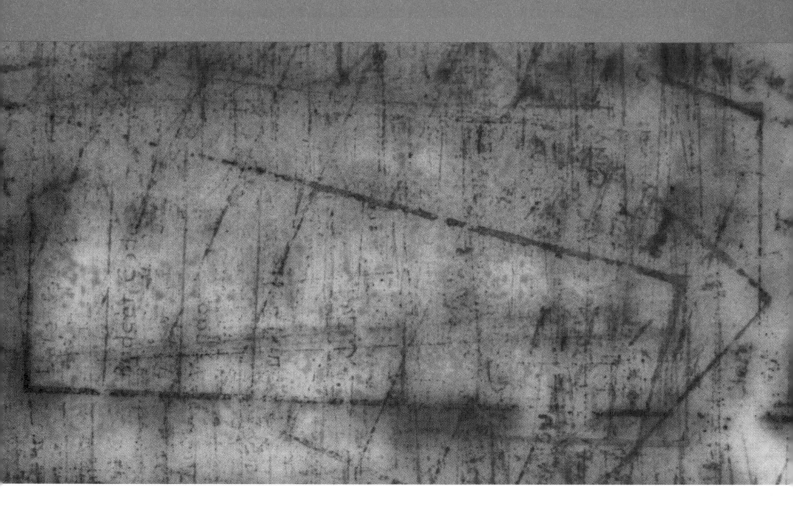

## CHAPTER CONTENTS

## EXPECTED LEARNING OUTCOMES

**After completing this chapter, the student will be
able to:**

1. Discuss how the body responds to stress.
2. Define crisis.
3. Identify the characteristics of crisis.
4. Explain the factors that impact an individual's
   response to stress and development of crisis.
5. Differentiate between the types and magnitudes of
   crisis.
6. Describe crisis intervention.
7. Trace the historical and current role of the psychiatric-mental health nurse in crisis intervention and
   stress management.

# CHAPTER 6
# CRISIS AND CRISIS INTERVENTION

Katherine R. Casale

8. Apply the nursing process for crisis intervention to develop a plan of care for a person experiencing crisis.

9. Explain the methods used to assist psychiatric-mental health nurses to deal with effects of providing crisis care.

## KEY TERMS

Crisis

Crisis intervention

Debriefing

Maturational crisis

Situational crisis

Social crisis

Stress

Nurses have many opportunities to interact with patients while engaged in the interpersonal relationship for delivering psychiatric-mental health nursing care. It is inevitable that many of these interactions will occur during moments of crisis. Crisis in mental health may range from violent out-of-control behavior to withdrawal and suicidal ideation, affecting individuals, families, communities, and the world. Understanding the nature of crisis and how to best intervene is crucial to a nurse's skill set. Nurses have the ability and moral obligation to prepare for and respond to these critical moments of human need. With knowledge in crisis intervention, nurses are thus empowered to make a difference during these pivotal moments.

This chapter briefly reviews the stress response and how it relates to crisis. It discusses the characteristics and types of crises and the factors that can affect an individual's response to a crisis. Integrating the interpersonal relationship and therapeutic use of self, the nurse's role in crisis intervention is explored by applying the nursing process.

## STRESS RESPONSE

**STRESS** is an increase in an individual's level of arousal created by a stimulus. Initially, as stress levels increase, a person's performance and ability to focus may actually improve. Attention to detail sharpens and the person is in a heightened state of readiness to take in the world around him. Immediately, the body physiologically responds to stress via the brain, which alerts the adrenal glands to produce adrenaline (McEwan & Lasley, 2002). This classic "fight or flight" reaction can ensure one's safety. However, once a stress threshold is crossed, these benefits are lost and performance and health deteriorate. A sustained stress response can cause damage to the cardiovascular, immune, and nervous systems, causing chronic illness and maladaptation (U.S. Department of Health and Human Services [DHHS], 2005). **Evidence-Based Practice 6-1** provides information of the potential effects of stress.

> *Stress is a stimulus that increases an individual's level of arousal.*

### General Adaptation Syndrome

Hans Selye first identified the body's reaction to physiologic stress through research he performed in 1956 on laboratory animals. Termed the general adaptation syndrome, he identified three stages of a person's reaction to stress and the accompanying responses experienced. Since his initial research, additional studies have shown that this response occurs not only when a person is subjected to physiologic stress but also when subjected to psychologic or emotional stress.

### Alarm Stage

In this stage, the body is stimulated by a stressor. This causes the hypothalamus, in turn, to stimulate the sympathetic nervous system, which leads to innervation of the glands, such as the pituitary and adrenal glands and various body systems to prepare the body to defend itself against the stressor. **Table 6-1** summarizes the major events that occur in the body during the alarm stage.

### Resistance and Recovery Stage

In the resistance and recovery stage, the body continues to maintain its preparedness against the stressor and adapt to the situation. If the person is able to adapt, the stressor abates and the body recovers, returning to its normal state. However, if the stress continues, the person progresses to the next stage.

### Exhaustion Stage

The exhaustion stage occurs when the person is no longer able to adapt to the continued stress. The defense mechanisms and reserves of the body are depleted. If intervention does not occur, exhaustion continues, which can lead to death.

> *The three stages of stress response are: alarm, resistance and recovery, and exhaustion.*

## CRISIS

**CRISIS** is a time-limited event, usually lasting no more than 4 to 6 weeks, that results from extended periods of stress unrelieved by adaptive coping mechanisms. Many different types of stress can lead to crisis. Modern science recognizes the biopsychosocial components of crisis from its examination of the reaction of people to global natural disasters such as the devastating tsunami in Phuket, Thailand, during the holiday season of 2004, followed by Hurricane Katrina the following summer in New Orleans.

**EVIDENCE-BASED PRACTICE 6-1:**
**EFFECTS OF STRESS**

### STUDY

Can prolonged stress affect whether breast cancer returns? *NIH Medline Plus* Magazine, *3*(1): 6, Winter 2008.

### SUMMARY

In a study funded by National Institute on Aging (NIA) and the National Cancer Institute (NCI), a group of 94 women in whom breast cancer had spread (metastatic) or returned (recurrent) were asked to determine if they ever experienced stressful or traumatic life events. The categories ranged from traumatic stress to some stress to no significant stress. Responses to the questions were markedly different. A comparison of the data revealed a significantly longer disease-free interval among women reporting no traumatic or stressful life events. Results also showed that a history of traumatic events early in life can have many physical and emotional effects, including changing the hormonal stress response system. The research also demonstrated that individuals function better after exposure to traumatic stress if they deal with it directly, facing it rather than avoiding or fleeing from it.

### APPLICATION TO PRACTICE

These findings support the need for nurses working in all areas, especially in psychiatric-mental health, to implement interventions to assist patients in dealing with stress rather than avoiding it. Such interventions could help prevent an individual from crossing over his or her stress threshold, thereby minimizing the effects of stress on the person's health status.

### QUESTIONS TO PONDER

1. *What types of interventions might be appropriate to institute for this group?*
2. *How would the interventions proposed be different and/or similar for different populations?*

Man-made disasters, such as the attacks on the World Trade Center and the U.S. Pentagon in 2001 and the 2004 train bombing in Madrid, also created crisis responses in citizens around the world.

These disasters, whether created by man or nature, affect many thousands of individuals simultaneously. They are abrupt interruptions in the usual way of life, creating disequilibrium and a sense of helplessness. Feelings of vulnerability result. Nurses have a unique opportunity to plan for and intervene to support individuals, groups, and communities during times of crisis.

> *Crisis is a time-limited event that usually lasts no longer than 4 to 6 weeks in which the person is unable to relieve prolonged stress through adaptive coping mechanisms.*

**TABLE 6-1: THE BODY'S RESPONSE TO STRESS IN THE ALARM STAGE**

| SYSTEM OR ORGAN INVOLVEMENT | RESPONSE |
| --- | --- |
| Posterior pituitary gland | ↑ secretion of antidiuretic hormone (ADH) ➔ ↑ water reabsorption and ↓ urine output |
| Anterior pituitary gland ➔ adrenal cortex | ↑ secretion of adrenocorticotropic hormone (ACTH) ➔ ↑ cortisol and aldosterone secretion<br>↑ aldosterone secretion ➔ to ↑ sodium reabsorption, ↑ water reabsorption, ↑ potassium excretion, and ↓ urine output<br>↑ cortisol secretion ➔ ↑ gluconeogensis, ↑ protein catabolism, ↑ fat catabolism |
| Adrenal cortex and sympathetic nervous system stimulation | Release of norepinephrine and epinephrine<br>Epinephrine ➔ ↑ heart rate, ↑ oxygen consumption, ↑ blood glucose, and ↑ mental acuity<br>Norepinephrine ➔ ↑ blood flow to skeletal muscles, ↑ arterial blood pressure |
| Eye | Pupillary dilation |
| Lacrimal glands | ↑ secretions |
| Respiratory system | Bronchodilation<br>↑ respiratory rate |
| Cardiovascular system | ↑ myocardial contractility<br>↑ cardiac output and heart rate<br>↑ blood pressure |
| Gastrointestinal system | ↓ motility<br>↑ sphincter contraction |
| Liver | ↑ glycogenolysis<br>↑ gluconeogenesis<br>↓ glycogen synthesis |
| Urinary system | ↑ motility of ureters<br>Bladder contraction<br>Sphincter relaxation |
| Sweat glands | ↑ secretions |

## Characteristics of a Crisis

For many individuals, modern everyday life is a series of events strung together with stress and anxiety. A crisis occurs when there is a real or perceived threat to a person's physical, social, or psychological self. Additionally, witnessing a trauma of another individual or of an entire community can also lead to crisis (Everly & Lating, 1995; **Figure 6-1**).

In crisis, an individual confronts a stressor and his or her coping mechanisms fail to resolve the perceived stress. Crisis is a time-limited state of disequilibrium accompanied by increased anxiety that can trigger adaptive or non-adaptive bio-psychosocial responses to maturational, situational, or interpersonal experiences (Boyd, 2008). Typically, a crisis interrupts psychological balance or homeostasis. Subsequently, this disruption overwhelms a person's ability to deal with the challenge or threat at hand (Fortinash & Holoday Worret, 2007). Regardless of whether the stressor is internal or external, the change in the environment causes disequilibrium, interrupting the individual's coping patterns and usual behaviors.

Often, crisis is viewed as a negative occurrence. However, the experience of a crisis does not mean that a psychopathology exists. Crisis can also provide an opportunity for personal growth and positive change (Flannery & Everly, 2000). For example, adaptation by the person during crisis allows the person to act and resolve the situation. The person can be supported to consider the incident from a fresh perspective and can develop new coping skills for use during future periods of stress. Mounting an adaptive response allows individuals to seek and implement solutions, thus restoring homeostasis and promoting personal growth. When an individual's responses are maladaptive, he or she feels a sense of helplessness, unable to harness the internal or external resources needed to resolve the all-encompassing anxiety and stress. This individual needs support from health care professionals to work through the crisis and restore homeostasis.

Individuals and families experience crises every day. Across the lifespan, from infancy to death, many situations in an individual's life can lead to stress and precipitate a crisis. For some, a single event, such as the unexpected

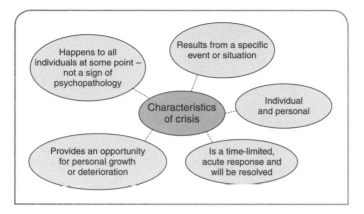

Figure 6-1 *Characteristics of crisis.*

death of a child, can cause a person to lose complete control and become unable to follow through with the simplest daily functions. For others, a series of stressors such as loss of a job followed by illness of a parent and then death of a loved one, can compound the anxiety. This series of events leads to feelings of loss of control, becoming more than the individual can handle.

> *Crisis can have positive or negative results for a person.*

During a period of crisis, new emotional and physiological symptoms, such as nausea and/or emesis, head and body aches, and bowel changes, may emerge. These symptoms, in combination with extreme impairment in daily functioning, signal crisis and need for professional intervention (Boyd, 2008). The *Diagnostic and Statistical Manual of Mental Disorders, Fourth Edition, Text Revision* (*DSM-IV-TR*, American Psychiatric Association, 2000), associates crisis with several different psychiatric diagnoses and disorders including depression, anxiety, and post-traumatic stress disorder. However, it does not categorize crisis as a distinct diagnosis (Fortinash & Holoday Worret, 2007).

> *Crisis is not an established psychiatric diagnosis. It is, however, associated with numerous psychiatric disorders classified by the* DSM-IV-TR.

## Factors Impacting an Individual's Response to Crisis

Each individual's response to crisis is unique. Not every person experiencing stress will go on to experience crisis. Additionally, individuals exposed to the same crisis will exhibit completely different responses. According to research by Aguilera (1998), individuals develop balancing factors that determine the manner in which they will respond to crisis. These balancing factors include: the individual's perception of the event; availability of situational supports; and availability of adequate coping strategies. Table 6-2 describes these balancing factors and how they impact the development of crisis.

Developmental factors also can impact a person's response to stress and development of crisis. For adults, a crisis can be difficult to accept and impossible to understand, eroding feelings of personal and community safety. Adolescents and children may be even more deeply affected (Davidhizar & Shearer, 2002). The effects of disaster and crisis on a child may interfere with normal growth and development, leading to negative long-term physical and psychological health outcomes (Crane, 2005). Therefore, both physical and psychological emergency interventions must be addressed promptly in crisis, including natural and man-made disasters.

## Development of Crisis

When examining the ways in which crisis unfolds, it is helpful to separate the phenomenon into four distinct phases. These phases, depicted in **Figure 6-2**, were first identified by Gerald Caplan in 1964.

### Phase 1

Phase one begins with exposure to a significant precipitating stressor. This stressor can be large or small in scale (affecting a single individual or many persons), a natural- or human-initiated disaster, or an accident or an intentional affront.

Large scale stressors such as disasters affect millions of people annually. Some of the more publicly recognized events include such natural disasters as earthquakes, tornadoes, hurricanes, and floods. However, equally stressful are man-made disasters such as acts of terrorism and school shootings. For days and weeks after these events, the video tapes are repeated over and over again int hemedia. People are repeatedly exposed to the horror and stress that these depictions evoke. Small scale stressors, individual stressors, such as a murdered family member or the terminal illness of a spouse, can also affect

### TABLE 6-2: BALANCING FACTORS IN RESPONSE TO CRISIS

| BALANCING FACTOR | DEVELOPMENT OF CRISIS | NO CRISIS |
|---|---|---|
| Perception of event | Distorted perception → ineffective problem solving → failure to restore homeostasis | Realistic perception → use of adequate resources → restoration of homeostasis |
| Availability of situational supports | Inadequate supports → feelings of being overwhelmed and isolated | Use of available persons in environment → assistance in solving problem |
| Availability of adequate coping skills | Inability to use strategies from previous experiences or strategies used unsuccessful → continued disequilibrium, tension and anxiety | Use of strategies from the past successful → diversion of crisis |

the lives of individuals in overwhelming ways (Davidhizar & Shearer, 2002).

During this phase, the individual experiences anxiety and begins to use previous problem-solving strategies used for coping. For some individuals with strong coping skills, the crisis ends at this point. When the stress level is manageable, the brain may initiate actions to restore internal balance and resolve the threat or stress. How is this possible for some? The brain does a computer-like search: "Have I encountered this problem before? How did I deal with it then? Do I possess internal resources that I can use to deal with this problem? Do I have friends of family to count on?" Most people are resilient and can rebound from a transient stressor. This stress response becomes problematic, however, when it cannot be resolved by the individual and the crisis begins to interrupt daily functioning (DHHS, 2005).

## Phase 2

The individual moves into the second phase of crisis when anxiety exacerbates to a level where problem-solving ability is arrested or becomes unsuccessful. Stress interferes with daily activities and the person becomes increasingly uncomfortable. The person struggles to find a previously used coping strategy. The lack of success with its use or the inability to find an appropriate coping strategy leads to a sense of restlessness, confusion, and helplessness.

## Phase 3

Upon moving into the third phase, the individual expands the search for helpful resources in an effort to relieve the psychological discomfort caused by the stressor. He or she draws upon all available resources, internal and external, in an attempt to relieve the stress and discomfort. For example, the person may try to look at the situation from a different perspective or possibly ignore certain aspects of the situation in an attempt to cope. At this juncture, the individual searches for possible new methods for solutions, and may seek the assistance of professionals such as services of a nurse, psychologist, crisis worker, or some other external source for possible answers and resolution. If the new methods are effective, the crisis will resolve, allowing the individual to return to a functional level, which may be the same, higher, or lower than the person's previous level of functioning.

## Phase 4

If individuals cannot find resolution in the second or third phases, their anxiety levels continue to build. Either they build "beyond a further threshold" or the "burden increases to a breaking point" (Caplan, 1964). Here, the level of anxiety can approach panic or despair, the hallmark of this phase. Emotions are fragile and labile, thought processes are disrupted, possibly even with psychotic thinking, and external supports are necessary.

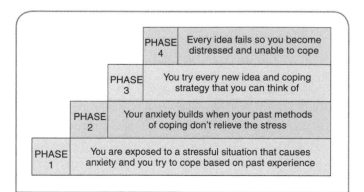

**Figure 6-2** *Phases of crisis.*

*A crisis develops over four phases. If the crisis is not resolved during the second or third phase, panic or despair can occur in the fourth phase.*

## Classification of Crises

During the last 30 years, many experts have categorized acute emotional crises in several different ways. Some organize them by type while others categorize them by increasing severity. At the low end of the continuum are crises that develop because of external interruptions or problems. Crises induced by psychopathology and psychiatric emergencies are at the most intense and complex end of the crisis continuum. Many psychiatric diagnoses prevent individuals from resolving internal conflicts, leaving them panicked, dysfunctional, and unable to safely live in an unsupervised community setting. These individuals, regardless of age, lack the ability to maintain their own personal safety during the crisis and must rely on others to help them make responsible decisions and choices (Davidhizar, 2005).

Regardless of the severity, a simple way to categorize crises that occur in reaction to life events is by considering their point of origin. Using this method, three categories of emotional crisis are identified as: maturational, situational, and social (also called adventitious).

### Maturational Crisis

A **MATURATIONAL CRISIS** occurs during an individual's normal growth and development at any point of change. Examples of maturational crises include leaving home for college (for either the child who is leaving or the parent who is left behind), getting married, having children, or retirement. These normal events occur in everyone's life, but can be identified as an actual or perceived threat that could lead to crisis. When the response to these life transitions is negative or overwhelming and the individual feels a lack of control, crisis occurs and professional intervention may become necessary. In this instance, an internal arrest of development stalls the person's journey through Maslow's (1968) hierarchy of needs, which progress from the most basic level (physiologic needs) to the highest level of actualization (see also Chapter 10 for a more in-depth discussion of Maslow; Gorman, 2008). The priority is to assist the individuals to recognize the specific point of conflict and readjust their capacity to resolve the conflict and move along life's path. Providing support, helping to define the problem and develop an action plan, and connecting the person to appropriate community resources are important interventions.

### Situational Crisis

A **SITUATIONAL CRISIS** stems from an unanticipated life event that threatens one's sense of self or security. The threat can be internal such as a disease. Or it can be external such as family illness, the unexpected death of a loved one, foreclosure on a home, death of a pet, and being fired from a job. Any of these examples could lead to an individual's inability to cope. A person's ability to resolve this type of crisis depends on his or her unique perception of the event, adequacy of a support system, and his or her repertoire of coping mechanisms (Aguilera, 1998). The loss of personal control associated with situational crises may leave the person unable to complete tasks of everyday living. In this instance, the use of past coping skills along with new alternative coping strategies, support, active listening, and connection to community resources are helpful.

### Social Crisis

A **SOCIAL CRISIS**, also called an adventitious crisis, results from an unexpected and unusual social or environmental catastrophe that can either be a natural or man-made disaster. The crisis can affect an individual, families, communities, a specific geographic area, or millions of people. Earthquakes, tsunamis, and hurricanes are all natural disasters that have left thousands, perhaps millions, of people facing crisis. Man-made crises include crimes of rape and murder, city-wide riots, terrorist attacks, or global wars. In these instances, the individuals are overwhelmed by the events that typically involve trauma, injury, destruction or sacrifice (Boyd, 2008). The widespread media coverage of various disasters can result in crisis for persons who are far removed from the area but subsequently are exposed to the repeated depictions of the injuries and devastation.

*Crises may be categorized as maturational, situational, or social.*

## CRISIS INTERVENTION

Crisis, defined as being self-limiting, requires prompt intervention to achieve a positive outcome. With effective professional intervention, psychosocial homeostasis can be restored and the individual can resume or even exceed the pre-crisis level of functioning. A negative outcome, in which the individual stabilizes at a lower level of functioning, is also possible. The likelihood of this outcome increases when the individual has a history of psychiatric instability or illness.

CRISIS INTERVENTION is a time-limited professional strategy designed to address an immediate problem, resolve acute feelings of distress or panic, and restore independent problem-solving skills (Fortinash & Holoday Worret, 2008). As noted by Hoff (2001), the three goals of crisis intervention are: (a) alleviation of the acute distress; (b) restoration of independent functioning; and (c) prevention or resolution of psychological trauma. The psychiatric-mental health nurse engaged in the interpersonal relationship can serve as the vehicle for achieving these goals.

> *Crisis intervention is a strategy used to combat the immediate issue of the crisis and work to resolve it.*

services to the immigrants of New York's lower east side. Wald established the country's first visiting nurse organization. Visiting pregnant women, the elderly, and the disabled in their homes, Wald encountered daily crises in need of immediate attention and advocated for the downtrodden and poor.(Chitty, 2005).

During the latter half of the twentieth century, Hildegard Peplau, a pioneer in psychiatric-mental health nursing, published studies examining anxiety and its role in crisis management. She defined the stages of anxiety that can develop in response to a personal, community, or global crisis. Peplau stressed that nurses must recognize anxiety as a state of being that emerges from unmet expectations or needs. Peplau defined nursing as a therapeutic interpersonal relationship in which the nurse assumes one of six professional roles: counselor, resource person, teacher, leader, technical expert, or surrogate. By assuming these roles, the nurse is able to facilitate crisis resolution for an individual, family, or community (Boyd, 2008).

These nursing visionaries have paved the way for today's nurses to be at the forefront of individual and community crisis management. Organized crisis response teams rapidly recognize and intervene to enhance the delivery of best practices in crisis intervention (Nursing Best Practice Guideline, 2006).

## Nurses and Crisis Intervention: Historical Perspectives

Since the middle 1800s, nurses have assumed an active role in managing crises. Florence Nightingale, considered by many to be the founder of modern nursing, was an innovative thinker and change agent who consistently showed an interest in the welfare of those affected by crisis. During the Crimean War, she led 38 nurses into a battlefield hospital in Scutari, Turkey, encountering thousands of wounded soldiers lying on blood-soaked straw mats crawling with lice and vermin (Tye, 2009).

Nightingale was a compassionate nurse leader who met crisis directly by providing compassionate nursing care, consoling despondent amputees, and writing letters to families of patients who had died. She revolutionized the profession of nursing by incorporating a culture of accountability, emphasizing that patients be treated with dignity in a clean environment regardless of social standing. She developed the concept of nursing triage, which addressed the need for group crisis interventions still used by nurses today (Cohen, 1984).

In the early 1900s, Lillian Wald emerged as another community nursing leader who provided crisis intervention

## Nurses and Crisis Intervention: Current Perspectives

The potential for disasters and violence in society has been a constant theme throughout history, with nurses leading the way as coordinators of the crisis healthcare team. Nurses possess the expertise to develop strategies for intervening in mental health crises. The psychiatric-mental health nurse recognizes that each individual's response to stress is unique; this variation in response is due to personality traits, environment, life experience, and coping skills. When a person encounters an internal or external stressor, the nurse is cognizant of the physiologic and psychological responses that either lead to the person's coping and adaptation, or require professional interventions. The psychiatric-mental health nurse can assist through the development of an interpersonal relationship during times of stress.

The new millennium has led to new ways to deliver crisis intervention, and nurses play a key role in all of them. Computerized chat rooms and individual on-line capabilities allow for brief individualized crisis therapy. Despite risks of on-line therapy such as the lack of regulated professional qualifications and the reluctance of insurance companies to reimburse for on-line counseling (Fortinash & Holoday Worret, 2007), web-based resources offer global information to individuals with limited local resources.

Crisis interventions can be offered to families in their homes as well as in office-based practices. Through their interpersonal relationships, psychiatric-mental health nurses often counsel families and children who have ineffective coping skills. In the event of a community crisis, nurses and other members of the health care team often come to the disaster location and actively care for patients.

## Crisis Intervention and the Nursing Process

The psychiatric-mental health nurse uses the nursing process, integrating critical thinking, and clinical decision making to provide the highest quality of nursing care. The psychiatric-mental health nurse begins with assessment of the patient. During assessment, the nurse typically asks the person to describe the precipitating incident and when it occurred. This information provides the nurse with clues as to how the person perceives and interprets the incident. Throughout the assessment, the nurse observes the person's physical and mental status closely for changes. The nurse gathers information about the person's history of previous stressors and how and what the person used to cope with them while developing the interpersonal relationship. The nurse also investigates if the person has tried any of these past methods for the current situation and whether or not they were successful. Other important areas to address during assessment include the person's pre-crisis level of functioning, strengths and weaknesses, usual coping strategies, and problem solving skills and available support systems.

The nurse analyzes the information gained from the assessment to identify the person's priority needs, which form the basis for the nursing diagnoses. Common examples of applicable nursing diagnoses may include anxiety, ineffective coping, powerlessness, risk for self-directed violence, and interrupted family processes. From there, the nurse determines the appropriate outcomes based on the priority nursing diagnoses and plans appropriate interventions. The nurse integrates critical thinking and clinical decision making in developing the plan, taking into consideration the type of crisis the person is experiencing and the individual's strengths, weaknesses, and support systems available.

The implementation of the care is to facilitate crisis resolution. However, when implementing care, the nurse must immediately address any life-threatening injuries or conditions first.

Once the immediate threats to life are controlled, then the nurse can begin to using therapeutic communication and therapeutic use of self to continue establishing the interpersonal relationship. The nurse actively listens, observes, and encourages the person to express his or her thoughts and feelings. Doing so helps the individual to understand the significance of the crisis. The nurse also helps the individual in confronting reality to avoid denial, which is an ineffective coping mechanism. Throughout the process, the nurse avoids giving false reassurance and provides accurate information to assist with problem solving and begin to integrate the effects of the crisis into reality.

The nurse focuses on reinforcing previous successful coping skills and encourages their use. In addition, the nurse assists the individual in developing new strategies to aid in adaptation to the current situation and encourages the use of available support systems. If necessary, the nurse can provide referrals to appropriate services to help enhance the individual's social network, thereby diminishing the effect of the crisis.

Evaluation, in general, focuses on whether the crisis has been resolved. The nurse reassesses the situation, looking for the following:
- Positive behavioral changes
- Use of effective adaptive coping methods
- Individual's growth with insight into the crisis and precipitating events
- Belief in ability to respond to future stressors to avoid crisis development
- Anticipatory plan of action for future responses to similar stressors

In addition, evaluation also serves as the time for scheduling follow-up for the individual and linking him or her with appropriate external support systems that the person may use in times of stress.

## Nurse's Role During and After Community and Global Disasters

Nurses are witnesses to a world of crises on an extraordinary scale. Never before have we had the ability to observe moments of crisis on all seven continents simultaneously. Television, the Internet, Facebook, and Twitter allow us to interface in real time with people enmeshed in disasters of a local, national, and global scale. As noted by Richards (2009), the Chinese word for crisis incorporates the symbols for "danger" and "critical moment." As nurses, we have the ability and moral obligation to prepare for and respond to these critical moments of human need. Nurses are empowered to make a difference during these pivotal moments, when individuals are vulnerable and communities are crumbling. See **How Would You Respond? 6-1** for a crisis scenario involving a natural disaster.

To intervene effectively during any crisis, nurses must develop expertise to identify persons in crisis and prioritize their needs. This is especially true when the scope of the disaster encompasses hundreds or thousands of victims. The most effective plan mirrors the priorities of Maslow's (1968) hierarchy of human needs. (See Chapter 10 for further information.)

First, nurses should connect the individual to resources that meet his or her basic physiologic needs of food, water, and rest (**Figure 6-3**). Until these fundamental needs are met, the person cannot focus elsewhere in a situation that is likely overwhelming. The primary initial goal should be clear and straight-forward: Provide nutrition, hydration, and rest that will enable the individual to cope with the intimidating obstacles that will follow.

Next, safety and security needs should be addressed. Housing is frequently an urgent concern in the face of a natural disaster, such as a hurricane, flood, or earthquake. The individual's home may be damaged, uninhabitable, or simply gone. The nurse's priority focus is to help the individual and family regain a sense of control and organization by providing alternative housing or connecting them with resources such as friends and family who can temporarily meet that need.

Throughout the interaction with the victims of the disaster, nurses must set an example for professionals and volunteer disaster workers by remaining flexible and providing practical assistance. Lives have

---

### HOW WOULD YOU RESPOND? 6-1:
### THE CRISIS OF A NATURAL DISASTER

Calista, a 19-year-old single mother of Asia, 18 months, and Jake, age 3, is a resident of New Orleans. Prior to Hurricane Katrina, she lived with her mother in a trailer in St. Bernard Parish. Calista's mother watched Asia and Jake, who has cerebral palsy, while Calista worked at a convenience store and attended the local community college.

Hurricane Katrina destroyed Calista's neighborhood on August 29, 2005. While Calista was at work, the storm flattened their trailer, killing her mother instantly. Neighbors pulled Jake and Asia from the wreckage. They were uninjured but the floodwaters were rising so rapidly that the neighbors were evacuated by bus to Houston, with the two children in tow. Because all lines of communication were knocked out by the storm, the neighbors were unable to contact Calista to notify her of her mother's death and her children's safety. Shortly after the neighborhood evacuation, Calista left her job and waded through waist-deep water to return to her home. She found it submerged and empty. No one remained to tell her about the fate of her mother or children. Sobbing, she made her way to a nearby first aid station, and met a disaster nurse, who offered to help.

#### CRITICAL THINKING QUESTIONS

1. *What types of crises are Calista, Jake, and Asia facing in this scenario?*

2. *Which actual and potential symptoms of traumatic stress might the nurse expect?*

3. *What would be the priority nursing diagnoses for Calista?*

4. *Which therapeutic interventions should the nurse initiate and how should they be prioritized?*

5. *How should the nurse develop an interpersonal relationship with Calista?*

*(cont.)*

**HOW WOULD YOU RESPOND? 6-1: (*CONT.*)**
**THE CRISIS OF A NATURAL DISASTER**

The disaster nurse completes a brief physical and psychosocial assessment. The nurse ensures that Calista is safe and uninjured, except for weakness from lack of nutrition and acute panic. The nurse establishes an interpersonal relationship with her, and identifies Calista's priority problems. Through this process, the nurse recognizes that Calista's priority needs are to find out the location and condition of her mother and children, make a plan to reunite with them, and obtain food and safe shelter for herself and her family. The nurse discovers that Calista's mother is listed on a casualty report as being deceased. Calista sees an acquaintance at the first aid station who reports seeing her children board a bus traveling to safer ground in Houston.

### CRITICAL THINKING QUESTIONS

1. *What verbal and non-verbal communication techniques should the nurse use to establish rapport with Calista?*

2. *Which key pieces of information must the nurse convey to Calista?*

3. *Applying the steps of the Nursing Process, develop a plan of therapeutic intervention that:*
   *a. identifies Calista's strengths*
   *b. explores available resources*
   *c. sets realistic short-term goals*

The disaster nurse brings Calista to a quiet corner and prepares tea and sandwiches that they share together. The disaster nurse uses a reality-oriented approach and tells Calista that her mother has died in the flood. She offers to take Calista to the make-shift morgue in the school auditorium to help her find her mother's body, but Calista insists that her primary concern is to be reunited with her children. The nurse asks Calista for a brief health history of Asia and Jake. She locates a Red Cross volunteer and delegates the responsibility of finding a bus that will take Calista to Houston. Meanwhile, the Nurse contacts multiple shelters and learns the location of Jake and Asia, and provides information regarding the children's medical issues to the emergency workers at the shelter. When Calista learns that her children are safe, she collapses on the floor in tears.

### CRITICAL THINKING QUESTION

1. *What would be the priority physiological, psychosocial, and spiritual nursing interventions appropriate to implement during this two hour window of time?*

*(cont.)*

### HOW WOULD YOU RESPOND? 6-1: (*CONT.*)
### THE CRISIS OF A NATURAL DISASTER

Fourteen hours later, Calista is reunited with Asia and Jake at the Astrodome Amphitheater. Jake asks her where Grandma is and when can they go back to their house. Calista is exhausted but is determined to appear strong and in control. Another disaster nurse meets the family and offers to help.

#### CRITICAL THINKING QUESTIONS

1. *Why does the second disaster nurse expect Calista's anxiety level to continue to rise?*

2. *Considering the maturational stages of her two children, what would be an appropriate way to explain the following issues:*
   a. *death of grandmother*
   b. *loss of their home*
   c. *effects of the natural disaster*

3. *To which community resources should the second disaster nurse refer the family?*

4. *Using Maslow's (1968) Hierarchy of Needs, develop short- and long-term goals for Calista and her children.*

5. *Describe the advantages of estabilshing a therapeutic interpersonal relationship with Calista and her children.*

#### APPLYING THE CONCEPTS

Calista and her family are experiencing several crises here; for example, the social crisis of a natural disaster and situational crises involving the death of the grandmother and the loss of their home. The phases of crisis development and factors impacting Calista's response to the crises are illustrated as the disaster nurses intervene with her. The disaster nurse deals with the immediate needs of Calista and her family while carefully planning for needs as they are presented and arise. Additionally, the nurse anticipates future needs and tries to set up further assistance as the crisis unfolds. Certainly, Calista and her family will have need of further assistance but the initial crisis has been handled and a pathway to healing can begin.

been permanently altered in an instant, and feelings of panic and loss of control have replaced the orderly life once known. The disaster workers may also need to be reminded to care for themselves as well as the victims. Responders may need a break away from the disasters, and may need to be encouraged to eat and sleep before

*Nurses must remember to be flexible and set a professional example during crises.*

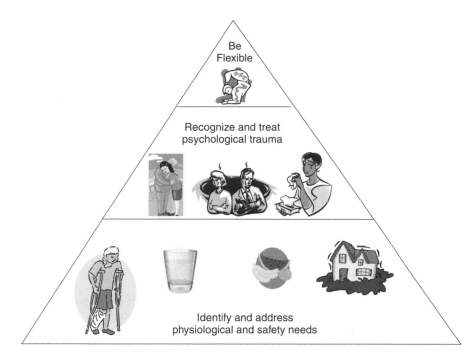

Figure 6-3 *Nursing Response to Community and Global Disaster.*

they collapse and become ineffective care providers (Bornemann, 2005).

After the individual is safe and rested, the momentary relief may allow for feelings of thankfulness and control. However, the psychiatric-mental health nurse is aware that likely this sequence of events will be followed by anger and frustration, when the scope of their loss is realized. The sheer weight of the work that will be needed to rebuild a normal life may feel overwhelming and untenable. Outreach workers on site should actively seek out victims, rather than wait to be contacted, because the anxiety and fear may be paralyzing. Families may not know where to turn or what steps to take to rebuild what has been taken from them. Psychiatric-mental health nurses recognize that, once the initial crisis has passed, the aftermath can leave people emotionally depleted. Caregivers, including members of the health care team, may also need nurturing, comfort, and support. Health care workers may need to take breaks or leave the scene of the disaster in order to regain strength and focus.

> *It is imperative that crisis workers, including nurses, take care of their own emotional well-being to remain effective.*

Stress management is key to coping with disasters (Litz, 2004). A depleted care provider becomes ineffective. After the 2010 earthquake in Haiti, collaborative teams of health care providers rotated through makeshift mobile hospitals. International teams provided medical care for a week or two, and then left to allow fresh, rested nurses and doctors to take their places.

During global disasters, nurses should recognize that everyone is potentially touched by the scope of the incident. In this electronic age, visual images of those suffering, injured, and killed are broadcast on every television channel and across the Internet. We can hear the screams and feel the pain as if we were at the scene. Unlike previous generations, we are all touched and impacted by the trauma and we may grieve with the victims. Grief may be displayed in numerous ways, such as anxiety, anger, fear, numbness, heightened arousal, sleep disturbances, or substance abuse. Signs of dysfunction may appear immediately or may be delayed, emerging months or years later. And while the scope of reactions to disasters is broad, the reactions also may vary across the lifespan.

Disasters and crises are difficult for adults to assimilate and understand, leaving them unable to cope or rebuild their lives without help. The crisis may affect a child even more deeply, because children are in the midst of moving through the stages of development. Changes in children's behavior that arise from crisis are usually reversible with appropriate, prompt intervention. However, prolonged or extreme stress may have a permanent impact on

## TABLE 6-3: NURSING CRISIS SUPPORT STRATEGIES FOR CHILDREN

| SUPPORT STRATEGY | NURSING INTERVENTION |
|---|---|
| Assess for signs of physiologic or psychosocial stress | • Be alert for deviation from normal patterns of eating, sleeping, coping, and activity level<br>• Communicate with children, parents, and teachers<br>• Compare ego competency development pre- and post-disaster, noting regression |
| Provide verbal and non-verbal reassurance | • Use reassuring truthful language, such as "I am going to help you" or "Mommy is not going to leave you"<br>• Offer a security blanket or similar object that the child used to self-soothe at an earlier age<br>• Tell the child that adults are doing everything they can to make the situation better<br>• Provide hugs and physical closeness |
| Foster expression of feelings | • Ask children how the crisis makes them feel<br>• Provide toys and art supplies to promote non-verbal expression of emotion and play-acting<br>• Answer questions honestly at the child's developmental level<br>• Reassure children that the disaster was not their fault |
| Encourage behaviors and rituals that promote stability and security | • Re-establish family traditions, such as doing homework together or having pancakes for Sunday breakfast<br>• Decrease or eliminate the child's exposure to television and other media cover of the crisis<br>• If parents are struggling to cope, have relatives or friends step in for support |
| Act as a role model | • Demonstrate behaviors that the child can emulate<br>• Verbalize the steps you are taking to help yourself heal/recover from the tragedy<br>• Encourage interactions with mental health counselors<br>• Use humor as a stress-buster |
| Evaluate for Post Traumatic Stress Disorder (acute, chronic, or delayed-onset) | • Recognize the diagnostic criteria for PTSD<br>• Observe for signs of depression, altered sleep, behavior and appetite patterns, and increasing anxiety or acting-out behavior |

*From Davidhizar, R., & Shearer, R. (2002). Helping children cope with public disasters. American Journal of Nursing, 102(3), 26-33.*

development and may lead to psychiatric illness (Hamblin, 2001). Strategies for supporting children in the face of disaster, as noted by Davidhizar and Shearer (2002) are summarized in **Table 6-3.**

## IMPACT OF DEALING WITH CRISES ON PSYCHIATRIC-MENTAL HEALTH NURSES

Nurses working in psychiatric-mental health in-patient or out-patient settings need to be educated about crisis intervention. Dealing with the stress of crisis on a day-to-day basis can affect a nurse's or care provider's mental well being. For psychiatric-mental health nurses, programs such as Crisis Prevention Intervention (CPI) or equivalent type programs are taught to the registered nurses during orientation. Neither nurses nor other staff members are allowed to engage into a crisis incident until they have been through the facility's training program. It is imperative that nurses are trained to deal with crisis so that the patient and the staff remain free from physical and emotional harm.

Another aspect of dealing with crisis is the emotional toll that can take place for the care givers. Institutions provide **DEBRIEFING**, a method used following a crisis incident to allow staff to verbalize their feelings and thoughts about the event. It is critical that debriefing is conducted by a staff member who approaches the incident in a non-judgmental manner and that it take place in a safe and supportive environment. This is not to say that staff may not discuss how things may have been handled differently and make suggestions for change. This should take place as soon as possible following the incident usually within 24–48 hours.

There has been increased interest in conducting research on health care providers who have been involved in disasters such as post 9/11 and Hurricane Katrina and the burnout they can experience. If a nurse is involved in a situation where her or she feels the needs for assistance with handling a post-crisis situation, most institutions have employee assistance programs (EAP) where you as a provider can seek additional services.

## SUMMARY POINTS

- Stress is an increase in an indivdidual's level of arousal created by a stimulus. The body responds to stress in three stages. If the body is not able to adapt to stress, exhaustion occurs.

- Crisis is a time-limited event usually lasting no longer than 4 to 6 weeks. It occurs when an individual experiences a real or perceived threat to his or her physical, social, or psychological self.

- With crisis, the individual confronts a stressor but is unable to use his or her coping mechanisms to resolve the perceived stress. Disequilibrium occurs, interrupting the person's coping patterns and usual behaviors.

- Crisis can be a negative or positive force. It can provide an opportunity for personal growth and positive change, but it can also lead to a sense of helplessness.

- Crisis is associated with several different psychiatric disorders classified by the *DSM-IV-TR* but crisis is not considered a distinct psychiatric diagnosis.

- An individual's response to crisis is unique and not everyone who experiences stress will develop crisis. Individuals develop balancing factors that determine how they will respond to crisis. These balancing factors are: the individual's perception of the event, availability of situational supports, and availability of adequate coping strategies.

- Crisis develops over four phases beginning with exposure to a significant precipitating stressor. During the second phase, the individual attempts to adapt to the stressor but the usual coping strategies become ineffective. In the third phase, the individual seeks out resources to relieve the increased discomfort. If the crisis is not resolved, the individual progresses to the fourth phase characterized by panic or despair levels of anxiety.

- Crisis can be classified in several ways. Crisis classification based on point of origin include: maturational, situational, and social.

- Psychiatric-mental health nurses integrate the concepts of critical thinking, clinical decision making, and therapeutic use of self when using the nursing process to provide care to a person in crisis to promote crisis resolution and restoration of the person's homestasis.

- Dealing with the stress of crisis on a day-to-day basis can affect a nurse's or care provider's mental well being. Nurses need to be mindful of the potential for this strain and use adaptive coping skills to maintain their own well being. Debriefing following a crisis incident is one method to allow staff to verbalize their feelings and thoughts about the event.

**NCLEX-PREP***

1. While interviewing a middle-aged woman who has come to the mental health care facility, the woman states, "My oldest son just left for college last week. I'm so lost without him. The house seems so empty." The nurse would interpret the woman's statement as suggesting which type of crisis?

   a. Maturational
   b. Situational
   c. Social
   d. Adventitious

2. A nurse assesses a patient and determines that the patient is in the alarm stage of responding to stress. Which of the following would the nurse most likely assess?

   a. Pupil constriction
   b. Decrease in heart rate
   c. Rapid respirations
   d. Dry skin

3. A group of psychiatric-mental health nurses are preparing an inservice presentation about stress and crisis. Which of the following would the group most likely include in the presentation?

   a. Crisis can be a chronic situation due to stress.
   b. An unknown stimulus is responsible for the crisis.
   c. The stress associated with crisis must be real.
   d. Crisis is not considered a mental illness.

4. The following are phases associated with a crisis. Which of the following occurs first?

   a. Distress occurs as every method of coping fails.
   b. Anxiety increases as past coping methods are ineffective.
   c. Exposure to a stressor leads to use of past coping mechanisms.
   d. New and different coping strategies are tried.

5. When providing care to individuals involved in a community disaster, which of the following would be the priority?

   a. Food and water
   b. Safety
   c. Shelter
   d. Referrals

*Answers to these questions appear on page 639.

## REFERENCES

Aguilera, D.C. (1998). *Crisis intervention: Theory and methodology* (8th ed.) St Louis: Mosby.

American Psychiatric Association. (2000). *Diagnostic and statistical manual of mental disorders* (4th ed., text rev.). Washington, DC: American Psychiatric Association.

Bornemann, T.H. (2005). Disaster response for mental health professionals. *Journal of Psychosocial Nursing, 43*(11),18–21.

Boyd, M. A. (2008). *Psychiatric nursing: Contemporary practice* (4th ed) Philadelphia: Lippincott Williams & Wilkin.

Can prolonged stress affect whether breast cancer returns. NIH Medline Plus the Magazine, 3(1): 6, Winter 2008. Available at: http://www.nlm.nih.gov/medlineplus/magazine/issues/winter08 Accessed January 2011.

Caplan, G. (1964). *Principles of preventive psychiatry.* New York: Basic Books.

Chitty, K.K. (2005). *Professional nursing concepts and challenges* (4th ed.). St. Louis, MO: Elsevier Saunders.

Cohen, I. (1984) "Florence Nightingale". *Scientific American,* 250, 136.

Crane, P., & Clements, P. (2005). Psychological response to disasters: Focus on adolescents. *Journal of Psychosocial Nursing, 43*(8), 31–38.

Davidhizar, R., & Shearer, R. (2002). Helping children cope with public disasters. *American Journal of Nursing, 102*(3), 26–33.

Doenges, M. E. et al. (2008). *Nursing Diagnosis Manual: Planning, individualizing, and documenting client care.* Philadelphia: F.A. Davis.

Everly, G., & Lating, J. (1995). *Psychotraumatology: Key papers and core concepts in posttraumatic stress.* New York, NY: Plenum.

Flannery, R. B., & Everly, G. S. (2000). Crisis intervention: a review. *International Journal of Emergency Mental Health, 2,*: 119–125.

Fortinash, K. M., & Holoday Worret, P.A. (2008). *Psychiatric mental health nursing* (4th ed.) St. Louis, MO: Mosby Elsevier.

Gorman, L. M., & Sultan, D. F. (2008). *Psychosocial nursing for general patient care* (3rd ed). Philadelphia, PA: F.A.Davis.

Hoff, L. (2001). *People in crisis: Clinical and public health perspective.* San Francisco, CA: Jossey-Bass Publishers.

Litz, B. T. (2004). *Early intervention for trauma and traumatic loss.* New York, NY: Guilford Press.

Maslow, A. (1968). *Toward a psychology of being.* 2nd ed. New York, NY: D. Van Nostrand.

McEwan, B. S., & Lasley, Z. E. N. (2002), *The end of stress as we know it.* Washington, DC: Joseph Henry Press.

Registered Nurse Association of Ontario. (2006). *Nursing Best Practice Guideline: Crisis intervention supplement.* Toronto, Canada.

Richards, J. (2009). Times of crisis, times of action. *Nursing Leadership, 22*(1), 22 23.

Selye, H. (1956). *The stress of life.* New York: McGraw-Hill.

Tye, J. (2009). Florence Nightingale's Lessons for Cultural Transformation. *Hospitals and Health Networks Magazine.* Accessed September 2010. Available at: http://www.hhnmag.com/hhnmag_app/jsp/articledisplay.jsp?dcrpath=HHNMAG/Article/data/05MAY2009/090504HHN_Online_Tye&domain=HHNMAG

U.S. Department of Health and Human Services. (2005). A guide to managing stress in crisis response professions. DHHS Publication No. SMA 4113. Rockville, MD: Center for Mental Health Services, Substance Abuse and Mental Health Services Administration.

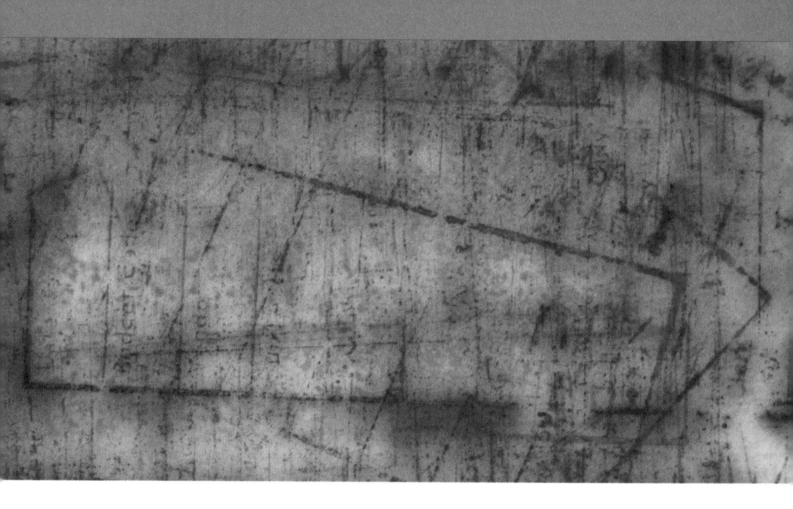

## CHAPTER CONTENTS

Definition of Case Management

Historical Evolution of Psychiatric Case Management

Case Management Process

Interpersonal Perspectives for Case Management

Measurement of Quality in Case Management

## EXPECTED LEARNING OUTCOMES

**After completing this chapter, the student will be able to:**

1. Define case management.
2. Trace the historical evolution of psychiatric case management.
3. Identify the prominent case management models.
4. Describe the specific role case management has in mental health care.
5. Discuss the functions and activities involved in case management.
6. Identify the goals and principles associated with case management.

# CHAPTER 7
# PSYCHIATRIC CASE MANAGEMENT

E. J. Ernst

7. List the skills needed to function as a psychiatric-mental health nurse case manager.

8. Explain the roles assumed by psychiatric-mental health nurse case manager.

9. Correlate how the interpersonal process relates to case management.

## KEY TERMS

Broker case management model

Case management

Clinical case management

Colorado model

In-patient psychiatric case management model

Managed care agent (MCA)

Managed care organization

Case management has evolved over the decades in an attempt to meet the needs of patients in varied settings. Psychiatric nursing case management, which has developed through its blending and adaptations of the definitions of case management, has a rich history not exclusive to the psychiatric-mental health nurse. Nor is it exclusive to the discipline of nursing because it often includes other disciplines such as social workers and other mental health professions. However, the psychiatric-mental health nurse (PMHN) has played an important role for patients with wide-ranging psychiatric diagnoses that can span multiple settings. As the therapeutic interpersonal relationship is the foundation of psychiatric-mental health nursing, it is important for the PMHN case manager to integrate interpersonal relationships throughout the case management process and build on the strength of the existing relationship.

This chapter addresses the topic of case management and the role of the case manager in psychiatric-mental health nursing practice. This chapter provides a definition for case management and traces the historical evolution of psychiatric case management. It reviews the key psychiatric case management models and the goals, principles, and skills involved in the case management process. The chapter integrates the interpersonal process with case management, describing the roles of the PMHN case manager. The chapter concludes with a description of how case management relates to quality of care.

## DEFINITION OF CASE MANAGEMENT

CASE MANAGEMENT refers to an outcome-oriented process that coordinates care and advocates for patients and patient populations across the health care continuum. While other definitions of case management also exist, Box 7-1 presents two definitions by key professional organizations. The underlying theme for all the definitions is collaborative action for outcome achievement. The results are reduced cost, decreased use of resources, and improved quality of care.

In general, case management spans health care to include not only multi-disciplinary health professionals but also insurance companies and MANAGED CARE ORGANIZATIONS. Case management, however, is not managed care. Managed care is a system of health care delivery and financing that is designed to control health care costs. Health care clinicians may approach case management as a method to provide continuity of care for patients. However, insurance companies and managed care organizations may view case management as an opportunity to regulate the services provided to individuals, thereby controlling costs. Thus, conflict in case management may occur because of the ideological difference in the perception of the role of case management (Belcher, 1993).

The American Nurses Association (ANA) approved a definition of case management that was later adopted by the American Nurses Credentialing Center (ANCC). The ANCC is the certifying body in nursing that provides certification for many nursing specialties, including the practice of case management in nursing. The ANA defines nursing case management as:

*"a dynamic and systematic collaborative approach to providing and coordinating health care services to a defined population. It is a participative process to identify*

---

### BOX 7-1: **DEFINITIONS OF CASE MANAGEMENT**

"A collaborative process of assessment, planning, facilitation, care coordination, evaluation, and advocacy for options and services to meet an individual's health needs through communication and available resources to promote quality, cost-effective outcomes."

"An intervention in which health care is integrated, coordinated, and advocated for individuals, families, and groups who require services. The aim of case management is to decrease fragmentation and ensure access to appropriate, individualized, and cost-effective care. As a case manager, the nurse has the authority and accountability required to negotiate with multiple clinicians and obtain diverse services."

—The American Nurses Association, American Psychiatric Nurses Association, and International Society of Psychiatric-Mental Nurses, Psychiatric-Mental Health Nursing: Scope and Standards of Practice, 2007, all have adopted these definitions.

*From Standards of Practice for Case Management, published by the Case Management Society of America (CMSA). Retrieved June 6, 2011, from http://www.cmsa.org/SOP*

*and facilitate options and services for meeting individuals' health needs, while decreasing fragmentation and duplication of care, and enhancing quality, cost-effective clinical outcomes. The framework for nursing case management includes five components: assessment, planning, implementation, evaluation, and interaction." (ANCC, 2000, p. 27)*

ANA (2000) further narrowed the definition of case management for the psychiatric-mental health setting. The ANA in conjunction with the American Psychiatric Nurses Association (APNA) and the International Society of Psychiatric-Mental Health Nurses (ISPN) defined case management as:

*"a clinical component of the psychiatric-mental health nurse's role in both inpatient and outpatient settings. Nurses who are functioning in the case manager role support the patient's highest level of functioning through interventions that are designed to enhance self-sufficiency and progress toward optimal health. These interventions may include risk assessment, supportive counseling, problem solving, teaching, medication and health status monitoring, comprehensive care planning, and linkage to, and identification and coordination of, various other health and human services." (ANA, APNA, and ISPN, 2007, p. 90)*

This definition became part of the *Scope and Standards of Psychiatric-Mental Health Nursing Practice* published in 2007.

> *Case management refers to an outcome-oriented process that coordinates care and advocates for patients and patient populations across the health care continuum. Although not exclusive to psychiatric-mental health nursing, it is an important component of psychiatric-mental health nursing.*

## HISTORICAL EVOLUTION OF PSYCHIATRIC CASE MANAGEMENT

Case management is a practice strategy that has been in existence for more than half a century. Early on, case management occurred primarily in public health settings, eventually expanding into the insurance industry. In the 1980s, the establishment of diagnosis related groups (DRGs) created a prospective payment system based on categories of patient diagnoses. Thus, institutions were being paid a predetermined amount based on the diagnosis rather than being paid for the actual cost of care. DRGs fueled further growth as case management began being implemented in acute care facilities.

Psychiatric-mental health case management and the role of the PMHN case manager have evolved significantly over the past decades. Two events in the mid-20th century spurred the use of case management in psychiatric-mental health nursing. These two events were the return of World War II veterans experiencing psychiatric conditions and the deinstitutionalization of chronic mentally ill individuals.

The return of World War II service members with psychiatric conditions changed the way mental health services were offered by the Veterans Administration. The concept of caring for patients across a continuum evolved after World War II to describe the extended community services needed for mental health patients. The Veterans Administration developed a model of case management that addressed not only the psychiatric needs of the veterans but also their health and social service needs (Kersbergen, 1996).

Deinstitutionalization of psychiatric inpatients in the 1950s and 1960s resulted from the development of medications targeting the chronically mentally ill individuals' most troubling symptoms. Pharmacological advancements prompted the movement of individuals from large, locked psychiatric in-patient institutions to community settings. Case management services expanded and were refined in the 1970s to include community mental health centers. These centers offered supportive community-based services to chronic mentally ill persons living in community settings after having been institutionalized for many years or in some cases decades (Herrick & Bartlett, 2004). The case manager in a community mental health setting provided a wide range of services such as helping the patient with housing needs, linking them with workforce re-entry services, assuring they had adequate food resources, assisting them with transportation needs, assessing medication compliance, and assessing daily functioning. Case management became an important means to ensure the delivery and coordination of community services for these individuals with chronic mental health conditions (Lee, Mackenzie, Dudley-Brown, & Chin, 1998; Yamashita, Forchuk, & Mound, 2005). The goal of case management programs in community mental health settings was to keep the mentally ill out of locked, in-patient hospitals and in the least restrictive community setting.

Case management received U.S. government support in the 1970s. A major stipulation of this support was that community mental health settings assign an individual to mentally ill patients to coordinate their care (Herrick & Bartlett, 2004). Case managers were to assist patients in setting and achieving realistic goals and in utilizing resources appropriately so that patients could live, learn, and work in the social systems of their choice.

> *Returning World War II veterans experiencing psychiatric conditions and the deinstitutionalization of chronic mentally ill patients are two key events that prompted the evolution of psychiatric- mental health case management.*

## Case Management Models

As case management evolved in the general health care arena and psychiatric-mental health nursing, the models for delivery of case management also have grown. These models developed in response to the diverse needs of a wide range of mentally ill patients. Currently, multiple case management models exist, with the PMHN providing services to patients in in-patient and out-patient settings. The PMHN may assume the role of primary case manager or function as part of a case management team in collaboration with other health professionals. The spectrum of case management services ranges from the least intensive services that of the case management service initiator, to the most intensive case management services, that of the clinical case manager. The level of service ideally is based on the patient's acuity level and psychiatric stability. Patients at high risk for homelessness, substance abuse, incarceration, decompensation, and/or rehospitalization require a more intensive model of clinical case management (Malone, Workneh, Butchart, & Clark, 1999).

Case management models vary significantly in methodology. However, most research has credited case management for increased psychiatric stability (Malone, et al., 1999). The increased psychiatric stability has been evidenced by increased independence, residential stability, vocational and social functions, decreased inappropriate use of emergency services, appropriate use of community

services, and increased adherence of clients to medication and aftercare regimens (Malone et al., 1999).

Although there are numerous case management models in existence, four important models related to psychiatric-mental health nursing are presented here.

> *Multiple case management models exist with the PMHN assuming the role of primary case manager or functioning as part of a case management team in collaboration with other health professionals. Services provided by the PMHN case manager can range from initiating the service to providing clinical case management.*

### In-Patient Model

The **IN-PATIENT PSYCHIATRIC CASE MANAGEMENT MODEL** originated at Waltham Weston Hospital in the emergency department (Herrick & Bartlett, 2004). In this model, psychiatric patients presenting to the hospital's emergency department were assigned to a **MANAGED CARE AGENT**. This agent, who was a psychiatrist, therapist, or other psychiatric clinician performed the initial assessment and initiated the treatment plan. The managed care agent also became part of a treatment team. In addition, the agent acted as the patient's advocate, assisting with accessing appropriate in-patient or out-patient services, including crisis intervention, in-patient hospitalization, respite care, or partial hospitalization. These services were based on the needs of the patient. At the same time, the managed care agent also had to balance care costs and quality. Moreover, the agent was responsible for the patient 24 hours a day, 7 days a week. The sustained consistent relationship associated with this case management model required strong interpersonal process skills.

### Continuum of Care Model

The continuum of care model, also known as the **COLORADO MODEL**, was developed at the University of Colorado Health Sciences Center (Herrick & Bartlett, 2004). This psychiatric case management model combined focused therapy (therapy aimed at intense frequent therapeutic engagement of the individual patient), assertive community treatment (ACT; individualized services available 24 hours a day based on needs delivered by a team of practitioners to the patients where they live) and family-centered interventions (services aimed at working with the patient from family systems perspective). Its goal was to rapidly transition hospitalized patients back into the community setting. The patient's treatment plan was developed by the patient, the patient's family, and treatment team and was based on the assessed needs of the patient. The case manager guides the patient and family across the continuum of care, assisting the patient in accessing appropriate treatment. The case manager also coordinates the multidisciplinary team and monitors and documents the patient's progress.

## Broker Case Management Model

Community mental health centers employ multiple case management models. The **BROKER CASE MANAGEMENT MODEL** was developed in the 1960s and 1970s. With this model, brokering case managers, typically single individuals, are responsible for referral, placement, and monitoring of patients (Neale & Rosenheck, 1995). They provide little services themselves. Rather, they assess a patient's needs and arrange for services from other providers to meet the patient's needs. Brokering case managers may have large caseloads—100 patients or more (Malone et al., 1999). Many community mental health centers have combined the broker model with the disease management model to provide service to the chronic mentally ill (Herrick & Bartlett, 2004). The disease management model focuses on medical or somatic management of symptoms and relies on early detection of decompensation by the medical or somatic team.

Community mental health psychiatric case management services target patients' needs to support independent living across the life span. Psychiatric services include crisis intervention, psychotherapy, family support, and medication management. Community mental health psychiatric case management recognizes the integrated role non-psychiatric case management services play in chronic mentally ill clients' well-being. Accordingly, assistance with housing, vocational training, and rehabilitative services are included under the model's umbrella of services (Herrick & Bartlett, 2004).

## Clinical Case Management

**CLINICAL CASE MANAGEMENT** is a worker-intensive, clinical case management model. The individuals commonly have the greatest need for services. The PMHN may work as the primary clinician or in collaboration with other health professionals in the community setting. The clinical case manager's care is based on the level and type of services provided (Malone et al., 1999). Research suggests that the optimal case manager-to-client ratio ranges from 1:12 to 1:15 (Harris & Bergman, 1988).

Intensive clinical case management may include multidisciplinary, assertive, team-based support services in the community. Although services may vary, typically 24-hours-a-day, 7-days-a-week access to a multi-disciplinary staff is provided. Round-the-clock, supportive telephone access and crisis intervention may be included (Borland, McRae, & Lycan, 1989; McRae, Higgins, Lycan, & Sherman, 1990).

> *Four models of psychiatric-mental health case management include: in-patient psychiatric case management model; continuum of care psychiatric case management model; the broker model; and clinical case management model.*

## CASE MANAGEMENT PROCESS

For case management to be successful, individuals at risk must be identified early and then appropriately stratified according to need (Moreo & Llewellyn, 2005). Case management services, therefore, must focus on the needs of the individual. Cooperation and partnership between the case manager and the individual and his or her family are essential to the case management process to promote increased compliance with the treatment plan (Moreo & Llewellyn, 2005). **Box 7-2** highlights the key characteristics of case management.

In response to an individual's health care problem, case managers are able to organize and sequence services (Knollmueller, 1989). Ultimately, case management should enhance self-care and self-determination, provide continuity of appropriate care, maximize independence by enhancing functional capacity, and coordinate existing and new services to best serve the patient's needs (White, 1986).

> *The case management process requires an interactive relationship that views the patient holistically and fosters empowerment through advocacy and education.*

**BOX 7-2: KEY CHARACTERISTICS OF CASE MANAGEMENT**

- Relationship based
- Interactive with patient and others
- Holistic
- Patient empowerment through advocacy
- Information provision through education

**BOX 7-3: PRINCIPLES OF CASE MANAGEMENT FOR ADULTS WITH SEVERE AND PERSISTENT MENTAL ILLNESS**

According to the NACM, to achieve the goal of case management, services provided should be:

- Consumer-focused
- Empowering for patients
- Racially and culturally appropriate
- Flexible
- Strength-focused
- Normalizing, incorporating natural supports
- Capable of meeting special needs
- Accountable

*From the National Association of Case Management (NACM).*

## Goals and Principles of Case Management

The goal of case management is to provide individualized and holistic services to individuals at risk. The services should enhance self-care across the continuum of all health care services provided to a patient (Moreo & Llewellyn, 2005). Spanning the continuum of services provided, the discipline of case management is dynamic and interactive. It requires a high level of interaction with the patient and his or her family as well as among clinicians from multiple disciplines. Strong interpersonal skills are essential for building relationships with diverse individuals to provide service (Moreo & Llewellyn).

Overall, case management should "ensure the continuity of care between all points of care" (Mayer, 1996). Components of this overall goal include early detection and intervention, interdisciplinary communication and care planning, resource use to meet patient's needs, formation of strong alliances between families and health care professionals, and social support and health education. To achieve this outcome, the National Association of Case Management (1997) identified principles for service provision that addressed consumer-focused case management and other community support for adults with severe and persistent mental illness. These principles are highlighted in **Box 7-3**.

The end result of case management would be achievement of positive health outcomes through the delivery of coordinated, cost-effective, high-quality care. This care "enhances independent living capability and maximizes the quality of life of patients" (Mayer, 1996).

## Necessary Skills for Case Management

The psychiatric-mental health case manager integrates four critical skills to carry out the process of case management. These skills are critical thinking, communication, negotiation, and collaboration.

### Critical Thinking

Critical thinking, as described in Chapter 5, refers to a purposeful method of reasoning that is systematic, reflective, rational, and outcome oriented. Psychiatric-mental health nurses use critical thinking as a basis for clinical decision making to plan and implement the most effective interventions for a patient.

PMHN case managers use critical thinking to sort through the myriad of information about a patient and the situation. Critical thinking is reflected by determining what information is pertinent and relevant, what, if any, additional information is needed, why certain events occurred or did not occur, and what the potential issues and problems are. For example, after sorting through information from the medical record and patient interview, the case manager realizes that information about the patient's medication use has gaps. The case manager would investigate further to determine exactly what information is missing, such as if a medication was prescribed but not taken, and why.

From the information gathered, the PMHN case manager prioritizes the information and identifies relevant problems. Together with the patient, family, and other disciplines, options are explored, planned and put into action. Throughout the process, the PMHN case manager continually evaluates the plan and activities, adapting, readjusting, or altering the plan based on changes that have occurred.

### Communication

Communication is essential for the case management process (see Chapter 3 for a more in-depth discussion of communication skills). The PMHN case manager requires astute communication skills to obtain from and deliver information to the patient, patient's family, other disciplines, and service providers. A sample interaction is illustrated in **Therapeutic Interaction 7-1**. For example, as a case manager for a patient with a chemical dependency history, the case manager may be involved in transporting the patient to the dentist for some procedures. The patient says, "If I get my tooth pulled, I hope they give some pain meds." The psychiatric case manager might respond, "Well, I think they are likely to offer you something. With your history of addiction, what do you think would be best to accept?"

The PMHN case manager needs to be succinct and clearly articulate both verbally and in writing essential information. He or she acts as the central hub for communication, ensuring that information is shared clearly, accurately, and in a timely and efficient manner among all parties involved.

### Negotiation

Negotiation is another essential skill required for effective case management. The PMHN case manager interacts with numerous individuals and parties involved in the

---

### THERAPEUTIC INTERACTION 7-1: EXPLAINING THE CASE MANAGER'S ROLE

J. is a young adult male who has been diagnosed with depression. He is visiting the community mental health center for the first time since his discharge from an acute care facility.

| | |
|---|---|
| **C.M.:** "Hello, J.,  I'm H. and I will be your case manager here at the agency." | Establishment of who you are and your role |
| **Patient:** "You will be my what?" | Seeking clarification |
| **C.M.:** "A case manager. Here at this facilty, a case manager is someone who will help make sure that you have access to all the things you need to help you live successfully in the community." | Providing clarification; identifying his or her role through explanation |
| **Patient:** "Are you gonna control my money and how I spend it?" | Feels threatened by possible loss of independence |
| **C.M.:** "Do you need help with managing your money? If so I am glad to assist." | Offers support to decrease perception of threat |
| **Patient:** "My dad is my payee, can you make it so I have my own money?" | Seeks more independence |
| **C.M.:** "That's important to you?" | Validate/clarify |
| **Patient:** "You bet it is, I'm not a child." | Feels embarrassed by the circumstances |
| **C.M.:** "I can arrange a meeting between you, your father, and myself. That way I can get to know you and your father better and try to understand how and why he became your payee in the first place." | Offers an option for gathering information that will also possibly strengthen the interpersonal relationship |

patient's care. He or she must be able to look at the "big picture" fairly and objectively, balancing the demands and needs of all the parties involved to ensure that the best outcome for the patient is achieved. For example, a case manager for a patient who needs to attend ten Alcoholic Anonymous meetings a month per court order may negotiate transportation to and from five of the meetings each month with the patient's sponsor. Or the case manager may be able to obtain bus tokens from the local transportation office so that the patient can ride the bus to and from the meetings. Mediation and compromise are fundamental to negotiation and resolution of the issues and problems.

## Collaboration

The case manager is one of several members of a team. This team commonly includes the patient, patient's family, other health care professionals, administrative staff, other agencies, and service providers to name just a few. The PMHN case manager works closely with the many different team members. Cooperative interaction among members is essential to promote positive outcomes. Collaboration is further emphasized by the Standards of Professional Performance (Standard 11) of the Psychiatric-Mental Health Nurse: Scope and Standards of Practice (ANA, APNA, & ISPN, 2007, p. 50). Therefore, the PMHN case manager must work cooperatively with others to ensure the best patient outcomes.

> *A PMHN case manager must be skilled in critical thinking, communication, negotiation, and collaboration.*

## Essential Functions of the Case Management Process

The case management process involves the following functions: assessment, planning, implementation, coordination, monitoring, and evaluation. These functions are essential for ensuring outcomes that are holistic and individualized to the patient's needs. The cooperation of the patient, as well as all members of the team, is crucial to the success of the case management process. Cooperation of the patient and the family allows the patient the best opportunity for a successful outcome of the treatment plan (Moreo & Llewellyn, 2005).

## Assessment

The foundation of the case management process is assessment. Assessment is a systematic multidimensional approach to the collection of data from the patient, family, significant others, and health care providers. A written release of information to the case manager and organization must be obtained prior to collection of patient data to ensure adherence to patient privacy regulations (Moreo & Llewellyn, 2005).

Sources of patient data important to the case management assessment process may include the patient, family members, health care institutions, employers, schools, and military records. Data collected are not limited to the patient's physical and psychosocial dimensions but also includes spiritual, cognitive, functional, and developmental abilities as well as economic and lifestyle issues (Moreo & Llewellyn, 2005). Collection of patient data allows the case manager to critically analyze elements essential to subsequent functions in the case management process.

Thorough analysis by the case manager of all collateral data collected allows the case manager the best information set from which to make decisions about formulating a case management treatment plan (Moreo & Llewellyn, 2005). Collateral data may provide insight into the patient's past and present utilization of health care and/or case management services. Often, services accessed by patients are not appropriate and/or are not contributing to a long-term solution for a patient's stability. Many institutions have standardized case management assessment screening and scoring tools to ensure uniformity of data collected during interviews of the patient, family, and significant others (Moreo & Llewellyn, 2005).

In some settings, a screening assessment may be done initially to determine if the patient would benefit from case management. Areas related to screening may include factors such as age, diagnoses, frequency of hospitalizations, numbers of providers, instability of home environment, substance abuse, and risk for complications. If appropriate, then the patient is referred for case management.

## Planning

The planning function allows the case manager to make decisions based on collected data to formulate an appropriate plan of action. During this time, the case manager works in concert with all team members to develop a patient-centered, evidence-based, outcome-oriented, collaborative, and interdisciplinary plan of action. The individualized treatment plan should embody the patient's immediate, intermediate, and long-term needs (Moreo & Llewellyn, 2005). The plan is action-oriented, detailing the specific steps and sequence, and time-specific, identifying the duration and frequency of the actions.

Time frame benchmarks should be developed to later assist with evaluation of the goals identified in the plan. Planning should allow for the possibility that case management may start in one setting such as the acute care setting until the patient is discharged and then transferred to the outpatient setting. Continuity of case management is highest when one individual provides case management services across the continuum of health care settings. However, if transfer is necessary, the case manager should ensure that his or her written records and documents are created in a manner that would facilitate the transfer of care to another case manager should that be necessary (Moreo & Llewellyn, 2005).

Including the family in the plan of care has been identified as crucial in developing a therapeutic alliance (Yamashita et al., 2005). However, doing so may require reconnection with family after a prolonged period of time. In such cases, the case manager should educate the family to correct any misconceptions or misunderstandings they may have regarding the patient's needs (Yamashita et al., 2005).

## Implementation

Implementation is the execution of the case management treatment plan tailored to the individual patient's needs. Upon the approval of the treatment plan by the patient, family, physician, and payer, the case manager ensures that the established multi-disciplinary team work toward a mutual goal. The effectiveness of the plan's implementation is significantly related to the case manager's ability to plan care that is cost effective, timely, and appropriate. The patient and all individuals involved in the case management process should have a clear understanding of their role and the goals established (Moreo & Llewellyn, 2005). Patient participation is important to prepare him or her for the changes that may occur with the ultimate outcome of promoting self-advocacy, self-determination, and autonomy.

## Coordination

Coordination is essential to the case management process. The multitude of information, activities, and resources needed for achieving the ultimate outcome require organization, integration, and modification to ensure that there is a smooth flow and efficient follow through of the plan. Essential competencies needed for coordination include communication, collaboration, assertiveness, and cooperation. These competencies are reflected in activities such as updating involved participants, following up

with team members and service providers, and advocating for the patient's needs. Moreover, a case manager needs to understand how health care organizations and insurance systems work. He or she must be able to navigate the myriad of delivery systems, reimbursement methods, and benefit programs to facilitate the plan of care to meet the patient's needs.

During the coordination process, the case manager validates that the plans in place are being implemented in a timely and safe manner. The case manager also ensures that patient confidentiality is maintained. Should a problem with the case management plan arise, the case manager needs to assess the situation and determine the best changes to the plan that will rectify the situation. A case manager must be able to anticipate situations and proactively modify or correct elements essential to a smooth provision of care to the patient (Moreo & Llewellyn, 2005).

## Monitoring

The case manager ensures the treatment plan is effective by monitoring the plan of care on a continuing and regular basis. The interval for monitoring is dependent upon the individual's needs because each person is unique. Thus, monitoring is performed as often as appropriate based on the individual's needs and progress. For example, a person living alone most likely would require more frequent monitoring than one who is living at home with extended family support.

The case manager assesses and reassesses data from the patient, family, and health care providers to ascertain whether the treatment plan is on target to meet the goals established in the plan. Monitoring is patient-focused, that is, it is done from the patient's viewpoint. It looks at areas that reflect the patient, such as medications, functional level, compliance with instructions, and adherence to follow-up visits. The case manager is able to modify segments of the treatment plan or the treatment plan as a whole if needed to promote patient progress toward the treatment goals (Moreo & Llewellyn, 2005).

## Evaluation

The evaluation of the case management treatment plan is the final function associated with case management. Evaluation, like monitoring, occurs continuously. It also can occur at specific designated frequencies and when needed. Additionally, evaluation always is done when the plan has been completed.

Evaluation is based on assessment of the patient's ability to work toward and accomplish goals delineated in the plan. It allows the case manager to critically analyze and determine if each health care provider's participation in the treatment plan has been consistent with the organization's standards and appropriate for the patient's needs (Moreo & Llewellyn, 2005).

> *The case management process involves the functions of assessment, planning, implementation, coordination, monitoring, and evaluation.*

## INTERPERSONAL PERSPECTIVES FOR CASE MANAGEMENT

Hildegard Peplau delineated a theoretical basis from which an interpersonal perspective for providing case management services may be developed. Peplau (1962) described nursing as an "educative instrument, a maturing force that aims to promote forward movement of the personality in the direction of creative, constructive, productive, personal, and community living" (p. 53). Links between the work of Peplau and the case management model underscore the importance of the "interactive interpersonal relationship" between the case manager and the patient (Forchuk et al., 1989, p. 36). Therefore, establishing a one-to-one therapeutic interpersonal relationship is essential to the case management process (Forchuk, Beaton, Crawford, Ide, Voorberg, & Bethune, 1989). **Evidence-Based Practice** 7-1 emphasizes the importance of the interpersonal relationship for psychiatric case management.

The case manager, initially, is a stranger to the patient. Through interaction, the case manager and patient develop a professional relationship based on the process of the case management. This relationship is more than simply the focused content of interactions between the two parties involved. The patient's needs are at the foundation of this process. Thus, the patient and nurse, in conjunction with other disciplines and services, identify the needs, develop mutual goals, and work to meet these needs and goals. The PMHN case manager uses critical thinking, communication, negotiation and collaboration throughout the relationship.

Several of the functions of case management, including assessment, planning, implementation and evaluation, closely resemble the steps of the nursing process and the stages of the therapeutic relationship

as described by Peplau (1952, 1991; see Chapter 2 for more information about Peplau's stages of the therapeutic relationship and Chapter 5 for a comparison of Peplau's stages and the nursing process). These parallels reinforce the significance of the interpersonal process in case management.

Research also substantiates the interpersonal nature of case management. A study by Forchuk et al. (1989) asserted that trust building and establishment of rapport are essential to the interpersonal connection between the case manager and the patient. Additionally, the case manager must assume multiple roles and be able to adapt to changes in the relationship with the patient (Forchuk et al. 1989). Moreover, appropriate humor, touch, and recognition by the case manager that each patient is a unique individual are characteristics and qualities important to the case manager (Hellwig, 1993).

> *The case management process closely resembles the steps of the nursing process and the stages of the therapeutic relationship.*

### Roles of the Psychiatric-Mental Health Nurse Case Manager

The *Scope and Standards of Psychiatric-Mental Health Nursing Practice* (ANA, APNA, & ISPN, 2007) provides standards for all aspects of psychiatric-mental health nursing care. These standards apply to basic and advanced practice registered nurses. Case management is specifically addressed in Standards of Care, Standard Vf: Case Management (**Box** 7-4). Typically, the desired qualifications of the psychiatric-mental health case manager include earned degrees in higher education (baccalaureate or graduate degree) and professional licensure along with certification by the ANCC.

The role of the PMHN case manager varies depending on the case management model used and the institution. The role is further defined by the population served, the setting, and the situation. Although the role of the case manager may vary, all roles have the common goal of improving the quality of health care every individual receives by collaborating with patient's to access, facilitate, plan, and advocate for their needs (Moreo & Llewellyn, 2005).

---

**EVIDENCE-BASED PRACTICE 7-1:**
**THE PROCESS OF CASE MANAGEMENT**

STUDY

Yamashita, M., Forshuk, C., & Mound, B. (2005). Nurse Case Management: Negotiating care together within a developing relationship. *Perspectives in Psychiatric Care, 41* (2): 62–70.

SUMMARY

The purpose of this study was to explain the process of nurse case management involving patients experiencing chronic mental illness. The authors were attempting to define psychiatric-mental health nursing case management, to elucidate characteristics, and to identify common themes between mental health care sites. The authors conducted interviews with nurses in in-patient, transitional, and community settings in four cities in southern Ontario, Canada. The findings identified that negotiating care together within a developing relationship was the basic social process. A common theme of greatest importance emerged, that of "building a trusting relationship" as the foundation of case management. A need for a holistic approach was identified as crucial throughout the relationship. By employing the holistic approach to the therapeutic relationship, the best "negotiation" can proceed on behalf of the patient.

APPLICATION TO PRACTICE

Regardless of the setting, the study demonstrated consistency in the basic social process as key to case management. The establishment of mutual respect and a holistic approach are significant to ensure that the best outcomes for the patient are achieved. This study helps to further emphasize the therapeutic relationship as the basis for psychiatric-mental health nursing case management.

QUESTIONS TO PONDER

1. *How would the roles of the psychiatric-mental health nurse case manager correlate with building a trusting relationship?*
2. *What barriers might impact the psychiatric-mental health nurse case manager's ability to develop a therapeutic relationship with the patient and thus interfere with the case management process?*

---

The PMHN case manager is charged with the responsibility to initiate and tailor a patient needs-based treatment plan that spans the continuum of care. Case manager roles may include: advocate, consultant, educator, liaison, facilitator, mentor, and researcher (Moreo & Llewellyn, 2005). Although these roles are not specific to psychiatric-mental health nursing case management, all of them do apply. The interpersonal process involving the PMHN and patient further enhance these roles. These roles also are similar in focus to those roles identified by Peplau in 1952 (see Chapter 2 for more information about Peplau and roles of the psychiatric-mental health nurse), thus reinforcing the interpersonal process emphasis of case management.

> ## Q BOX 7-4: STANDARD Vf: CASE MANAGEMENT
>
> The psychiatric-mental health nurse provides case management to coordinate comprehensive health services and ensure continuity of care.
>
> ### MEASUREMENT CRITERIA
>
> 1. Case management services are based on a comprehensive approach to the patient's physical, mental, emotional, and social health problems and resource availability.
> 2. Case management services are provided in terms of the patient's needs and the accessibility, availability, quality, and cost-effectiveness of care.
> 3. Health-related services and more specialized care are negotiated on behalf of the patient with the appropriate agencies and providers as needed.
> 4. Relationships with agencies and providers are maintained throughout the patient's use of the health care services to ensure continuity of care.
>
> *From the American Nurses Association, American Psychiatric Nurses Association, International Society of Psychiatric-Mental Health Nurses. (2007). Psychiatric-Mental Health Nursing: Scope and Standards of Practice. Silver Springs, MD: American Nurses Association Publishing Program.*

> *When engaged in the case management process, the PMHN case manager can assume seven different roles: advocate, consultant, educator, liaison, facilitator, mentor, and researcher.*

## Advocate

As an advocate, the PMHN case manager ensures that the patient's individualized needs are addressed and that all members of the team providing services work collaboratively across the continuum of care. As an advocate, he or she helps to identify what the patient wants and needs and to balance these with the available resources. Advocacy ensures patient access to treatment alternatives that are safe, coordinated, and the least restrictive (Moreo & Llewellyn, 2005).

## Consultant

The PMHN case manager's role as a consultant is demonstrated by the nurse acting as a resource for members of the team during the course of treatment. He or she collaborates and coordinates with team members and/or the patient and his or her family to assist them in accessing the needed services, including specialty or hard-to-find resources. As a consultant, the PMHN case manager is able to make recommendations about the suitability of

vocational resources or training that may be incorporated into the patient's short-term or long-term treatment goals (Moreo & Llewellyn, 2005).

## Educator

The PMHN case manager teaches the team about the dynamic role of the case manager and how his or her role interfaces across the continuum of care. Additionally, the PMHN case manager educates the patient and family about the specific condition or treatment and assists them in obtaining more information about it. Teaching areas may include specific issues targeting the disease processes and patient's wellness as well as symptom management, disease prognosis, injury and relapse prevention, and adherence to treatment recommendations including medication adherence (Moreo & Llewellyn, 2005). In addition, the PMHN case manager provides patients and families with information about the health care system and how it works, as well as insurance regulations, reimbursement policies, and appropriate resources and services.

Active participation by the patient and family is essential to the psychiatric stability of the patient. The PMHN case manager is able to assist the patient and family in better understanding technical medical terms, complexities in care, and what to expect across the continuum of care. The education provided allows the patient and family the opportunity to make informed care decisions regarding treatment and care (Moreo & Llewellyn, 2005). Informed decision making promotes empowerment.

## Liaison

The PMHN case manager's role as a liaison unites the patient and family, the health care team, and the payer with the community. He or she acts as the central point for communication, negotiation, and collaboration among the patient, family, health care providers, agencies, and other non-medical providers of services. Strong interpersonal skills are needed to build positive relationships and affect change. Assertiveness, empathy, and a high degree of organization are qualities necessary for this role (Moreo & Llewellyn, 2005).

## Facilitator

The PMHN case manager's role as a facilitator ensures that the patient's plan of care moves in the proper direction. He or she has the requisite knowledge and skills to proactively identify barriers to care and to identify system problems that may be common to the organization and affect multiple patients. The PMHN case manager can approach identified problems and bring them to the attention of the appropriate decision makers and committees. In addition, he or she works to ensure that the patient's transition from different levels of care occurs seamlessly, using the best possible resources and level of care based on cost, value, outcomes and patient factors. Thus, the PMHN case manager plays a significant role in the continuous quality improvement of an organization (Moreo & Llewellyn, 2005).

## Mentor

The PMHN case manager's role as a mentor allows novice case managers (those new to the role) the opportunity to be mentored by more experienced case managers. The experienced case manager not only introduces the novice case manager to the role and the practice of case management, but also introduces him or her to the philosophy, systems, and resources in place at a particular institution (Moreo & Llewellyn, 2005). More experienced PMHN case managers offer their expertise, support, guidance, leadership, knowledge, and skills to the novice case manager as well as to the patient, family, and others involved in the case management plan.

## Researcher

The role as a researcher allows the PMHN case manager to enhance the body of knowledge that provides the basis of care. This individual typically has a graduate degree, such as a masters or doctoral degree in nursing, which included significant coursework in literature review, research methodologies, and statistics. Case management is a dynamic role in nursing and research must keep pace with the advancements of the profession. Research findings should be formally disseminated to add to the body of evidence, and PMHN case managers should incorporate research findings into evidence-based case management practice (Moreo & Llewellyn, 2005).

## Practice Guidelines

The National Association of Case Management ([NACM] 1997) developed guidelines for case management practice with adults with severe and persistent mental illness. The development of the guidelines published in a monograph was funded by the Center for Mental Services within the Substance Abuse and Mental Health Service Administration (SAMHSA). NACM asserted that with the growth of outcome-oriented case management services, the guidelines developed would serve as a framework to promote consistency. The guidelines set parameters for case management practice. However, they do not follow any one particular case management model. While nurses were not described in these guidelines as the primary case manager, the importance of including the discipline of nursing was emphasized (NACM, 1997).

The case management guideline development process was undertaken by using focus group guidance from an expert review panel, feedback from people with serious mental illness, and case managers from across the United States (NACM, 1997). The case management guidelines also included feedback from telephone interviews with managed behavioral health organizations and state offices implementing state-managed care programs for the serious and persistently mentally ill. Crisis prevention, access to medical and psychiatric services, and access to community resources were identified as the most important issues by the focus groups. Engagement and relationship building were also identified as important elements in case management (NACM, 1997).

The guidelines reflected three levels of intensity for case management services (NACM, 1997). Crisis prevention was a top priority for each of the levels of case management.

- Level One case management services were described as the most extensive services for individuals with the greatest need and disability.
- Level Two case management services were described as supportive to promote recovery and rehabilitation.
- Level Three case management services were described as the least extensive providing a basic link to crisis management services for individuals who were more independent and were self-managing their lives.

> *Case management services range in intensity from the most extensive support for individuals with the greatest need (Level One) to the least extensive support providing a basic link to crisis management services (Level Three).*

The risk for no case management services was discussed, and it was agreed that level three case management would provide access to services in times of urgent need (NACM, 1997).

The NACM (1997) also delineated critical elements of case management that shape practice. These critical elements must exist regardless of the level of case management service being provided. The critical elements include: coordination; consumer choice; determination of strengths and preferences; comprehensive, outcome-oriented service planning; collaboration with psychiatrists and other service providers; continuity of care; and family and kindred support.

> *At any level of service, case management must include the critical elements of coordination, consumer choice, determination of strengths and preferences, comprehensive, outcome-oriented service planning, collaboration with psychiatrists and other service providers, continuity of care, and family and kindred support.*

## Admission and Assignment to Case Management Services

The NACM (1997) identified admission criteria based on the patient meeting the criteria for serious and persistent mental illness. The serious and persistent mentally ill individuals were often those individuals with high utilization of inpatient or state hospital services. The following are the admission criteria authored by the NACM:

1. Diagnosable Axis I *Diagnostic and Statistical Manual of Mental Disorders, Fourth Edition, Text Revision*

(*DSM-IV-TR*) psychiatric disorder; Axis II psychiatric disorder if there is sufficient functional difficulties, an extended duration of problems/illness, and continued reliance upon publicly funded services and supports present.
2. Clinically necessary treatment or service due to presence of medical and psychosocial needs.
3. A reasonable expectation for remediation of symptoms, behavior improvement, and increased potential for recovery with case management intervention/support or decompensation or relapse due to no case management.
4. Level assignment based on: collaborative conversations between the consumer (and family member, with consumer concurrence) to determine preferences, self-assessment of needs, clinician assessment of needs, strengths on which to build, and expectations for change or support; an assessment tool adopted by the provider, funder, or managed care organization which is consistent with current knowledge and acceptable to both consumers and practitioners; and a second clinical opinion for final recommendation when there is substantial disagreement between the collaborative effort and the assessment process (NACM, 1997).

According to the NACM, "admission to case management does not necessarily mean that the consumer should or must have access to all community support services; it does require a thorough assessment of needs with access to the least intrusive or restrictive services available, as well as special assistance in meeting individual needs" (NACM, 1997, p. 16).

The assessment tool used for the level assignment process may be based on state mental health authorities or managed care organizations. However, attention to the individual's identified needs, the social resources they have on admission, and their strengths is crucial to the assignment of mental health care needs (NACM, 1997).

In addition, determining the level of case management is based on evaluation of seven specific areas. These areas are: consumer choice; willingness; social resources and natural supports available to consumers; safety; culture; co-occurring conditions; and any legal issues (NACM, 1997).

## Transition Between Levels and Discharge From Case Management

The patient's desires and input must be a primary consideration for the transition between case management levels and/or discharge from case management services (NACM, 1997). A patient's level of stability is established by evaluating symptoms, personal resources, and supports. The NACM recommends that, when possible, there should be an overlap including continuity of staff and psychiatrist in order to transition a patient between levels.

## Personal Practice Guidelines

In addition to guidelines that shape case management practice, individuals acting in the role of case manager also should adhere to practice guidelines on the personal level. The personal practice guidelines established by the NACM are summarized in **Box 7-5**.

## MEASUREMENT OF QUALITY IN CASE MANAGEMENT

The foundation that is central to case management regardless of the setting or model used is the philosophy that "when an individual reaches the optimum level of wellness and functional capability, everyone benefits: the individuals being served, their support systems, the health care delivery systems and the various reimbursement services" (Case Management Society of America [CSMA], 2010). The case management process is goal-directed and depends upon the case manager's ability to identify and change practice patterns and plans of care as needed to allow produce outcomes. The case manager "should maximize the client's health, wellness, safety, adaptation, and self-care through quality case management, client satisfaction, and cost-efficiency" and "facilitate coordination, communication, and collaboration with the client and other stakeholders in order to achieve goals and maximize positive client outcomes" (CMSA, 2010, pp. 17–18). Guidelines for measuring the outcomes dictate that the case manager use the goal-oriented process to move a patient toward wellness, safety, self-care, and/or rehabilitation (CMSA, 2010).

---

### BOX 7-5: NACM'S PERSONAL PRACTICE GUIDELINES

AS A CASE MANAGER, I...

- Am committed to respect the dignity and autonomy of all persons and to behave in a manner that communicates this respect,
- Am committed to each individual's right to self-determination, and the rights of people to make their own life choices,
- Am committed to fight stigma wherever I find it, to educate the community, and to promote community integration for the people I serve,
- Do not allow my words or actions to reflect prejudice or discrimination regarding a person's race, culture, creed, gender or sexual orientation,
- Strive to both seek and provide culturally-sensitive services for each person and to continually increase my cultural competence,
- Am committed to helping persons find or acknowledge their strengths and to use these strengths to achieve their goals,
- Am committed to helping persons achieve maximum self-responsibility and to find and use services that promote increased knowledge, skills and competencies,
- Acknowledge the power of self-help and peer support and encourage participation in these activities with those I serve,
- Am honest with myself, my colleagues, the people I serve, and others involved in their care,
- Keep confidential all information entrusted to me by those I serve except when to do so puts the person or others at grave risk. I am obligated to explain the limits of confidentiality to the persons I serve at the beginning of our working together,
- Am committed to a holistic perspective, seeing each person I serve in the context of their family, friends, other significant other people in their lives, their community, and their culture, and working within the context of this natural support system.

*From the National Association of Case Management (NACM).*

Case management services promote quality, targeted, effective outcomes for the patient and/or family (CMSA, 2010). To ensure the quality of care, specific indicators related to the case manager and case management process are used to measure the quality of care and improvements implemented by the case manager. Outcome standards are demonstrated by the following:

- Evaluation of documented goals as to the level of achievement

- Demonstration of efficacy, quality and cost-effectiveness in achieving documented goals

- Measurement and reporting of how the documented goals impacted the plan of care

- Use of appropriate adherence guidelines, standardized tools, and proven process to determine individuals' preferences for and understanding of the plan, need for and willingness to change, and available support to maintain healthy change

- Employment of evidence-based guidelines

- Evaluation of patient satisfaction (CMSA, 2010).

Outcomes measurement can be difficult because mental health stability must be quantified. The NACM (1997) stated that one of the most quantifiable outcomes of case management is the reduction in hospitalizations and use of expensive mental health services. The NACM further stated that symptom reduction and improved quality of life indicators, such as health, living situation, work, relationships with friends and family, and social opportunities, should be evaluated.

Several research studies have evaluated the quality of life for patients receiving psychiatric-mental health case management services. The results indicate varying levels of reported quality of life (Malone et al., 1999). A study by Stein and Test (1980) asserted that patients enrolled in a specialized model of case management reported an increased level of independent functioning as well as a decrease in symptomology when compared against standard treatment. In another study, Bigelow and Young (1991) reported case-managed patients asserted a greater sense of well-being and less psychological distress compared to the control group. Moreover, a third study by Neale and Rosenheck (1995) reported that an intensive case management program at the Veteran's Administration

that provided a strong patient-case manager alliance increased global assessment of functioning (GAF) scores and decreased symptom severity.

> *The underlying premise of all case management is that everyone benefits when the patient reaches his or her optimum level of wellness and capability.*

Although the research described demonstrates measurement of positive outcomes, social, financial, cognitive, and psychological problems create barriers for outcome achievement, measurement, and, subsequently, the quality of care. One of the most significant barriers for case management results from medication non-compliance. Medication adherence is dramatically influenced by the patient's knowledge, motivation, and attitude toward pharmacologic interventions (CMSA, 2006). Based on a document authored by the World Health Organization (WHO), the CMSA developed guidelines targeting medication adherence (WHO, 2003).

According to the CMSA (2006), the ultimate goal of the medication adherence guidelines is to provide an environment where structured-interaction based on patient-specific needs result in increased motivation and knowledge targeting medication adherence. The CMSA further stated that although the guidelines developed by the organization target medication adherence, the guidelines could be readily adapted to any situation where the goal of case management was to increase adherence to a specific therapeutic treatment plan. The organization developed several case management assessment tools, including the "readiness ruler" to assist case managers in tailoring their interactions to the level appropriate to the patient's readiness and to gauge the level of patient engagement in the process, thereby providing a measureable means for evaluation of outcomes and quality of care.

## SUMMARY POINTS

- Case management refers to an outcome-oriented process that coordinates care and advocates for patients and patient populations across the health care continuum. Although many definitions of case management may exist, the underlying theme is collaborative action for outcome achievement.

- The role of the PMI IN case manager is guided by the Scope and Standards of Psychiatric-Mental Health Nursing Practice (2007). Psychiatric-mental health nursing case management is dynamic, capable of adapting to patient-centered needs that vary widely.

- Multiple case management models exist and these models vary significantly in their methodology. Important models related to psychiatric-mental health nursing include the in-patient psychiatric case management model; continuum of care psychiatric case management model; the broker case management model; and the clinical case management model.

- PMHN case managers use the skills of critical thinking, communication, negotiation, and collaboration to provide coordinated, cost-effective, high-quality care to meet the needs of patients.

- The case management process involves assessment, planning, implementation, coordination, monitoring, and evaluation to ensure outcome achievement that is holistic and individualized to the patient's needs.

- Establishment of a one-to-one therapeutic interpersonal relationship is essential to the case management process. The patient's needs are the foundation of the therapeutic process and of case management.

- The role of the PMHN case manager varies depending on the case management model used, the institution, the population being served, the setting, and the situation. Case manager roles typically include: advocate, consultant, educator, liaison, facilitator, mentor, and researcher. The interpersonal process involving the PMHN and patient further enhance these roles, which are similar in focus to those roles identified by Hildegard Peplau in 1952.

- Guidelines for case management practice with adults with severe and persistent mental illness have been developed to serve as a framework to promote consistency. In addition, individuals acting in the role of case manager also should adhere to practice guidelines on the personal level.

- Quality in case management is measured by outcomes such as reduction in hospitalizations, use of expensive mental health services, symptom reduction, and improved quality of life indicators such as health, living situation, work, relationships with friends and family, and social opportunities. Medication adherence is also used.

**NCLEX-PREP***

1. A nursing instructor is preparing a class for a group of students about case management in psychiatric-mental health nursing. Which of the following would the instructor most likely include about psychiatric-mental health case management?

   a. It is a method of care delivery that is unique to psychiatric-mental health nursing.
   b. It is a health care financing strategy aimed at reducing costs.
   c. It involves multi-disciplinary collaboration to achieve outcomes.
   d. It involves reducing fragmentation of care during illness episodes.

2. A psychiatric-mental health nurse is working as a case manager and has a caseload of 120 patients. The nurse is responsible for assessing the patients' needs and arranging for services. The nurse is functioning within which case management model?

   a. Broker case management
   b. Clinical case management
   c. Intensive case management
   d. Continuum of care

3. A psychiatric-mental health nurse case manager is reviewing a patient's assessment information and determines that more information is needed to determine why the patient stopped coming to the clinic for his medication prescription. The nurse is demonstrating which of the following?

   a. Communication
   b. Critical thinking
   c. Negotiation
   d. Collaboration

4. Which of the following best depicts a psychiatric-mental health nurse case manager acting in the role of a consultant?

   a. Instructing the patient about the need for adhering to his medication schedule.
   b. Promoting patient access to the least restrictive treatment method.
   c. Recommending possible vocational services that would be appropriate.
   d. Proactively identifying potential barriers that may affect the patient.

5. A psychiatric-mental health patient requires level two case management services. Which of the following most likely would be involved?

   a. Crisis prevention
   b. Extensive services
   c. Crisis management
   d. Supportive services

*Answers to these questions appear on page 639.

## REFERENCES

American Nurses Association (ANA), American Psychiatric Nurses Association (APNA), International Society of Psychiatric-Mental Health Nurses (ISPN). (2007). *Psychiatric-Mental Health Nursing: Scope and Standards of Practice.* Silver Springs, MD: American Nurses Association Publishing Program.

American Nursing Credentialing Center ([ANCC] 2000). *ANCC Board Certification.* Washington, DC: ANCC. 27–28.

Belcher, J. (1993). The trade-offs of developing a case management model for chronically mentally ill people. *Health & Social Work, 18,* 20–31.

Bigelow, D., & Young, D. (1991). Effectiveness of a case management program. *Community Mental Health Journal, 27,* 115–123.

Borland, A., McRae, J., & Lycan, C. (1989). Outcomes of five years of continuous intensive case management. *Hospital & Community Psychiatry, 40,* 369–376.

Case Management Society of America ([CMSA] 2006). *Case Management Adherence Guidelines (v. 2.0).* Retrieved June 10, 2009, from http://www.cmsa.org/portals/0/pdf/cmag2.pdf

Case Management Society of America ([CMSA] 2010). Standards of Practice for Case Management. Retrieved from: http://cmsa.org/portals/0/pdf/memberonly/StandardsOfPractice.pdf (accessed 1/3/2011).

Forchuk, C., Beaton, S., Crawford, L., Ide, L., Voorberg, N., & Bethune, J. (1989). Incorporating Peplau's theory and case management. *Journal of Psychosocial Nursing, 27,* 35–38.

Harris, M., & Bergman, H. (1988). Misconceptions about use of case management services by the chronically mentally ill: A utilization analysis. *Hospital & Community Psychiatry, 39,* 1276–1280.

Hellwig, K. (1993). Psychiatric home care nursing: Managing patients in the community setting. *Journal of Psychosocial Nursing & Mental Health Service, 31,* 21.

Herrick, C., & Bartlett, R. (2004). Psychiatric nursing case management: Past, present, and future. *Issues in Mental Health Nursing, 25,* 589–602.

Kersbergen, A. (1996). Case management: A rich history of coordinating care to control costs. *Nursing Outlook, 44,* 169–172.

Knollmeuller, R. (1989). Case management: What's in a name? *Nursing Management, 20,* 38–42.

Lamb, G., & Stempel, J. (1994). Nurse case management from the client's view: Growing as insider-expert. *Nursing Outlook, 42,* 7–13.

Lee, D., Mackenzie, A., Dudley-Brown, S., & Chin, T. (1998). Case management: a review of the definitions and practice. *Journal of Advance Nursing, 27,* 933–939.

Ling, Cindy (2009) Case management basics. Retrieved from: http://ce.nurse.com/PageNotFound.aspx?404;http://ce.nurse.com:80/60102/CoursePage (accessed 1/3/2011).

Malone, S., Worknch, F., Butchart, J., & Clark, C. (1999). Team case management of chronically mentally ill veterans: A group therapy approach. *Nursing Case Management, 4,* 158–166.

Mayer, G. (1996). Case management as a mindset. *Quality Management in Health Care, 5,* 7–16.

McRae, J., Higgins, M., Lycan, C., & Sherman, W. (1990). What happens to patients after fie years of intensive case management stops? *Hospital & Community Psychiatry, 41,* 175–179.

Moreo, K., & Llewellyn, A. (2005). *Case Management Review and Resource Manual: The Essence of Case Management, 2nd Ed.* Silver Spring, MD: ANCC.

National Association of Case Management ([NACM] 1997). *Case management practice guidelines for adults with severe and persistent mental illness.* Retrieved May 20, 2009 from http://www.your-nacm.com/CMguidelines.pdf

National Association of Case Management ([NACM] 2005). *Personal practice guidelines.* Retrieved May 20, 2009 from http://www.yournacm.com/guidelines.html

Neale, M., & Rosenheck, R. (1995). Therapeutic alliance and outcome in a VA intensive case management program. *Psychiatric Services, 46,* 719–721.

Peplau, H. (1962). Interpersonal technique: The crux of psychiatric nursing. *American Journal of Nursing, 62,* 53.

Peplau, H. (1952). *Interpersonal relations in nursing.* NY: G.P. Putnam and Sons.

Peplau, H. E. (1991). *Interpersonal relations in nursing: A conceptual framework of reference for psychodynamic nursing.* New York: Springer Publishing Co., Inc.

Stein, L., & Test, M. (1980). Alternative to mental hospital treatment. *Archives of General Psychiatry, 37,* 392–397.

Stroul, B. (1988). *Community support systems for persons with long-term mental illness: Questions and answers.* In National Association of Case Management (1997). *Case management practice guidelines for adults with severe and persistent mental illness.* Retrieved May 20, 2009 from http://www.yournacm.com/CMguidelines.pdf

Vanderplassen, W., et al. (2007). Effectiveness of different models of case management for substance-abusing populations. *Journal of Psychoactive Drugs, 39*(1): 81–95.

White, M. (1986). Case management. In *The Encyclopedia of Aging,* edited by G. Maddox. New York: Springer.

World Health Organization (2003). World Health Organization Report: Adherence to long-term therapies: Evidence for action. Available at: http://whqlibdoc.who.int/publications/2003/9241545992.pdf (accessed 1/10/2011).

Yamashita, M., Forshuk, C., & Mound, B. (2005). Nurse case management: Negotiating care together within a developing relationship. *Perspectives in Psychiatric Care, 41,* 62–70.

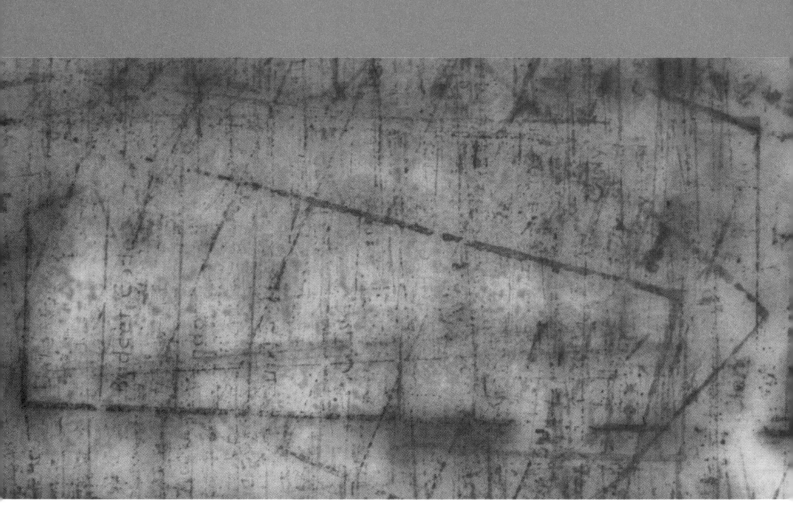

## CHAPTER CONTENTS

## CHAPTER 8

# KNOWN RISK FACTORS FOR PREVALENT MENTAL ILLNESS AND NURSING INTERVENTIONS FOR PREVENTION

Kathleen L. Patusky

## EXPECTED LEARNING OUTCOMES

**After completing this chapter, the student will be able to:**

1. Define the term, risk factor.
2. Explain how risk factors may be grouped or categorized.
3. Describe the significance of protective factors.
4. Identify the major risk factors associated with schizophrenia, affective disorders, substance-related disorders, anxiety disorders, and personality disorders.
5. Describe interventions appropriate for primary and secondary prevention.
6. Integrate the interpersonal process with primary, secondary, and tertiary prevention activities.

## KEY TERMS

Primary prevention

Protective factor

Psychomimetic disorders

Resilience

Risk factor

Secondary prevention

Stress-vulnerability-coping model

Temperament

Tertiary prevention

Why does a patient develop a mental disorder? What makes one person more susceptible to developing mental illness than another? The answers to these questions are important to psychiatric-mental health nurses because they provide the foundation for implementing preventive strategies.

Some individuals have RISK FACTORS that increase their chances of developing mental illness. Risk factors are those characteristics, variables, or hazards that, if present for a given individual, make it more likely that this individual, rather than someone selected at random from the general population, will develop a disorder (United States Department of Health and Human Services [DHHS], 1999, p. 1). Thus, a risk factor *might* predispose an individual to develop a mental illness. However, risk factors do not guarantee that a mental illness will occur. Knowledge about risk factors is important to psychiatric-mental health nurses as they develop interventions focused on preventing mental illness.

This chapter provides an overview of risk factors and how they are categorized. It also describes the impact of protective factors on the development of a mental illness. The chapter addresses the important risk factors associated with major classifications of psychiatric-mental health disorders and describes preventive strategies to reduce the impact of risk factors for developing a psychiatric-mental health disorder.

> *Risk factors are characteristics, variables, or hazards that increase the probability that an individual will develop a disorder.*

## THE NATURE OF RISK FACTORS

The underlying cause(s) of mental illness continues to be elusive. However, extensive research into the biology of mental illness has led to the belief that there is a disruption in neurotransmission in the brain. Links between specific neurotransmitters such as serotonin, dopamine, and norepinephrine and the development of psychiatric disorders such as depression and schizophrenia have been postulated leading to the development of drug therapy to control the disorders. Unfortunately, biology alone is not enough to explain the development of mental illness. Currently, scientists believe that mental illness is due to a combination of influences, not just the person's biologic makeup.

One major influence impacting mental health and the development of mental illness is a risk factor. As defined earlier, risk factors are those variables that might predispose an individual to develop a mental illness. A single risk factor is rarely enough to initiate a mental disorder. However, its presence makes the patient vulnerable to the effects of additional risk factors. As risk factors accumulate, the likelihood of a disorder increases. The existence of multiple risk factors is common to many psychiatric-mental health disorders.

## Categories of Risk Factors

Risk factors can be categorized or classified in different ways. One method divides risk factors as individual, family, or community risk factors (**Table 8-1**). Another way of categorizing risk factors is within biological and psychosocial categories, or intrapersonal and environmental categories. A third approach delineates risk factors into more specific categories, such as genetic, biological, psychological, social, and environmental factors. For example, biologic factors may include head injury, poor nutrition, and exposure to toxins or viruses. Social factors may include parental mental illness or criminality, economic hardship, abuse, neglect, exposure to violence, or death of a family member or close friend.

Many psychiatric disorders share risk factors that can be differentiated as biological/genetic or personal/social/environmental. Questions raised include:

- Do individuals develop a mental illness because they inherit it?
- Is it built into their physiology?
- Or is mental illness cultivated as a learned phenomenon, an interaction between the person, family members and significant others, and the community?

The current perspective is that both genetics and environment play a role. For example, the person might have a genetic predisposition toward schizophrenia, but does not experience life traumas that activate the tendency. Therefore, schizophrenia will not emerge. On the other hand, a person might have a low genetic propensity for depression, but experiences major traumas, loss of loved ones, and financial instability within a short time span. Thus, a depressive episode may result. An understanding of the convergence of possible risk factors is important when evaluating patients for psychiatric-mental health disorders.

Some risk factors can be changed while others cannot. In addition, some risk factors are more responsive to treatment than others are. Age and gender, for example, are risk factors for many disorders that cannot be changed. Another

| TABLE 8-1: **TYPES OF RISK FACTORS** | | |
|---|---|---|
| INDIVIDUAL RISK FACTORS | FAMILY RISK FACTORS | COMMUNITY RISK FACTORS |
| • Neurological deficits<br>• Temperament<br>• Physical illness, chronic medical conditions (DHHS, 1999; Mayo Clinic, 2010)<br>• Below-average intelligence (DHHS, 1999)<br>• Psychoactive drug use during adolescence<br>• Childhood abuse or neglect<br>• Lack of friendships or healthy relationships<br>• Combat (Mayo Clinic, 2010)<br>• Genetics | • Biological relatives with a mental disorder (Mayo Clinic, 2010)<br>• Marital discord<br>• Social disadvantage<br>• Overcrowding or large family size<br>• Father/mother's criminality<br>• Father/mother's mental disorder<br>• Foster care (DHHS, 1999) | • High crime rate/violence<br>• Inadequate schools<br>• Poverty<br>• Inadequate housing<br>• Poor access to health care |

risk factor, stress, may prompt the initial onset of a disorder and can be addressed so that stress levels are reduced.

Risk factors can be identified prior to the emergence of a psychiatric-mental health disorder. Risk factors also can change in response to a new developmental stage or a new stressor. For example, starting college at age 45 may raise the issue of stresses related to self-image, family responsibilities, or financial resources. In addition, risk factors may develop as a consequence of a psychiatric-mental health disorder, thus increasing the person's susceptibility for further difficulties or future problems.

> Risk factors may be classified in different ways. Possible categories include: individual, family, and community; biological and psychosocial; intrapersonal and environmental; or genetic, biological, psychological, social, and environmental. Many psychiatric disorders share risk factors that can be differentiated as biological and/or genetic or personal/social/environmental.

## Protective Factors

The risk factors for each individual are unique. What is a risk factor for one person may not be a risk factor for another. Thus, the one person may have protective factors to mitigate the effects of risk factors.

**PROTECTIVE FACTORS** are characteristics, variables, or traits that guard against or buffer the effect of risk factors. They promote adaptation, thereby improving the individual's response to a risk factor. Protective factors may actually reduce the probability that a person will develop a psychiatric-mental health disorder or may decrease the severity of a problem.

Protective factors may be classified as internal or external. Examples of internal protective factors include: good health, high stress tolerance, positive coping skills, average or better intelligence, flexibility, and a positive outlook on life. Examples of external protective factors include: supportive and positive family, social and community relationships, adequate economic resources, and recreational activities.

> Individuals possess characteristics, variables, or traits that guard against or buffer the effect of risk factors. These are known as protective factors.

Generally, people feel more secure and better able to cope with life situations when their health is good; they have a sense of control over what is happening around them; and they have a sense of connectedness to others, including family and community members. Knowing that others are available and willing to provide social support is also protective. Spiritual beliefs and a sense of meaning and purpose in life help individuals during difficult times. Economic resources can provide security to individuals, especially older adults.

**RESILIENCE** is a personal trait of individuals that serves as a protective mechanism. Resilience is the process of adapting well in the face of adversity, trauma, tragedy, threats or even significant sources of stress (American Psychological Association [APA], 2011). People are not born with resilience. It is something that is learned over time and involves behaviors, thoughts, and actions. Resilient people have a sense that they are able to cope with chronic stress or recover from trauma through skills such as communication skills, problem-solving skills, and positive coping styles. Skills that help an individual cope with life's problems can strengthen resilience and foster a belief in the self and in one's ability to cope.

> *Resilience is a protective function that is learned over time.*

## The Stress-Vulnerability-Coping Model

An individual's risk and protective factors determine how well he or she will cope with stressors. If risk factors are high and protective factors are low, the individual will have more difficulty coping and an increased chance of developing a psychiatric-mental health disorder. The **STRESS-VULNERABILITY-COPING MODEL** of mental illness presents one way of understanding how risk factors are involved with the development of psychiatric-mental health disorders (Mental Illness Fellowship Victoria [MIFV], 2008).

The stress-vulnerability-coping model identifies risk factors according to three categories: biological, personal, and environmental. Biological risk factors include a family history of mental illness, brain abnormalities, neurodevelopmental problems, and diseases of a medical nature. Personal risk factors include poor social skills, poor coping skills, and communication difficulties. Environmental risk factors include substance abuse, work or school problems, rejection by other people, stressful relationships, poor social support, and the occurrence of major life events (MIFV, 2008).

This model also identifies protective factors for psychiatric-mental health disorders. These include good physical health, no family history of mental illness, good coping and communication skills, good levels of social support, medication, and talk therapy when indicated.

Although the stress-vulnerability-coping model was originally developed to explain the development of schizophrenia, it is now used to understand other psychiatric disorders as well (MIFV, 2008).

According to the stress-vulnerability-coping model, mental illness arises from the interplay of the three dominant factors, that is, stress, vulnerability, and coping. Good coping skills protect the individual from developing a mental illness even when they are in high-stress situations and vulnerable. This vulnerability increases as the number and intensity of risk factors increase.

## RISK FACTORS FOR MAJOR PSYCHIATRIC-MENTAL HEALTH DISORDERS

The probability that an individual will develop a psychiatric-mental health disorder is dependent on that person's risk and protective factors. Although these factors are unique to the individual, some of these factors, such as genetics, often are seen as playing a role in the development of several different psychiatric-mental health disorders. The risk factors for the major classes of psychiatric-mental health disorders are addressed.

## Disorders of Infancy, Childhood, or Adolescence

Genetics/biology and temperament are two important intrapersonal risk factors for the development of psychiatric-mental health disorders occurring from infancy to adolescence (**Box 8-1**). Genetics refers to the complex makeup of genes and deoxyribonucleic acid (DNA) that will contribute to the biology of the child's brain. Biology also includes any birth traumas, exposure to infections or toxins while in utero, or other insults that affect brain structures or chemistry.

> **Q BOX 8-1: RISK FACTORS FOR DISORDERS OF INFANCY, CHILDHOOD, OR ADOLESCENCE**
>
> Genetics/biology
> - Genes/DNA and brain development
> - Birth traumas
> - Intrauterine exposure to drugs
> - Exposure to infections, toxins (such as lead poisoning), or other insults affecting brain structures or chemistry
>
> Temperament

TEMPERAMENT has been viewed as a precursor to personality. Researchers have suggested that temperament is "hard-wired" into each child at birth, not learned. Temperament represents innate aspects of personality that determine how a child tends to respond to the world. It is the distinctive behavior involved with activity and adaptation.

Several studies have been done to describe temperament. A classic landmark study by Thomas, Chess, and Birch (1968) identified three patterns of temperament:

- *Easy or flexible:* Positive mood and approach to new situations, low emotional intensity, and regular eating and sleeping patterns. Children are generally calm, happy, and not easily upset.
- *Difficult, active, or feisty:* Negative mood and response to new situations, high emotional intensity, irregular sleeping and eating patterns. Children are often fussy, fearful of new people or situations, easily upset by noise or commotion, and intense in their reactions.
- *Slow-to-warm-up or cautious:* Negative but mild emotional response to new situations that are intense and initially slow in adapting but eventually become positive. Children are inactive and fussy, tend to withdraw or react negatively to new situations but become more positive with continued exposure.

Another study described children as challenging (fitting a typology of high maintenance, cautious, and slow-to-warm-up) or easy (industrious, social, and eager to try; McClowery, 2002). Neither challenging nor easy temperaments are necessarily risk factors on their own. The issue is one of "goodness of fit" (Thomas, Chess, & Birch, 1968). For example, if an infant is fussy and cranky, he or she will likely be fine if the mother is easy going and not overly disturbed by the infant's agitation. However, if the mother is anxious and stressed, both she and the infant are likely to irritate each other further. As children age, temperament is assimilated into personality and the issue of goodness of fit can continue to determine the quality of a child's social relationships (Thomas & Chess, 1984; Maziade et al., 1985; Werner & Smith, 1992).

*Genetics/biology and temperament are two important intrapersonal risk factors for the development of psychiatric-mental health disorders occurring from infancy to adolescence.*

In addition to genetics/biology and temperament, other general risk factors during childhood may lead to a variety of psychiatric-mental health problems. These include the individual factors of neurophysiological deficits such as attention deficit disorders (ADD), hyperactivity and autism, difficult temperament, chronic physical illness, and below-average intelligence. In addition, children are especially sensitive to family issues such as severe marital discord, social disadvantage, overcrowding or large family size, paternal criminality, maternal mental disorder, and admission into foster care. Community factors such as living in an area with a high rate of crime and inadequate schools also can have a major effect (DHHS, 1999).

Moreover, some individual risk factors can lead to a state of vulnerability in which other risk factors can have a greater effect. For example, while low birthweight is a general risk factor for multiple physical and mental outcomes, when combined with a high-risk environment, it often results in poorer outcomes (McGauhey, Starfield, Alexander, & Ensminger, 1991).

## Schizophrenia

Experts have concluded that genetic and environmental risk factors interact in the development of schizophrenia (**Box 8-2**). Studies have shown that the correlation of schizophrenia between identical twins is less than 50%, supporting the claim that genetics alone is insufficient as a cause. However, the high correlation supports a strong genetic component. This strong relationship decreases gradually among relatives of the patient with schizophrenia. Moreover, second-degree relatives are several times more likely to develop schizophrenia than someone in the general population, while third-degree relatives are twice as likely to develop schizophrenia. Although a specific

---

**Q  BOX 8-2: RISK FACTORS FOR SCHIZOPHRENIA**

Genetic/familial patterns

Gestational and birth complications
- Maternal malnutrition
- Rh incompatibility

Birth during late winter or early spring

Major life changes

Lower socioeconomic status (poverty)

Stress

Substance abuse

causal gene has not been identified, several possibilities are being explored. Experts believe that there are at least as many as 10 gene variations that can result in symptoms (Schizophrenia.com, 2009).

A long history of research has considered gestational and birth complications as biological risk factors for schizophrenia. Closely associated with these complications are maternal malnutrition and Rh incompatibility. In addition, a late winter or early spring birth (particularly during the months of February and March) has been identified as a risk factor due to maternal exposure to influenza or viral infections, especially during the 2nd trimester (Buchanan & Carpenter, 2004; Meltzer & Fatemi, 2008).

The stress-vulnerability-coping model, described earlier in this chapter, was developed initially to explain schizophrenia. This model included poverty as a risk factor, although some researchers view poverty as a result of illness rather than part of the cause. Meltzer and Fatemi (2008) concluded that patients with schizophrenia are at high risk for poverty because they face difficulties with unemployment, homelessness, inadequate housing, poor health, and poor access to health care—labeled the "downward drift" in socioeconomic status. Especially tragic is the fact that first episodes often occur during late adolescence or the early twenties. Major life changes, another risk factor, are relevant at this time as individuals leave home for the first time, go to college, start a first job, or marry. Additional risk factors include substance abuse and stressors of everyday life.

Researchers have attempted to identify risk factors that would predict psychosis in young adults before a full-blown episode, permitting earlier interventions (Cannon et al., 2008). The factors identified were accurate in predicting psychosis 35% of the time. This number rose to 65%–80% if specific combinations of risk factors were found in study participants. These combinations included: (a) decline in social functioning, withdrawal, and inactivity; (b) family history of psychosis with recent deterioration of function (e.g., drop in grades, withdrawal from school activities); (c) increase in unusual thoughts; and (d) increase in suspiciousness or paranoia and past or current drug abuse.

> *Risk factors for schizophrenia include the interaction between genetics and environment. In addition, gestational and birth complications are associated biological risk factors.*

## Affective Disorders

Affective disorders include major depression and bipolar disorder. Decades of research support the heritability of major depression, which shows an increased risk for depression among first-degree relatives who have depression. Identical twin studies show a concordance rate or the presence of the trait in both of the twins of 45%–60%, while studies of non-identical twins show a concordance rate of only 12% (Kelsoe, 2005). Similar rates are found for bipolar disorder, supporting its heritability. With genetics serving as a risk factor for both depression and bipolar disorder, new findings indicate a genetic "hotspot" that identifies risk for both disorders (Bipolar Disorder Genome Study [BIGS] Consortium, 2010). The search for additional genetic risk factors for depression or bipolar disorder continues. **Table 8-2** identifies the risk factors associated with affective disorders.

Gender is an additional risk factor for developing affective disorders. Bipolar I Disorder occurs equally in men and women, whereas Bipolar II Disorder is more common in women (Baldassano et al., 2005). Researchers also have shown the prevalence of depression in women as 1½–3 times that of men, with lifetime prevalence ranging from 6%–17% (Kessler, 2003).

Brain imaging has revealed a biological risk factor of abnormal mood regulation circuitry in the brain. This abnormality is present even when the patient with depression feels well. It reasserts itself during relapse when levels of certain neurotransmitters drop (Hasler et al., 2008). Given the cyclical nature of depression, this risk factor offers an explanation for both the initiation and the relapses of major depressive disorders.

The potentially cyclical nature of depression indicates that a history of past episodes is a risk factor. Life stressors also are known to play a role in the emergence of depression. Substance use, particularly central nervous system (CNS) depressants, can result in depression. Individuals with few social supports, especially the elderly or those with a medical illness, are at high risk for depression.

Family history is an important area of discovery with bipolar disorder. Children having a parent or sibling with bipolar disorder are 4 to 6 times more likely to develop the disorder than the average person. However, most children with a family history of bipolar disorder do not develop the illness (Nurnberger & Foroud, 2000). Studies have shown that certain traits, including a history of hospitalizations, co-morbid obsessive-compulsive disorder, age at first manic episode, and number and frequency of manic episodes, are present in families with a bipolar member

| TABLE 8-2: RISK FACTORS FOR AFFECTIVE DISORDERS | |
| --- | --- |
| **MAJOR DEPRESSION** | **BIPOLAR DISORDER** |
| Gender | Attention deficit hyperactivity disorder (ADHD) |
| Genetics/familial patterns | Genetics/familial patterns |
| History of depressive episodes | Substance use/abuse |
| Biological: Abnormal mood regulation circuitry | |
| Stress | |
| Substance use | |
| Few social supports | |
| Medical illness | |

(Potash et al., 2007). These traits serve as risk factors for the child's development of bipolar disorders.

> *Genetics is a risk factor for both depression and bipolar disorders. Gender, life stressors, substance abuse, and inadequate social supports are additional risk factors.*

## Substance-Related Disorders

Genetics and neurophysiology are now viewed as exerting a strong influence on the abuse of substances, especially alcohol. Specific genes have been identified that increase the risk for alcoholism (Edenberg, 2003). Areas of the brain linked to cravings or vulnerability to substance use, reward pathways, mechanisms of drugs and their effects on neurotransmitters are a few of the research findings that aid the current understanding of substance abuse (Liu et al., 2005; Kreek, Bart, Lilly, LaForge, & Nielsen, 2005).

While substance use disorders are strongly linked to familial patterns (Thompson, Lande, & Kalapatapu, 2009), genetics, biology, and learning from the environment also probably play intrinsically connected roles (**Box 8-3**). The child who sees a parent drink a beer and tries one for him/her- self is responding to modeled behavior. If the child goes on to sneak a beer two or three times a week, at what point do genetics and biology take over to create dependence? Similar familial patterning and genetic connections have been seen with heroin (Pickens et al., 2001; Trafton, Tracy, Oliva, & Humphreys, 2007).

The existence of a medical disorder can also combine with biology and genetics to serve as a risk factor. Consider the current focus on addiction to prescription medications. The patient who experiences a painful injury but has no previous history of substance abuse and is prescribed oxycodone (Oxycontin) or hydrocodone and acetaminophen (Vicodin), may find that the stimulation of the brain's reward pathways and the activation of craving sites lead to a substance use disorder.

Age is another risk factor. Individuals who use substances at an early age—16 years old or younger—are more prone to substance abuse or dependence (Mayo Clinic, 2010). Gender, however, is somewhat equivocal. Men are more likely to abuse or become dependent on substances, although this pattern may depend on the type of substance. Personality factors of impulsivity or risk taking place a person at greater risk of substance abuse or dependence. Mood instability, particularly the presence of depression or anxiety, serves as an additional risk factor (Jackson, Sher, & Park, 2005), as does a perception that one is under extreme stress (Sinha, Garcia, Paliwal, Kreek, & Rounsaville, 2006).

**BOX 8-3: RISK FACTORS FOR SUBSTANCE-RELATED DISORDERS**

Genetics/familial pattern

Age

Gender

Personality factors: impulsivity, risk taking

Depression, anxiety

Post-traumatic stress disorder (PTSD)

Stress

*Substance use disorders are strongly linked to familial patterns. Genetics, biology, and learning from the environment are also thought to be intrinsically connected.*

## Anxiety Disorders

The expansive category of anxiety disorders contains several specific diagnoses that share many of the same risk factors, although with some variation. In general, anxiety disorders are viewed as arising in individuals with a biologically low response threshold to circumstances that generate anxiety. The autonomic nervous system creates a more intense response to the experience of anxiety or fear. The regulation of the neurotransmitters, gamma-aminobutyric acid (GABA) and serotonin, are implicated (Neumeister, Bonne, & Charney, 2005). From individual and environmental perspectives, patients with low self-esteem who demonstrate timidity and discomfort with aggression and who describe their parents as critical or angry are more likely to develop an anxiety disorder (**Box 8-4**).

Specific diagnoses within the anxiety disorders category have been studied for their genetic risk factors. Heritability of panic disorder has been established (Smoller, Gardner-Schuster, & Covino, 2008). Approximately 50% of persons with this disorder have a similarly affected relative. Twin studies also support genetic risk factors for panic disorders and other anxiety disorders. Obsessive-compulsive disorder has been linked with a genetic mutation (Ozaki et al., 2003).

The genetics of post-traumatic stress disorder (PTSD) is also under investigation. With PTSD, classified as an anxiety disorder, a person develops distressing symptoms after exposure to a traumatic life event. The person persistently re-experiences the trauma of the event and avoids any stimuli associated with the trauma. (See Chapter 13 for a more detailed discussion of PTSD.) Currently, research is considering certain substances that contribute to fear memories. These biological risk factors include stathmin (a protein necessary for fear formation [Shumyatsky et al., 2005]) and gastrin-releasing peptide (GRP; a brain chemical that seems to control the fear response [Shumayatsky et al., 2002]). Serotonin has also been found to play a role in fueling the fear response (Hariri et al., 2002). At the same time, environmental factors such as childhood trauma, history of abuse, head injury, or existing mental

> **Q** **BOX 8-4: RISK FACTORS FOR ANXIETY DISORDERS**
>
> Biological propensity: low response threshold
>
> Childhood trauma
>
> Genetics/familial patterns
>
> Childhood trauma
>
> Head injury
>
> History of abuse
>
> History of other mental illness
>
> Low self-esteem/timidity; discomfort with aggression
>
> Critical or angry parents
>
> Violence, disasters
>
> Stress

illness have been noted to predispose a person to PTSD (Gurvits et al., 2000; Holt, Montesinos, & Christense, 2007). Situational risk factors also have been identified and include: "survival of natural and man-made disasters such as floods; violent crimes such as kidnapping, rape or murder of a parent, sniper fire and school shootings; motor vehicle accidents such as automobile and plane crashes; severe burns; exposure to community violence; war; peer suicide; and sexual or physical abuse" (Hamblin & Barnett, 2009, p. 1).

In contrast to risk factors, an optimistic outlook, an ability to frame negative circumstances as challenges, and availability of social support can serve as protective factors (Brewin, 2005). Additionally, developing resilience also is important. Reducing PTSD is possible if the individual actively seeks support from friends and family. Joining a support group after a traumatic event can be helpful, although some experts warn against poorly facilitated groups that can re-traumatize the members. Being able to view one's actions in response to the event positively, having a positive coping strategy, learning from the situation, and being able to overcome fear with effective action reduces the likelihood of a negative outcome (Brewin, Andrews, & Valentine, 2000).

*An optimistic outlook, social support, and resilience are protective factors for anxiety disorders.*

## Personality Disorders

Risk factors related to personality disorders have received little research attention generally. Historically, these disorders were viewed as a learned problem involving an individual's character. More recent research has shown that a physiological basis exists. A genetic basis is assumed, although specific mechanisms have not been detailed. Biological components are suggestive of frontal lobe deficits and vague, inconsistent, or non-specific neurological findings (McCabe, 2003).

Based on the limited amount of research available, overall risk factors for personality disorders include a family history of personality disorders or other mental illness; verbal, physical, or sexual abuse, neglect, or trauma during childhood; a chaotic family life during childhood; diagnosis of a childhood conduct disorder; and death or divorce of parents during childhood (Carter, Peter, Mulder, & Luty, 2001; Mayo Clinic, 2010; Reich & Zanarini, 2001; Shiner & Caspi, 2003; Tackett, 2006; **Box 8-5**). Although personality disorders may begin in childhood and continue into adulthood, personality disorders are seldom diagnosed in a child because the behavioral pattern may be part of a developmental phase.

Certain types of personality disorders are associated with specific risk factors. For example, gender is a risk factor for borderline, antisocial, and narcissistic personality disorders. It is estimated that 77% of patients with a diagnosis of borderline personality diagnosis are female (McCabe, 2003). About 3%–5% of men and 1% of women are diagnosed with antisocial personality disorder. More men than women are diagnosed with narcissistic personality disorder (Mayo Clinic, 2010).

Additionally, some types of personality disorders have distinctive risk factors that vary from the general list. For example, narcissistic personality disorder more often begins in early adulthood and is associated with risk factors including parental neglect, in which the parents ignore the child's expressed fears and needs. Praise and affection are withheld, while neglect and emotional abuse may occur. Parental caregiving is unpredictable or unreliable with the parents modeling manipulative behavior.

Patients are at greater risk of developing schizoid personality disorder if they have a parent or other relative with schizoid or schizotypal personality disorder, or schizophrenia. Risk is also increased if their childhood included experiences of neglect or scorn, abuse or mistreatment, or an emotionally detached parent. Patients at risk of schizotypal personality often have a relative with schizophrenia or an emotionally detached parent. Childhood abuse or mistreatment, childhood trauma, and living in a childhood home of deprivation and neglect are additional risk factors of schizotypal personality disorder (Mayo Clinic, 2010).

> *In general, risk factors for personality disorders include a family history of personality disorders or other mental illness; verbal, physical, or sexual abuse, neglect, or trauma during childhood; a chaotic family life during childhood; diagnosis of a childhood conduct disorder; and death or divorce of parents during childhood.*

## THE INTERFACE OF PSYCHIATRIC-MENTAL HEALTH DISORDERS AND MEDICAL CONDITIONS

Medical conditions can act as risk factors, also playing a role in the development of a psychiatric-mental health disorder. Consider the average patient with a medical problem. The patient's reaction to a basic procedure might be influenced by psychological risk factors, such as fear, anxiety, or depression that can complicate care. The impact may lead to the patient's inability to participate in care or to make decisions about care. The existence of psychiatric-mental health issues such as substance abuse or obsessive compulsive behavior could complicate the picture further. Any medical disorder could be a risk factor for a psychiatric-mental health disorder. Any psychiatric-mental health disorder might place a patient at greater risk for a medical

---

**BOX 8-5: RISK FACTORS FOR PERSONALITY DISORDERS**

Gender

Genetics/familial pattern (family history)

Abuse/neglect during childhood

Trauma during childhood

- Chaotic family life
- Parental death or divorce

Diagnosis of conduct disorder as a child

disorder. Some, if not all, medical and psychiatric-mental health disorders may represent a circular risk relationship. Therefore, a firm knowledge base about the impact of psychiatric-mental health disorders on patients with medical conditions and the influence of medical conditions on psychiatric-mental health problems is needed.

## Factors Influencing Risk

Demographics reveal that the aging population is growing. The projected increases in the aging population suggest that the incidence and prevalence of dementias, delirium, and late-onset psychiatric-mental health disorders will also increase. Secondly, the population of mentally ill older adults is growing such that it is the largest that it has been in history. Individuals who might have died previously due to nonspecific treatments, or even side effects of the medications, are now living longer. Psychiatric illnesses are chronic conditions; just as many persons are living longer with chronic medical illnesses, the same is true for psychiatric illnesses. No longer are psychiatric patients dying in the back wards of out-dated institutions. Rather, most psychiatric-mental health patients reside in communities. These patients are not only coping with their psychiatric-mental health disorders, but they also are presenting with the common disorders associated with aging such as arthritis, hypertension, diabetes, or chronic obstructive pulmonary disease. The average patient on a medical or surgical unit might also have schizophrenia, bipolar disorder, or an anxiety disorder.

Medically induced pathology is another area of concern. Patients with no previous psychiatric history can experience medication reactions that reveal an underlying psychiatric-mental health problem, such as a hypomanic phase of bipolar disorder in response to the use of corticosteroids. Patients with preexisting psychiatric-mental health disorders might find that their psychotropic medications react unfavorably with medications used to treat the medical condition. The reaction may be an additive or synergistic effect or an adverse effect, including a return of psychiatric symptoms. If given a medication that causes psychiatric symptoms in some individuals, patients with a psychiatric-mental health history of problems may be at greater risk for a reaction. Additionally, psychotropic medications can serve as risk factors, demonstrating idiosyncratic or toxic effects unrelated to the medical picture. Unless these effects are accurately identified and properly treated, the patient can experience serious harm or even death. Moreover, discontinuation of certain psychotropic medications without tapering can lead to very uncomfortable symptoms for the patient.

Lastly, medical disorders may mimic psychiatric disorders. The term **PSYCHOMIMETIC DISORDERS** could be misleading, presenting as a seizure disorder or another medical condition such as Cushing's syndrome. Medications such as reserpine, lidocaine, procainamide, L-dopa, and many others produce effects that are similar to psychiatric-mental health disorder symptoms (Evans et al., 2005). Awareness of physical illness and the complications that might serve as psychiatric-mental health risk factors is necessary to assist in recognizing and preventing patient difficulties before they occur.

> *Any medical disorder could be a risk factor for a psychiatric-mental health disorder. Any psychiatric-mental health disorder might place a patient at greater risk for a medical disorder.*

## Medical and Psychiatric-Mental Health Disorders as Risk Factors

Multiple medical disorders have been associated with the development of psychiatric-mental health disorders (**Table 8-3**). In particular, major depression is of primary concern because of the associated increased morbidity and mortality that occurs when a patient with a medical disorder develops depression.

Depression in patients with cancer can compromise adherence to a treatment regimen, or prompt risky health behaviors. Depression has also been associated with immunosuppression, which might increase cancer risk. Depression in patients who have had a stroke has been shown to limit the return of activities of daily living (ADLs) and impair cognitive function. Mortality rates for patients with stroke and depression also show a three- to four-fold increase (Evans et.al., 2005). In patients with heart disease, depression is strongly associated with a poor prognosis after a myocardial infarction prognosis and the risk of death is also increased, even years later. Heart disease is common in patients with bipolar disorder who also experience an increased risk of death (Evans et al., 2005).

Depression also is considered a risk factor in HIV/AIDS. Depression is associated with poor adherence to medication treatment, deterioration in psychological function, more rapid progression of HIV/AIDS, and higher

## TABLE 8-3: MEDICAL DISORDERS AND CONDITIONS THAT PRESENT RISK OF PSYCHIATRIC COMORBIDITY

| MEDICAL DISORDERS AND CONDITIONS | PSYCHIATRIC-MENTAL HEALTH DISORDER (OFTEN SEEN AS CO-MORBIDITY) |
| --- | --- |
| Fibromyalgia<br>Risk for hypertension<br>Smoking | Psychiatric illness |
| Acute coronary syndrome<br>Alzheimer's disease<br>Cancer<br>Chronic obstructive pulmonary disease<br>Congestive heart failure<br>Coronary artery bypass graft<br>Coronary/ischemic heart disease<br>Cystic fibrosis<br>Diabetes mellitus<br>End-stage renal disease<br>Epilepsy<br>Fibromyalgia<br>HIV/AIDS<br>Interpersonal violence<br>Menopause<br>Multiple sclerosis<br>Musculoskeletal conditions<br>Myocardial infarction<br>Obesity<br>Osteopenia/osteoporosis<br>Otorhinolaryngic conditions<br>Pain<br>Parkinson's disease<br>Postpartum (depressive disorders)<br>Rheumatic disorders<br>Stroke<br>Thyroid disease | Depressive disorders |
| Acute coronary syndrome<br>Chronic obstructive pulmonary disease<br>Elevated serum cholesterol<br>Fibromyalgia<br>Hyperthyroidism<br>Rheumatic disorders | Panic and other anxiety disorders |
| Coronary heart disease | Psychosis/schizophrenia |
| Diabetes insipidus<br>Diabetes mellitus, type 2<br>Dyslipidemia<br>HIV/AIDS<br>Hypertension<br>Hypertriglyceridemia<br>Infectious hepatitis<br>Metabolic syndrome<br>Obesity | Bipolar disorder |
| Myocardial infarction<br>Diabetes mellitus, type 2<br>Dyslipidemia<br>Heart disease<br>Hypertension<br>Obesity<br>Osteoporosis<br>Smoking<br>Thyroid disease | Acute stress disorder |

*(cont.)*

**TABLE 8-3: MEDICAL DISORDERS AND CONDITIONS THAT PRESENT RISK OF PSYCHIATRIC COMORBIDITY (*CONT.*)**

| MEDICAL DISORDERS AND CONDITIONS | PSYCHIATRIC-MENTAL HEALTH DISORDER (OFTEN SEEN AS CO-MORBIDITY) |
| --- | --- |
| Alcoholic hepatitis<br>Cardiovascular disease<br>Cirrhosis of the liver<br>Gastric ulcer/gastritis<br>Hematologic problems<br>Pancreatitis | Substance abuse |
| Otorhinolaryngic conditions | Dementia |
| Cardiovascular disease<br>Infectious diseases<br>Liver/renal disease<br>Otorhinolaryngic conditions | Delirium |
| Epilepsy<br>Low cholesterol levels | Violent death/suicide |

mortality rates (Evans et al., 2005). For example, posttraumatic stress disorder (PTSD) and depression have been shown to influence medication adherence and HIV disease markers (Boarts, Buckley-Fischer, Armelie, Bogart, & Delahanty, 2009). A study by Cruess et al. (2003) concluded that the immune system changes prompted by depression might affect entry and replication of the virus in the body. Additionally, bipolar disorder is considered a risk factor with HIV/AIDS because it might promote high risk behaviors.

Diabetes and depression demonstrate a circular risk relationship. Both can present with symptoms of weight loss, fatigue, hypersomnia, and decreased libido (Lustman & Clouse, 2005). Depression also may be linked with poor glucose control through the hypothalamus-pituitary-thyroid axis. In a study of patients with diabetes, approximately 26% of patients self-reported symptoms of depression (Evans et al., 2005). However, other sources suggest the incidence may be even higher. Among patients with diabetes, depression has been associated with nonadherence to the treatment regimen, poor glycemic control, increased health care costs, progression and earlier onset of micro- and macrovascular complications, disability, and death.

## THE INTERPERSONAL PROCESS FOR RISK REDUCTION

The nurse is his or her own best instrument of care when approaching risk factors. Through the interpersonal relationship that the nurse develops with the patient, he or she can best assist the patient in understanding the various risk factors and in building on the patient's strengths to prevent illness and promote health. The personal qualities of awareness, judgment, and initiative are paramount.

- Awareness is necessary to identify when a risk factor is part of the patient's assessment information. It presumes that the nurse has a knowledge base of risk factors that includes an appreciation of the psychiatric-mental health and medical components and their potential consequences.
- Judgment is required to determine the importance of the risk factor, and to prioritize the multiple risk factors present. It helps the nurse identify appropriate responses and recognize how quickly the responses should begin.
- Initiative prompts the nurse to take action and address the risk factor. Some risk factors may be more responsive to intervention than others. Unless an emergency is identified, the nurse will have the greatest and most immediate impact on the patient by addressing risks first that are more easily and quickly changed.

The development of the interpersonal relationship with the patient is a key component of the therapy. Many of the risk factors for psychiatric-mental health disorders involve emotional isolation and lack of support. The nurse is in a position to provide therapeutic interpersonal experiences for the patient, maintaining appropriate boundaries while offering support and validation for the patient's emotional state. The effectively managed interpersonal relationship serves as a protective factor for the patient in illness prevention and health promotion. The nurse's therapeutic use of self is no less relevant or important than any other medical instrument.

Prevention identifies risk factors to target for intervention. Interventions focus on changing those risk factors that can be changed, and enhancing protective factors. It is the nurse who performs these functions and thus has the greatest impact on the patient. The nurse applies the interpersonal process at the primary, secondary, and tertiary levels of prevention. **PRIMARY PREVENTION** refers to interventions that delay or avoid the onset of illness; **SECONDARY PREVENTION** refers to treatment, including identifying persons with disorders and standardizing treatment for disorders; and **TERTIARY PREVENTION** refers to maintenance including decreasing relapse or recurrence, and providing rehabilitation (DHHS, 1999).

*Integrating the interpersonal process at the primary, secondary, and tertiary levels of prevention can help to minimize risk factors and enhance protective factors. Establishing a therapeutic nurse-patient relationship also acts as a protective factor.*

## Primary Prevention

Primary prevention is aimed at avoiding or delaying the onset of illness. Nurses perform primary prevention of mental illness by intervening to address and neutralize the influence of risk factors. The emphasis is on health promotion and disease prevention, focusing on reducing the occurrence of a condition, most often at the community level. A key primary preventive strategy is psychoeducation geared to individuals, families, and communities. Examples of primary prevention strategies include teaching about:

- Drug awareness programs; ways to prevent substance abuse; early signs of substance abuse
- Positive coping methods; ways to promote resilience (**Patient and Family Teaching 8-1** highlights ways to build resilience)
- Ways to reduce stress and cope with situational and maturational changes
- Parenting skills for prospective new parents
- Stress management techniques

For patients who have not yet entered the mental health system, community outreach is ideal. The public needs to learn more about psychiatric-mental health

disorders so that individuals can assess their own risk. In addition, educated persons might be less prone to stigmatize patients with psychiatric-mental health disorders, thereby reducing the risks of the stigma and rejection associated with psychiatric-mental health disorders that keep individuals from seeking treatment. Even individuals who may never need to see a mental health professional can benefit from the stress reduction and problem-solving techniques that can be taught, thus increasing protective factors available.

In neighborhoods with high crime rates, stress is particularly high. Community-wide prevention programs aimed at teaching how to reduce stress and minimize violence would be helpful. One study addressed a psychoeducational program that was conducted at a community "safe house" with children ages 6–12. The study demonstrated how to promote effective coping among children living in a violent community (Jones & Selder, 1996).

*Primary prevention interventions address and neutralize the influence of risk factors to avoid or delay the onset of illness.*

## Secondary Prevention

Nurses perform secondary prevention by identifying the existence of risk factors, assessing for the presence of the disorder, and initiating appropriate and early treatment according to evidence-based standards of care. Early treatment helps to reduce the possible duration of the disorder and its associated complications. Examples of secondary prevention activities include:

- Ongoing assessments of patients at risk for a disorder with prompt identification of symptoms when they occur
- Initiating appropriate treatment and referrals for treatment
- Teaching the patient about the disorder and treatment plan, including areas such as medication adherence, counseling, and available support services.

Stress also is a major risk factor of many disorders. Removing this risk through education about ways to minimize stress serves a preventive function. Parent education groups are prime examples of interventions that can relieve stress and improve the family situation. One such group working with abusive or potentially abusive parents used a systematic training workbook to focus on

**PATIENT AND FAMILY TEACHING 8-1:
BUILDING RESILIENCE**

The way a person develops resilience is highly individualized. Here are some suggestions about how to develop resilience:

- Make connections with and accept help and support from close family members, friends, or others

- View crises as problems that can be dealt with to change your interpretation and response to crises

- Accept that change is part of life and focus on things that can be changed rather than those that cannot be changed

- Develop realistic goals, no matter how small

- Decisively act rather than avoid or detach from the problem

- Develop self-confidence and trusting instincts

- Look for opportunities for self-discovery (learning something as a result of the struggle or problem)

- Keep things in perspective

- Maintain a positive outlook, focusing on the expectation that good things will happen rather than being fearful

- Take care of yourself, physically and emotionally

- Use journaling, meditation, spiritual practices, or other ways to deal with stress and build or restore hope

*From American Psychological Association[2011]. The road to resilience. Available at: http://www.apa.org/helpcenter/road-resilience.aspx Accessed 1/13/2011.*

effective problem solving. After nine weeks of discussion groups, role playing, exercises on hypothetical parenting situations, and homework assignments, the parents demonstrated more positive perceptions of their children and scored lower on a measure of abuse potential. An unintended consequence of the group was increased social support and contact among the parents, resulting in a positive influence on the risk factor of isolationism associated with child abuse (Fennell & Fishel, 1998).

Psychoeducation plays an important role here as well. It can address a number of risk factors on a group or individual basis. Patients' understanding of their own risk factors, their disorders, and their treatments can help them regain a sense of control over their situation. This understanding can demystify their experience and correct inaccurate perceptions. For example, many patients assume that a diagnosis of major depression means that they are "crazy," with all the attendant fears, misconceptions, and stigmatizing characterizations that exist in society. This assumption and associated feelings can be reduced with an adequate understanding of the condition.

Nurses can counter stress and major life changes with psychoeducational instruction and role playing

on problem solving, coping, and relaxation techniques. Specific education and discussion on the physical consequences of substance use or habit may lead to a reduction in the inappropriate use of substances or unhealthy lifestyle habits. Nurses can use health promotion theory to support the patient's ability to follow through with commitments to a healthier lifestyle. A study of an educational intervention around antipsychotic-induced weight gain demonstrated that patients with the diagnosis of schizophrenia or schizoaffective disorder were able to participate in the program and gain less weight than a standard care group (Littrell, Hilligos, Kirshner, Petty, & Johnson, 2003). **Evidence-Based Practice 8-1** describes this study.

The effects of non-modifiable risk factors, such as gender or genetic makeup, can be mitigated with psychoeducation. By explaining these factors, nurses can help patients and family members understand that their disorders have real causes and that they are not to blame for their condition. Thus, guilt and fear are lessened. Parents especially may assume blame when their children have disorders with a genetic component. Parents need to hear and understand that the environment and their nurturing and parenting attitudes will also influence how well

## EVIDENCE-BASED PRACTICE 8-1:
## SCHIZOPHRENIA, WEIGHT GAIN, AND PSYCHOEDUCATION

### STUDY

Littrell, K.H., Hilligos, N.M., Kirshner, C.D., Petty, R.G., & Johnson, C.G. (2003). The effects of an educational intervention on antipsychotic-induced weight gain. *Journal of Nursing Scholarship, 35*, 237–241.

### SUMMARY

A quasi-experimental study was conducted with 70 patients who had a diagnosis of schizophrenia or schizoaffective disorder. Patients were randomly assigned to an intervention or standard care group. The intervention group received four months of psychoeducation including content on nutrition, exercise, and how to lead a healthy life style. All patients were followed for two months after the intervention was concluded. Findings revealed a statistically significant difference in weight change between the two groups, demonstrating that the group receiving the psychoeducation gained less weight.

### APPLICATION TO PRACTICE

Psychiatric-mental health nurses need to be cognizant that individuals with schizophrenia have an increased risk of weight gain due to inactivity and as a possible side effect of prescribed antipsychotic medication. This weight gain has the potential to impact the patient's overall health status. Thus, implementing a psychoeducational program that focuses on a healthy lifestyle can help reduce the risk of weight gain in patients taking antipsychotic medications, thereby promoting improved health and well-being for the patient along with better outcomes.

### QUESTIONS TO PONDER

1. *The study addressed psychoeducation focusing on nutrition, exercise, and a healthy lifestyle. What other topics might be appropriate to address in a future research study?*
2. *How might the psychoeducation described in this study impact medication adherence?*

their child does. This topic naturally leads to further education about how to cope with their child's behaviors. In an intervention study aimed at increasing parents' ability to manage the problem behaviors of children with Asperger syndrome, parental training sessions were able to decrease the number and intensity of problem behaviors and increase the children's social interaction (Sofronoff, Leslie, & Brown, 2004).

> *Secondary prevention activities focus on early detection and intervention in an effort to reduce the possible duration of the disorder and its associated complications.*

## Tertiary Prevention

Tertiary prevention focuses on activities to reduce the residual effects of the disorder and promote rehabilitation and restoration of function. Nurses institute actions to prevent complications associated with the disorder and to promote a return to the patient's maximum level of functioning possible. Examples of tertiary prevention strategies include:

- Teaching the patient about the side effects of medications
- Intervening when the patient show signs of exacerbation of symptoms
- Referring the patient to the primary therapist when he or she shows signs of escalating illness

These tertiary prevention activities aid in reducing the stress and in providing support, thus reducing the risk factors associated with the illness. For example, if the patient needs to be in a protected environment, such as an in-patient facility, referral by the nurse helps to reduce the environmental risk factors. The nurse may have noted that the patient is in danger of self-harm. As with primary and secondary interventions, the nurse uses a wide range of psychoeducational interventions. For this patient, psychoeducation would focus on helping the patient learn new ways of behaving and coping.

> *Tertiary prevention activities focus on minimizing complications and promoting the patient's return to his or her maximum level of functioning.*

### SUMMARY POINTS

- Although the exact cause of psychiatric-mental health disorders is not known, certain risk factors have been identified that increase a person's chance for developing a psychiatric-mental health disorder. However, the presence of risk factors does not guarantee that a disorder will occur.

- Many psychiatric-mental health disorders share risk factors that can be differentiated as biological/genetic or personal/social/environmental.

- Protective factors guard against or buffer the effect of risk factors. They may be internal, such as good health, high stress tolerance, and positive coping skills, or external, such as supportive family and social relationships, adequate economic resources, and recreational activities.

- Resilience is a protective factor that refers to the process of adapting well in the face of adversity, trauma, tragedy, threats, or even significant sources of stress. It is learned over time.

- The stress-vulnerability-coping model, initially developed to explain schizophrenia,

can be adapted to aid in understanding other psychiatric-mental health disorders.

- Psychiatric-mental health disorders occurring during infancy, childhood, and adolescence can be linked to genetics/biology and temperament as risk factors. Temperament refers to the innate aspects of an individual's personality and how he or she responds to the world. The issue of temperament as a risk factor focuses on the "goodness of fit."

- Genetic and environmental risk factors are identified as risk factors interacting in the development of schizophrenia. Heredity, gender, and life stressors have been demonstrated scientifically to be risk factors for affective disorders such as major depression and bipolar disorder.

- Genetics and neurophysiology are viewed as exerting a strong influence on the abuse of substances, especially alcohol. Specific genes have been identified to show an increased risk for alcoholism. Substance use disorders also are strongly linked to familial patterns.

*(cont.)*

## SUMMARY POINTS (*CONT.*)

- Anxiety disorders are associated with risk factors involving altered neurotransmitters, genetics, the environment, and situational stressors.

- Family history of psychiatric-mental health disorders, abuse/neglect/trauma, chaotic family life, diagnosis of a childhood conduct disorder, and parental death or divorce are considered risk factors for the development of personality disorders.

- Any medical disorder could be a risk factor for the development of a psychiatric-mental health disorder and any psychiatric-mental health disorder can place a patient at greater risk for a medical problem. Some medical and psychiatric-mental health disorders represent a circular risk relationship.

- The aging of the general population, the growing of the population of older mentally ill adults, medically induced pathology, and psychomimetic disorders are issues impacting a person's risk.

- Prevention identifies risk factors to target for intervention. Interventions focus on changing those risk factors that can be changed, and enhancing protective factors. It is the nurse who performs these functions and thus has the greatest impact on the patient. The nurse applies the interpersonal process at the primary level to delay or prevent the onset of illness, at the secondary level to identify persons with disorders and initiate early treatment, and at the tertiary level to decrease relapse or recurrence, and provide rehabilitation.

## NCLEX-PREP*

1. A group of nursing students are reviewing the various risk factors associated with psychiatric-mental health disorders. The students demonstrate understanding of the information when they identify which of the following as a family risk factor?

   a. Poverty
   b. High crime rate
   c. Placement in foster care
   d. Temperament

2. A nurse is providing primary prevention to a local community group about psychiatric-mental health disorders. Which of the following would the nurse include as a protective factor? Select all that apply.

   a. Flexibility
   b. High intelligence
   c. Limited social relationships
   d. Absence of recreational activities
   e. Adequate economic resources

3. When describing the possibility of developing a psychiatric-mental health disorder related to a medical condition, which disorder would the nurse identify as most common and problematic?

   a. Schizophrenia
   b. Acute stress disorder
   c. Personality disorder
   d. Depression

4. When implementing secondary prevention strategies, which of the following would the psychiatric-mental health nurse do first?

   a. Conduct community screening
   b. Identify existence of risk factors
   c. Teach about coping skills
   d. Make referrals for immediate treatment

(*cont.*)

⬛ **NCLEX-PREP\*** *(CONT.)*

5. After teaching a group of students about risk and protective factors, the nursing instructor determines that additional teaching is needed when the students state which of the following about resilience?

    a. "Everyone is born with resilience but not everybody uses it."

    b. "It is a protective factor that helps balance out the risk factors."

    c. "Individuals need time to develop resilience."

    d. "Resilience promotes better coping with trauma or stress."

\*Answers to these questions appear on page 639.

## REFERENCES

American Psychological Association (2011). The road to resilience. Available at: http://www.apa.org/helpcenter/road-resilience.aspx (accessed 1/13/2011).

Baldassano, C.F., Marangell, L.B., Gyulai, L., Ghaemi, S.N., Joffe, H., Kim, D.R., ... Cohen, L.S. (2005). Gender differences in bipolar disorder: Retrospective data from the first 500 STEP-BD participants. *Bipolar Disorders, 7*(5), 465–470.

Bipolar Disorder Genome Study (BiGS) Consortium. (2010). Meta-analysis of genome-wide association data identifies a risk locus for major mood disorders. *Nature Genetics,* Jan 17. [Epub ahead of print] PMID: 20081856.

Boarts, J.M., Buckley-Fischer, B.A., Armelie, A.P., Bogart, L.M., & Delahanty, D.L. (2009). The impact of HIV diagnosis-related vs. non-diagnosis related trauma on PTSD, depression, medication adherence, and HIV disease markers. *Journal of Evidence-Based Social Work, 6*(1), 4–16.

Brewin, C.R. (2005). Risk factor effect sizes in PTSD: What this means for intervention. *Journal of Trauma & Dissociation, 6*(2), 123–130.

Brewin, C.R., Andrews, B., & Valentine, J.D. (2000). Meta-analysis of risk factors for posttraumatic stress disorder in trauma-exposed adults. *Journal of Consulting & Clinical Psychology, 68*(5), 748–766.

Buchanan, R.W., & Carpenter, W.T. (2004). Schizophrenia: Introduction and overview and other psychotic disorders. In B. Sadock & V. Sadock (Eds.), *Kaplan & Sadock's comprehensive textbook of psychiatry* (8th ed.), pp. 1096–1109. Philadelphia: Lippincott Williams & Wilkins.

Cannon, T.D., Cadenhead, K., Cornblatt, B., Woods, S.W., Addington, J., Walker, E., & Heinssen, R. (2008). Prediction of psychosis in high risk youth: A multi-site longitudinal study in North America. *Archives of General Psychiatry, 65*(1), 28–37.

Carter, J.J., Peter, R., Mulder, R.T., & Luty, S.E. (2001). The contribution of temperament, childhood neglect, and abuse to the development of personality dysfunction: A comparison of three models. *Journal of Personality Disorders, 15*(2), 123–135.

Cruess, D.G., Douglas, S.D., Petitto, J.M., Leserman, J., Ten Have, T., Gettes, D., ... Evans, D.L. (2003). Association of depression, CD8+ T lymphocytes, and natural killer cell activity: Implications for morbidity and mortality in human immunodeficiency virus disease. *Current Psychiatry Reports, 5*, 445–450.

Edenberg, H.J. (2003). *The collaborative study on the genetics of alcoholism: An update.* Retrieved from http://pubs. niaaa.nih.gov/publications/arh26–3/214–218.htm

Evans, D.L., Charney, D.S., Lewis, L., Golden, R.N., Gorman, J.M., Krishnan, K.R., Valvo, W.J. (2005). Mood disorders in the medically ill: Scientific review and recommendations. *Biological Psychiatry, 58*(3), 175–189.

Fennell, D.C., & Fishel, A.H. (1998). Parent education: An evaluation of STEP on abusive parents' perceptions and abuse potential. *Journal of Child and Adolescent Psychiatric Nursing, 11*(3), 107–120.

Gurvits, T.V., Gilbertson, M.W., Lasko, N.B., Tarhan, A.S., Simeon, D., Macklin, M.W., Pitman, R.K. (2000). Neurologic soft signs in chronic posttraumatic stress disorder. *Archives of General Psychiatry, 57*(2), 181–186.

Hamblin, J., & Barnett, E. (2009). *PTSD in children and adolescents.* Retrieved from http://www.ptsd.va.gov/professional/pages/ptsd_in_children_and_adolescents_overview_for_professionals.asp

Hariri, A.R., Mattay, V.S., Tessitore, A., Kolachana, B., Fera, F., Goldman, D., ... Weinberger, D.R. (2002). Serotonin transporter genetic variation and the response of the human amygdala. *Science, 297*(5580), 400–403.

Hasler, G., Fromm, S., Carlson, P.J., Luckenbaugh, D.A., Waldeck, T., Geraci, M., ... Drevets, W.C. (2008). Neural response to catecholamine depletion in unmedicated subjects with major depressive disorder in remission and healthy subjects. *Archives of General Psychiatry, 65*(5), 521–531.

Holt, R.L., Montesinos, S., & Christense, R.C. (2007). Physical and sexual abuse history in women seeking treatment at a psychiatric clinic for the homeless. *Journal of Psychiatric Practice, 13*, 58–60.

Jackson, K.M., Sher, K.J., & Park, A. (2005). Drinking among college students: Consumption and consequences. In M. Galanter (Ed.), *Recent developments in alcoholism: Alcohol problems in adolescents and young adults,* pp. 85–117. New York: Springer.

Jones, F.C., & Selder, F. (1996). Psychoeducational groups to promote effective coping in school-age children living in violent communities. *Issues in Mental Health Nursing, 17*, 559–71.

Kelsoe, J.E. (2005). Mood disorders: Genetics. In B. Sadock & V. Sadock (Eds.), *Kaplan & Sadock's comprehensive textbook of psychiatry* (8th ed.), pp. 1582–1594. Philadelphia: Lippincott Williams & Wilkins.

Kessler, R.C. (2003). Epidemiology of women and depression. *Journal of Affective Disorders, 74*, 5–13.

Kreek, M.J., Bart, G., Lilly, C., LaForge, K.S., & Nielsen, D.A. (2005). Pharmacogenetics and human molecular genetics of opiate and cocaine addictions and their treatments. *Pharmacology Review, 57*(1), 1–26.

Littrell, K.H., Hilligos, N.M., Kirshner, C.D., Petty, R.G., & Johnson, C.G. (2003). The effects of an educational intervention on antipsychotic-induced weight gain. *Journal of Nursing Scholarship, 35*, 237–241.

Liu, Q.R., Drgon, T., Walther, D., Johnson, C., Poleskaya, O., Hess, J., & Uhl, G.R. (2005). Pooled association genome scanning: Validation and use to identify addiction vulnerability loci in two samples. *Proceedings of the National Academy of Sciences of the United States of America, 102*(33), 11864–11869.

Lustman, P.J., & Clouse, R.E. (2005). Depression in diabetic patients: The relationship between mood and glycemic control. *Journal of Diabetes & Its Complications, 19*(2), 113–122.

Mayo Clinic, (2010). *Mental illness: Risk factors.* Retrieved from http://www.mayoclinic.com/health/mental-illness/DS01104/DSECTION=risk-factors

Maziade, M., Caperaa, P., Laplante, B., Boudreault, M., Thivierge, J., Cote, R., & Boutin, P. (1985). Value of difficult temperament among 7-year-olds in the general population for predicting psychiatric diagnosis at age 12. *American Journal of Psychiatry, 142*, 943–946.

McCabe, S. (2003, May). *A new equation for understanding and treating depression.* Presentation at MAAPPNG meeting, Atlanta, Georgia.

McClowry, S.G. (2002). The temperament profiles of school-age children. *Journal of Pediatric Nursing, 17*, 3–10.

McGauhey, P., Starfield, B., Alexander, C., & Ensminger, M.E. (1991). Social environment and vulnerability of low birth weight children. *Pediatrics, 88*, 943–953.

Meltzer, H.Y., & Fatemi, H.S. (2008). Schizophrenia. In M.H. Ebert, P.T. Loosen, B. Nurcombe, & J.F. Leckman (Eds.), *Current Diagnosis & Treatment: Psychiatry* (2nd ed.), pp. 260–277. New York: McGraw-Hill.

Mental Illness Fellowship Victoria (MIFV) (2008). *Recognising possible triggers of mental illness onset or relapse: The stress-vulnerability-coping model of mental illness.* Retrieved from http://www.mifellowship.org/documents/StressVulnerabilityCoping Model.pdf

Neumeister, A., Bonne, O., & Charney, D.S. (2005). Anxiety disorders: Neurochemical aspects. In B. Sadock & V. Sadock (Eds.), *Kaplan & Sadock's comprehensive textbook of psychiatry* (8th ed.), pp. 1739–1747. Philadelphia: Lippincott Williams & Wilkins.

Nurnberger, J.I., Jr., & Foroud, T. (2000). Genetics of bipolar affective disorder. *Current Psychiatry Reports, 2*(2), 147–157.

Ozaki, N., Goldman, D., Kaye, W., Plotnicov, K., Greenberg, B., Lappaleinen, J., ... Murphy, D.L. (2003). Serotonin transporter missense mutation associated with a complex neuropsychiatric phenotype. *Molecular Psychiatry, 8*, 933–936.

Pickens, R.W., Preston, K.L., Miles, D.R., Gupton, A.E., Johnson, E.O., Newlin, D.B., ... Umbricht, A. (2001). Family history influence on drug abuse severity and treatment outcome. *Drug and Alcohol Dependence, 61*, 261–270.

Potash, J.B., Toolan, J., Steele, J., Miller, E.B., Pearl, J., Zandi, P.P., ... McMahon, F.J. (2007). The bipolar disorder phenome database: A resource for genetic studies. *American Journal of Psychiatry, 164*(8), 1229–1237.

Reich, D.B., & Zanarini, M.C. (2001). Developmental aspects of borderline personality disorder. *Harvard Review of Psychiatry, 9*, 294–301.

Risch, N., Herrell, R., Lehner, T., Liang, K.Y., Eaves, L., Hoh, J., ... Merikangas, K.R. (2009). Interaction between the serotonin transporter gene, stressful life events and risk of depression: A meta-analysis. *Journal of the American Medical Association, 301*(23), 2462–71.

Schizophrenia.com. (2009). *The causes of schizophrenia.* Retrieved from http://schizophrenia.com/hypo.php

Shiner, R., & Caspi, A. (2003). Personality differences in childhood and adolescence: Measurement, development, and consequences. *Journal of Child Psychology and Psychiatry, 44*(1), 2–32.

Shumyatsky, G.P., Malleret, G., Shin, R.M., Takizawa, S., Tully, K., Tsvetkov, E., Bolshakov, V.Y. (2005). Stathmin, a gene enriched in the amygdala, controls both learned and innate fear. *Cell, 123*(4), 697–709.

Shumyatsky, G.P., Tsvetkov, E., Malleret, G., Vronskaya, S., Hatton, M., Hampton, L., ... Bolshakov, V.Y. (2002). Identification of a signaling network in lateral nucleus of amygdala important for inhibiting memory specifically related to learned fear. *Cell, 111* (6), 905–918.

Sinha, R., Garcia, M., Paliwal, P., Kreek, M.J., & Rounsaville, B.J. (2006). Stress-induced cocaine craving and hypothalamic-pituitary-adrenal responses are predictive of cocaine relapse outcomes. *Archives of General Psychiatry, 63*, 324–331.

Smoller, J. W., Gardner-Schuster, E., & Covino, J. (2008). The genetic basis of panic and phobic anxiety disorders. *American Journal of Medical Genetics, 148*: 118–126.

Sofronoff, K., Leslie, A., & Brown, W. (2004). Parent management training and Asperger syndrome: A randomized controlled trial to evaluate a parent based intervention. *Autism, 8*, 301–317.

Tackett, J.L. (2006). Evaluating models of the personality-psychopathology relationship in children and adolescents. *Clinical Psychology Review, 26*(5), 584–599.

Thomas, A., & Chess, S. (1984). Genesis and evolution of behavioral disorders: From infancy to early adult life. *American Journal of Psychiatry, 141*, 1–9.

Thomas, A., Chess, S., & Birch, H.G. (1968). *Temperament and behavior disorders in childhood.* New York: New York University Press.

Thompson, W., Lande, R.G., & Kalapatapu, R.K. (2009). *Alcoholism.* Retrieved from http://www.emedicine.com/med/topic98.htm

Trafton, J.A., Tracy, S.W., Oliva, E.M., & Humphreys, K. (2007). Different components of opioid-substitution treatment predict outcomes of patients with and without a parent with substance-use problems. *Journal of Studies on Alcohol and Drugs, 68*(2), 165–172.

U.S. Dept. of Health and Human Services. (1999). *Mental health: A report of the Surgeon General.* Rockville, MD: USDHHS. Retrieved March 2, 2010, from http://www.surgeongeneral.gov/library/mentalhealth/chapter2/sec5.html

Werner, E.E., & Smith, R.S. (1992). *Overcoming the odds: High risk children from birth to adulthood.* New York: Cornell University Press.

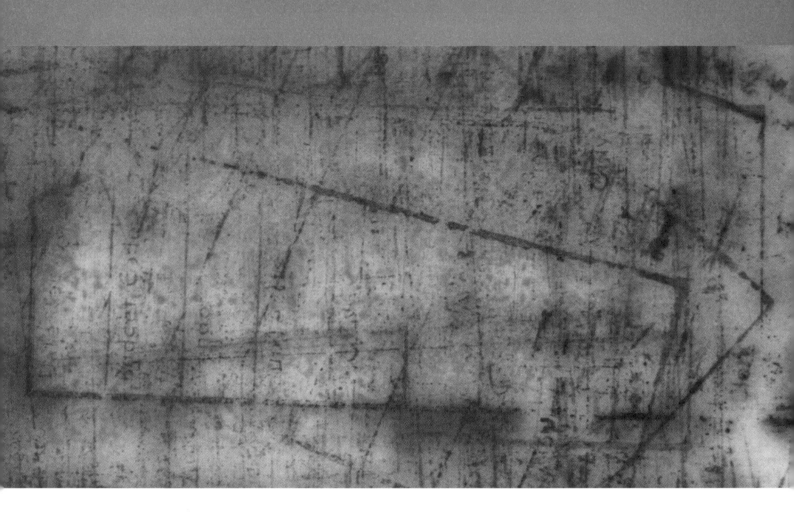

## CHAPTER CONTENTS

General Systems Theory

Groups and Group Therapy

Family Psychotherapy

The Interpersonal Process and Group
and Family Therapy

## EXPECTED LEARNING OUTCOMES

**After completing this chapter, the student will be able to:**

1. Describe systems theory, including the major concepts.
2. Discuss the relationship of general systems theory to nursing theories.
3. Apply systems theory thinking to psychiatric-mental health nursing.
4. Define group therapy.
5. Identify key concepts related to group therapy, including those from systems theory.
6. Explain the eleven curative factors of a therapeutic group.

# CHAPTER 9
# SYSTEMS CONCEPTS AND WORKING IN GROUPS

Kathleen Tusaie

7. Describe the content of a supportive and insight-oriented group.

8. Discuss how family is considered a specialized type of group.

9. Describe the use of a genogram in family assessment.

10. Identify the relationship between interpersonal based therapy and group and family therapy.

## KEY TERMS

Curative factors

Family therapy

Genogram

Group

Group dynamics

Group process

Group therapy

Lines of resistance

Normal line of defense

System

Therapeutic groups

Consider the following situation:

*Three blind people encountered an elephant. The first touching an ear stated, "It is a large, rough thing, wide, and broad like a rug." The second holding the trunk stated, "No, it is a straight hollow pipe." While the third holding the front leg replied, "It is mighty and firm like a pillar." Given these individuals' ways of knowing, they will never know an elephant. (Old Sufi story)*

From the individual perspective, each person's statement is correct. Yet, instinctively, the individuals know that the truths expressed by each person are incomplete truths and cannot ever wholly describe the elephant. Systems theory provides a framework to see the whole elephant.

Using systems theory or systems thinking provides a means for thinking about the larger picture and holds the potential for treatment planning leading to higher levels of functioning. It does not produce "quick fixes." How an individual thinks not only determines what he or she sees, but also what he or she does. This chapter provides an overview of General Systems Theory and exposes the reader to systems thinking. It reviews examples of how systems theory is reflected in nursing theory. The chapter discusses groups, group therapy, and family therapy as they relate to systems theory and systems thinking with examples of applications to each. Exercises are integrated throughout this chapter to facilitate understanding of personal experiences within systems thinking and its relevance to psychiatric-mental health nursing practice.

## GENERAL SYSTEMS THEORY

Biologist Ludwig von Bertalanffy proposed a General Systems Theory in 1928 to provide a way of thinking that could be applied across professional boundaries and promote holistic thinking. Rather than reducing a system (human body) to the components of its parts (cells), systems theory focuses on the interactions of its parts and the nonlinear, dynamic pattern of those interactions. General Systems Theory has diverse applications, including engineering, philosophy, mathematics, computer modeling, ecology, management, nursing, psychotherapy, and others.

A **SYSTEM** is any group of components sufficiently related to identify patterns of interaction (Kuhn, 1996). A change in any component induces change in one or more other components of the system and in the system as a whole. No component of the system can be understood out of the context of the way it interacts with other components. Thus the system is more than a sum of its parts (**Figure 9-1**).

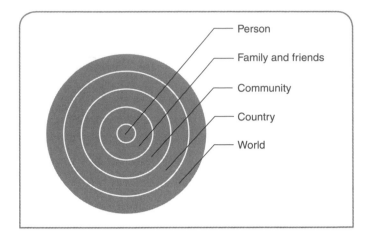

Figure 9-1 *Person as part of the world system.*

von Bertalanffy (1968) described two major types of systems: closed and open. Closed systems are those in which the components are isolated from the environment. In contrast, open systems are those in which the components interact with the environment and with the other components of the system. Thus the system is dynamic and ever-changing. **How Would You Respond? 9-1** provides an example of an open system.

*A system is a group of components that interact, such that a change in one component affects the other components and the system overall. Using systems theory or systems thinking provides an opportunity to look at the "bigger picture" and promotes treatment planning that ultimately can lead to higher levels of functioning.*

### Systems Theory and Nursing Theory

Theory provides a systematic way of viewing the world to describe, explain, predict, or control it. Theories are created by experienced practitioners who make abstractions from large collections of facts and concepts. The practice of psychiatric-mental health nursing is derived from theory that has been tested through research to produce evidence for practice. There is an intertwining, circular relationship among theory, practice, and research. Nursing theorists

**HOW WOULD YOU RESPOND? 9-1: THINKING IN SYSTEMS**

Review Figure 9-1. Place yourself as the person at the center of the system. Then insert the names of people or groups to complete the surrounding circles for family and friends, community, country, and the world.

Now think of a recent event in your community, country, or the world.

**CRITICAL THINKING QUESTIONS**

1. *How did you respond to this event? What affect did it have on you? How were others affected?*

2. *Was the system stressed, disturbing the usual balance and homeostasis?*

3. *What did you notice about coping and adaptation for yourself? For others in the system? For the system overall?*

4. *If the imbalance or disruption was too great, what developed or occurred?*

who have built upon General Systems Theory are briefly reviewed here.

Systems thinking is not new to nursing. The basic elements in any description of nursing include not only person and health, but also the environment (Fawcett, 1984). The environment the person emerges from and returns to is considered across several nursing theories. For example, Florence Nightingale's (1859) broad view of nursing included creating the right environment for the patient's natural, reparative powers to act, as well as awareness of the influences of socio-political-religious issues upon nursing practice (Reed & Zurakowski, 1996). As nursing continued to evolve, other theorists began to address environment as having a major impact on a person. *The Science of Unitary Man* published by Martha Rogers (1970, 1992), reflects an open system model. In her model, Rogers describes the person as an energy field inseparable from the environment with continuous and mutual interaction between the two. As a result, both the person and environment experience changes at the same time and in the same manner. The person is described

in the context of an environment resulting in constant change as well as the continuous evolution of the change itself. Thus, the person is viewed as a unified whole that is more than and different from the sum of the parts. Rogers (1970) describes the professional practice of nursing as seeking to understand patterns of interactions between person and environment and working "with" the patient for "…realization of maximum health potential" (p.122). This is an important statement because it emphasizes that patients are active participants who make choices rather than passive recipients of nursing care.

> *Systems thinking is not new to nursing. The environment has been a major component of many nursing theories.*

Another nursing model that applies systems theory is Neuman's Systems Model (2002). This model is based upon concepts of stress and coping (Lazarus & Folkman, 1984) and General Systems Theory (von Bertalanffy, 1968). The whole person (client) system is defined as the person in interaction with the internal and external environment. Each client system is a unique composite of factors and characteristics within a given range of possible responses. The central core of the client system includes basic survival factors common to all, such as normal temperature, genetic structure, and organ functioning. This central core is surrounded by circles that function as **LINES OF RESISTANCE**. These lines represent the internal factors that an individual uses to help defend against stressors. Extending out further from the core is the next level of circles, or the **NORMAL LINE OF DEFENSE**. This normal line of defense, or usual response to stressors, represents the individual's usual state of wellness. According to Neuman, the normal line of defense is flexible and dynamic with the ability to expand or contract as needed in response to stressors. She further describes stressors as known, unknown, and/or universal. Each differing stressor has the potential, alone or in combination, to disturb the stability of the system. When a stressor penetrates the normal lines of defense, protective factors within the lines of resistance are activated to protect the central core's functioning. In other words, the entire client system is constantly in a dynamic process of input, output, feedback, and compensation with the goal of maintaining balance.

Neuman identified specific nursing interventions to retain or maintain system stability. Thus, primary, secondary, or tertiary prevention are possible interventions that can be used in the model (Neuman, 2002). Primary prevention, or wellness promotion and disease prevention, represents expanding the normal line of defense, strengthening the flexible line of defense, or decreasing the possibility of encountering stressors before their invasion. Interventions described as secondary prevention, or treatment of symptoms, are focused upon strengthening the lines of resistance to protect the core of the system. Interventions such as prompt detection of symptoms and early treatment are examples. Tertiary prevention indicates adjustive processes or readaptation, such as sleeping or learning new coping skills, taking place as the system begins to return to a balanced state of wellness. Once balance is achieved, these processes then begin to function as primary prevention interventions, demonstrating a circular pattern of interventions.

The system described by Neuman's model may be the individual person, a family, a group, or a community. In addition, application of this model has been described across all nursing specialties, as well as across disciplines and internationally (Neuman, 2002).

## Systems Theory and Psychiatric-Mental Health Nursing

The brief overview of systems thinking previously provided argues that a system perspective has always been present in the discipline of nursing. However, the definition of system and environment has varied. These broad theorists have provided a framework for thinking about psychiatric-mental health nursing.

Consider this example. During an in-patient hospitalization, Mr. Davis, an individual experiencing auditory and visual hallucinations, has been stabilized with medications, a structured environment, and one-to-one interactions with nurses. The primary focus of the nurse-patient interactions has been to establish trust and to emphasize the importance of medication to minimize the distress experienced with the hallucinations. This is a very appropriate, evidence-based approach and Mr. Davis is discharged with decreased symptoms. However, within several weeks, he is readmitted to the in-patient unit. How is this exacerbation of symptoms explained? From a snapshot or reductionist explanation, the individual stopped taking his medications and symptoms returned. This would not be incorrect. However, this view is limiting because it only provides a narrowed view or "quick fix" for the problem. It does not explain the whole experience for this patient. Using systems thinking, Mr. Davis would be viewed as a person who does not live in isolation. Rather he is part of the family system, the community, and world as a whole. There would be awareness of the interactions among the family who have been encouraging the patient to not take his medications, possibly because they are too expensive or because they cause adverse effects. In addition, Mr. Davis has resumed chain-smoking cigarettes, which interferes with the absorption of the medications. His lack of any daily routine, the consumption of only fast food and snacks at home, combined with living in a high crime neighborhood are all possible interacting factors leading to his current situation. Thus, the use of systems thinking promotes comprehensive, holistic care.

## GROUPS AND GROUP THERAPY

Individuals are members of multiple groups. A **GROUP** refers to any collection of two or more individuals who share at least one commonality or goal, such that the relationship is interdependent. Applying systems theory, a group is a set of components that work together to achieve a function or purpose. Groups may be formal or informal. Formal groups are structured and have authority. Informal groups typically address personal needs.

Psychiatric-mental health nurses are members of multiple groups, both formal and informal. Professional or more formal group affiliations may include the clinical group of students in the psychiatric-mental health nursing rotation, the student body of a college of nursing, all student nurses belonging to Student Nurses Association, club memberships, as well as work-related groups such as the treatment team in the place of employment. More informal group memberships focus on casualness and personal needs. These include family, friends, or even a small informal group in the work setting. (Note that the family is a specialized type of group and is discussed later in the chapter using Bowen's Family Systems Theory [1978] as the framework. The focus of the discussion here is on **THERAPEUTIC GROUPS**, groups used to promote psychologic growth, development, and transformation.) **GROUP THERAPY** is the process by which group leaders with advanced educational degrees and experience provide psychotherapy with members to improve their interpersonal functioning.

> *Two or more people together functioning interdependently form a group. Family is a specialized type of group.*

## Types of Therapeutic Groups

Therapeutic groups may be categorized as open or closed systems based on membership. Open groups are ones in which new members can join and old members can leave at different times. Members are welcome to attend the group meetings at any time in the individual's recovery as well as at any stage of the group's development. Open groups typically are ongoing, which permits their availability of access to a greater number of individuals. Unfortunately, new members joining an open group face a disadvantage in that they have yet to form relationships already present in existing group members. Thus, cohesiveness may be less. An example of an open group is Alcoholics Anonymous (AA), one of the most successful approaches for maintaining sobriety today.

Closed groups are ones in which membership is limited to those members involved when the group initially forms. No new group members can join. If an old member leaves, no new member comes in to take his or her place. For example, if a closed group initially started out with eight members, and two members leave the group, the group remains with only six members. This approach facilitates more group cohesiveness, safety, and interpersonal learning. An example of a closed group is an insight-oriented psychotherapy group meeting for 90 minutes a week for 12 weeks as part of an out-patient practice. When the 12 weeks are over, the group disbands. Then another group starts again, with new members being accepted for the specified time frame.

Another way to classify groups is related to the group's purpose and goals. These may include therapeutic insight-oriented groups and supportive groups. Insight-oriented groups are characterized by increased process, focusing on the interpersonal relationships among members and their communication patterns and styles to foster the development of better perception into one's self. Generally, these groups are less structured and require leaders prepared at the gradual level of education (Puskar, McClure, & McGinnis, 2007).

Supportive groups have a specific content and structure and are often lead by nurses (Hsiao, Lin, & Lai, 2004). More structure and less process characterize the supportive group. Some of these include education groups, recreation groups, socialization groups, or reality orientation with older adults (Kavanagh, Duncan-McConnell, Greenwood, Trivedi, & Wykes, 2003; O'Donald & O'Mahoney, 2009). In structured environments such as in-patient or partial hospitalization programs, goal-planning groups, which meet in the morning to set goals for the day and then again before bedtime to review goal achievement, are examples of supportive groups.

Self-help groups are also considered a supportive group. This type of group usually consists of persons coping with a particular problem. Some self-help groups include Alcoholics Anonymous (AA), National Alliance for the Mentally Ill (NAMI), Overeaters Anonymous (OA), groups of individuals with a specific diagnosis such as cancer support group (Moyer, Sohl, Oliver, & Schneider, 2009), Alzheimer's support group for caretakers, or diabetic support groups. Self-help groups offer acceptance, mutual support, and help in overcoming maladaptive behaviors. Although controversial, web-based self-help groups are showing promising results. Issues involving problem drinking, smoking, depression, anxiety, and work-related stress have all demonstrated positive change following involvement in a web-based self-help program (Griffiths, Farrer, & Christensen, 2010; Van Straten, Cuijpers, & Smits, 2008).

A final classification for types of groups is based on setting, an important consideration for group therapy. Therapeutic groups classified by setting are in-patient or out-patient. Current in-patient treatment has shifted dramatically from the history of prolonged stays in remote state hospitals to brief, often repeated hospitalizations in small acute general hospital units. Although the core of group therapy remains the same, adaptations are necessary for the acute in-patient setting. Yalom (2005) has discussed these adaptations in great detail and are summarized in **Table 9-1**.

Several methods have been used to adjust to these issues. Often, in-patient groups are categorized by level of functioning, organizing the groups as lower functioning and higher functioning groups. Shifting the time frame is another adjustment strategy. This shift necessitates that the group leader provides structure and participation by members in each session. There is no time to be passive and allow group cohesion to develop. In-patient groups also may be influenced by incidents on the unit because group members are living together. Thus, by shifting the time frame, an aftercare group available immediately after discharge from the in-patient setting could be developed. Then the in-patient, aftercare, and out-patient groups would be seen as continuous and complementary.

> *Groups may be classified by membership as open or closed, by purpose as insight-oriented or supportive, and by setting as in-patient or out-patient.*

| TABLE 9-1: COMPARISON OF IN-PATIENT AND OUT-PATIENT THERAPEUTIC GROUPS | |
| --- | --- |
| **IN-PATIENT THERAPEUTIC GROUPS** | **OUT-PATIENT THERAPEUTIC GROUPS** |
| Overlap of therapies may result in competition for patients. Administrative staff makes decisions about group frequency, duration, optional or mandatory attendance, and group leadership | Leader makes decisions about group membership, procedures, and functions independently |
| Patient acuity is greater, which limits the cognitive abilities of patients to participate | Patients are better able to participate due to a lessened illness acuity |
| Shorter or briefer lengths of stay lead to a new patient in every group session | Group membership is more consistent |

## Group Process and Group Dynamics

Individuals participate in group process even if they are unaware of that participation. **GROUP PROCESS** refers to interaction among group members. **GROUP DYNAMICS** refers to the forces that produce patterns within the groups as the group moves toward its goals. As mentioned previously, a group results any time two or more people are together and interdependent. Interdependence of group members is the key difference between a group and a collection or aggregate of individuals. Interdependence involves a common task or purpose that has brought the people together, some characteristic shared in common, and a pattern of interaction established among the people.

## Curative Factors of Groups

Expectations are different for each type of group member. However, common factors operate in all types of groups. These factors, called **CURATIVE FACTORS** (Yalom, 2005), describe the patterns of interaction in a therapeutic group. Using Neuman's model and the group as the system of focus, the curative factors are the central core necessary for the survival of the group.

Yalom (2005) identified eleven categories of curative factors:

1. Instillation of hope
2. Universality
3. Imparting of information
4. Altruism
5. Corrective recapitulation of the primary family group
6. Development of socialization techniques
7. Imitative behavior
8. Interpersonal learning
9. Group cohesiveness
10. Catharsis
11. Existential factors

These curative factors are interdependent. However, some factors take on a more significant role at different times during the group process depending on the group's purpose, time frame, and stage of development.

> *Yalom identified eleven curative factors that are interdependent within a group. They are the central core necessary for group survival.*

### Instillation of Hope

Feeling hopeful is necessary in all types of therapy. In group therapy, hope or optimism that the therapy will be helpful often keeps the person involved until the other curative factors develop. Literature on the mechanisms by which optimism promotes mental and physical health and studies indicating that optimism can be increased through psychotherapy—individual as well as group—is extensive (Alloy, Abramson, & Chiara, 2000; Seligman, 1998; Tusaie & Patterson, 2006).

Being hopeful is also an important factor in the group leader or facilitator. Believing that the group process is beneficial and important is necessary for an effective outcome. During the first group meeting or preceding the meeting, the leader may share positive expectations and enthusiasm for the group experience with prospective members. However, this optimism must be genuine to be effective.

In addition to the group leader or facilitator's optimism, other techniques are used to encourage optimism. When identifying group members, including individuals who are further along in the process of treatment and recovery as well as individuals who are in their initial session may be beneficial. This allows more experienced members to offer encouragement and advice as well as to role model healthier behavior during the group process. Self-help groups such as Alcoholics Anonymous place emphasis upon instillation of hope in several ways. For example, all members tell their stories of falling into alcoholism and the awful consequences, followed by recovery and healthier, happier living without alcohol. Instillation of hope is very influential in the beginning group to maintain attendance and participation.

## Universality

As group members continue to feel hopeful, they begin to develop the belief they are not alone and not so different from others in the group. This belief leads to a feeling of connectedness and safeness within the group sessions. Often patients have poor social skills and experience interpersonal conflicts within many settings, thus leading to lack of personal connectedness and validation in their lives. The experience of universality has been described as a "welcome to the human race" (Yalom, 2005). For example, in an adolescent out-patient psychotherapy group, one young girl who was crying disclosed that she had been arrested for shoplifting. The group members validated her embarrassment and then several shared that they had also attempted to shoplift to see if they could get away with it and stated, "That's what we do, we push the limits, that's part of being a kid." The sharing of information helped the patient feel less distressed. It then led to a discussion involving the importance of thinking about consequences before acting and what could be learned from this experience.

The experience of universality may also happen during individual therapy, but there is less opportunity for validation. For example, a patient shares information about his inability to keep up with his employment responsibilities following the death of his mother. Following a discussion of the experienced difficulties, the nurse normalizes the difficulties by stating that "it is common to have difficulty functioning when grieving" and the patient begins to feel less self-critical. A similar message from not only the nurse but also group members is often more powerful. Thus, the patient experiences universality and maintains hope.

## Imparting of information

This curative factor includes didactic information provided by the leader or facilitator, as well as advice and suggestions offered by group members. Providing information about mental health and illness or other topics is an important factor. The discussion at the beginning of this chapter presented the innate need of all people to explain experiences in some way. The ability to understand the source and meaning of symptoms provides a sense of cognitive control and relieves some of the uncertainty and anxiety experienced by an individual with symptoms of psychiatric-mental health disorders. Knowledge is power. Providing information also conveys a sense of interest and caring that contributes to this curative factor.

Undergraduate nurses are often leading educational groups that focus on diagnoses, medications, or coping skills. Although imparting information is an important curative factor, no factor operates in isolation. In other words, using part of the group session to provide information and part of the session for discussion to encourage activation of other curative factors such as altruism, hope, socialization techniques, interpersonal learning, group cohesiveness, and catharsis is most effective. Activation of curative factors is necessary for an effective outcome from the group therapy session.

## Altruism

Patients are enormously helpful to each other during group therapy sessions. They offer support, suggestions, insight, and share similar issues. Frequently, patients will listen more readily to another group member than the nurse or therapist because the therapist is considered a paid professional. However, another member can be counted on to be more truthful and practical (Yalom, 2005). Sometimes, an individual will resist suggestions or even participation in a group because "we will pull each other down" or "I won't have time to talk." However, this usually represents a hidden message that the individual believes he or she has nothing to offer and may require additional work in individual sessions.

Altruism also is associated with the belief that helping others increases one's self-esteem. If an individual can offer something of use to another, his or her feelings of uselessness are decreased. In addition, self-preoccupation and absorption with one's own problems may be decreased. The therapeutic group teaches the lesson that decreasing self-absorption provides a different view of their world.

## The Corrective Recapitulation of the Primary Family Group

Patients come to group being shaped by their experiences in their families. Group therapy resembles family structure: Group members may interact with leaders as they did with parents and interact with members as they did with siblings. Often, these communication patterns are dysfunctional. Using the therapeutic group format, members can learn more effective and functional communication patterns. (Family patterns will be discussed in more detail at the end of this chapter.)

## Development of Socialization Techniques

The development of basic social skills is a curative factor present in all groups to varying degrees. For example, a group session with individuals who have been institutionalized for years preparing for community reintegration would directly address the development and practice of social skills such as maintaining eye contact, carrying on a conversation, and use of polite comments. However, a group of divorced women planning to re-enter the dating scene would focus on different issues. Involvement in any group holds the potential to learn how to communicate and interact with sensitivity and empathy, and with less judgmental approaches. These skills can only improve social functioning in the world.

## Imitative Behavior

Individuals commonly pick up or imitate behaviors of social groups. This may involve walking, talking, dressing, or thinking like others. Sometimes, it may involve something as simple as a haircut or something more involved such as adding coping strategies observed in the group. A group member may try on a new behavior to break up old patterns during the process of change.

## Interpersonal Learning

Interpersonal learning is an important and complex curative factor. Frequently referred to as insight, interpersonal learning reflects an understanding of the patterns in behavior, and thinking and working through feelings.

Interpersonal learning is bi-directional. In other words, what is learned in the world is carried into the group and what is learned in the group is carried into the world. Thus, an adaptive spiral is set into motion as described by Neuman's circular pattern of interventions. More specifically, Yalom (2005) described a pattern of interpersonal learning in a therapeutic group. First, a member displays a behavior. Next, through feedback and self-observation, the impact of the behavior upon others' feelings and opinions about him are recognized. The person also recognizes the impact of the behavior on the opinion that he has of himself. Finally, the individual takes responsibility for the creation of his interpersonal relationships in conjunction with an awareness that he can make changes.

A group leader can use specific techniques when intervening to facilitate interpersonal growth. These include offering feedback on a specific behavior in the group, encouraging self-observation, and reinforcing the transfer of learning.

## Group Cohesiveness

Cohesiveness in group therapy is similar to the therapeutic relationship in individual therapy. This sense of "we-ness," solidarity, or attractiveness of the group for its members is not only a curative factor, but a necessary condition for effective group therapy. Groups differ in the degree of cohesiveness. Factors that promote group cohesiveness are highlighted in **Box 9-1**. Those with higher levels of cohesiveness will attend regularly, provide support, defend the group rules, be more accepting of members, and feel greater security and relief from tension in the group.

The group leader can do much to promote cohesiveness. Selection of members and discussing group rules, being a technical expert and serving a role model of therapeutic communication are a few examples for fostering group cohesiveness.

## Catharsis

Members of a group learning how to express feelings and being able to verbalize what is bothering them is a powerful aspect of a therapeutic group. Without catharsis, a group would be more of an academic, sterile experience. However, it is important to remember that catharsis alone is not adequate for an effective group. Interaction of the curative factors is necessary.

## Existential Factors

The final curative factor, existential factors, involves recognition and acceptance of some universal truths about life experience. These include recognizing that sometimes life is unfair, setting priorities and being less caught up in trivialities, and learning that an individual must take responsibility for him- or herself no matter how much guidance and connection are felt with others. Yalom (2005) described this recognition using the following analogy—"being a ship floating in the dark…even though no physical mooring could be made, it was comforting to see the lights of other ships in the same water" (p. 91).

---

**BOX 9-1: FACTORS THAT PROMOTE GROUP COHESIVENESS**

- Sharing of similar values and beliefs
- Commitment to the group's existence
- Clearly defined group goals
- Cooperative interaction among members
- Democratic leadership with equal participation of members
- Size appropriate for the intended goal
- Atmosphere of value and acceptance

> *Cohesiveness in a group reflects the solidarity of the group. It is a curative factor essential for ensuring the effectiveness of group therapy.*

## Group Development

One pattern seen in all groups, regardless of the type, is the movement through phases as the group develops. These phases of group development are similar to those in the nurse-patient relationship: orientation, working, and termination.

The orientation or beginning phase of the group is characterized by the group leader and members getting to know one another. The duration of this phase varies depending on numerous factors such as the size of the group and its purpose. Initially, members participate hesitantly and search to define how the group is going to help them. Members also determine how they will interact with other members. The group leader or facilitator orients the members and promotes an environment of trust. The leader and members work together to establish the group's rules and goals. During this phase, it is important for the leader to set structure with clear expectations, including confidentiality, respect, and safety.

In the beginning, members may be reluctant to verbalize their true feelings because they have yet to develop trust and fear not being accepted by the group. Thus they often display polite and conforming behaviors, playing the role of the "good patient" and not wishing to offend anyone. As the group progresses, conflicts commonly ensue as power struggles occur and members become more comfortable in the group.

As the group moves into the working phase, group cohesiveness begins to increase as the group engages in activities to achieve the goals. Problem solving, decision making, education, and sharing of feelings and experiences occur. Conflict is managed by the members. The members increase their reliance on each other rather than the leader for guidance. The leader's major role during this phase is one of facilitating the group and keeping the group on track.

During termination phase, the group reviews the work done and how that work can be applied in the future. Preparation for separation and ending the group takes place. Members may experience grief over the loss of the group, especially if the group has been established for a long time. Feelings such as abandonment, guilt, fear, and anger may arise. The leader encourages the members to look back on what has occurred and discuss their feelings of loss associated with the ending of the group.

> *A group progresses through three phases of development: orientation, working, and termination.*

## Role of the Group Leader or Facilitator

The group leader or facilitator plays a very important role in promoting the effectiveness of the group. The specific interventions by the leader shift with the purpose and the stage of the group's development. **Table 9-2** identifies the role of the leader for each phase of group development.

Preparation for the group is essential and includes clearly identifying the purpose and the procedures to be followed in the group, preparing any materials needed, arranging the room to encourage communication (chairs in circle, closed door, or private room), and selecting patients. These strategies represent normal lines of defense identified in Neuman's theory, to protect the group from outside interruptions. Once the leader or facilitator clearly understands the purpose of the group, this information is shared with prospective members. Group members should be at similar levels of acuity and cognitive functioning.

Most importantly, the group leader or facilitator must maintain a constant awareness of the differences between individual therapy and group therapy. This includes not doing individual therapy with members during the group session. Rather, interventions must be directed toward the development of the curative factors in the group. Members' participation is necessary. Furthermore, confidence in the effectiveness of group therapy and nonjudgmental comments encourage effectiveness.

At the completion of each group, the leader is responsible for reviewing and documenting the session. If co-leaders are present, this task is simplified. The dynamics as well as the content must be documented. One method for documenting dynamics is the interaction chronogram (**Figure 9-2**; Cox, 1973). The most effective groups show crossed lines of communication and not simply the leader talking to each member. Documentation usually involves each member's type of participation and the themes of the content (i.e., "participated actively by supporting group members and discussing anxiety about marital conflicts").

**TABLE 9-2: PHASE OF GROUP DEVELOPMENT WITH GROUP'S TASK AND LEADER'S ROLE**

| GROUP PHASE | GROUP TASK | LEADER'S ROLE |
| --- | --- | --- |
| Orientation | Define goals | Provide structure by describing group purpose and expectations. |
| | Ways of interacting | Role model respectful communication. Emphasize positives: "It took a lot of courage to talk about that. I believe everyone here feels a little scared to talk about themselves." |
| | | Use nonverbal reinforcement of therapeutic communication; e.g., bending forward, smiling, nodding after member's comments. |
| | Build universality, cohesiveness, and optimism | Emphasize similarities among members: "It is interesting to notice that everyone in this group has been in therapy before...everyone has at least one significant relationship in their lives." |
| | | "Ken you are being discharged tomorrow, would you tell the group what has been helpful for you?" |
| Working | Accomplish group purpose | Keep the group on task with gentle confrontation: "I notice we have been talking about last evening's meal for 10 minutes; do you want to continue this or focus upon...(group purpose)? Let's get back to talking about..." |
| | Encourage interpersonal learning | Comment on what you see happening in the group process for clarification: "I'm not sure what is happening in our discussion today, but I notice Joe keeps tapping his foot, Sue has not talked to anyone, and Mary moved her chair away from the group—what do you all think about this?" |
| | | Encourage communication by questioning: "Would you talk more about that?" |
| Termination | Prepare for separation | Review group accomplishments and support members by summarizing and paraphrasing. |
| | Plan for future | "What stands out for you about the group? What have you learned? What are your feelings about ending the group? How will you apply what you have learned?" |

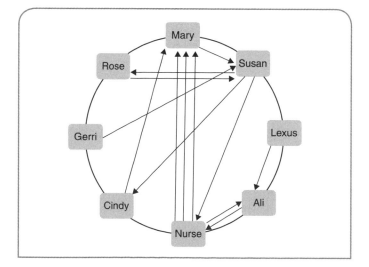

Figure 9-2 *Interaction chronogram of a stress management group.*

Applying Neuman's theory, the leader's or facilitator's role is to develop and maintain the lines of defense and resistance to stressors that threaten the core factors or group development. As such, the leader's interventions shift in response to members' participation, which can either facilitate or interfere with the group process.

*The group leader or facilitator assumes different roles depending on the phase of the group's development and in response to the members' participation.*

## Roles of Group Members

Members of the group may interact in a manner that supports or interferes with the development and maintenance of curative factors and group purpose (Benne & Sheats, 1948). Typically, the roles of group members can be divided into three categories: roles that keep the group on task and focused, roles that maintain the group, and roles that threaten curative factors and group functioning. **Table 9-3** describes these roles.

The group leader or facilitator needs to engage in minimal intervention when dealing with roles that keep the group on task and focused and those that maintain the group because the members are encouraging the group process. However, with roles that threaten curative factors, the members are more self than group focused. Therefore, the leader must interrupt these behaviors in a therapeutic manner. **Therapeutic Interaction 9-1** provides an example of how to address the disruptive behavior of a group member. In a well-developed working group, the members may intervene themselves, not allowing the self-centered behaviors to continue.

For example, when a group member is monopolizing the session in the role of help seeker, self-confessor, or recognition seeker, the behavior must be checked. However, the leader cannot simply tell the person to stop. This has little therapeutic value for the member or the group. The member's anxiety will continue and he or she most likely will resume the same behavior because no learning has taken place. The other group members may feel threatened by the leader's comments and fear their contributions

may also be silenced. This of course does not promote a sense of safety and cohesiveness. Possible effective interventions include summarization and mild confrontation such as "I notice that Mike seems to be doing most of the talking so far today. Can the rest of you identify with his comments or is there something else to be discussed?" Or, "Sue, I wonder if you noticed that group members are not involved today. It may be best for you to stop speaking because it may be important for you to hear what others are thinking now." If the monopolizing individual is losing touch with reality and exhibiting psychotic behavior, such as responding to hallucinations or describing bizarre delusions, it is best to remove the member from the group and spend individual time with him or her to decrease the anxiety. Of course, this is possible only if there is a co-leader who is available to leave the group with the member. This example speaks to the importance of screening potential group members for cognitive functioning and ability to participate in the group session.

At the opposite end of member participation is the silent group member. A general rule is to allow a person to participate as much or as little as they wish. However, it has also been reported that individuals participating more in the group process make more therapeutic change (Yalom, 2005). Therefore, before intervening, the group leader needs to assess the reasons for the silence. Some members may be afraid of disclosing too much or are fearful of losing their temper or crying. Another may be feeling intimidated by a certain member or may be sulking to have the group attend to them. This may need to be explored individually outside of the group. The leader may also ask the member

---

**TABLE 9-3: ROLES OF GROUP MEMBERS**

| ROLES FOR KEEPING THE GROUP ON TASK AND FOCUSED | ROLES THAT MAINTAIN THE GROUP | ROLES THAT THREATEN CURATIVE FACTORS AND GROUP FUNCTIONING |
|---|---|---|
| • Coordinator who connects ideas and suggestions<br>• Elaborator who expands on ideas discussed<br>• Energizer who encourages group participation and action<br>• Information giver or seeker who offers information or asks the group questions<br>• Opinion giver who offers personal opinions | • Encourager who praises others<br>• Compromiser who gives in during a conflict<br>• Follower who agrees with the group<br>• Harmonizer who works at settling conflicts<br>• Standard setter who verbalizes group standards | • Self-confessor who talks about own issues or feelings that are unrelated to the group discussion<br>• Recognition seeker who attempts to have the group focus on his/her achievements by bragging<br>• Blocker who disagrees with everything<br>• Dominator who works at controlling members by interrupting<br>• Help seeker who seeks group sympathy excessively without concern for other members<br>• Aggressor who criticizes and attacks other group members<br>• Playboy who acts disinterested and bored |

> ### THERAPEUTIC INTERACTION 9-1:
> ### INTERACTION BETWEEN GROUP LEADER (GL) AND DISRUPTIVE GROUP MEMBER
>
> T. is a newly admitted patient who is hypomanic and is attending group for the first time. T. keeps disrupting the group by monopolizing the conversation.

| | |
|---|---|
| **GL:** "T., thank you for sharing but let us hear from someone else now." | Setting limits |
| **T.:** "But I am not finished talking. I have lots more to say and what I have to say is more important than what they have to say." | Intrusive and grandiose statements |
| **GL:** "It is also important for you to listen in group because you can learn something from other group members that may help you with your problem." | Trying to help the patient maintain proper behavior in group setting and also to explain purpose |
| **T.:** "Can I have another turn talking later?" | Testing the boundaries and limits established by the GL |
| **GL:** "If we have time today you can talk again; if not, you can attend tomorrow and talk more about what is going on with you. C., I see you have your hand raised; let's hear from you." | Continuing to set limits in a kind but firm matter-of-fact manner<br><br>Facilitating group process by calling on another patient to share |

to respond to comments about body language or questions such as, "What is the best question to ask today to bring you into group involvement?" Or, "Is this a meeting where you are going to need prodding?" "How did that question make you feel?" It is important to remember that silence in itself is communication. **How Would You Respond? 9-2** provides a practical example of a group session and the roles assumed by the group members.

> *Group members can assume roles that keep the group on task and focused, that maintain the group, and that threaten curative factors and group functioning.*

## Examples of Group Therapy

As described earlier in the chapter, various types of groups can develop. The basic structure for a lower functioning in-patient therapy group was presented by Yalom (1983). The basic plan of a session is: 2–5 minutes of orientation, 5–10 minutes of warm-up, 20–30 minutes of a structured exercise, and 5–10 minutes of session review.

- Orientation involves providing the names of the leader, co-leader, and each member; the purpose of the session; the length of the session; and the rules. Rules may include such information as only one person speaks at a time or each member must stay for entire group.
- Warm-up may involve a brief physical activity such as a ring toss, muscle relaxation exercise, or an easy chair yoga or breathing exercises.
- Structured activity may include items such as sentence completion (**Box 9-2**), an art project such as creating a collage from magazine pictures on any topic, creating a painting using a piece of newspaper covered with tempera paint brush strokes followed by the group naming the painting, reading of a poem followed by discussion of the meaning and reactions to the poem, or writing poems using a template (Leedy, 1973).

• Session review follows the activity in which there is a discussion focused on impressions of the session—"What did you like or dislike about this session? What surprised you in this session?"

It is important to remember that as the functioning level of group members decreases, structure and leader activity increase.

Another type of group frequently led by nursing generalists is psychoeducational groups. These groups focus on topics such as medications or a specific diagnosis. Information usually is provided in the form of handouts or videos followed by general discussion of the content. Psychoeducational groups are more than just the leader simply providing information. The discussion must involve activation of curative factors.

> *A psychoeducational group is one example of a group led by psychiatric-mental health nurses prepared at the basic (generalist) level.*

## FAMILY PSYCHOTHERAPY

**FAMILY THERAPY** can be defined as insight-oriented therapy with the goal of altering interactions between or among family members, thus improving the functioning of the family as a unit or any individual within the family.

### HOW WOULD YOU RESPOND? 9-2: NURSE-LED STRESS MANAGEMENT GROUP

This is the third meeting of a group of seven women who had bariatric surgery about 6 months ago. They have all lost large amounts of weight, but are having difficulty coping with stress in their lives without overeating. The purpose of this 8-week, closed, outpatient group is to identify alternate ways of coping with stress. The group is in the working phase. Each session lasts 90 minutes and meets weekly.

First, the nurse leader asks if there are any comments about the previous session, then sets the agenda for the session—exploring situations, thoughts, and feelings that trigger overeating. Mary begins by describing the birthday party yesterday where she overate. Then Cindy states she also had a similar experience with her family. Next, Susan looks at Cindy and states that she just gets the urge to eat and is not aware of what preceeds that. Then Susan asks the leader why it is important to understand

this; she simply measures her food and refuses to eat more because she doesn't want to gain weight back. The group leader refers the question back to the group, "What does everyone else think about that?" Mary looks at Susan and begins to explain her thinking, then Rose and Gerri also respond. Susan looks irritated and states that she is not going to change anything because measuring food is working. Lexus and Ali are looking at the floor and not speaking. The leader looks around the group and states, "It takes a lot of courage to make such a change as to have bariatric surgery and it seems like the adjustments after the surgery are also challenging. What does the group think about Susan's comment?" Ali speaks next, stating that not everyone agrees that we are courageous, some people think it is the "lazy way to lose weight." Then Lexus agrees and provides some examples of comments made to her.

### CRITICAL THINKING QUESTIONS

Refer to Figure 9-2, the Interaction Chronogram, to answer the following questions:

1. Would you classify this group as insight oriented or supportive?

2. What role did each member play in this session segment?

3. What curative factors may be active in this session?

👍 **APPLYING THE CONCEPTS**

This would be considered an insight-oriented group for several reasons. First, there was not a lecture or presentation by the facilitator. The general agenda was set and then opened to the group for discussion. The purpose was to have the group discuss their own situations and then, by group interaction, identify triggers and feelings. As the group continued, the focus shifted more from information to feelings and the leader respected and encouraged that direction of discussion.

There was movement among multiple roles in this session, with the majority facilitating curative factors. The nurse leader was in the role of facilitator and agenda setter. Initially, two members were in roles that interfered with building curative factors. Both Ali and Lexus were silent and avoidant, but later moved into roles of information providers. The other group members moved among several roles which facilitated development of curative factors. These included the role of elaborator by expanding on each other's comments, information giver and seeker, follower by agreeing with comments, and opinion giver. At one point, there was almost a conflict, with Susan taking the role of blocker by questioning the importance of the discussion. This was countered by Mary, Rose, and Gerri assuming the roles of harmonizers and then Susan as the compromiser.

The curative factors most likely present in this session would include catharsis and imparting information, interpersonal learning, development of socialization techniques, cohesiveness, and universality. Although there is overlap among these factors, each factor can be identified in this group. Several group members shared information and expressed their feelings (catharsis). During this sharing, there was agreement among most members and a sense of experiencing the same difficulties (we are not alone), which is cohesiveness and universality. During this process, individuals listened, watched, and interacted appropriately, indicating the learning of socialization techniques. There was also most likely general existential factors indicated by participants "enjoying" the group as well as instillation of hope that there are additional strategies available and they are not hopeless.

---

The family is viewed as the patient. At one time, the term family referred only to those relationships of blood, marriage, or adoption. However, the wide-ranging family configurations of today have led to much broader definitions of what constitutes a family.

Family therapy is considered a specialized type of group therapy based on the understanding that the family has a multigenerational history and patterns of interacting already in place. Family members may or may not live together but depend upon each other for physical and emotional well-being. **Box 9-3** lists the characteristics of optimal family functioning. The family is a natural system, not one created specifically for a period of time to address with therapy.

of a larger community system. Thus, a change in one system impacts all of the other components.

Family therapy aims to reduce pathological conflict and anxiety, to promote the abilities of individuals and the family as a whole to cope with destructive forces within the environment, and to promote integration into society, extended family, and the community. Many models of family therapy exist and the approach used depends upon the training, environment, and personality of the therapist and family. Combinations of theories have been discussed as one way of understanding both the individual and the family simultaneously. An overview of Bowen Family Systems is provided as the framework for understanding families.

## Models of Family Therapy

Models of family therapy commonly view families as open systems comprised of individual members interacting within the family system and within the environment. Within the family system are various subsystems, such as the parental subsystem, parent-child subsystem, and sibling subsystems. The family also is considered a subsystem

> *Family therapy is a specialized form of group therapy that focuses on the family as an open system to alter the interactions between or among members.*

---

**Q BOX 9-2: EXAMPLES OF SENTENCE COMPLETION ACTIVITIES**

*Examples of sentence completion may include sentences encouraging self disclosure:*

One thing people would be surprised to know about me is _____. *or*

One thing I really enjoy is _____.

Someone I really miss is _____.

I handle separation by _____.

The last time I was angry was _____.

What really irritates me is _____.

*Other types of sentence completion may include a focus upon change, such as:*

One thing I really want to change about myself is _____.

Two things I like about myself and do not want to change are _____.

The reason it is hard for me to change is _____.

These completed sentences can then be discussed and elaborated on in the whole group or in pairs first and then summarized in the whole group. Group leaders may pair up with members who are having a hard time with the activity or the leaders may roam around the room checking on each pair's discussion.

---

**Q BOX 9-3: OPTIMAL FAMILY FUNCTIONING**

- Open, trusting relationships
- High respect for individuality and autonomy
- Open, clear, honest communication
- Parental coalition with shared power
- Flexible rules
- Spontaneous interaction with use of humor
- High levels of initiative as opposed to passivity
- Uniqueness and differences encouraged and appreciated

*From Walsh, F. (2003). Normal Family Processes. New York: Guilford Press.*

## Bowen Family Systems

Bowen (1978) described several concepts important to family functioning. A person's level of differentiation or ability to be his or her true self within family pressures and expectations is a key concept. Differentiation of self involves the ability to remain emotionally present, engaged, and nonreactive in emotionally charged situations, while also expressing one's own goals, values, and principles. This must be accomplished without expecting others to change. If differentiation of self is low, anxiety and symptoms are high. In response to intense anxiety, families make decisions based on emotions, not logical thinking. Throughout family therapy, the therapist uses a logical, somewhat distant approach, attempting to balance logic and emotion. In other words, a decrease in emotional reactivity about family issues leads to more logical thinking and higher levels of differentiation.

Increasing differentiation of self also requires an understanding of emotional triangles and multigenerational transmission of anxiety. The concept of emotional triangles involves a three-party system, where two of the members are close with resultant exclusion of a third person. There are multiple, shifting triangles in every family. The triangle functions to decrease anxiety by sharing the emotional load. For example, if there is excessive conflict between a husband and wife, the wife may pull in a child and focus most of her attention on childcare. The husband then becomes the outsider and focuses upon work. Although anxiety may be relieved, the conflict is not resolved.

Bowen also believed that patterns of interaction are transmitted from one generation to the next. Thus a family's ways of dealing or coping with conflicts, their attitudes, beliefs, conflicts, and emotional processes can be traced from parents to children over several generations. One method useful in evaluating multigenerational transmission of anxiety is a genogram.

> *Key concepts associated with the Bowen Family Systems include: differentiation of self, emotional triangles, and multigenerational transmission of anxiety.*

## Genogram

A **GENOGRAM** is a tool developed to show a map of the multigenerational family structure and process. This family history tool is invaluable, especially for those with psychiatric-mental health disorders, in light of the increased understanding of genetics. The genogram can concisely record important information about family history (McGuinness, Noonan, & Dyer, 2009).

Genograms were first developed by Bowen. He used them to assist family therapy trainees in understanding their own families and functioning patterns.

Constructing a genogram involves specific steps and is described in great detail by McGoldrick, Gerson, and Shellenberger (1999). The backbone of the genogram is the representation of how different family members are related to one another from one generation to another. Specific symbols are used to depict these relationships (**Table 9-4**).

Genograms may be drawn by hand or computer generated with special software that can be purchased online. When done by hand, the paper is divided into thirds horizontally for a three-generation family history. Typically, the genogram begins on the left with the husband. As much or as little detail may be included.

The first step in constructing a genogram is to ask questions to obtain the basic facts about the family, such as names, births, marriages, deaths, and birth order of children. Then additional information is collected based on the purpose of the family history. For example, a patient, Mary, was having difficulty understanding the reasons for developing a serious mental illness and feeling so different from her family. By obtaining a three-generation family history and drawing a genogram indicating health problems, the family history of mental illness becomes clearer (**Figure 9-3**). Thus, a map of health problems in Mary's family is depicted for three generations.

The genogram can be expanded with other facts as well as symbols to indicate relationships, such as very close, conflicted, distant, or estranged or cutoff (McGoldrick, Gerson, and Shellenberger, 1999). Consider your own family and create a personal three-generational family genogram with as much or as little information available.

## THE INTERPERSONAL PROCESS AND GROUP AND FAMILY THERAPY

The interpersonal process is key to group and family therapy. Throughout, there is a need for the development of trust with a focus on the family's needs. Additionally, the phases of group development parallel those of the interpersonal process. This correlation is highlighted in **Table 9-5**.

Nurses who lead groups have informally recognized the effectiveness of group work. Recently, there have been more structured evaluations such as meta-analysis. For example, McDermut, Miller, and Brown (2001) provided a review of studies examining the effectiveness of group psychotherapy for the treatment of depression. Group treatment was found to be as effective as individual therapy in 75% of the studies and more effective in the remaining 25%. **Evidence-Based Practice 9-1** highlights this research involving group therapy.

As an adjunctive treatment for schizophrenia, group therapy has been successful in reducing social isolation and improving adaptive coping strategies (Kapur, 1993). However, group therapy is rarely available for this population due to the growing trend of "medication management" of individuals with long-term mental illness, rather than therapy in the community. (More detailed discussion about treatments can be found in later chapters on specific psychiatric-mental health disorders.)

There are several similarities involved in interpersonal therapy and group therapy. During the working and resolution phases of the interpersonal relationship and during the working and termination phases of group therapy, evaluation occurs. Group leaders can evaluate the group by asking members specific questions. These may include: "How do you think the group is going?" "What was important to you in today's group?" "Was there something you wanted to discuss that was not covered?" "Have you noticed any differences in how you feel about yourself or in your relationships?" This ongoing feedback not only provides information on group effectiveness but also direction for shifts in the group planning and content.

This evaluation process usually reveals that change takes place at different rates in each individual. Some group members enter the group ready to change and change feelings about themselves, their environments, and how they relate to others. For example, a woman who has been depressed decides to end an abusive relationship. Others listen and take information in but do not change. Some may develop an understanding of their problems and plan to change but do not do so for many months or even years. The readiness and timing of change varies across individuals.

**TABLE 9-4: GENOGRAM SYMBOLS**

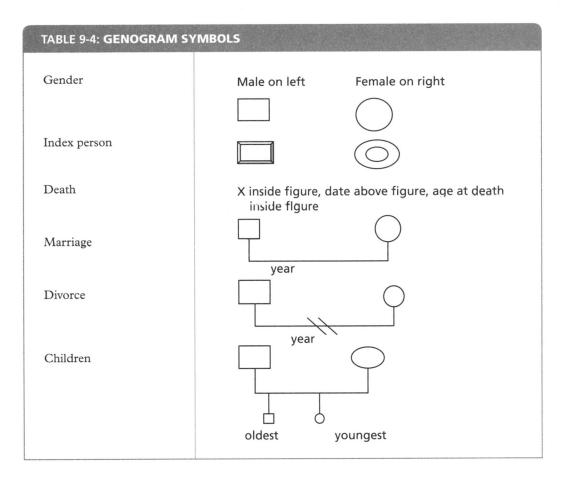

Integrating both group and individual therapy may be appropriate for a patient. The therapist is usually the same for both individual and group. Flexibility in planning treatment is a vital component for effectiveness.

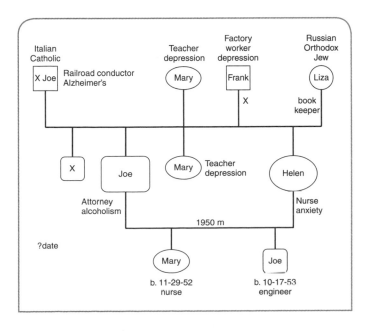

Figure 9–3 *A family genogram.*

Group therapy provides a range of individuals for interpersonal learning and holds the potential to work through family influences in the microcosm of the group. Other advantages include cost effectiveness and the ability to provide treatment to more patients in the same time period. Of course, there are disadvantages of group therapy, including possible breeches of confidentiality and group leaders lacking skills to facilitate the curative factors.

Although family psychotherapy is not within the scope of practice for undergraduate nurses, an awareness of family dynamics is important for all levels of psychiatric-mental health nursing. At the undergraduate level, the family is seen as the context or environment for the individual. Using this awareness, nurses can provide support and education to families formally and informally. One example of a family group is a psycho-education group. For example, the nurse would meet with several families who have a member experiencing depression. During the psychoeducation group, the nurse would provide information about depression, treatment options, and strategies for coping along with the consequences of the illness. This could then be followed by an open discussion among family members about what they have learned.

## TABLE 9-5: COMPARISON OF INTERPERSONAL PROCESS AND GROUP PSYCHOTHERAPY

| | PEPLAU INTERPERSONAL THERAPY | YALOM GROUP PSYCHOTHERAPY |
|---|---|---|
| Patient addressed | Individual | Group |
| Goals | Decreased anxiety<br>Self-maintenance | Creation and maintenance of curative factors |
| Phases of development | Orientation, identification, exploitation, resolution | Orientation, work, termination |
| Explanation of anxiety during therapy | Due to unmet needs | Inevitable experience during initial stages of group formation |
| Role of nurse | To manage the nurse-patient relationship | To facilitate curative factors in group process |
| Diagnostic process | First step in understanding patient | Behavior in group is important, not diagnosis |

### EVIDENCE-BASED PRACTICE 9-1: GROUP THERAPY FOR DEPRESSION

#### STUDY

McDermut, W., Miller, I., & Brown, R. (2001). The efficacy of group psychotherapy for depression: A meta-analysis and review of empirical research. *Clinical Psychology: Science and Practice, 8,* 98–116.

#### SUMMARY

The researchers examined studies published in the English language from 1970 to 1998, selecting studies that tested the efficacy of group therapy for depressive disorders, used well-known self-report or interviewer-based measures of depression and reported pre-treatment and post-treatment scores on depression tools for the participants. They examined 48 studies, collecting information on diagnostic criteria, inclusion and exclusion criteria, depression measures, and results. Forty-five of the 48 studies reported that group psychotherapy was effective for reducing depressive symptoms. Forty-three studies showed statistically significant decreases in depressive symptoms for those receiving group psychotherapy; two of the studies did not report statistical analyses.

#### APPLICATION TO PRACTICE

Group therapy is a valid and effective intervention for patients with depression. Based on this knowledge, nurses can advocate for this treatment when their patients are experiencing depression. The sharing in group therapy can help to foster positive coping strategies. Additionally, nurses can apply the concepts of group therapy when conducting psychoeducational groups for patients with depression, thereby strengthening the interpersonal relationship.

#### QUESTIONS TO PONDER

1. *What issues might arise related to group roles during group therapy for patients with depression?*
2. *Which of Yalom's 11 curative factors would be most important when engaged in a psychoeducational group focusing on medication therapy for patients with depression?*

**SUMMARY POINTS**

- A system is a group of components related sufficiently to identify patterns of interaction such that a change in any component leads to a change in one or more of the other components and in the system as a whole.

- In an open system, the components interact with the environment and with each other, making the system dynamic and ever-changing. The components in a closed system are isolated from the environment.

- Systems thinking in nursing can be traced back to Florence Nightingale who identified the need for creating the appropriate environment for the patient. Betty Neuman applied systems theory to her model, identifying the person as interacting with the internal and external environment. Neuman viewed the patient as a unique system composed of factors and characteristics.

- Applying systems theory or systems thinking in psychiatric-mental health nursing encourages psychiatric-mental health nurses to look at the bigger picture, thereby promoting comprehensive, holistic care.

- A group is any collection of two or more individuals who are interdependent and share at least one commonality or goal. Applying systems theory, a group is a set of components that work together to achieve a function or purpose.

- Groups may be formal or informal. Other classifications include: open or closed (based on membership), therapeutic insight-oriented or supportive (based on purpose), or in-patient or out-patient (based on setting).

- Group process refers to the interaction among group members; group dynamics refers to the forces that produce the patterns within the group as the group moves toward its goals.

- All groups share common factors called curative factors. These factors include: instillation of hope; universality; imparting of information; altruism; corrective recapitulation of the primary family group; development of socialization techniques; imitative behavior; interpersonal learning; group cohesiveness; catharsis; and existential factors.

- Group development occurs through phases that are similar to those in the nurse-patient relationship. The phases of group development are: orientation, working, and termination.

- The group leader or facilitator plays an important role in promoting the effectiveness of the group. The role shifts with the purpose of the group and the phase of the group's development.

- The role of group members can be divided into three categories: roles that keep the group on task and focused; roles that maintain the group; and roles that threaten curative factors and group functioning.

- Family psychotherapy is a specialized form of group therapy. It is an insight-oriented therapy with the goal of altering interactions between or among family members to improve the functioning of the family as a unit or any individual within the family.

- Many models of family therapy exist. One model, the Bowen Family Systems Model, addresses concepts important to family function: differentiation of self, emotional triangles, and multigenerational transmission of anxiety.

- A genogram is a tool that can be created to show a map of multigenerational family structure and process. Through the use of symbols, it depicts the relationships

*(cont.)*

## SUMMARY POINTS (*CONT.*)

among different family members from one generation to another.

• Change occurs at varying rates in each individual and each group. Evaluation of the patient's

perception during group therapy is important to encourage patient involvement and influence the direction of the group sessions.

## NCLEX-PREP*

1. A group of nursing students are reviewing information about systems theory. The students demonstrate the need for additional review when they identify which of the following?

   a. The interactions of a system are viewed in a linear fashion.
   b. The parts of a closed system are isolated from the environment.
   c. A change in one component affects other components.
   d. An open system is dynamic and constantly changing.

2. A nursing instructor is preparing a teaching plan for a class about nursing theories. Which of the following would the instructor include when describing the Neuman Systems Model?

   a. The person is an energy field continually interacting with the environment.
   b. Each patient has a central core that includes survival factors common to all.
   c. A proper environment is necessary to promote the patient's reparative powers.
   d. The nurse and patient engage in an interpersonal process to reach a desired goal.

3. A psychiatric-mental health nurse is a member of several groups. Which of the following would be considered an informal group?

   a. Treatment team
   b. Specialty nursing association
   c. Friends from work
   d. Nurses working on the unit

4. A group is in the orientation phase of development. The group facilitator would be involved with which of the following?

   a. Keeping the group on task
   b. Clarifying what is happening in the group
   c. Reviewing group accomplishments
   d. Describing group expectations

5. During a group session, the group leader notices that a member is boasting about his accomplishments in an effort to get the group to focus on him rather than focus on the task of the group. The leader would identify this behavior as reflecting which role?

   a. Encourager
   b. Energizer
   c. Recognition seeker
   d. Standard setter

6. During a group session, a member states that she feels embarrassed about being arrested for trying to steal clothing from a department store. Several other group members then share similar feelings about their involvement with law enforcement, which then leads to a discussion about thinking about consequences and learning from the experience.
The leader interprets this interaction as reflecting which curative factor?

   a. Instillation of hope
   b. Universality
   c. Altruism
   d. Imitative behavior

(*cont.*)

**NCLEX-PREP\* (CONT.)**

7. A mother and her adult daughter are experiencing a conflict. As a result, the mother turns to her sister and focuses her attention on her. The adult daughter then begins to focus on her work role. Applying the Bowen Family Systems Model, which of the following is present?

a. Differentiation of self
b. Emotional triangle
c. Multigenerational transmission
d. Corrective recapitulation of the primary family group

\*Answers to these questions appear on page 639.

## REFERENCES

Alloy, L., Abramson, L., & Chiara, M. (2000). On the mechanisms by which optimism promotes positive mental and physical health. In J. Gillham (Ed.), *The Science of Optimism and Hope*. Philadelphia: Templeton Foundation Press.

American Group Psychotherapy Association (2007). Practice guidelines for group psychotherapy. http://www.agpa.org/guidelines/groupprocess.html (accessed 1/22/2011).

Benne, K., & Sheats, P. (1948). Functional roles of group members. *Journal of Social Issues*, 4(2), 41.

Bowen, M. (1978). *Family therapy in clinical practice*. New York: Jason Aronson.

Cox, M. (1973). The group therapy interaction chronogram. *British Journal of Social Work*, 3, 243–256.

Fawcett, J. (1984). *Analysis and evaluation of conceptual models of nursing*. Philadelphia: F.A. Davis.

Forchuk, C., & Dorsay, J. (1995). Hildegard Peplau meets family systems nursing: Innovation in theory-based practice. *Journal of Advanced Nursing*, 21, 110–115.

Griffiths, K., Farrer, I.., & Christensen, H. (2010). Efficacy of internet interventions for depression and anxiety disorders: A review of randomized controlled trials. *Medical Journal of Australia*, 92 (11 Supplement), s4–11.

Hsiao, F., Lin, S., Liao, H., & Lai, M. (2004). Chinese inpatients' subjective experience of the helping process as viewed through examination of a nurses' focused, structured therapy group. *Journal of Clinical Nursing*, 13(7), 886–94.

Kapur, R. (1993). The effects of group interventions with the severely mentally ill. *Group Analysis*, 26(4), 339–351.

Kavanagh, K., Duncan-McConnell, D., Greenwood, K., Trivedi, P., & Wykes, T. (2003). Educating acute inpatients about medication: Is it worth it? An exploratory study of group education on a psychiatric intensive care unit. *Journal of Mental Health*, 12(1), 71–80.

Kuhn, T. (1996). *The Structure of Scientific Revolutions* (3rd ed). Chicago: University of Chicago Press.

Lazarus, R., & Folkman, S. (1984). *Stress, Appraisal and Coping*. New York: Springer.

Leedy, J. (1973). Poetry therapy: The use of poetry in the treatment of emotional disorders. Philadelphia: Lippincott.

McDermut, W., Miller, I., & Brown, R. (2001). The efficacy of group psychotherapy for depression: A metaanalysis and review of empirical research. *Clinical Psychology: Science and Practice*, 8, 98–116.

McGuinness, T., Noonan, P., & Dyer, J. (2009). Family history as a tool for psychiatric nurses. *Archives of Psychiatric Nursing*, 19(3), 116–124.

McGoldrick, M., Gerson, R., & Shellenberger, S. (1999). *Genograms in family assessment*. New York: W.W. Norton.

Moyer, A., Sohl, S., Oliver, S., & Schneider, S. (2009). Characteristics and methodological quality of 25 years of research investigating psychosocial interventions for cancer. *Cancer Treatment*, 35(5), 475–484.

Neuman, B. (2002). The Neuman systems model. In B. Neuman and J. Fawcett (Eds)., *The Neuman Systems Model* (4th ed.). Upper Saddle River, NJ: Prentice-Hall.

Nightingale, F. (1969). *Notes on nursing: What it is and is not*. New York: Dover (Originally published, 1859).

O'Donald, A., & O'Mahoney, J. (2009). Service users experience of a therapeutic group program in an acute psychiatric inpatient unit. *Journal of Psychiatric and Mental Health Nursing*, 16(6), 323–330.

Puskar, K., McClure, E., & McGinniss, K. (2007). Advanced practice nurses' role in alcohol abuse group therapy. *Australian Journal of Nursing*, 25(1), 64–9.

Reed, P., & Zurakowski, T. (1996). Nightingale: Foundations of nursing. In J. Fitzpatrick & A. Whall (Eds.), *Conceptual models of nursing: Analysis and application* (3d ed). Stamford, CT: Appleton and Lange.

Rogers, M.E. (1970). *The theoretical basis of nursing*. Philadelphia: F.A. Davis.

Rogers, M.E. (1992). Nursing science and the space age. *Nursing Science Quarterly*, 27–34.

Seligman, M. (1998). *Learner Optimism*. NY: Knopf, Inc.

Tusaie, K., & Patterson, K. (2006). Relationships among trait, situational, and comparative optimism: Clarifying concepts for a theory and evidence-based intervention to maximize resilience. *Archives of Psychiatric Nursing*, 20(3), 144–150.

Van Stratten, A., Cuijpers, P., & Smits, N. (2008). Web-based self-help for symptoms of depression, anxiety, and stress. *Journal of Internet Research*, 10(1), e7.

Von Bertalanffy, L. (1968). *General Systems Theory: Foundations, Developments, Applications*. New York: Braziller.

Walsh, F. (2003). *Normal Family Processes*. New York: Guilford Press.

Yalom, I. (1983). *Inpatient Group Psychotherapy*. New York: Basic Books.

Yalom, I. (2005). *The Theory and Practice of Group Psychotherapy*. 5th ed. NY: Basic Books.

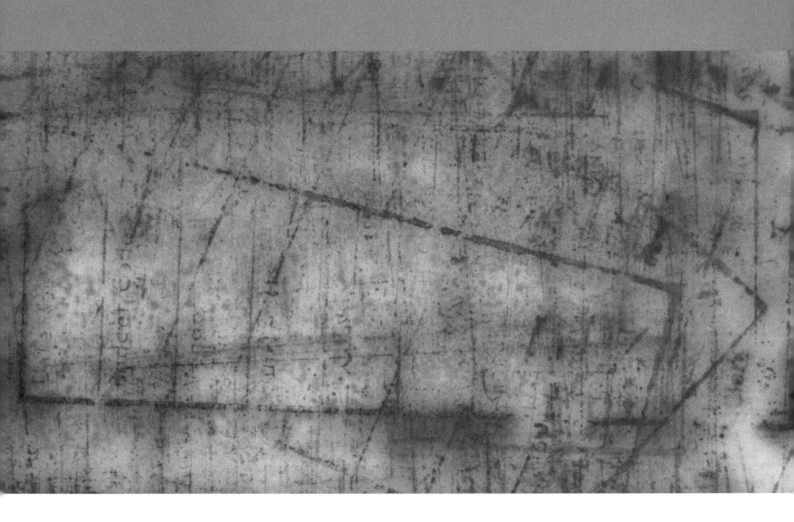

## CHAPTER CONTENTS

Mental Illness

Theories and mental illness

## EXPECTED LEARNING OUTCOMES

**After completing this chapter, the student will be able to:**

1. Describe how the definitions of mental illness have developed through the years.
2. Discuss the different disciplinary perspectives of mental illness.
3. Define six major grand theories used to explain mental health and illness.
4. Identify the major theorists associated with the psychodynamic, behavioral, cognitive, social, humanistic, and biological theories of mental health and illness.

## CHAPTER 10

# THEORIES OF MENTAL HEALTH AND ILLNESS: PSYCHODYNAMIC, SOCIAL, COGNITIVE, BEHAVIORAL, HUMANISTIC, AND BIOLOGICAL INFLUENCES

Patti Hart O'Regan

5. Discuss the concepts or beliefs of one theorist associated with the psychodynamic, behavioral, cognitive, social, and humanistic theories of mental health and illness.

6. Explain the current areas of research reflecting biological psychology theory.

## KEY TERMS

Behavioral psychology theory

Biological psychology theory

Classical conditioning

Cognitive dissonance

Cognitive psychology theory

Ego defense mechanisms

Gestalt

Grand theories

Humanistic psychology theory

Mental illness

Micro-level theories

Middle-range theories

Operant conditioning

Psychodynamic theory

Self-efficacy

Social psychological theory

Systematic desensitization

Theory

Psychiatric-mental health nurses (PMHNs) need to have a comprehensive knowledge foundation about mental illness and the theoretical underpinnings associated with it. Definitions of theory, theories of mental health, and theories of mental illness abound. The variation in these definitions is often contingent upon the disciplinary perspective. Presently, theory development in psychiatric-mental health and mental illness is undergoing extensive change, and the implications for psychiatric-mental health nursing practice are many. The PMHN needs a firm grasp of theoretical understandings, evidence-based research, and clinical practice standards, to provide PMHNs and other psychiatric-mental health professionals a basis for developing appropriate interventions for and with patients diagnosed with psychiatric-mental health disorders. These theoretical, epidemiological, translational research and clinical practice outcomes,' together with the clinical knowledge garnered through the interpersonal relationship that the nurse has developed with the patient, provide a foundation for an efficacious, patient-centered therapeutic intervention.

This chapter provides an overview of various prominent theories of mental illness. The work of influential theorists, researchers, and practitioners from several disciplines, including but not limited to nursing, medicine, and psychology, is described. Theoretical concepts and explanations of the potential etiology of mental illness from within the framework of psychodynamic, behavioral, cognitive, social, humanistic, and biological theory also are presented. Pertinent definitions, historical background, epidemiological incidence and prevalence rates, and comparative disease burden (e.g., disability, economic cost) of mental illness also are included.

## MENTAL ILLNESS

The question is: What is mental illness? When asking mental health care providers or when researching mental health care disciplines, the result would reveal a wide variation in the definition of this term. Many mental health professionals would most likely define mental illness based on the *Diagnostic and Statistical Manual of Mental Disorders, Fourth Edition, Text Revision (DSM-IV-TR)*, which is the widely accepted resource for defining mental disorders. Additionally, nursing professionals may use the North American Nursing Diagnosis Association-International (NANDA-I) Definitions and Classification (NANDA-I, 2008) or the International Classification for Nursing Practice (ICNP) taxonomy for nursing-specific definitions that include mental illness.

The first U.S. Surgeon General's report on mental health and illness—*Mental Health: A Report of the Surgeon General* (U.S. Department of Health and Human Services [DHHS],

1999)—defined MENTAL ILLNESS as mental disorders that are diagnosable conditions characterized by abnormalities in cognition, emotion, or mood, or the highest integrative aspects of behavior, such as social interactions or planning of future activities. This definition is consistent with concepts included in nursing diagnosis classification systems.

> *No one simple definition of mental illness exists. The DMS-IV-TR and NANDA classifications offer widely accepted descriptions of mental illness.*

## Evolution of Thinking About Mental Illness

The mind and mental illness have been subjects of concern, philosophical and theoretical debate, and research for more than two millennia. The quest for knowledge and understanding of the human mind is evident in the writings of early philosophers and scientists such as Aristotle, Descartes, Locke, Hume, and Kant. They explored concepts of the human mind, emotions, thoughts, and behaviors, and how the mind relates to the material or physical body and human condition along the continuum of health. The early philosophical questions included whether a mind actually existed, and if it did, where was it located and was it a force for good or evil? Others asked, if there was a mind, was it separate from or a part of the physical body that could be objectified, would expand with space, and be experienced, and did it contain all the biological senses of sight, hearing, smell, touch, and taste?

An important and enduring question is that of nature versus nurture. Is an individual born with a mind and body that are destined to become the product of its nature, or are there some other internal or external influences that affect how well or poorly the mind and body will perform after the individual is born? These questions continue to be relevant today and remain part of the philosophical and theoretical dialogue and debate among researchers and practitioners. Research and practice based upon mind-body theories of monism (mind and body are of one thing, inseparable), dualism (mind and body are separate entities), interactionism, and positive empiricism that began centuries ago can still be found to lesser or greater degrees in contemporary theories. Questions, debates, theories, and research hypotheses that guided early experimental and empirical research studies are the foundation of what became known as the science of psychology and the art and science of psychiatric-mental health nursing and psychiatric medicine.

Contemporary literature on mental illness is replete with research guided by different theoretical frameworks. However, the theoretical descriptions of the etiology and treatment approaches within these theories differ.

> *Attempts to understand the human mind, body, and behavior can be traced as far back as Aristotle.*

## The Current State of Mental Illness

Comparative data from the 1996 and 2006 Medical Expenditure Panel Survey—Household Component (MEPS-HC), co-sponsored by the Agency for Health Care Research and Quality (AHRQ) and the National Center for Health Statistics (NCHS), indicate that mental disorder was ranked among the top five most costly medical conditions in the U.S. in both 1996 and 2006 (Soni, 2009). That same study revealed that the number of people with a mental disorder had risen from 19.3 million to 36.2 million. In addition, comparison of the time period between 1996 and 2006 demonstrated that mental disorders accounted for the largest increase in expenditure of all medical conditions, rising from $35.2 billion in 1996 (adjusted for inflation) to $57.5 billion in 2006 (Soni, 2009). Mental illness is considered to be epidemic based on recent studies and statistics. For example, prevalence rates and descriptive statistical data reported by the National Institute of Mental Health (NIMH) in 2009 indicate that 26.2% of Americans ages 18 and older suffer from a diagnosable mental disorder in a given year. This would be equivalent to 57.7 million people when applied to 2004 U.S. Census data. In addition, major depression, the most commonly diagnosed mental disorder, is the leading cause of disability in the United States for ages 15 to 44 (NIMH, 2009). Moreover, the Centers for Disease Control and Prevention National Vital Statistics Report (Heron et al., 2009) ranked suicide as the 11th leading cause of death in the United States. Thus, despite existing theory, research, and treatment options, mental illness remains epidemic in the United States and is a major health concern that requires public health initiatives to reduce the magnitude of human suffering and the costs associated with it.

Based on the results of these studies, more questions have come to light:

- How did we get to where we are today?
- Do we really know more about the mind, mental illness, and how to prevent it or alleviate the symptoms and causes of mental illness than our predecessors?
- Why hasn't increased access to and provision of mental health care in the United States, increased standardization of diagnostic criteria using the *DSM-IV -TR*, and increased use of evidenced based practices, particularly involving psychotropic medications, lessened the epidemic of mental illness in the United States?
- Do we have more mental illness in the United States now, or are we better at diagnosing it?
- Are there other influences, such as economic, political, and cultural, or research methodologies that contribute to the increased prevalence statistics of mental illness over time in the United States?

The answers to these questions are not simple. Contemporary literature has a plethora of information; for example, research results stating that there is indeed more scientific information about mental illness etiology, diagnoses, and possible treatments. It is known that economic influences play a role in selecting criteria to be used for diagnosis of mental illnesses. Insurance reimbursement to mental health providers often requires that a patient be diagnosed with a mental disorder that is included in the *DSM-IV-TR* Axis I only, or, to a lesser extent, the *International Classification of Diagnoses (ICD)-10*, which is the British and World Health Organization's (WHO) version of illness classification. However, despite this plethora of information, there is no full disciplinary, interdisciplinary, or subspecialty consensus on the value, validity, or reliability of the understandings of mental illness.

## THEORIES AND MENTAL ILLNESS

There are many definitions of **THEORY** in the literature. Some definitions are highly abstract while others are narrow and reductionistic. According to the American Psychological Association (APA, 2009), a theory is defined as **an** organized set of concepts that explains a phenomenon or set of phenomena. Nurse researchers Im and Meleis defined theory as an organized, coherent, and systematic articulation of a set of statements related to significant questions in a discipline that are communicated in a meaningful whole to describe or explain a phenomenon or set of phenomena (1999). For theory and research to become useful and contribute to the best evidence-based practices and quality outcomes in health care, theory-driven research must:

1. Be applied and outcomes measured in the clinical setting

2. Reciprocally and continuously inform each other, similar to the feedback mechanism of a heat thermostat or that of the hypothalamus-pituitary-adrenal gland stress response feedback mechanism

Mental health and psychology are associated with numerous theories. Theories can be organized into a framework involving their level of abstraction. **GRAND THEORIES**, such as the six that are addressed in this chapter, are the most abstract and broad in scope. **MIDDLE-RANGE THEORIES**, such as self-efficacy theory that is highlighted in Bandura's social cognitive theory later in this chapter, are less abstract (more concrete) than grand theories. The third category of theories is labeled **MICRO-LEVEL THEORIES**, which are the least abstract and narrow in scope (Smith & Liehr, 2003).

> *There are three main types of theory: grand, middle-range, and micro-level.*

Many different schools of thought also are prevalent in mental health and psychology but all share the same commonality—the study of the mind, body, and/or behavior. Six grand theories in mental health and psychology, often used in guiding mental health research, are explored here. They are: (a) psychodynamic theory, (b) behavioral theory, (c) cognitive theory, (d) social theory, (e) humanistic theory, and (f) biological theory. **Box 10-1** defines these six theories.

## Psychodynamic Theories

**PSYCHODYNAMIC THEORIES** focus on the unconscious and assert that underlying unconscious or repressed conflicts are responsible for conflicts, disruptions, and disturbances in behavior and personality. Actions are believed to be motivated by emotions and thoughts. Therefore, to understand and change behavior, a person needs to develop awareness and insight into his or her thoughts and emotions. Psychodynamic theories are based on Sigmund Freud's psychoanalytic theory.

### Sigmund Freud

Freud developed the first psychodynamic theory, called psychoanalytic theory. He is considered the father of psychoanalysis. He identified two major components of the mind: the conscious portion, which includes awareness of events, thoughts, and feelings that can be remembered, and the unconscious portion, which includes thought and feelings that are not accessible to an individual's conscious or

---

**Q BOX 10-1: GRAND THEORIES IN MENTAL HEALTH AND PSYCHOLOGY**

- **BEHAVIORAL PSYCHOLOGY THEORY:** Scientific approach that limits the study of psychology to measurable or observable behavior (APA, 2009).
- **COGNITIVE PSYCHOLOGY THEORY:** The study of higher mental processes such as attention, language use, memory, perception, problem solving, and thinking (APA, 2009).
- **SOCIAL PSYCHOLOGICAL THEORY:** The study of the effect of social variables on individual behavior, attitudes, perceptions, and motives; also includes group and intergroup phenomena (American Psychiatric Association [APA], 2009); social brain (neuro) psychology theory (more specific social psychological theory) as the means for understanding the connection between the mind and body through the study of social influences (understanding the effect of society on the brain that is the seat of emotions and behavior; Cacioppo, 2002).
- **HUMANISTIC PSYCHOLOGY:** A group of psychologies that include early and emerging orientations and perspectives, including Rogerian, existential, transpersonal, phenomenological, hermeneutic, feminist, and other psychologies (APA, 2010).
- **BIOLOGICAL PSYCHOLOGY (OR BIOPSYCHOLOGY) THEORY:** The study of human or animal psychology using a biological approach in order to understand human behavior; involving brain physiology, genetics, and evolution as means for understanding behavior (Wickens, 2005).
- **PSYCHODYNAMIC THEORY:** A psychological model in which behavior is explained in terms of past experiences and motivational forces; actions are viewed as stemming from inherited instincts, biological drives, and attempts to resolve conflicts between personal needs and social requirements (APA, 2009).

subconscious awareness. Freud also described the personality as consisting of three continuously interacting parts: the id, ego, and superego. The id represents the impulsive part of the self based on unconscious drives and primitive instincts. It is based on pleasure and involved with satisfying needs to attain immediate gratification. The superego represents the moral self associated with ethics, standards, and self-criticism. It develops as the individual internalizes values and morals learned from the interaction with parents and other primary caretakers. The ego can be viewed as the mediator between the id and superego, the rational decision maker based in reality and used to reduce tension and anxiety (Carver & Scheier, 2004).

According to Freud, an individual's personality develops over five stages from birth through approximately 20 years of age. Termed the psychosexual phases of personality development, the phases include oral, anal, phallic, latency, and genital. Each phase is associated with a specific developmental task. Failure to achieve the task during any of the first three early childhood psychosexual stages may lead to fixation in that stage, unconscious sexual or aggressive conflicts, and to mental illness.

### TABLE 10-1: FREUD'S DEFENSE MECHANISMS

| DEFENSE MECHANISM | DESCRIPTION | EXAMPLE |
| --- | --- | --- |
| Denial | Refusal to acknowledge a reality or feelings associated with the reality | A person uses cocaine every day but refuses to admit that he has a problem with substance abuse |
| Displacement | Transfer of feelings or a response from one object or person to another less threatening substitute object, person, or activity | A husband who is angry with his wife yells at his son<br>A woman who is upset about her work situation kicks a chair |
| Intellectualization | Use of logic, reasoning, and analysis to avoid expression of actual feelings related to a stressful situation | A woman details specific problems in her work environment as the reason for her being fired rather than verbalizing her upset over losing her job |
| Projection | Attribution of unacceptable feelings, impulses, or thoughts to another | An female adolescent is angry with a close friend but states that the friend is the one who is angry at her |
| Rationalization | Use of incorrect explanations, excuses, or logical reasoning to explain unacceptable thoughts, actions, or feelings | A doctor makes a medication error in prescribing for a terminally ill patient. He thinks, "Why tell anyone? They were going to die anyway" |
| Reaction formation | Exaggeration of thoughts, feelings, or actions that are in direct opposition to those being felt in an attempt to prevent expression of unacceptable or undesirable thoughts, feelings, or behaviors | A religious man who is aroused by sexually explicit images may take on an attitude of criticism toward the topic. He may end up sacrificing many of the positive things in his life, including family relationships, by traveling around the country to anti-pornography rallies |
| Regression | Retreat to an earlier stage of development for comfort measures associated with it in response to stress | A 3-year-old child with a new baby brother in the house begins to suck his thumb |
| Repression | Involuntary blocking or removal from conscious awareness of disturbing or unpleasant feelings, thoughts, or experiences | A woman who was raped cannot remember the events of the rape |
| Sublimation | Directing of personally or socially unacceptable feelings and impulses into ones that are constructive | A person with homicidal urges goes to school and becomes a judge and deals with murder trials |
| Suppression | Intentional blocking of disturbing feelings or experiences from one's awareness | A person who is overwhelmed with work responsibilities says, "Tomorrow is another day" |

Freud developed the theory of EGO DEFENSE MECHANISMS, which are conscious and unconscious tools used to protect and defend the ego. The mechanisms are used to reduce anxiety when confronted with conflict between libido energy drives of the id and superego. Psychoanalytic defense mechanisms outlined by Freud include: denial, displacement, intellectualization, projection, rationalization, reaction formation, regression, repression, sublimation, and suppression (**Table 10-1**). Defense mechanisms are used by everyone at times. They can be helpful and healthy, especially when used temporarily over a short time to deal with a conflict. However, excessive use, or overuse of defense mechanisms has the potential to lead to distortion or blurring of reality, leading to inappropriate aggressive or socially unacceptable behaviors or psychosis.

Freud believed that most conflicts originate as a result of sexual aggression or aggression-related, unresolved unconscious conflicts originating during childhood years. These conflicts lead to tension, developmental disruption, and mental illness, particularly anxiety spectrum disorders. Freud's theory is often labeled the "will to pleasure" theory. He developed psychoanalysis as the means to unlock the unconscious and resolve these childhood conflicts.

## Other Psychodynamic Theorists

Alfred Adler and Carl Jung knew and became students of Freud. Adler, Jung, and Viktor Frankl were among the early psychoanalytic leaders. However, each of them branched out from Freud's initial precepts, identifying other theoretical constructs and strategies for understanding etiology and effective treatment of mental health conditions. Additionally, other psychodynamic leaders like Eric Erickson and Karen Horney broke off from traditional Freudian psychoanalytic concepts, veering away from the belief that sexual desires and conflicts in childhood were the major cause of later conflicts and mental illnesses. **Table 10-2** summarizes the major beliefs for each of these theorists.

Although these theorists maintained a largely psychodynamic orientation, each built upon their background in psychoanalytic theory and developed their own new theories. Some of these theorists could be included in more than one category of grand psychological theory, as they incorporated theoretical concepts and constructs from behavioral, social, and/or biological theory into their theories.

Psychoanalysis is conducted one or more times a week over several years. Techniques such as free association (spontaneously saying whatever comes to mind), introspection, and sometimes dream analysis are used to facilitate insight into repressed conflicts. The therapy is

believed to reduce tension and anxiety, resolve conflict, and restore mental health.

> *Psychodynamic theories focus on the unconsciousness involving repressed conflicts. Sigmund Freud developed the first psychodynamic theory called psychoanalytic theory.*

## Behavioral Theories

Behavioral theory, also called behaviorism, assumes that only observable, measurable, and objective criteria are important to understand human behavior and effect behavioral change. It attempts to explain an individual's actions, that is, how a person acts. According to behavioral theory, a person's behavior is the result of learning that has occurred in response to a stimulus. Behavioral theory does not include the concept of the unconscious in explaining mental health and illness.

Ivan Pavlov is credited with discovering the behavioral theory of classical conditioning. Other individuals have been credited with the title, father of behavioral psychology. They include Edward L. Thorndike, John B. Watson, and B.F. Skinner.

> *Behavioral theory proposes that a person's behavior is the result of learning that is a response to a stimulus.*

### Ivan Pavlov

Ivan Pavlov is a Nobel prize–winning physiologist who discovered the phenomenon of associative stimulus-response behavior while studying digestive processes in dogs. He noticed a curious association occurring during his experiments. The dogs in his sample began to salivate before food was placed in their mouths by the assistants. The dogs began drooling (an unconditioned response) at the sight of food or upon hearing the sound of food being prepared (an unconditioned stimulus). These observations led him to conduct experiments to understand these curious, unexplained behaviors. During those

### TABLE 10-2: OTHER PSYCHOANALYTICAL THEORISTS

| THEORIST | MAJOR BELIEFS |
| --- | --- |
| Alfred Adler | "Will to power" theory<br>Conflict between feelings of inferiority and superiority rooted in an infant's dependent role |
| Viktor Frankl | Theory of meaning: "Will to meaning"<br>Later development of an existential form of therapy called logotherapy to help patients survive by learning to attach (positive and purposeful) meaning to their circumstances and give purpose to their lives<br>Major influence on Joyce Travelbee |
| Carl Jung | Concept of individuation<br>Theory of the personal and collective unconscious |
| Erik Erikson | Eight stages of psychosocial development (ego) theory; included some concepts from psychoanalytic theory (e.g., ego development, albeit present from birth as viewed by Erikson versus Freud)<br>1. Trust versus mistrust (birth to 18 months)<br>2. Autonomy versus shame (18 months to 3 years)<br>3. Initiative versus guilt (3–5 years)<br>4. Industry versus inferiority (6–12 years)<br>5. Identity versus role confusion (12–18 years)<br>6. Affiliation and love (18–35 years)<br>7. Generativity versus self-absorption or stagnation (35–55 years)<br>8. Integrity versus despair (age 55 to end of life)<br>Mastery of the tasks—Success or failure to manage the polar conflicts or tasks inherent within each developmental stage is considered a determinant of continued social and psychological growth and mental health.<br>Effect of social experiences, or culture, on development of an individual's personality (enduring patterns of behavior over time), throughout their lifetime |
| Karen Horney | Belief that neurosis was an ongoing process and that the key was in understanding parental indifference toward children<br>Identification of ten neurotic needs; classified into three categories:<br>*Moving Toward People*<br>1. The need for affection and approval; pleasing others and being liked by them<br>2. The need for a partner; one whom they can love and who will solve all problems<br>*Moving Against People*<br>3. The need for power; the ability to bend wills and achieve control over others—while most persons seek strength, the neurotic may be desperate for it<br>4. The need to exploit others; to get the better of them. To become manipulative, fostering the belief that people are there simply to be used<br>5. The need for social recognition; prestige and limelight<br>6. The need for personal admiration; for both inner and outer qualities—to be valued<br>7. The need for personal achievement; though virtually all persons wish to make achievements, as with No. 3, the neurotic may be desperate for achievement<br>*Moving Away From People*<br>8. The need for self sufficiency and independence; while most people desire some autonomy, the neurotic may simply wish to discard other individuals entirely<br>9. The need for perfection; while many people are driven to perfect their lives in the form of well-being, the neurotic may display a fear of being slightly flawed<br>10. The need to restrict life practices to within narrow borders; to live as inconspicuous a life as possible |

experiments, Pavlov discovered that after several trials of ringing a bell (conditioned stimuli) just prior to putting food into the dogs' mouths, the dogs began associating the sound of the bell with food. Subsequently, the dogs began to drool (a conditioned response). Continued experiments revealed that the dogs salivated with just the bell ringing, even without the presence of food. The learned associative behavioral stimulus-response discovered by

Pavlov (1927), called **CLASSICAL CONDITIONING**, was later applied to human learning involved in the etiology and treatment of mental illnesses.

### John B. Watson

John B. Watson, a psychologist and theorist pioneer of radical behaviorism, rejected the existence or influence of the then-dominant psychodynamic theory concepts of "consciousness" and the "mind." Around the same time as Pavlov was conducting his experiments, Watson began to introduce his behavioral theory in the United States. He viewed learning and animal behavior (not differentiating human from other animal behavior) as dependent upon three things—muscles, organs, and glands. Watson also believed that the more often a response to a stimulus occurs (principle of frequency) and the more recently a response is made (recency), the chances are that the response will be repeated.

### Martin Seligman

Several decades following Pavlov's discoveries, Martin Seligman conducted animal lab experiments involving Pavlovian harness restraints and electric shock on canines. He studied the use of conditioned stimulus-response theory related to learning and avoidance behaviors. His findings led to his theory of learned helplessness.

Seligman discovered that the sustained, uncontrollable nature of a negative inescapable event was a factor that interfered with learning. In his experiments, harnessed canines were exposed to a sustained electric shock. The dogs were unable to avoid or escape the shock because they were harnessed. Seligman then conducted additional experiments in which the dogs were exposed to the electric shock but were unharnessed and free to escape or avoid it. His findings revealed that even with the opportunity to avoid the shock, the canines did not try to escape. This led to his theory of "learned helplessness." Later, Seligman adapted his laboratory discoveries to humans by adding the human dimension of attribution of meaning (cognitive explanations) to negative events in a person's life using an optimistic versus pessimistic lens (self-explanation). Seligman's theory of Learned Helplessness, and later his theory of Learned Optimism, propose that prior inescapable negative events, negative cognition, and locus of control are important contributors to depression and anxiety in humans (Abramson, Seligman, & Teasdale, 1978; Beck, Rush, & Shaw et al., 1979; Seligman, 1992). Others have proposed competing theories to that of Seligman's about the relationship between uncontrollable, inescapable, negative events and depression in humans. For example, pathophysiologic events involving changes in neurochemical hormonal balance such as with epinephrine and gamma-aminobutyric acid (GABA) occur during and in response to the inescapable, stressful event, or chronic negative stressor. These, rather than cognitive mediators alone, are important contributors to learning and future behaviors or modulators of behavior in depression (Weiss, Glazer, Pohorecky, Brick, & Miller, 1975).

### Edward L. Thorndike

Edward L. Thorndike discovered the theory of "law of effect" (the effect of consequences on future behaviors) and the behavior modification method of **OPERANT CONDITIONING** (also called instrumental conditioning). Operant conditioning, in contrast to Pavlov's classical conditioning, attends to consequences (or responses) and the modification of future behavior based upon the (positive or negative) reinforcement, punishment, or extinction associated with the consequence (response). Thorndike's discoveries were conducted through experimental studies of cat behavior. Thorndike placed a cat in an enclosed box with open slats on one side and placed a bowl of food outside the box within the cat's view. The cat would repeatedly put their front leg through the slats to reach for the food, finding the food to be out of reach. The cat, by accident, would eventually knock down a lever inside the cage that opened the door of the box. When the door opened, the cat escaped from the box. Thorndike continued to put the cat back in the box under the same conditions numerous times. He observed that initially the cat continued to reach his leg through the slats in the box, trying unsuccessfully to reach the food outside the box. However, with each accidental knocking down of the lever inside and escape from the box, the time spent inside the box before the lever opened the door lessened. After numerous trials, the cat ultimately learned to intentionally hit the lever to escape the box, without food being present outside the box. Escape from the box became the reward for pressing the lever that opened the door from inside the box. Operant conditioning is a process and method for exerting influence over our environment and changing our behavior (or that of others), thus increasing, decreasing, or extinguishing behaviors through the use of rewards and consequences. Operant conditioning has been widely used in educational institutions for decades to assist in promoting student learning and behavioral change (Deutsch & Krauss, 1965).

### B.F. Skinner

B.F. Skinner developed several theories, one of which was "radical behaviorism," another was an operant conditioning chamber. Later known as the Skinner box, this is a laboratory structure for the experimental observation and analysis of animal behavior. He is considered by some to be the father of behavioral therapy. Skinner, like Thorndike, studied operant conditioning, focusing on the external environment and how consequences of those operations modify future behavior. Skinner rejected some of Thorndike's concepts and modified the theory of operant conditioning. Reinforcement or the consequence of the behavior is the key to whether a behavior would be repeated. His theory is reflected in the use of contingency rewards to reinforce or extinguish behaviors in residential institutional settings such as psychiatric hospitals and facilities serving severely mentally retarded people for half a century (Deutsch & Krauss, 1965).

> *Classical and operant conditioning are two key behavioral theories.*

### Joseph Wolpe

Joseph Wolpe developed the (subset) theory and methodology for behavioral change. Wolpe (1958) believed that behavior was learned and that behavior in response to anxiety could be unlearned. Additionally, he believed that the anxiety response inhibits other responses such as relaxation. Thus, if a person could increase the responses that were inhibited due to anxiety, then the anxiety response would diminish. Through a process he called counter-conditioning, individuals were taught relaxation techniques and encouraged to use these techniques while being systematically exposed to the anxiety-producing stimulus. Initially, the individual was exposed to the lowest level stimulus that would produce anxiety. Then gradually, as the person maintained relaxation, the stimulus intensity increased. Ultimately, the individual learned to use relaxation to overcome the stimulus. Wolpe's work is the basis for **SYSTEMATIC DESENSITIZATION**. In systematic desensitization, the subject is gradually introduced to the source of the fear or anxiety over the course of time and under controlled conditions. This methodology is based on Pavlov's theory of classical conditioning (Wolpe, 1976) and has been widely used as a psychotherapeutic tool applicable to office or other settings in the treatment of multiple mental health conditions, particularly with phobias, panic disorders, and other anxiety spectrum disorders.

### Cognitive Theories

Cognitive theories arose out of the need to explain more complex behaviors that could not be explained by observable actions alone. These theories focus on how a person's thinking about a situation or event affects the stimulus and response.

### Aaron Beck

Aaron Beck is known as the founder of cognitive theory and therapy. Later, as a number of behaviorists began incorporating some of Beck's cognitive concepts into behavioral theory and therapy, acclaiming Beck as the father of cognitive behavioral therapy (CBT). Beck began his career as a psychiatrist practicing psychoanalytic theory. Later, he began his systematic research on the influence of a person's cognitions, thoughts, and beliefs on their behavior and in the development and treatment of depression. Cognitive theory and therapy has been used for half a century in the research and treatment of affective disorders such as depression and anxiety, as well as substance abuse and personality disorders (Beck, Rush, Shaw et al., 1979).

Later research and clinical treatment were expanded from affective, personality, and substance abuse disorders to include what are classified as thought disorders, (e.g., schizophrenia, delusional disorders). This continued research led Beck et al. (2008) to develop a theory and framework, using a neurobiopsychosocial model to address thought disorders. They incorporated neurobiological science with cognitive behavioral therapy to reduce thought distortions and psychotic symptoms. Doing so was found to improve emotional, social, and behavioral functioning in people with thought disorders such as schizophrenia. Until the last few years, symptoms of schizophrenia, including psychosis (which includes delusions and/or hallucinations), and negative symptoms such as avolition, alogia, flat affect, anergia, and social isolation, were largely thought to be non-responsive to psychotherapy. These symptoms, which had previously been treated with only psychotropic drugs or psychosocial education and milieu therapy to help patients maintain basic activities of daily living, were found to be reduced with psychotherapy.

### Albert Ellis

Albert Ellis began his career training in psychoanalytical theory and practice. Later, due to observations made through many years of clinical practice, dismissing the need to see patients daily over the course of years to effect change, Ellis developed the cognitive rational-emotive theory and therapy of behavior change (Ellis, 2004). Ellis theorizes an individual's irrational beliefs, attitudes, and faulty thinking create and maintain dysfunctional emotional and behavioral imbalance. Thus, an awareness and changing of irrational beliefs to rational beliefs restores mental health. Ellis's theory assumes that an event (experience), followed by irrational beliefs about the experience and the resultant consequences of those faulty beliefs are the cause of depression, panic, obsessive-compulsive disorder, substance abuse, as well as other mental disorders.

> *Cognitive theories address a person's thinking about an event or situation as having an effect on his or her response to a stimulus (behavior).*

## Social Theories

Social mental health and psychology theorists agree that understanding social, cultural, and other environmental factors is important to understand human behavior. The focus is on how these factors are influenced by or influence individual or group behavior and learning processes. Theories, concepts, and techniques such as classical and operant conditioning, reinforcement theory, insight, genetics, and perception from psychodynamic, behavioral, biological, and cognitive grand theories are used by social psychology theorists. In addition to generating new social learning or psychology theories, concepts, and techniques, social psychology theorists use theory and techniques from multiple grand psychology theories to investigate how people and groups effect or are affected by each other, thereby enhancing the understanding of normal and abnormal behavior. Albert Bandura, Kurt Lewin, Leon Festinger (Lewin's student), Neal Miller, John Dollard, Robert Merton, and Alfred Allport are but a few of the renowned social learning or psychology theorists whose work continues to be cited in contemporary research. Bandura, Lewin, and Festinger are discussed here. Some nurse theorists who synthesized existential or interpersonal theories of mental health could also be included as social mental health and psychology theorists. However, they will be discussed with humanistic theories.

### Albert Bandura

Bandura (1963, 1966, 1997) developed social cognitive theory, which assumes that human beings influence and are influenced by their environment, and that a reciprocal relationship between an individual and their social environment exists. Bandura labeled this concept as reciprocal determinism. Bandura's theory is still often categorized as a social psychology or social learning theory despite Bandura having changed the title of his theory to social cognitive

theory after recognizing the important reciprocal influence of personal (cognitive, affective, and biological), behavioral, and environmental events. According to Bandura, the ability of humans to change their behaviors and interactions in their social environment can be influenced by observing others' behaviors and selecting those observed behaviors they believe they can and want to change in themselves. This is what Bandura describes as imitating and selecting new behaviors observed in other humans or caricatures. This process and concept is called behavior modeling.

Behavioral modeling is influenced by **SELF-EFFICACY**. Bandura (1977) began introducing the construct of self-efficacy in mid-1970, later integrating his middle-range theory of self-efficacy as a main component of social cognitive theory. Self-efficacy involves the beliefs people hold about their ability to accomplish something and their belief about what the outcomes will be.

Bandura's model has been studied extensively and used to help persons diagnosed with depression, anxiety, substance abuse, and personality disorders. Additionally, Bandura studied the relationship between adolescents' experience of vicarious violence, including watching violence on TV or observing adults modeling aggressive or non-aggressive behavior, and subsequent rewarding of each type of behavior. Bandura's study showed that children who watched more violence on TV are more aggressive as adults and that those children who watched adult role models discouraging aggressive behaviors exhibited less aggressive behavior as adults.

### Kurt Lewin

Kurt Lewin is viewed by some as the father of social psychology due to his early work in utilizing the scientific and experimental methods in the study of human social behavior. Lewin developed field and valence theory and the concepts of stages of group dynamics, sensitivity training, and action research (Deutsch & Krauss, 1965; Lewin, 1951; Sansone, Morf, & Panter, 2004). Lewin, like many social psychologists, viewed the interaction of a person's situational environment combined with their personality or past learning experience, and strength and weakness of motivation as critical mediators of behavior. His theory is helpful in understanding a person's motivation for changing behavior.

> *Social theories focus on understanding the influences of and interaction between the environment, cognition, and a person's behavior.*

## Leon Festinger

Leon Festinger (1962, 1964; Deutsch & Krauss, 1965), a student of Kurt Lewin, is credited with the development of cognitive dissonance theory, an extension of Festinger's theory of social comparison. COGNITIVE DISSONANCE refers to the inability of the human mind to contain two disparate, conflicting thoughts or beliefs simultaneously. It also includes the process of how a person will engage in rationalization, change their beliefs or behavior to eliminate the tension or imbalance associated with cognitive dissonance, and restore cognitive or mental balance. For example, a person is having chest pains and believes that he or she may be having a heart attack and needs to go to the local hospital for medical help. Simultaneously, the person believes that the local hospital provides very poor care and that he or she may be harmed by the poor care. Thus, a state of cognitive dissonance could arise. In the above scenario, the person will make a decision, changing one of the two disparate beliefs or intended behaviors, to reduce cognitive dissonance and restore cognitive balance: The person might decide to go to a different hospital where he or she believes that no harm would result, or might rationalize the severity and meaning of the chest pain, thus changing the belief about the pain. For example, the person might believe that the chest pain was indigestion, thereby dismissing the potential urgency and waiting to see if the symptoms lessen or stop over the next few hours. In doing so, the person would not go to the hospital.

## Humanistic Theories

Humanism, as related to humanist mental health and psychological theory, is considered to have emerged in the early 1950s. The belief was developed by those who were not content with the existing psychoanalytic and behavioral theories and concepts. Social, cognitive, and existential mental health and illness theorists are many times included under the rubric of cognitive, social, and/ or humanistic mental health grand theory. Existential, phenomenological, and interpersonal humanistic mental health theory and practice became prominent humanistic perspectives and orientations.

Humanistic theory moved traditional concepts of mental health and illness from a focus on illness, determinism, the unconscious, and reductionism to a focus on health. Health included: mental illness as part of health continuum; free will, individual choice, and responsibility; subjective, interpersonal, and reciprocal experience; meaning, purpose, and patterns; human potential; holistic care; and the human experience of being whole (GESTALT). Many with earlier training and practice in traditional

psychoanalytic and behavior theory later synthesized their own theories and therapies and became part of the humanism movement during the 1950s and throughout the subsequent half century.

Theorists from multiple disciplines played a role in the development of the humanistic mental health movement. Nurse theorists included Hildegard Peplau (see Chapter 2), Joyce Fitzpatrick, Rosemarie Parse, Patricia Starck, Joyce Travelbee (see Chapter 2), and Jean Watson. Physician theorists included Viktor Frankl and Fritz Perls. Psychological theorists Carl Rogers, Abraham Maslow, and Everett Shostrom are among those who influenced the development of humanistic mental health theory and practice. These theories reflected the theoretical shift toward a more holistic, interpersonal, positive perspective.

## Carl Rogers

Carl Rogers (1961) developed the theory of non-directive therapy called client-centered therapy, which was later called person-centered therapy (Rogers, 1961). Rogers began his writing in the 1940s and became a leader of the humanistic psychologists in the 1960s. Some of Rogers's theoretical concepts (and part of the therapeutic process) include the here-and-now, therapeutic relationship, interpersonal relationships, empathy, unconditional positive regard, humans as individuals, person as subject versus object (Koch, 1959).

## Viktor Frankl

Viktor Frankl (1962, 1978), a holocaust survivor and psychiatric physician, trained and practiced during his early years as a psychoanalyst. Later, Frankl rejected some of the psychodynamic concepts established by Freud and developed his own (existential) theory of meaning and therapeutic techniques of logotherapy. Frankl's (1962, 1969, 1978) theory of meaning included three major concepts: life purpose, freedom of choice, and human suffering. According to Frankl, individuals look for purpose and meaning in their lives and experiences. He believed that all life, even in the most desperate of situations, has meaning and it is the meaning a person ascribes to these situations that can increase suffering or gives a person purpose and reason to live. Frankl used his theory and logotherapeutic interventions mainly to treat patients with psychiatric disorders. His work became a foundational component of the existential humanistic movement. Research using Frankl's theory of meaning is summarized in **Evidence-Based Practice 10-1**.

## Patricia Starck

Patricia Starck, a nurse theorist, contacted Viktor Frankl while working on her doctoral dissertation and they

> ### EVIDENCE-BASED PRACTICE 10-1:
> ### LOGOTHERAPY IN PRACTICE
>
> #### STUDY
>
> Kang, K., Im, J., Kim, H., Kim, S., Song, M., & Sim., S. (2009). Effect of logotherapy on the suffering: Finding meaning, and spiritual well-being of adolescents with terminal cancer. *Journal of the Korean Academy of Child Health Nursing*, *15*(2), 136–144.
>
> #### SUMMARY
>
> The researchers conducted an experimental study to evaluate the effects of psychological interventions by nurses on hospitalized adolescents with terminal cancer. They used Viktor Frankl's theory of meaning and logotherapeutic interventions. Study results showed that the group of patients who received logotherapeutic interventions showed significant reduction in suffering and improvement in meaning in life versus those patients who did not receive logotherapeutic interventions.
>
> #### APPLICATION TO PRACTICE
>
> Although this study focuses on adolescents with terminal cancer, the findings could be applied to any patient experiencing distress, be it physical, mental, or emotional. Assisting patients to find meaning in their illness can help promote feelings of control over situations in which they may have felt hopeless and powerless. The positive effects of this empowerment can strengthen a person's resolve and decision-making capabilities, which, in turn, can promote better outcomes including adherence to treatment regimens.
>
> #### QUESTIONS TO PONDER
>
> 1. *How could the results of this study apply to your nursing practice?*
> 2. *Could logotherapeutic interventions be used to help prevent, as well as treat, existential distress, depression, substance abuse, or mental illness?*

remained in contact over the subsequent 20 years (Smith & Liehr, 2003). Frankl's theory of meaning, his three concepts of life purpose, freedom to choose, and human suffering and logotherapeutic interventions were traditionally used to treat individuals with psychiatric disorders. Starck expanded Frankl's works and has been noted as the first to use the theory of meaning and logotherapy to treat the human suffering of the physically disabled. She developed the Meaning In Suffering Test (MIST), a research instrument used to quantify meaning and in clinical practice to guide logotherapeutic interventions. Stark applied the theory of meaning in her work with spinal cord injured patients and physically disabled persons (Smith & Liehr, 2003).

## Abraham Maslow

Abraham Maslow (1970), a theorist mentored by Adler, developed a holistic-dynamic theory of motivation and a hierarchy of human needs. Maslow's method of study was in contrast to the earlier traditional methodology for researching mental health and illness through study of psychopathology of humans considered mentally ill. Rather, Maslow studied individuals considered to be the healthiest. That is, he studied those without strong traits or diagnoses of neurosis, psychosis, or psychopathic personality. According to Maslow, needs provide the motivation for human beings. He developed a hierarchy of needs, which progresses from most basic to the highest level of actualization. This hierarchy includes: physiological needs, safety needs, belongingness and love needs, esteem needs, and the need for self-actualization. Satisfaction of these needs, however, does not always occur in a linear fashion because they are contingent upon mediating life circumstances.

## Jean Watson

Jean Watson, a nurse theorist, developed the theory of human caring. Watson's theory includes many assumptions and concepts central to humanistic mental health theory, including holistic care, congruence, respect, subject as person versus object, individual perception of experience, authenticity, and gestalt or harmony among the mind/body/spirit. Watson's theory is similar to the therapeutic relationship concept applied to person-centered (mental health) therapy of Rogers and Peplau's therapeutic relationship concept applied to the interpersonal nurse-patient relationship. Watson's caring theory includes the concepts of unconditional acceptance, positive regard, and subjective (lived) experience in a (mutually) therapeutic, restorative (transpersonal) relationship between nurse and patient. Watson's view of nurses facilitating patients' discovery of meaning (in their situation, illness, or suffering) to promote improvement in mind, body, and spirit health reflects phenomenology and existential humanistic mental health theory described in Frankl's theory of meaning. Watson's early work included 10 carative factors, later expanded, revised, and named 10 clinical caritas processes that can be applied by nurses when promoting positive therapeutic outcomes of patients experiencing hopelessness, depression, anxiety, and other mental health and illness conditions. Her original eighth carative factor contains specific reference to the role of the nurse in regard to mental health, identifying the need for nurses to provide for a "...corrective mental, physical, societal, and spiritual environment" (University of Colorado at Denver and Health Sciences Center, School of Nursing, 2006; Watson, 1988). In her most updated version of clinical caritas processes, this factor has been refined to "create a healing environment for the physical and spiritual self which respects human dignity" (Watson, 2007).

> *Humanistic theories reflected the theoretical shift toward a more holistic, interpersonal, positive perspective.*

## Biological Theories

Biological psychology theory or biopsychology refers to the study of human or animal psychology using a biological approach to understand human behavior. It includes brain physiology, genetics, and evolution as means for understanding behavior (Wilkens, 2005). Frameworks such as neuropsychology, psychoneuroendocrinology, psychoneuroimmunology, psychosomatic medicine, and others have evolved and all have in common the study of how the mind affects biological processes, or vice versa, in relation to disease states and behaviors. Over the past 40 years, interest in integrative psychobiology has substantially increased (Azar, 1999).

Beginning in 1970, Robert Ader conducted experimental studies with rats to explore if and how the brain, particularly mental states including stress and anxiety, influence the immune system (Ader, 1995; Azar, 1999). If placed in the current language and lexicon of neurobehavioral or neurobiological science, this could be conceptualized as an "internal human behavior." Results of many of Ader's studies indicate a relationship between the brain, mind, and the functioning of the immune system related to disease progression or healing. Ader is credited with coining the term psychoneuroimmunology and is considered by some the father of psychoneuroimmunology.

Also, considerable research has been conducted on relationships between psychological variables, including emotions and stress (Yehuda, Levengood, Schmeidler, & Wilson, 1996), and biological variables, including molecular changes and somatic diseases, in humans (Everson, Kaplan, Goldberg, Salonen, & Salonen, 1997; Levine & Ursin, 1991). Various principles describing the relationship between psychological stimuli and the endocrine system continue to be supported in psychoneuroimmunoendocrinology research. One example is a set of principles developed by J.W. Mason (1968) that included the principle reflecting the role of psychological stimuli on pituitary-adrenal-cortical activity.

Significant research has been conducted on the biological variables contributing to or resulting from depression. Major depression is the most commonly diagnosed mental disorder, a contributor to the eleventh-leading cause of death (suicide), and the leading cause of disability in the United States for ages 15–44 (NIMH, 2009). The literature offers evidence that atherosclerosis and atherosclerotic progression, known risk factors for cerebrovascular accidents, coronary heart disease, peripheral vascular disease, and mortality, are positively correlated with hopelessness and depression. In addition, research shows that depression may be a risk factor for atherogenesis (Everson et al., 1997; O'Regan, 2000).

Additional studies provide further evidence of the connection between atherosclerosis and depression. For example, results of the seminal population-based study conducted by Everson et al. (1997), referred to as the Finland Kuopio Study, indicate a significant positive relationship between atherosclerosis progression in the intima-media lining of the carotid artery and hopelessness. Coffey et al. (1990) identified a relationship between cerebrovascular atherosclerotic changes and depression. Inspired by the results of the Finland Kuopio Study (1997), O'Regan (2000) explored the relationship between atherosclerosis and hopelessness and depression. Although the O'Regan study sample size was small, results of the study support previous research indicating a relationship between depression and atherosclerosis. The results of O'Regan's study also indicate that there is a linear predictive relationship between the severity of depression and the severity of atherosclerosis, and that depression individually accounted for approximately 20% of the variance in atherosclerosis severity.

Molecular genetics, neuron receptors, and neurotransmitters also continue to receive attention. A dysregulation in neurotransmitters is a proposed cause of primary mental disorders such as depression, anxiety, attention deficit disorders, schizophrenia, dementia, and symptoms of mental illness. Most psychotropic medications are designed to work based on the neurobehavioral theory supporting this dysregulation. Over the past two decades, molecular genetics and randomized, double-blinded placebo-controlled experimental research on drugs that target specific neuron receptors and neurotransmitters, increasing or inhibiting the level of catecholamines such as dopamine, serotonin, and norepinephrine in the brain, have been dominant theories of mental illness etiology, research methods, and treatment. In addition, molecular genetics research is being coupled with magnetic

*Biological psychology theory includes brain physiology, genetics, and evolution as means for understanding behavior. Although numerous frameworks have evolved, they all address the effect of the mind on biological processes (or vice versa), disease states, and/or behaviors.*

resonance imaging (MRI), functional magnetic resonance imaging (fMRI), positron emission tomography (PET) scans, and, recently, computer programmed brain scans to study normal and abnormal brain structure and function in people with and without mental disorders.

The NIMH has issued a grant to study a new method for measuring areas of the brain to determine early and longitudinal differences and changes in the brains of people diagnosed with a mental disorder in comparison to those not diagnosed with a mental disorder (Wang et. al., 2008). Subjects currently are being enrolled in a study that will use a computer programmed to map brain structure size and shape. The use of the computer program replaces traditional manual measurement of brain scans in hopes of developing a tool to more accurately, quickly, and cost-effectively diagnose and treat mental disorders, including schizophrenia and mood disorders. In addition, computerized measurement photographs will provide image depiction of composite, longitudinal abnormal shrinkage in certain areas of the brain, including the thalamus, caudate, and amygdala, over a two-year period in individuals with schizophrenia.

Research is also investigating possible genetic links to mental illness. A team of researchers at the University of Edinburg had previously found a gene, *DISC1*, that is a risk factor for schizophrenia, bipolar affective disorder, and major depression. They identified additional psychiatric disorder and psychotropic treatment-specific relationships in a 2007 molecular genetics study (University of Edinburg, 2007). The follow-up study found two types of damage on the same *DISC1* gene. Treatment efficacy for patients taking antipsychotic medication was associated with one area of *DISC1* gene damage, while treatment efficacy for patients taking antidepressant medications was specific to the other identified *DISC1* gene damage area.

Research on genetic links is continuing. In January 2010, a group of researchers with the NIMH unit on the Genetic Basis of Mood and Anxiety Disorders, published results of the meta-analyses conducted on major mood disorders (McMahon et al., 2010). Their results indicate that people diagnosed with major depression or bipolar disorder have a significantly higher level of a gene overexpression or underexpression in certain areas of the brain than control subjects not diagnosed with these disorders. The gene identified, *PBRM1*, chromosome 3, is responsible for communicating upregulation or downregulation signals to cell components. The gene acts like a lightbulb switch, influencing whether or not to increase (turn on) or decrease (shut off) gene expression, and thus, potentially, play a role in affecting mood regulation.

The biological-molecular genetics neuroscience theory movement is on an accelerated trajectory with the potential to change (redesign) all existing classification systems for mental health and illness. It also may change the diagnostics and, perhaps, the acceptable (thus reimbursable) prescribed treatment methods and providers of mental illness treatment in the future. In the first quarter of 2010, the NIMH (2010) announced that it was launching an initiative, the Research Domain Criteria Project, to study and develop a classification of mental illness through a new lens. This new lens would be different from that of the traditional classification lens using clinical observation. It is expected to result in mental health treatments that are based on research-identified genetic factors and that incorporate similarities among and across existing diagnoses. The NIMH reports that, unlike conventional classification systems like that of the *DSM-IV-TR* or *ICD-10*, which are based upon "clinical observation," they will study and develop a mental illness classification system based on genetics and neuroscience while not excluding clinical observation. The NIMH acknowledges that it may, over time, affect the existing dominant classification systems for mental health diagnoses and treatment. Since 1952, the major (provider-reimbursement friendly) classification system used for diagnosis, research, and treatment of mental illnesses has been the American Psychiatric Association's *DSM-IV-TR*. Following a decade of draft revisions and publishing of the new proposed revisions online for public review and comments (view online at http://www.dsm5.org/Pages/Default.aspx), the fifth edition of the DSM is currently projected to be published in May of 2013.

## SUMMARY POINTS

- Theories associated with mental health and mental illness can be classified as grand theories (abstract and broad in scope), middle-range theories (usually subspecialty oriented), or micro-level (least abstract and narrow in scope). Six grand theories in mental health and psychology include: social, behavioral, psychodynamic, cognitive, humanistic, and biological.

- Psychodynamic theories focus on the unconscious and assert that underlying unconscious or repressed conflicts are responsible for conflicts, disruptions, and disturbances in behavior and personality. Freud is considered the father of psychoanalysis.

- The underlying belief of behavioral theory is that observable criteria are important to understand and change human behavior. Behavioral theorists include Pavlov, Seligman, Thorndike, Watson, and Skinner.

- Aaron Beck is considered the founder of cognitive theory, which focuses on how a person's thinking affects behavior.

- Social theories reflect an understanding that social and cultural environmental factors are important to understand human behavior. Social theorists include Bandura, Lewin, and Festinger.

- Humanistic theories focus on health rather than on illness, determinism, the unconscious, and reductionism. Humanistic nurse theorists include Peplau, Fitzpatrick, Parse, Starck, Travelbee, and Watson.

- Maslow, a humanistic theorist, developed a holistic-dynamic theory of motivation and hierarchy of human needs. Watson, a nurse theorist, developed the theory of human caring.

- Biological theories focus on brain physiology, genetics, and evolution for understanding behavior. All the frameworks share a commonality, that is, how the mind affects biological processes or vice versa.

**NCLEX-PREP***

1. A nursing instructor is developing a class for a group of students about the theories of mental health and illness. When gathering information for a discussion on cognitive theories, which of the following would the instructor most likely include?
   a. Development of psychoanalytic theory
   b. Thorndike
   c. Seligman
   d. Beck
   e. Bandura

2. Applying Freud's theory, which of the following stages would occur first in the development of personality?
   a. Oral
   b. Phallic
   c. Latency
   d. Anal

3. After engaging in an argument with a friend at work, a person becomes angry. Moments later, upon returning to his/her office, he punches the wall. The person is demonstrating which defense mechanism?
   a. Suppression
   b. Rationalization
   c. Denial
   d. Displacement

4. A group of nursing students are reviewing information about theories of mental illness. The students demonstrate a need for additional review when they attribute which of the following as a concept identified by Albert Bandura?
   a. Reciprocal determination
   b. Behavior modeling
   c. Cognitive dissonance
   d. Self-efficacy

5. When applying Maslow's hierarchy of needs, which needs category would be the highest level to be achieved?
   a. Safety
   b. Self-actualization
   c. Love
   d. Self-esteem

*Answers to these questions appear on page 639.

# REFERENCES

Abramson, L.-Y., Seligman, M.-E.-P., & Teasdale, J.-D. (1978). Learned helplessness in humans: Critique and reformulation. *Journal of Abnormal Psychology, 87,* 32–48.

Ader, R. (1995). Historical perspectives on psychoneuroimmunology. In H. Friedman, T. L. Klein, & A.L. Friedman (Eds.), Psychoneuroimmunology, stress and infection, p. 1–21. Boca Raton: CRC Press.

American Psychiatric Association. (1994). *Diagnostic and statistical manual of mental disorders, (4th ed).* Washington, DC: Author.

American Psychological Association (APA). (2009). APA Online. Retrieved October 30, 2009, from http://www.psychology matters.org/glossary.html

American Psychological Association (APA). (2010). APA Online. Retrieved January 20, 2010, from http://www.apa.org/divisions/div32/

Azar, B. (1999). Father of PNI reflects on the field's growth. *APA Monitor, 30,* (6). Retrieved Nov 1, 2009, from http://www.apa.org/monitor/jun99/pni.html

Beck, A.T., Rector, N.A., Stolar, N., & Grant, P. (2008). *Schizophrenia: Cognitive theory, research and therapy.* Gilford Press: New York.

Beck, A.T., Rush, A.J., Shaw, B.F., & Emery, G. (1979). *Cognitive therapy of depression.* New York: Guilford

Bandura, A. (1966). *Behavioristic psychotherapy.* New York: Holt, Rinehart and Winston.

Bandura, A. (1963). *Social learning and personality* development. New York: Holt, Rinehart and Winston.

Bandura, A. (1977). Self-efficacy: Toward a unifying theory of behavioral change. *Psychological Review, 84,* 191–215.

Bandura, A. (1997). *Self-efficacy: The exercise of control.* New York: Freeman.

Cacioppo, J. (2002). Social neuroscience: Understanding the pieces fosters understanding the whole and vice versa. *American Psychologist. 57*(11): 819–831. http://www.cdc.gov/nchs/data/nhsr/nhsr007.pdf

Carver, C., & Scheier, M. (2004). *Perspectives on personality* (5th ed.). Boston: Pearson.

Deutsch, M., & Krauss, R. M. (1965). *Theories in social psychology.* New York: Basic Books.

Ellis, A. (2004). *Rational emotive behavior therapy: It works for me—It can work for you.* Amherst, NY: Prometheus Books.

Everson, S.A., Kaplan, G.A., Goldberg, D.E., Salonen, R., & Salonen, J.T. (1997). Hopelessness and 4-year progression of carotid atherosclerosis: The Kuopio ischemic heat disease study. *Atherosclerosis, Thrombosis & Vascular Biology, 17*(8): 1490–1495.

Festinger, L. (1962). *A theory of cognitive dissonance.* Stanford, CA: Stanford University Press.

Festinger, L. (1964). *Conflict, decision and dissonance.* Stanford, CA: Stanford University Press.

Frankl, V. (1978). *The unheard cry for meaning: Psychotherapy and humanism.* New York: Simon and Shuster.

Frankl, V. (1969). *The will to meaning.* New York: World Publishing.

Frankl, V. E. (1962). *Man's search for meaning.* New York: Simon and Schuster.

Heron, M.P., Hoyert, D.L., Murphy, S.L., Xu, J.Q., Kochanek, K.D., & Tejada-Vera, B. (2009). Deaths: Final data for 2006. *National vital statistics reports, 57*(14). Centers for Disease Control and Prevention, National Center for Health Statistics.

Im, E., & Meleis, A.L. (1999). Situation-specific theories: Philosophical roots, properties and approach. *Advances in Nursing Science, 22(2)*, p 11.

Kang, K., Im, J., Kim, H., Kim, S., Song, M., & Sim, S. (2009). Effect of logotherapy on the suffering, finding meaning, and spiritual well-being of adolescents with terminal cancer. *Journal of the Korean Academy of Child Health Nursing, 15*(2): 136–144.

Koch, S. (Ed.). (1959). *Psychology: A study of a science. Formulations of the person and the social context,* 184–256. New York: McGraw-Hill.

Levine, S., & Ursin, H. (1991). What is stress? In Brown, M.R., Rivier, C., & Koob, G. (eds.). *Stress Neurobiology and neuroendocrinology.* New York: Marcel Decker, p 3–21.

Lewin, K. (1951). Field theory in social science: Selected theoretical papers. D. Cartwright (Ed.) New York: Harpers.

Liebert, R.M., Poulos, R.W., & Marmor, G.S. (1977). Developmental psychology. Englewood Cliffs, NJ: Prentice-Hall.

Maslow, A. (1970). *Motivation and Personality.* New York: Harper and Row.

Mason, J.W. (1968). A review of psychoneuroendocrine research on the pituitary-adrenal-cortical system. *Psychosomatic Medicine, 30,* 576–607.

McMahon, F.J., Akula, N., Schulze, T.G., Muglia, P., Tozzi, F., Detera-Wadleigh, S.D., et al. (2010). Meta-analysis of genome-wide association data identifies a risk locus for major mood disorders on 3p21.1. *Nature Genetics, 42*(2), 126–31.

National Institute of Mental Health. (2009). Statistics. Retrieved November 2, 2009, from http://www.nimh.nih.gov/topics/statistics/index.shtml

National Institute of Mental Health. (2010). Genes and circuitry, not just clinical observation, to guide classification for research. *Science Update.* National Institute of Mental Health online. Retrieved February 2, 2010 from http://www.nimh.nih.gov/science-news/2010/genes-and-circuitry-not-just-clinical-observation-to-guide-classification-for-research.shtml

NANDA International. (2008). *Nursing diagnoses: Definitions and classification 2009–2011.* Hoboken, NJ: Wiley-Blackwell.

Northwestern University (2009, July 10). Map of your brain may reveal early mental illness. *ScienceDaily.* Retrieved November 1, 2009, from http://www.sciencedaily.com/releases/2009/07/090709095431.htm

O'Regan, P. (2000). Psychological links to atherosclerosis: Hopelessness and depression predict atherogenesis risk and severity. Unpublished master's thesis. University of South Florida, Tampa, Florida.

Pavlov, I.P. (1927). Conditioned reflexes. London: Oxford University Press.

Sansone, C., Morf, C.C., & Panter, A.T. (2004). *Handbook of methods in social psychology.* California: Sage Publications.

Seligman, M. (1992). *Helplessness: On depression, development, and death.* New York: Freeman.

Smith, M.J., & Liehr, P.R. (2003). Middle range theory for nursing. Springer: New York.

Soni, A. (2009). The five most costly conditions, 1996 and 2006: Estimates for the U.S. civilian noninstitutionalized population. *Statistical Brief,* 248. Agency for Health care Research and Quality. Retrieved Nov 10, 2009 from http://www.meps.ahrq.gov/mepsweb/data_files/publications/st248/stat248.pdf

University of Colorado at Denver and Health Sciences Center, School of Nursing. (2006). Watson's Caring Theory. Retrieved January 15, 2010 from http://nursing.ucdenver.edu/faculty/j_watson_about.htm

University of Edinburgh, (2007). Study of damaged gene gives insight into causes of mental illness. *ScienceDaily.* Retrieved November 22, 2009, from http://www.sciencedaily.com/releases/2007/05/070502143813.htm

U.S. Department of Health and Human Services. (1999). *Mental Health: A Report of the Surgeon General.* Washington, D.C. Retrieved October 15, 2009 from www.surgeongeneral.gov

Wang, L., Mamah, D., Harms, M., Karnik, M., Price, M., Gado, M., et al. (2008). Progressive deformation of deep brain nuclei and hippocampal-amygdala formation in schizophrenia. *Biological Psychiatry, 64,* (2).

Watson, J. (1988). *Nursing: Human science and human care. A theory of nursing.* New York: National League for Nursing.

Watson, J. (2007). Dr. Jean Watson's Human Caring Theory: Ten Caritas Processes Caritas Processes refined. Available at: http://www.watsoncaringscience.org/caring_science/10caritas.html (accessed 1/27/2011).

Watson, J.B. (1913). Psychology as the behaviorist views it. *Psychological Review, 20,* 158–177.

Wickens, A. (2005). *Foundations of biopsychology.* Prentice Hall.

Weiss, J.M., Glazer, H.L., Pohorecky, L. A., Brick, J., & Miller, N.E. (1975). Effects of chronic exposure to stressors on avoidance-escape behavior and on brain norepinephrine. *Psychosomatic Medicine, 37,* 522–533.

Wolpe, J. (1976). Behavior therapy and its malcontents–II. Multimodal eclecticism, cognitive exclusivism and "exposure" empiricism. *Journal of Behavior Therapy and Experimental Psychiatry, 7,* 109–116.

Wolpe, J. (1958). *Psychotherapy by reciprocal inhibition.* Stanford, CA: Stanford University Press.

Yehuda, R., Levengood, R.A., Schneidler, J., & Wilson, S. (1996). Increased pituitary activation following metyrapone administration in post-traumatic stress disorder. *Psychoneuroendocrinology, 21*(1): 1 16.

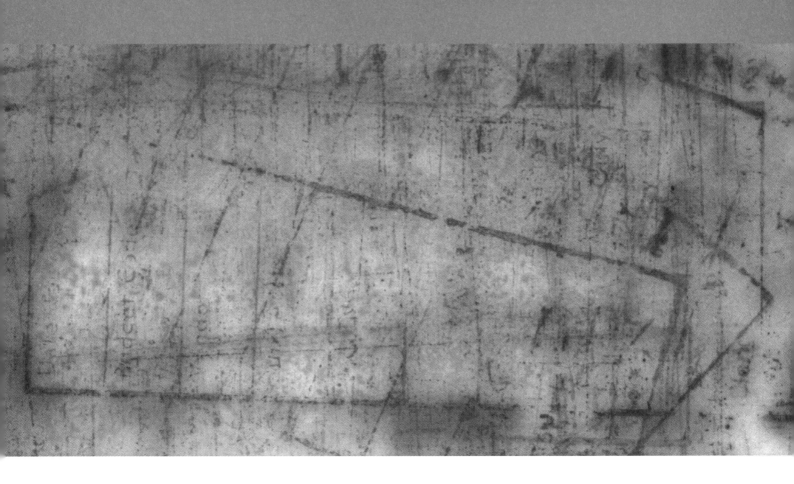

## CHAPTER CONTENTS

## EXPECTED LEARNING OUTCOMES

**After completing this chapter, the student will be able to:**

1. Define thought disorder.
2. Identify the disorders associated with Schizophrenia Spectrum Disorders (SSD).
3. Describe the history and epidemiology of thought disorders.
4. Discuss current scientific theories related to the etiology of thought disorders, including relevant biological and psychosocial theories.
5. Distinguish among the diagnostic criteria for thought disorders as identified by the *Diagnostic and*

# CHAPTER 11
# THOUGHT DISORDERS

Patricia A. Galon

*Statistical Manual of Mental Disorders, 4th edition, Text Revision (DSM-IV-TR).*

6. Describe common assessment strategies for individuals with thought disorders.
7. Explain treatment options for persons demonstrating thought disorders, emphasizing those that reflect evidence-based practices.
8. Apply the nursing process from an interpersonal perspective to the care of patients with thought disorders.

## KEY TERMS

Affective flattening
Alogia
Anhedonia
Anosognosia
Avolition
Delusion
Echolalia
Echopraxia
Erotomanic
Grandiose
Hallucination

Neuroleptic malignant syndrome
Psychosis
Schizophrenia
Thought disorder

THOUGHT DISORDER is a broad term applying to illnesses involving disordered thinking and disturbances in reality orientation and social involvement. Although symptoms of PSYCHOSIS (condition involving hallucinations, delusions, or disorganized thoughts, behavior, or speech) are often intermittently or continuously present, the underlying thought disorder is the most prominent cause of disability associated with this group of psychopathologies. Throughout this chapter this group of disorders will be referred to as Schizophrenia Spectrum Disorders (SSD). The term SCHIZOPHRENIA refers to a diagnostic category within the group of SSD.

This chapter covers the historical aspects and epidemiology of SSD and includes a detailed description of thought disorders as defined in the *Diagnostic and Statistical Manual, 4th edition, Text Revision (DSM-IV-TR, 2000)*. Relevant psychodynamic, cognitive behavioral, genetic, and neurobiological influences are described, along with common pharmacotherapy and nonpharmacotherapy strategies used in the treatment of SSD. Application of the nursing process from an interpersonal perspective is discussed, including a plan of care for a patient with a thought disorder.

## HISTORICAL PERSPECTIVES

References to madness in the Bible and in the Artharva Veda (sacred Hindu text) can be found. In addition, some of the symptoms of mental illness were described in ancient history. However, it was not until the beginning of the 19th century that SSD was clearly recorded in clinical literature. As a result, historians were left with two different interpretations: Either SSD is a relatively new plague of mankind, or, more simply, the descriptions of madness in ancient texts were too vague to identify the syndrome clearly. It should be noted, however, other mental disorders, particularly depression, mania, and dementia, were identifiable in very early historical documents (Torrey, 1980).

The two earliest clinical descriptions of the disorder(s) occurred nearly simultaneously in 1809. These descriptions were provided by Philip Pinel in France and John Haslam in England. Just three years later, in 1812, Benjamin Rush in the United States addressed the disorder. All three described SSD as a constellation of symptoms that included delusions, hallucinations, and paranoia. In 1860 a French physician, Benedict Morel, found that the disorder was associated with an early age of onset, leading him to believe that it was a type of early dementia. Thus, he named the syndrome dementia praecox. By 1876, Emil Kraeplin, a psychiatrist, began to note similarities in the descriptions of several neurological syndromes in the medical literature of the time. He proposed that all of these syndromes belonged to a group of disorders that shared an early onset, grave prognosis, and list of symptoms. Kraeplin was certain the symptoms were rooted in a yet-to-be identified neuroanatomical abnormality. Over thirty years later in 1911, Eugen Bleuler, a Swiss physician, renamed the disorder schizophrenia and described both core and associated symptoms of the disorder. Bleuler is credited with recognizing and identifying thought disorders as a primary cause of disability. Unlike his predecessors, Bleuler believed the origin of the disorder was psychological rather than neuroanatomical. These early clinicians influenced current conceptions of schizophrenia.

In 1959 Kurt Schneider, a German psychiatrist, defined a list of symptoms associated with schizophrenia, distinguishing it from other psychotic disorders. This list, which was considered quite reliable, was widely used by professionals and taught in clinical programs throughout Europe and the United States. In 1966, the World Health Organization (WHO) conducted a landmark study entitled International Pilot Study of Schizophrenia, establishing that the clinical picture of schizophrenia was clearly similar across cultures and political boundaries. This study served as a precursor to the revisions for the *DSM-III* in the United States in 1980, which narrowed the diagnostic criteria for schizophrenia (Lavretsky, 2008).

> *Schizophrenia was initially believed to be a type of early dementia. It was not until 1959 when it was defined with a specific list of symptoms by Kurt Schneider.*

The history of targeted and effective treatment for the SSD covers a much shorter period of time. Most persons with mental illnesses, presumably including SSD, were treated with banishment and cruelty for all but the last 200 years. Both Pinel and Rush were early advocates to improve the circumstances of persons in mental asylums. However, even in institutions where benevolent care was provided, effective treatment was not available. Early attempts at intervention included the use of restraints, opium, hydrotherapy, insulin, electroconvulsive therapy, and crude neurosurgical techniques. It was not until the early 1950s with the discovery of chlorpromazine by French researchers Pierre Deniken, Henri Laborit, and

Jean Delay that any effective treatment became available. Many credit the deinstitutionalization of the mentally ill as a major influence on the use of antipsychotic drugs, which rapidly became a mainstay of treatment. Others believe that the entitlement programs of the 1960s, such as Medicare and Medicaid, were a greater impetus to the deinstitutionalization process. Regardless, the use of antipsychotic drugs as treatment for SSD was an extremely influential development.

Psychoanalysis, based on Freud's theories, as a treatment for SSD was also important. It was the most widely used treatment technique for mental illness in the United States during the first half of the 20th century. Psychoanalysis was considered a legitimate treatment for SSD even beyond the discovery of antipsychotics. However, the number of mental health professionals using it began to dwindle. Its use as a treatment for mental disorders quickly declined in the later 1970s through the 1980s. Today, psychoanalysis is infrequently used as a therapeutic modality for any psychiatric disorder.

Psychoanalysis also was important to the development of psychiatric-mental health nursing. The psychoanalyst Harry Stack Sullivan and his Interpersonal Theory of Psychiatry greatly influenced Hildegard Peplau, often considered the "mother of psychiatric nursing." Both Sullivan and Peplau were associated with Chestnut Lodge, a private sanitarium outside Washington, DC. The facility staff there was committed to using psychoanalytic techniques. However, Sullivan and Peplau stressed the critical nature of interpersonal relations rather than intrapsychic processes (central to Freudian theory) in the development and treatment of mental disorders including SSD. They reported "good outcomes" for their clientele but it is not clear how the outcomes were determined.

Peplau continues to be an important figure in psychiatric-mental health nursing through her theory describing the development of the nurse-patient relationship as an interpersonal process, and her role in the development of advanced practice psychiatric nursing. Peplau understood the critical nature of communication and use of self when working with persons with SSD. She emphasized the importance of using the nurse-patient relationship to decrease symptoms, re-establish relatedness to the environment, and restore the boundaries of self identity. She believed that doing so should result in a more fully functioning person (Thelander, 1997). Peplau's Interpersonal Relations Theory continues to be relevant in relation to recovery in schizophrenia because she describes the helping relationship as one that brings strangers with differing perspectives together. These strangers then evolve into a collaborative dyad focused on the patient's goals.

> *Initially, patients with schizophrenia were treated cruelly with banishment from society. The discovery of the antipsychotic agent, chlorpromazine, in the early 1950s marked the first time effective treatment was available for schizophrenia.*

## EPIDEMIOLOGY

Understanding the epidemiology of a disease is critical to identifying risk factors and possible preventive strategies. It is also important to evaluate disease burden in order to set priorities for appropriate resource allocation.

In the past 10 years, there have been significant breakthroughs in epidemiologic methods and thus more is known about all disease processes, including SSD. Many of the old assumptions concerning the epidemiology of SSD have been challenged. Schizophrenia studies are plagued by issues that include an imprecise definition of the illness and changing diagnostic criteria (Castle & Morgan, 2008). A recent systematic review of epidemiologic studies of SSD over the past 50 years revealed some new information but also added some depth and detail to the current understanding of the disorders (McGrath, Saha, Chant, & Welham, 2008).

### Incidence

Incidence refers to the number of newly identified cases in a specific time period. According to McGrath (2008), who conducted a systematic review, the average incidence of schizophrenia across the world is approximately 15.2 per 100,000. Because the incidence in the study ranged from 7.7 to 43.0, it is safe to assume there is a fairly high variability in rates among locations. In addition, significant differences appeared in the incidence rate between males and females, with males having approximately a 1.4 times higher risk than women. In other words, for every 3 men affected with SSD, there are 2 women affected. The reason for this difference has not been clearly established. However, it has been attributed to the possible protective effect of female hormones (Castle & Morgan, 2008).

Statistics also reveal a significantly higher rate of the disorder among immigrants than in the native-born populations across societies. Again, the reasons for this difference are not clearly understood. One possible explanation is that vulnerable or disenfranchised individuals may choose to migrate more often. Another suggests that the disorder is a response to new biological and social risks in the adopted country (Castle & Morgan, 2008).

Economic status does not appear to be a factor. McGrath et al. (2008) found no difference in the incidence of schizophrenia based on economic status. However, those living in urban areas show a higher incidence rate than those living in rural or suburban settings.

## Prevalence

According to statistics, prevalence rates (the number of current cases) of the disorders do not vary by gender or urbanicity. Thus, the different findings for incidence and prevalence remain unexplained in the research literature and are considered as a direction for further study.

As mentioned, immigrant status does appear to be a factor. The prevalence rate for immigrants is 1.8 times higher than for those in the native-born population. Economic conditions do appear to influence prevalence rates, with developed countries estimating significantly higher rates of the disorder (3.3 per 1000) than that of less developed countries (2.6 per 1000). Prevalence estimates also differ significantly by latitude, with higher latitudes having significantly greater prevalence rates (7.5) than lower latitudes (3.3). Rate differences related to latitude are notable because they signify possible variation in a wide range of influential environmental and economic factors, such as temperature, ultraviolet exposure, precipitation, genetics, and socioeconomic status (McGrath, 2008).

## Mortality

Death is generally reported as standard mortality rate (SMR), which is calculated by dividing the observed mortality rate in the SSD population by the expected mortality rate in the general population matched in age and gender. The SMR for persons with SSD is 2.6 with no differences noted by gender. While suicide influences the SMR for this population, all major causes of death were elevated among those with SSD. A disturbing fact is that the mortality gap (the rate of death for the person with SSD compared to the standard mortality rate) for persons with SSD has increased significantly over the past 3 decades. Further, it is believed that the introduction of second-generation antipsychotics is likely to amplify the problem in coming decades by increasing the risk for metabolic syndrome (a condition associated with insulin resistance, central obesity, and altered serum lipid levels). When this condition occurs, the mortality rate from all causes has been shown to double (McGrath, 2008).

> *Schizophrenia occurs more commonly in men than in women, more often in immigrants than in the native-born population, and more often in those living in urban areas.*

## Remission/Recovery

Recovery in any chronic condition such as asthma, diabetes, or SSD, can be difficult to operationally define. No clear end state exists. The person remains vulnerable or the disease state continues despite a fading of the symptoms. Using recovery rates with SSD further complicates the definition because recognizing the concept of recovery from a consumer perspective may differ from the scientific definition. As a result, it may be clearer to discuss remission in this context. In the *DSM-IV-TR* (2000), remission is defined as a state of improvement in which clinically significant residual symptoms remain.

Studies of the course of schizophrenia have reported significantly varying rates of remission and widely different definitions. Auslander and Jeste (2004) found sustained remission rates of 8% in older community-dwelling adults. However, the sample of those with sustained remission was small ($n = 12$), so the results have limited generalizability. The authors speculate that remission rates could potentially be much higher (between 15% and 20%) if adequate psychosocial treatments and supports were in place for this population.

## DIAGNOSTIC CRITERIA

Thought disorders include the following: schizophrenia and its five subtypes, schizophreniform disorder, schizoaffective disorder, delusional disorder, brief psychotic disorder, and shared psychotic disorder. Each disorder has a specific set of diagnostic criteria that a patient must meet for diagnosis. **Box 11-1** highlights the major diagnostic criteria as identified by the *DSM-IV-TR*.

## Schizophrenia

**SCHIZOPHRENIA** is a thought disorder that involves bizarre behavior, thoughts, movement, perceptions, and emotions. There is no single symptom or sign that defines the disorder (Box 11-1). Symptoms experienced by the patient

**BOX 11-1: DIAGNOSTIC CRITERIA FOR THOUGHT DISORDERS**

**Schizophrenia**

Two or more of the following:

A. Characteristic symptoms
- Delusions
- Hallucinations
- Disorganized speech
- Grossly disorganized or catatonic behavior
- Negative symptoms

Only one of the above is necessary if bizarre delusions present or the hallucinatory experience is that of a running conversation or two people conversing.

B. Social or occupational dysfunction for a significant period since onset of the illness in one or more areas of work, interpersonal relations, or self-care

C. Duration continuing at least 6 months

D. Symptoms not the result of a mood disorder

E. Symptoms not the result of a substance abuse disorder or a general medical condition

F. If there is a history of autism or a pervasive developmental disorder, then an additional diagnosis is made of schizophrenia only if prominent delusions or hallucinations are also present for at least one month.

**Schizophrenia, Paranoid Type**
- Preoccupation with one or more delusions or frequent auditory hallucinations
- Disorganized speech, disorganized or catatonic behavior, or flat or inappropriate affect not prominent

**Schizophrenia, Disorganized Type**
- Prominent disorganized speech, disorganized behavior, flat or inappropriate affect
- The criteria for catatonic type not met

**Schizophrenia, Catatonic Type**
- Motoric immobility as evidenced by catalepsy or stupor
- Undirected excessive motor activity not influenced by external stimuli
- Extreme negativism consisting of motiveless resistance to all requests, instructions, or mutism
- Peculiar voluntary movement including stereotyped movements, prominent mannerisms, or grimacing
- Echolalia or echopraxia

**Schizophrenia, Undifferentiated Type**
- A type of schizophrenia that meets characteristics of schizophrenia (Criteria A) but not criteria for paranoid, disorganized, or catatonic type

**Schizophrenia, Residual Type**
- Absence of prominent delusions, hallucinations, disorganized speech, and grossly disorganized or catatonic behavior
- Continuing evidence of the disturbance as indicated by the presence of negative symptoms, or two or more symptoms listed as characteristics for schizophrenia (Criterion A) present in a lessened form such as odd beliefs or unusual perceptual experiences

*(cont.)*

## BOX 11-1: DIAGNOSTIC CRITERIA FOR THOUGHT DISORDERS (*CONT.*)

### Schizophreniform Disorder

- Characteristics of schizophrenia (Criterion A) that are not the result of a mood disorder (Criterion D), substance abuse, or general medical condition (Criterion E)
- An episode lasting at least 1 month but less than 6 months

It is specified further as with or without good prognostic features:

- Onset of prominent psychotic symptoms within 4 weeks of the first noticeable change in behavior or functioning
- Confusion or perplexity at height of the psychosis
- Good premorbid or occupational functioning
- Absence of blunted or flat affect

### Schizoaffective Disorder

An uninterrupted period of illness during which at some time there is either a major depressive disorder, a manic episode, or a mixed episode concurrent with symptoms that meet the characteristic symptoms for schizophrenia (Criterion A)

- Delusions or hallucinations for at least 2 weeks in the absence of prominent mood symptoms during the same period of illness
- Symptoms that meet criteria for a mood disorder present for a substantial portion of the total duration of the active and residual periods of the illness
- The disturbance not due to the direct physiological effects of a substance or a general medical condition
- Further specified as bipolar type if it includes a manic or mixed episode or as depressive type if the disturbance includes only depressive symptoms

### Delusional Disorder

- Nonbizarre delusions such as jealousy or having a disease of at least 1 month duration
- Characteristics for schizophrenia never been met
- Functioning not markedly impaired except for the impact of the delusion
- Mood episodes that may occur in conjunction with the delusions; if present, very brief in relation to the delusional periods
- Problem not due to the use of substances (marijuana) or a general medical condition
- Delusion type specified by theme as:
  - **EROTOMANIC** type: Delusions that another person, usually of higher status, is in love with the individual
  - **GRANDIOSE** type: Delusions of inflated worth, power or knowledge; possibly involving special relationships with a deity or famous person
  - Jealous type: Delusions that sexual partner is unfaithful
  - Persecutory type: Delusions that the person is being treated badly in some way
  - Somatic type: Delusion that the person has some physical defect or medical condition
  - Mixed type: Delusions that have characteristics of one or more categories noted above but no one theme predominates
  - Unspecified (delusions that do not fit one of the above categories)

### Brief Psychotic Disorder

- Presence of one or more of the following symptoms:
  - Delusions
  - Hallucinations
  - Disorganized speech
  - Grossly disorganized or psychotic behavior

*(cont.)*

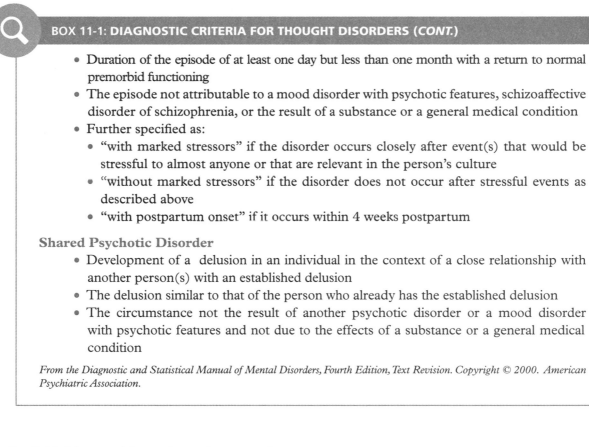

**BOX 11-1: DIAGNOSTIC CRITERIA FOR THOUGHT DISORDERS (*CONT.*)**

- Duration of the episode of at least one day but less than one month with a return to normal premorbid functioning
- The episode not attributable to a mood disorder with psychotic features, schizoaffective disorder of schizophrenia, or the result of a substance or a general medical condition
- Further specified as:
  - "with marked stressors" if the disorder occurs closely after event(s) that would be stressful to almost anyone or that are relevant in the person's culture
  - "without marked stressors" if the disorder does not occur after stressful events as described above
  - "with postpartum onset" if it occurs within 4 weeks postpartum

**Shared Psychotic Disorder**
- Development of a delusion in an individual in the context of a close relationship with another person(s) with an established delusion
- The delusion similar to that of the person who already has the established delusion
- The circumstance not the result of another psychotic disorder or a mood disorder with psychotic features and not due to the effects of a substance or a general medical condition

*From the Diagnostic and Statistical Manual of Mental Disorders, Fourth Edition, Text Revision. Copyright © 2000. American Psychiatric Association.*

are typically divided into positive and negative categories. Positive symptoms are excessive or amplified variations of normal functioning, such as:
- DELUSIONS (erroneous, false, fixed beliefs; a misinterpretation of an experience)
- HALLUCINATIONS, most commonly auditory or visual (erroneous or false sensory perceptions)
- Disorganized speech (Table 11-1 provides examples)
- Disorganized behavior such as aggression, agitation, regression, hypervigilance, waxy flexibility (odd or unusual fixed postural positions for an extended period of time), or ECHOPRAXIA (involuntary imitation of another's movements and gestures)

Negative symptoms reflect a diminished presentation of emotional expression and include:
- AFFECTIVE FLATTENING or blunting (restricted range and intensity of emotion)
- Decreased fluency of speech
- ALOGIA (decreased production of speech)
- AVOLITION (diminished goal directed activity)
- Ambivalence
- ANHEDONIA (inability to feel pleasure or joy from life)

For diagnosis, the disease must be present for at least six months. During this time frame, the patient must actively demonstrate the symptoms for a significant period of one month.

> *Schizophrenia is manifested by positive and negative symptoms. Positive symptoms are exaggerations of normal function; negative symptoms indicate decreased emotional expression.*

Schizophrenia is divided into five subtypes based on the prominent symptoms displayed. The five subtypes include: paranoid, disorganized, catatonic, undifferentiated, and residual (Box 11-1). Although specific information about prognosis is not known, persons with paranoid schizophrenia generally have the least disability, while those with disorganized schizophrenia have the greatest.

Schizophrenia, paranoid type is characterized by prominent delusions and hallucinations while affect and cognition are relatively preserved. Delusions typically are persecutory (the feeling that one is being watched, harmed, or plotted against) or grandiose (one has great wealth, power, or influence). Both types of delusions also may be present. Other common themes are jealousy, religiosity,

**TABLE 11-1: EXAMPLES OF DISTURBED SPEECH**

| DISTURBED SPEECH | DESCRIPTION | EXAMPLE |
|---|---|---|
| **ECHOLALIA** | Parrot-like repetition of another's words | *Nurse*: "Good morning, how are you today, John?" <br> *Patient*: "Good morning, how are you today, John?" |
| Circumstantiality | Detailed and lengthy talking about a subject | I would like to go to the recreation area; I know there are many things that I can do there. There are red balls, and blue balls, and yellow balls, and even a white ball on the pool table and I know how to play pool and I can hit the red ball, and the yellow ball, and the white ball is used to hit all of the other balls. |
| Loose associations | Sudden shifting from one topic to another without any connection | I wonder where my medication is. I know that it is not raining today. |
| Flight of ideas | Repeated and rapid changing of the subject | What time is it? Where is my medication? I want to go to recreation. I want to visit my friends. |
| Word salad | Words in succession without any connection or continuity of thought | Corn, paper, job, snow, swim, pickle. |
| Neologisms | Words made up by the patient | I have a farpart. Do you have a farpart? |
| Verbigeration | Repetition of words or phrases for no purpose | My part, my part, my part, my part … |
| Clang association | Repetition of words that sound alike or rhyme but are otherwise not connected | I have to run, but that's a pun, when it's no fun. |
| Stilted language | Language that is overly pompous, flowery, formal, or artificial | I am pleased to make acquaintances with such a precious and outstanding counterpart. |
| Perseveration | Repetition of word or phrases focusing on a single topic | It is snowing; it is snowing; it is snowing … |

or somatization. Delusions tend to be organized around a common theme and are sometimes referred to as systematized. Hallucinatory content is also related to the delusions. Persons with paranoid schizophrenia can be aloof, superior, and patronizing, and predisposed to suicide and violence. Based on the literature, age of onset is typically later than other subtypes of schizophrenia. Prognosis for occupational success and living independently is better than for other subtypes.

Schizophrenia, disorganized type is characterized by silliness and laughter not connected to speech content. Persons with this subtype often have trouble with organization and tasks. For example, the person may have difficulty with activities of daily living. Delusions and hallucinations, if present, are not organized around a central theme. This subtype is often associated with poor premorbid function, insidious, and early onset, and a course of illness without significant remission. This type of illness was previously labeled hebephrenic.

Schizophrenia, catatonic type is characterized by psychomotor disturbances, which may include immobility, excessive motor activity, extreme negativism, mutism, peculiar voluntary motor movement, echolalia, or echopraxia. Motor immobility may be manifested by catalepsy (waxy flexibility) or stupor. Voluntary movement may be peculiar and include assuming uncomfortable postures or grimacing. During periods of severe stupor or excitement, the person may require careful supervision to avoid injury to self or others. He or she is also at risk for dehydration, malnutrition, and exhaustion. To be diagnosed with this subtype, the manifestations must not be the result of neuroleptic-induced parkinsonism, a general medical condition, or a manic or depressive episode.

Schizophrenia, undifferentiated type is defined as schizophrenia that does not meet the criteria of the paranoid, disorganized, or catatonic type.

Schizophrenia, residual type is the term used when there has been at least one episode of schizophrenia, but the current clinical picture is without prominent positive psychotic symptoms. There is continuing evidence of negative symptoms or two or more less prominent positive symptoms. If delusions or hallucinations persist, they are not prominent or disturbing to the person. This may be a transition state from acute illness to full remission, but it also may be a state continuously present for many years without a new acute episode.

> *The five subtypes of schizophrenia are: paranoid, disorganized, catatonic, undifferentiated, and residual. Each is associated with characteristic symptoms.*

## Schizophreniform Disorder

Schizopheniform disorder shares identical essential features with schizophrenia with two differences (Box 11-1): First the total duration of the illness is at least one month but less than six months. Second, impaired social or occupational functioning during some part of the illness, although it may occur, is not required as a criterion. If the diagnosis persists beyond six months, it is changed to schizophrenia.

## Schizoaffective Disorder

Schizoaffective disorder occurs as an uninterrupted period of illness during which there is a major depressive, manic, or mixed episode concurrent with the characteristic symptoms of schizophrenia (Box 11-1). In addition, delusions or hallucinations are present. Persons with schizoaffective disorder may have marked difficulties in social contact and self-care. The risk for suicide also is increased. Residual symptoms may be less than in schizophrenia but **ANOSOGNOSIA** (poor insight) is often present and can result in poor treatment adherence. The incidence of this type of SSD is higher in women. The overall prognosis of schizoaffective disorder is better than that for schizophrenia. In addition, schizoaffective disorder also appears to increase the risk of schizophrenia and mood disorders in first-degree relatives. At times, it may be difficult to distinguish schizoaffective disorder from mood disorder with psychotic features. The distinguishing feature is that in mood disorder with psychotic features, the psychotic symptoms occur within the context of the mood disorder.

## Delusional Disorder

Delusional disorder is characterized by the presence of one or more non-bizarre delusions that persist for more than one month in a person who has never had a symptom presentation that met the diagnosis of schizophrenia. Hallucinations, if present, are not prominent. Evaluating delusions as non-bizarre can be problematic, especially in relation to cultural differences between the health care professional and the patient. In such cases, the determination can be made by considering plausibility, understandability, and the life experiences of the person. The individual's functional level may be variable because some behavior surrounding the delusions could diminish functioning. For example, if one believes he or she has a serious disease, he or she may self-isolate and seek medical treatments that could ultimately be harmful. More often, social and interpersonal functioning problems are greater than occupational functioning. The disorder tends to develop later in life compared to schizophrenia. Patients may experience periods when the disorder is fairly quiet. Additionally, the prognosis is often improved when the disorder occurs in response to a stressful event.

## Brief Psychotic Disorder

Brief psychotic disorder is a thought disorder that usually has an abrupt onset with at least one positive symptom associated with the characteristics of schizophrenia. This disorder, occurring most often during the second or third decade of life, commonly lasts between 1 and 30 days. The person has a full remission during the specified time period.

Although the duration of the disorder is brief, it may be quite intense and require a high level of supervision. The risk for suicide is especially high for younger persons. Individuals diagnosed with certain personality disorders such as borderline, paranoid, narcissistic, and histrionic personality disorders, may be at increased risk for this diagnosis. (See Chapter 14 for a discussion of personality disorders.)

## Shared Psychotic Disorder

Shared psychotic disorder (folie à deux) is a disorder in which a delusion develops in an individual who is involved in a close relationship with another person. The "primary case" or "the inducer" is the person who already has a psychotic disorder with prominent delusions. The delusions can range from ordinary to bizarre in nature. Generally the inducer is the dominant person in the relationship and gradually imparts the delusion to the more passive partner. Often, these persons are family members and have lived together for long periods in isolation. If the relationship with the inducer is interrupted, then the delusions of the other individual subside.*

The situation can involve more than two people, especially in a family situation where the inducer is the parent and the children adopt the delusional belief. These cases are not commonly seen in the treatment system so there is limited information on incidence, prevalence, or course of the disorder. There is a suggestion it is more common in women than in men.

> *Other thought disorders include: schizophreniform disorder, schizoaffective disorders, delusional disorder, brief psychotic disorder, and shared psychotic disorder.*

## ETIOLOGY OF SSD

The psychiatric syndromes whose prominent features involve disorders of thought are serious illnesses, occurring second only to heart disease in contributing to the existing world disease burden (Murray & Lopez, 1996). SSD affects individuals in nearly all aspects of their lives, including vocational, interpersonal, intrapsychic, and social competencies. These disorders tend to emerge in young adulthood and are lifelong conditions creating stress for families and communities. Unfortunately, the exact etiology of SSD is unknown.

Theories on the etiology of any disorder are important because ascertaining the cause of a disorder is helpful in developing treatment and prevention strategies. Psychosocial and biological theories are described here. However, since the discovery of antipsychotic drugs in the 1950s, the direction of research on the etiology of SSD has radically shifted in favor of biological theories.

### Psychosocial Theories

While the early psychosocial theories have been replaced, evolved, or discredited, their legacy may be important. These etiological conceptualizations of SSD continue to exert some influence on the current understanding. For example, the recognition of the importance of relationships

and communication, an appreciation of the conditions under which the diagnosis and treatment take place, and the recognition of family influence and distress in the face of a devastating illness are still viewed as important clinical factors that arose from earlier speculations about the origins of these serious disorders.

In the early years of the 20th century, psychoanalytic theory was used to explain the etiology of a wide range of psychiatric disorders, including SSD. Speculation was that the "schizophrenia process" began in the first few years of life as a result of a faulty maternal relationship. This pathologic relationship with the "first love object" created anxiety, leading to the expectation of a world that could not be trusted (Ferriera, 1961). Much of the support for this conceptualization came from case material obtained during the psychoanalysis of schizophrenic patients. The "schizophrenogenic mother" theory that resulted from these case reports negatively affected the relationship between mental health professionals and families during the period of this theory's acceptance. While this concept has dissipated considerably over the past 30 years, some lingering distrust remains.

In the 1920s, Harry Stack Sullivan, a psychoanalyst by training, began to integrate the theories of anthropology and the newly emerging field of social psychology into an evolving psychodynamic theory emphasizing interpersonal relationships in the etiology of schizophrenia. He theorized that the patient's observed maladaptive behaviors were the result of a history of faulty communication between the affected individual and the rest of society. Sullivan's contribution is important because he recognized the critical nature of the individual's relationships with others and his or her social and interpersonal environment to the development of pathology, rather than viewing it as the result of an intrapsychic experience (Evans, 1996).

During the mid-1950s, early family theories attributed the development of schizophrenia to disordered family communication. The speculation was that in the families of persons with SSD, homeostasis was maintained by a process called pseudomutuality. This process reflects a façade of family harmony maintained by a denial of problems. However, those problems later became manifested as troubled behaviors in the most vulnerable family member, the person who developed schizophrenia. While the family remained together, the burden of unresolved family issues was borne by the person with SSD (Ferriera, 1961). This theory is no longer accepted by mainstream clinicians.

Current research supports that psychological and social factors influence the emergence of symptoms of SSD in vulnerable individuals. No evidence exists to support the belief that psychosocial factors alone can

---

*\*From the Diagnostic and Statistical Manual of Mental Disorders, 4th Edition, Text Revision, Copyright © 2000 American Psychiatric Association.*

induce SSD in persons without a biological predisposition. Research has consistently supported that proximal stressful life events can influence the emergence of many psychiatric and physical conditions in humans, including SSD. Also, it may be true that early traumatic life events could increase the risk for mental health problems later in life, but again, this is not specific to SSD.

Special psychosocial contexts may exist in which SSD is more likely to emerge through a type of psychosocial "perfect storm." Here, stressful circumstances work together synergistically to influence symptom emergence. A possible example could be immigration. In such a context, individuals leave their country of origin as a result of fear or actual torture. They arrive in another culture where they do not speak the dominant language and are thus socially isolated and unable to validate their experiences. They may be made to feel unwelcome by officials (police) or neighbors. In addition, they commonly have the added stress of poverty due to poor employment opportunities. In such circumstances, a degree of paranoia may be adaptive for some but it may tip the balance toward illness in especially vulnerable persons.

Family interaction is another possible link to SSD. High levels of negative expressed emotion (EE) in family interaction appear to influence relapse in persons with SSD. Negative expressed emotion is characterized by communication that is hostile, critical, and emotionally over intrusive. Relapse rates for persons living in families with high negative expressed emotion is about 2.5 times as high as for those who live alone or in families with low negative expressed emotion. Studies involving high levels of expressed emotion have led to an increased understanding of the importance of family involvement in treatment. In addition, the studies have led to successful family interventions, which have reduced relapse rates (Kuipers, Bebbington, Dunn et al., 2006).

> *Early psychosocial theories identified a problematic maternal relationship as the cause of schizophrenia. Later, other theories addressed social context and unresolved family issues.*

## Biological Theories

Despite intense efforts in the recent past in this area, the specific biological etiology of SSD is still unknown.

However, two parallel avenues are providing current direction for continued study. Researchers continue to search for ways to combine their collective findings into a coherent theory of etiology and ultimately successful treatment (Downar & Kapur, 2008). The first avenue of discovery includes epidemiological/environmental, genetic, and neuroanatomical studies. The second addresses neurochemical aspects, using observations of evolving pharmacological treatment of SSD over the past 50 years as a basis for a theoretical understanding of its etiology.

Epidemiological studies of SSD point to a number of perinatal risk factors for schizophrenia. These include winter birth; urban birth setting and associated issues such as pollution or crowding; intrauterine infections such as rubella, influenza, or polio; pre-eclampsia (a pregnancy-related condition involving elevated blood pressure); low birth weight; or Rh incompatibility. In addition, maternal stress such as famine, depression, or an unwanted pregnancy is also associated with the later development of SSD. Unfortunately, no common mechanism of injury related to these multiple, contributing, antecedent conditions can account for the development of a disorder, nor do they provide an explanation for why the disease emerges decades after the original insults (Downar & Kapur, 2008).

### Genetics

Genetics is the greatest known risk factor predisposing an individual to develop SSD. In a meta-analysis of twin studies on schizophrenia, Sullivan and colleagues (2004) quantified the genetic and environmental contribution to the development of schizophrenia as 81% and 11%, respectively. Twin studies have also demonstrated that the concordance rate (presence of the same trait in each twin) for schizophrenia is about 40%–50% between monozygotic twins and about 10% between siblings, both highly suggestive of an inherited disorder. One particular gene has not been identified as causative; rather, a set of genes likely contributes to development of the disorder. The candidate genes for schizophrenia risk currently identified fall into two categories, those that contribute to neurotransmission and to neurodevelopment (Downar & Kapur, 2008).

### Neuroanatomic Factors

Various nonspecific macro- and micro-neuroanatomical findings are associated with SSD. The most common macro feature is enlargement of the cerebral lateral ventricles. In addition, the hippocampus and amygdala show decreased volume. The size of the prefrontal cortex appears diminished in persons with SSD who experience prominent negative symptoms. In monozygotic twins, the overall brain volume of the twin affected by SSD is decreased. Micro abnormalities have also been observed.

For example, alterations in the size, number, and structural organization of cells in the hippocampus and areas of the cortex have been reported in the literature. However, this significance is not clear (Downar & Kapur, 2008).

### Neurochemical Factors

Currently, two prominent neurochemical theories attempt to explain the etiology of SSD. The first, called the dopamine hypothesis, is supported by the 50-year history of treatment with antipsychotic medications that block dopamine. According to this theory, a disregulation of dopamine is the underlying etiologic mechanism responsible for SSD. This disregulation involves overactivity in the mesolimbic dopamine pathway, contributing to positive symptoms, and underactivity in the mesocortical dopamine pathway contributing to negative and cognitive symptoms. A second neurochemical theory of SSD is the glutamate hypothesis. This theory posits that alterations in the N-methyl-D-aspartate (NMDA) glutamate receptor are the mechanism responsible for all symptoms of SSD (positive, negative, and cognitive) due to its excitatory role in the central nervous system. One of the reasons that the NMDA glutamate hypothesis has captured the attention of researchers is that it plays an important role in neurodevelopmental processes both in utero and during adolescence, critical periods in development according to several current theories. It could prove to be a needed unifying concept in the understanding of the etiology of SSD (Downar & Kapur, 2008).

> *Biological theories suggest perinatal events, genetics, neuroanatomical abnormalities, and dysfunction of neurotransmitters as key risk factors for the development of schizophrenia.*

## TREATMENT OPTIONS

The treatment of SSD requires medical/pharmacological, environmental, psychosocial, and social interventions. None of these categories of treatment alone is sufficient to assist persons with SSD to live their lives to their fullest potential. Individuals living with SSD will require a combination of interventions across their lifetimes. Depending on their age and the severity and acuity of their condition at a given time, the priority of treatment interventions will vary.

The view of patients with SSD leading productive and satisfying lives traditionally has been pessimistic. Although newer treatment paradigms that combine pharmacological and psychosocial treatment modalities have proved helpful, some of the greatest strides forward are being attributed to the activities of the consumer movement that has given voice to persons with serious mental illnesses. Consumers have sought to de-emphasize the medical model that recognizes symptom reduction as the major goal of all treatment activities in favor of such concepts as empowerment, interpersonal and vocational competency, autonomy, and hope. Research indicates that perhaps 50% of persons with schizophrenia have achieved recovery for substantial periods of time (Bellack, 2006).

### Pharmacological Therapy

Following is an overview of pharmacological therapy for SSD; the reader is referred to other pharmacologic resources for more in-depth information. Medications used to treat SSD are called antipsychotic agents and typically are classified as first-generation or second-generation antipsychotics. They do not cure the disorder but research has shown that they are effective in managing the symptoms. Typically, medications used for psychiatric-mental health conditions are indicated for use in more than one disorder. For example, the drug olanzapine (Zyprexa) is indicated for use in psychosis and mood instability.

Generally, the therapeutic mechanism of action of antipsychotic drugs involves dopamine blockade in a number of central nervous system receptors. It is theorized that typical or first-generation antipsychotics block dopamine in the mesolimbic pathway, which likely dampens positive symptoms of the disorder. However, they also cause side effects by blocking dopamine in the nigrostriatal pathway and the tuberoinfundibular pathway leading to parkinsonism and increased prolactin secretion (resulting in galactorrhea, amenorrhea, and decreased libido) respectively. First-generation antipsychotic agents also cause other side effects such as sedation, seizures, arrhythmias, orthostatic hypotension. However, the most troubling side effects are the extrapyramidal symptoms, which include parkinsonism, akathisia, dystonias, and tardive dyskinesia and neuroleptic malignant syndrome (**Box 11-2**).

Atypical or second-generation antipsychotics are effective in treating positive symptoms of SSD, and perhaps negative symptoms as well. Their hypothesized action involves a simultaneous blockade of dopamine and serotonin receptors. Available serotonin then inhibits dopamine

## BOX 11-2: SIDE EFFECTS OF ANTIPSYCHOTIC AGENTS

### FIRST-GENERATION ANTIPSYCHOTIC DRUGS

- Sedation
- Extrapyramidal symptoms
  - Parkinsonism (tremor, shuffling gait, drooling, cogwheel rigidity)
  - Akathisia (muscle weakness, intense need to move about, restlessness with rigid posture or gait)
  - Dystonia (involuntary movements of muscles [spasms] and cramping, most commonly of the face, arms, legs, and neck)
  - Tardive dyskinesia (bizarre facial, tongue, and upper and lower extremity movements, lip smacking, blinking or grimacing, stiff neck, difficulty swallowing)
- Heatstroke
- Hyperprolactinemia
- **NEUROLEPTIC MALIGNANT SYNDROME** (muscle rigidity, high fever, unstable blood pressure, diaphoresis, pallor, delirium, tachycardia, tachypnea, rapid deterioration of mental status)
- Seizures
- Orthostatic hypotension
- Cardiac arrhythmias

### SECOND-GENERATION ANTIPSYCHOTIC DRUGS

- Extrapyramidal symptoms
  - Parkinsonism
  - Akathisia
  - Dystonia
  - Tardive dyskinesia
- Hyperprolactinemia
- Orthostatic hypotension
- Neuroleptic malignant syndrome
- Sedation
- Anticholinergic effects (dry mouth, blurred vision, constipation, urinary retention)
- Metabolic effects (weight gain, glucose intolerance or diabetes, hyperlipidemia)
- Sexual arousal difficulties
- Falls
- Agranulocytosis
- Prolongation of QTc interval

release to different degrees in different pathways. The greatest inhibition occurs in the desired mesolimbic pathway while decreasing the blockade in the nigrostriatal and tuberoinfundibular pathways. The decreased blockade in the latter two pathways leads to a decrease in the undesirable side effects noted previously. They may cause sedation, anticholinergic effects, orthostatic hypotension, prolongation of the QTc interval, difficulties of sexual arousal, and agranulocytosis. Additionally, second-generation agents are associated with the development of metabolic syndrome (central obesity weight gain, glucose intolerance, and hyperlipidemia) in many patients. **Drug Summary Table 11-1** lists first- and second-generation antipsychotics and implications for the interpersonal process.

While medications have the potential to diminish symptoms, they are ineffective if the patient does not take them. Working with patients to facilitate adherence to a prescribed medication regimen is essential.

Other medications may be used appropriately for persons with SSD. Mood stabilizers such as lithium and carbamazapine are indicated for persons with schizoaffective disorder as well as to treat aggression that may be a part of SSD. Antidepressants also are often prescribed for the depression associated with SSD after optimal response to antipsychotics is established. Benzodiazepines are commonly used together with antipsychotics to control acute agitation (Arey & Marder, 2008).

> *Antipsychotic agents are typically classified as first- or second-generation agents. Both are associated with extrapyramidal symptoms: parkinsonism, akathesia, dytonias, and tardive dyskinesia. Second-generation antipsychotics are associated with the development of metabolic syndrome.*

## Electroconvulsive Therapy

Electroconvulsive therapy (ECT) is regarded with great suspicion by the public and persons with psychiatric-mental health problems. In the United States, ECT is used mainly for the treatment of depression. In 2004, the American Psychiatric Association guidelines proposed that ECT can be used for persons with schizophrenia or schizoaffective disorder who have persistent

## DRUG SUMMARY 11-1: ANTIPSYCHOTIC AGENTS

### FIRST-GENERATION ANTIPSYCHOTIC DRUGS

| DRUG NAME | IMPLICATIONS FOR NURSING CARE |
|---|---|
| chlorpromazine (Thorazine)<br><br>perphenazine (Trilafon)<br><br>trifluoperazine (Stelazine)<br><br>fluphenazine (Prolixin)<br><br>thioridazine (Mellaril)<br><br>thiothixine (Navane)<br><br>haloperidol (Haloperidol)<br><br>loxapine (Loxitane) | • Work with patient on measures to reduce anticholinergic effects such as the use of sugarless gum or hard candy to alleviate dry mouth<br>• Institute safety measures to prevent falls<br>• Urge patient to report complaints of dizziness when rising from lying to sitting position or sitting to standing position<br>• Allow patient to verbalize feelings and issues related to drug therapy; work with patient and family to develop a method for ensuring adherence to drug therapy<br>• Monitor the patient for development of extrapyramidal side effects<br>• Be alert that neuroleptic malignant syndrome most often occurs during the first two weeks of therapy or after a dosage increase |

### SECOND-GENERATION ANTIPSYCHOTIC DRUGS

| DRUG NAME | IMPLICATIONS FOR THE INTERPERSONAL PROCESS |
|---|---|
| clozapine (Clozaril)<br><br>risperidone (Risperidone)<br><br>olanzapine (Zyprexa)<br><br>quetiapine (Seroquel)<br><br>ziprasidone (Geodon)<br><br>aripiprazole (Abilify)<br><br>paliperidone (Invega)<br><br>iloperidone (Fanapt)<br><br>asenapine (Saphris) | • Instruct the patient using aripiprazole (Abilify) not to take the drug with grapefruit juice<br>• For the patient taking clozapine, obtain baseline white blood cell counts to assess for agranulocytosis; explain to the patient that he or she will receive only a 1-week supply of the drug; assist the patient in arranging for follow-up weekly blood tests for the first 6 months of therapy; monitor the patient closely for signs and symptoms of infection; stress the need for not stopping the drug abruptly<br>• Allow patient to verbalize feelings and issues related to drug therapy; work with patient and family to develop a method for ensuring adherence to drug therapy<br>• Monitor the patient for development of extrapyramidal side effects<br>• Be alert that neuroleptic malignant syndrome most often occurs during the first two weeks of therapy or after a dosage increase |

severe psychosis and suicidal ideation, prominent catatonic features, and co-morbid depression. However, only 1% of the persons who receive ECT in the United States have a primary diagnosis of schizophrenia (McClintock, Ranginwala, & Husain, 2008). Despite its reputation, ECT is a safe treatment and used most often for persons who require a rapid response to treatment because of the severity of their condition. (See Chapter 12 for additional information on ECT.)

## Environmental Supports

Environmental supports broadly refer to compensatory mechanisms to address the cognitive deficits of persons with SSD. One such method is Cognitive Adaptive Training (CAT), a program of assessment and tailored interventions to assist the person to complete activities of daily living to improve the quality of life. Examples include the use of checklists for bathing or home maintenance activities, electronic pillboxes that sound an alarm to remind the individual to take medication, and arranging the person's clothes to promote appropriate and socially acceptable clothing choices (Velligan & Bow-Thomas, 2000).

## Psychological Therapies

Psychological therapies include those interventions that are derived primarily from the discipline of psychology. The most common psychological therapies used for persons with SSD are cognitive behavioral therapy and cognitive restructuring therapy.

### Cognitive Behavioral Therapy (CBT)

Cognitive behavioral therapy (CBT) is a form of psychotherapy that has been used successfully in depression and a number of other clinical syndromes since the mid-1970s. More recently, it has been used to treat persistent psychotic symptoms in persons with SSD in the United Kingdom. However, it has not been widely used in the United States.

CBT is based on the assumptions that the way individuals perceive situations influences their thoughts, emotions, and behaviors. In addition, persons may be influenced by core beliefs that result from life experiences. If the thoughts, emotions, behaviors, and core beliefs are negative, they are likely to exacerbate psychotic symptoms in persons with SSD. Some CBT experts believe that the way in which persons with SSD interpret the psychotic symptoms rather than the symptoms themselves is the cause of their distress. The aim is to assist the patient to reduce and master the distress (Morrison, 2005).

Although psychotherapy as a treatment for SSD has fallen out of favor in the United States due to a firmly rooted medical model, CBT is believed to be effective and well-tolerated by persons with SSD because it emphasizes a focus on the present, structures sessions through the use of homework and exercises, and is time limited. Research supports that CBT reduces the distress caused by residual psychotic symptoms more effectively than other psychological treatments such as supportive psychotherapy. This effectiveness is demonstrated when CBT is combined with other usual treatments such as medication and case management.

Briefly, the process of CBT begins with the establishment of a trusting therapeutic relationship as a foundation. The therapist and patient collaborate to build the problem list and formulate a treatment plan that addresses thoughts, feelings, and behaviors associated with problem areas. The therapist assists the patient to view his or her experience of psychotic symptoms from a normal perspective, collaboratively explores core beliefs that may be contributing to the problem, and formulates alternative explanations for their distress.

> *Cognitive behavioral therapy (CBT) is an effective treatment modality for schizophrenia because it focuses on the present, involves sessions requiring homework and exercises, and spans a limited time period.*

### Cognitive Rehabilitation or Restructuring Therapy (CRT)

As noted earlier, cognitive impairments are likely the most disabling aspects of thought disorders, contributing to the functional difficulties experienced by patients in work, social, and educational situations. Cognitive rehabilitation therapy (CRT) has been developed to assist patients in improving their memory and thinking styles. Such therapies are tailored to the specific patient problems identified after a careful assessment of the range and severity of individual cognitive impairments. The treatment is structured to involve pairs of patients, patients and therapists, patients and computers, or a combination of all three. CRT is often a manualized therapy, which means that it must be carefully delineated in a treatment manual and requires complete adherence to the description of the treatment to be successful. The goal is to improve cognition immediately through "exercises" and then transfer that improved cognitive ability to real-world situations to improve functional capacity. While CRT has not been established as an evidence-based practice, it has clear empirical support for its use (McGurk & Mueser, 2004).

## Assertive Community Treatment (ACT)

Assertive community treatment (ACT) is difficult to classify as it combines components of many different treatment modalities. ACT is a transdisciplinary treatment that is characterized by community treatment, low patient-to-staff ratios, and an indefinite duration of treatment. Services provided or available within an ACT program might include intensive case management, pharmacological treatment (with intense compliance monitoring), primary health care, housing/rental assistance, vocational services, substance abuse treatment (emphasizing a harm reduction approach), and enhanced socialization opportunities (Stein & Santos, 1998). ACT is supported by research indicating that it is successful in reducing the annual number of hospital days, arrests, and homelessness, while increasing employment and cost effectiveness.

Additional studies indicate that ACT is very well accepted by a sizable minority of patients. For example, in a study by Gerber and Prince (1999), up to 44% of clients are satisfied with ACT services and reported improvement in quality of life measures.

ACT has several unique characteristics that set it apart from other types of community care. ACT is not a time-limited form of intensive treatment. It requires a set of core professionals making up the team that include but are not limited to a nurse, psychiatrist, social worker, vocational rehabilitation specialist, substance abuse specialist, and a peer counselor. ACT teams have some service capabilities that are available 24 hours a day, seven days a week. Patients referred to ACT usually have been repeatedly unsuccessful with less intensive forms of treatment. Thus, when patients are admitted to an ACT model of care, they are assumed to need that level of care indefinitely. The patient is attached to a team rather than one staff person. While most teams have a primary worker assigned to each patient, that process is fluid. ACT teams encourage staff and patients to gradually develop relationships that best meet the patient's needs. (See Chapter 25 for additional information about ACT.)

## Social Therapies

Social therapies are those that are primarily focused on the social environment of the patient. Social therapies include family- and community-based interventions. Social support is a key component within social therapies, and may be offered to many members of the patient's social network.

### Family Psychoeducation

The long-term goal of family psychoeducation is to improve patient outcomes by promoting family well-being as an intermediate outcome. Family psychoeducation is not one specific model but a group of interventions that constitute a program that is professionally created and led, and lasting from 9 months to several years. It can be done individually, as a group, or as a combination of the two modalities. All methods of family psychoeducation share common characteristics:

- Education of families about psychopathologies
- Demonstration of concern and empathy for families dealing with a mental illness
- Avoidance of blaming relatives or pathologizing their efforts to cope
- Fostering of the development of all family members in their relationships with one another
- Enhancement of adherence
- Instillation of hope (Murray-Swank & Dixon, 2005)

The National Alliance for the Mentally Ill (NAMI) provides a 12-week program in many locations entitled Family to Family. This psychoeducational program includes many dimensions such as content about mental illnesses (including the latest research), workshops for teaching family members how to problem solve and deal with common symptoms and crises that may occur, strategies for intervention, and information about resources available for assistance. It is appropriate to incorporate the Family to Family curriculum (taught by NAMI members) into a longer-term professionally led family psychoeducation program.

Despite the robust research support for this intervention, long-term family psychoeducation has not been widely implemented. Murray-Swank and Dixon (2005) cite three reasons: lack of awareness of the research support, concerns about consumer confidentiality, and, finally, the lack of reimbursement for the program.

> *Family psychoeducation involves teaching the patient and family about the disorder as well as showing concern and empathy for the family, helping to improve the relationships among family members, promoting adherence to the regimen, and instilling hope.*

### Integrated Dual Diagnosis Treatment (IDDT)

Approximately 50% of individuals with SSD have a co-occurring substance abuse disorder. Therefore, all persons with SSD require routine screening for this problem. Despite the high level of co-existing substance abuse disorders and research documenting the success of integrated treatment (IDDT), especially for persons with serious mental illnesses, many communities still do not provide integrated services. The dire consequences of inadequate treatment in this fragile population have made this a matter of great concern because this group is particularly vulnerable to homelessness.

Traditional mental health and substance abuse treatment systems evolved simultaneously but separately within the health care system (Boyle, et al., 2005). The conjecture may be that these entities traditionally have had an antipathy for one another. That antipathy became even more intense as somatic treatments evolved as an increasingly critical part of mental health care. However, recently the two entities working together are producing impressive results for persons with SSD.

IDDT combines individualized treatment modalities and philosophies. Harm reduction is a concept that is often associated with this treatment modality. Harm reduction is a public health philosophy that purports that some human beings will always engage in risky behaviors. However, health care professionals are obligated to mitigate the harmful consequences to preserve life and health. This strategy is contrary to many of the traditional beliefs and practices of treatment systems, which advocate for total abstinence and self-responsibility as the only worthy path to success. An example demonstrating a harm-reduction philosophy is the policy of "damp housing." Instead of insisting on complete sobriety, a housing program allows formerly homeless persons with a dual diagnosis to reside there without the expectation of strict abstinence as long as they can be acceptable tenants (Boyle et al., 2005).

A more precise description of the philosophy of IDDT may be that of gradualism, the policy of working toward goals by gradual stages. Although health care professionals desire that patients stop using substances and adhere to treatment, they accept that cessation may occur over a period of time. In the example of "damp housing," the hope is that the individual will remain safe and be able to begin engaging with a caring health care professional. Should a window of opportunity present itself, more intense services would be readily available.

Another critical ingredient of IDDT is a sense of optimism. Many persons suffering from dual disorders have experienced multiple episodes of treatment failure in a fragmented treatment situation. Thus, they actively avoid interactions with the mental health and substance abuse treatment system. Subsequently, the methods of IDDT, which include assertive outreach, practical assistance, and an articulated belief in the individual's potential to recover, are essential.

IDDT teams consist of nurses, physicians, employment specialists, substance abuse counselors, and case managers. Core services provided include medication management (often long-acting antipsychotics), substance abuse counseling, housing assistance, and family psychoeducation. These services are not time limited. Other

> *Patients with schizophrenia often have a substance abuse disorder that requires treatment.*

services often used include outreach programs, motivational interventions, group treatment, representative payeeships, involuntary treatment, and coordination with the criminal justice system (parole or probation) when indicated (Boyle et al., 2005).

## Social Skills Training

Persons with SSD are at a disadvantage socially for a number of reasons. They experience cognitive disturbances and are exposed to limited opportunities to learn appropriate social behaviors because they often become ill at the time that adult social skills develop. Social skills training is a highly structured program that relies on didactic and experiential components to assist persons with SSD to master critical social skills. These skills may include areas such as starting a conversation, negotiation, and dating or sexual interactions. Skills are broken down into small discrete steps. Through the use of role playing, social modeling, and social reinforcement, individuals with SSD learn to overcome social awkwardness. Social skills training has some empirical support though it is difficult to generalize and further research is required (Tenhula & Bellack, 2008).

## Supported Employment

Employment rates for persons with serious mental illness are about 14% and represent the lowest employment rates of disabled persons, despite the availability of many prevocational programs in community mental health centers (Marwaha & Johnson, 2004). Engaging in meaningful work is an important part of the life of adults and a source of self-esteem, income, and socialization. The supported employment model, which is substantiated by evidence, allows persons with SSD to choose the type of work they would like to do, immediately places patients in competitive employment (working outside of a mental health agency), and supplies patients with a job coach (employed by the mental health system) to assist them to adjust to the employment situation.

A cardinal principle of supported employment is that it is integrated into the mental health services treatment plan. In the past, traditional mental health services and vocational services have not been closely associated with each other. While some patients are able to work full time, most choose part-time work. In addition, benefits counseling is needed to ensure that patients are able to maintain their entitlements (disability payments and medical insurance) when they are employed. This is critical because without continued treatment and access to medication, the person is likely to deteriorate and become unable to work.

The role of health care personnel in supported employment is crucial. Clinicians who prescribe medications, such as advanced practice nurses and physicians, and the psychiatric-mental health nurses who assist patients in managing medications, must do so in a manner that most enables patients to work. Management of medication dosing to minimize lethargy during work hours, simplification of medication regimes, and controlling and treating side effects are just some ways to promote supported employment. In addition, education concerning rest, hygiene, diet, and stress management may help patients maintain a job for a longer period of time.

## Illness Self-Management Training

As the name implies, with illness self-management training, the patient's role changes during the treatment process from one of passive recipient to that of active participant. It is now accepted that the long-term prognosis of SSD is not an inevitable downhill spiral. There is reason to believe that persons with SSD can improve and function as contributing members of society (Gingerich & Mueser, 2005).

Persons involved in the recovery movement have been working diligently to acquaint health care professionals to the idea that patients are willing and capable of collaborating in managing their symptoms and their lives. The goals of illness self-management training are to enable the patient to control symptoms and minimize episodes of relapse and hospitalization, thereby engendering a sense of hope (Resnik, Fontana, Lehman, & Rosenheck, 2005).

To that end, illness self-management training programs have been developed to provide an organized, comprehensive, and auditable approach to assist patients in developing their personal recovery skills. Four critical components of such programs include: elements of psychoeducation, enhancement of medication adherence, relapse prevention, and coping skills training. Trained professionals collaborate with patients to develop a personalized plan in individual or small group sessions over a period of 4 to 8 months. A key value is that of personalization; that is, striving to accomplish the goals of the client within the prescribed program.

## Supported Housing

Persons with SSD often have difficulty obtaining and maintaining adequate housing for a variety of reasons. Possible barriers include the stigma of the illness, poverty, unavailability of safe housing stock in the community, and the instability that accompanies periodic hospitalization. In the past, persons with SSD who were discharged from hospital settings were often required to progress through transitional housing programs or be transferred into nursing homes or other restrictive settings. Many individuals got bottlenecked into more restrictive programs than were necessary because of a lack of housing units on the less restrictive end of the spectrum. Currently, greater emphasis is on direct placement into supported housing settings rather than the step-by-step approach.

Supported housing is a concept that covers a number of program alternatives that promote housing as a priority within mental health treatment systems. Supported housing programs have treatment services readily available. These services may include case management, health services, or benefits assistance to persons living in their housing units. While tenants are not forced to participate in all services, the options approach allows patients both easy access and choice.

The evidence base for supported housing is increasing. Research supports a number of desirable outcomes from supportive housing including reductions in homelessness, hospitalization, incarceration, and psychiatric symptoms. In addition, there is evidence of greater life satisfaction, independent functioning, and a "sense of belonging" or having a place in society (Ridgeway, 2008).

> *Patients with schizophrenia may require social skills training, supported employment, illness self-management training, and supported housing.*

## Self-Help or Peer Assistance

Self-help or peer assistance for persons with mental illness have been developing over the past 40 years in the United States, with roots in the civil rights movement of the 1960s as well as the disability rights movement of the 1980s. Most current groups strive to provide individual assistance through peer-to-peer activities such as regular meetings, telephone warm lines (telephone contact with peers for support in difficult times), and advocacy to promote access to appropriate services, resources, and to decrease stigma. Groups may combine family and consumer advocacy activities, such as those of the National Alliance on Mental Illness and consumer and professional advocacy; for example, the Vet to Vet program within the Veterans Administration. Others are solely managed by individuals with mental illnesses, some of which are modeled after Alcoholics Anonymous, while others are clearly different, with educational and political goals. Still others are focused on separating themselves from what they see as a coercive mental health system, considering themselves "survivors" of the trauma of psychiatric care. Examples of widely used models include the Wellness Recovery Action Plan (WRAP) Program founded by Marianne Copeland, which offers patients a "toolbox" on how to deal with such issues as triggers and warning signs of impending illness (Copeland, 1999). Empirical evidence on the efficacy of self-help mental health groups is currently limited but the self-help experience or movement with other populations makes this a promising idea.

## APPLYING THE NURSING PROCESS FROM AN INTERPERSONAL PERSPECTIVE

Individuals with SSD can be found in many health care settings. Due to the severity of acute exacerbations of psychosis associated with these disorders, they account for 50% of psychiatric-mental health admissions to hospitals. They also represent a large portion of patients served in the public mental health system across the United States. Current estimates are that about 75% of services for patients with schizophrenia are covered by government sources such as Medicare and Medicaid (McDonald, Hertz, Lustik, & Unger, 2005). Many individuals with SSD also have co-morbidities including substance abuse, diabetes, and cardiovascular and respiratory disease. As a result, patients often can be encountered in general medical facilities, hospital emergency departments, and specialty clinics. Therefore, nurses need a firm understanding of the nursing process that integrates the interpersonal process when caring for patients with SSD. **Plan of Care 11-1** provides an example.

### Strategies for Optimal Assessment: Therapeutic Use of Self

Nurses engage in assessment using the interpersonal process, beginning with the initial encounter with the patient. Self-awareness and rapport are essential to establish trust and to develop a therapeutic nurse-patient relationship. These elements provide the foundation to allow assessment to progress so that important information about the patient, family, and his or her signs and symptoms can be obtained.

### Self-Awareness

Assessment of a patient with SSD requires the nurse to have a keen sense of self-awareness. Thus, the development of self-awareness is a critical task when working with this population. Persons with thought disorders are often stigmatized, that is, labeled or marked in a negative fashion. The labels frequently associated with SSD include: violent, incompetent, weak, and lazy. Additionally, patients with SSD may experience three levels of stigma as identified by Corrigan and Larson (2008): public, self, and structural.

- Public stigma describes society's negative beliefs, reactions, and behaviors toward people with SSD.
- Self stigma refers to the internalization of society's negative beliefs where persons with SSD begin to see themselves as incompetent or weak.
- Structural stigma refers to the political, economic, and historical structures that reinforce stigma, such as the inability of persons with SSD to hold public office or obtain professional licensure in some states.

All three types of stigma present barriers for persons with SSD and influence how they may be perceived within a therapeutic relationship as well. **Consumer Perspective 11-1** provides insight into what it is like to experience schizophrenia from the patient's viewpoint.

When beginning to work with this population, the following questions are helpful in promoting self-awareness:

1. How do I feel about an adult, physically healthy person who receives government assistance and has never worked?
2. How do I react when the person I am interviewing has a strong body odor, disheveled clothing, and is passively uncooperative?
3. How do I feel if the person I am admitting to the hospital came there directly from the county jail?

Unlike other illnesses, SSD may elicit feelings of alienation in others rather than sympathy toward the individual suffering from the disorder. Certainly, the association of these disorders with violence, often fueled by popular media, contributes to those feelings of alienation. However, some suggest that the lack of empathy directed at those with mental illness is a result of the difficulty encountered in putting oneself in the place of the victim and in perceiving the sometimes bizarre behavior as a genuine illness. It is easy to empathize with someone with cancer or diabetes because individuals can imagine themselves in those circumstances, but cannot see themselves as subject to "madness" (Torrey, 2006). The effect of this is to avoid contact with afflicted persons, thereby interfering with the nurse-patient relationship. In turn, this can add to feelings of isolation, inferiority, and social stigma for the person experiencing SSD.

Although identifying personal reactions can be uncomfortable, it is necessary to avoid adding to a

### PLAN OF CARE 11-1:
### THE PATIENT WITH SCHIZOPHRENIA SPECTRUM DISORDER

**NURSING DIAGNOSIS:** Disturbed sensory perception (auditory); related to neurological dysfunction; manifested by difficulty in cognitive processing and maintaining focus of attention

**OUTCOME IDENTIFICATION:** Patient will demonstrate a reduction in delusional thinking and hallucinations

| INTERVENTION | RATIONALE |
| --- | --- |
| Approach the patient in a calm, non threatening manner; demonstrate a caring and accepting attitude | Demonstrates caring and acceptance, which helps to foster trust, minimize self-stigma associated with the condition, and promote sharing of information |
| Maintain adequate interpersonal space between self and the patient | Respecting the patient's interpersonal space helps to minimize anxiety and threats patient may be feeling |
| Ensure the environment is safe and patient is free of hazards | Ensuring a safe environment is necessary to prevent injury related to disordered thinking |
| Administer prescribed antipsychotic agents; reinforce use of prescribed therapies, such as cognitive behavioral therapy | Antipsychotic agents help to control the positive and/or negative symptoms of the disorder; other therapies such as cognitive behavioral therapy help to promote reality-based thinking |
| Assess the patient for hallucinations and delusions; evaluate the content of the hallucinations | Assessing for disordered thinking provides information about context of the thinking from which to develop appropriate interventions |
| Acknowledge the existence of the delusions and hallucinations without reinforcing them; inform the patient that the nurse does not share the patient's perceptions | Acknowledging their presence validates what the patient is experiencing without confirming their reality; knowing that the nurse does not share the patient's perception may increase the chance that the patient will begin to question the "realness" of the experience |
| Work with the patient to determine what patient is feeling with the delusion; redirect patient to current reality | Focusing on the feelings of the delusion aid in fostering the understanding that the delusion(s) is (are) not real; redirecting the patient refocuses on the here and now |
| Encourage patient to discuss feelings related to the hallucinations instead of acting on those feelings | Discussing feelings of the hallucinations refocuses the patient on the reality and reduces the risk of acting on them |

*(cont.)*

**PLAN OF CARE 11-1:** (*CONT.*)
**THE PATIENT WITH SCHIZOPHRENIA SPECTRUM DISORDER**

| | |
|---|---|
| Employ reality-based diversional activities as much as possible | Participating in reality-based activities provides distraction and focuses thinking away from the delusions |
| Encourage the patient to connect the feelings with the delusions and hallucinations | Understanding the emotional connection can help the patient identify similar feelings in the future that can be addressed, thus helping to prevent delusions and hallucinations from reoccurring |
| Continue to monitor the patient for recurrence of delusions and hallucinations; provide supervision and surveillance in the least restrictive environment | Continuing to monitor the patient for recurrence is necessary to ensure the patient's overall safety |
| Encourage the patient to report any delusions or hallucinations to staff or others | Reporting of delusions or hallucinations provides opportunities to intervene early and prevent possible bizarre or violent behavior |

**NURSING DIAGNOSIS:** Risk for other-directed or self-directed violence related to lack of impulse control, command hallucinations, paranoia, agitation, aggressiveness

**OUTCOME IDENTIFICATION:** Patient will demonstrate control of behavior to remain safe, without harm to self or others

| INTERVENTION | RATIONALE |
|---|---|
| Assess the patient for indicators suggesting potential for harm to self or others, such as irritability, intimidation, restlessness, shouting or loud voices, or overt threats; ensure the safety of the patient and others | Identifying indicators of potential harm allows for early intervention |
| Question the patient directly about "voices" telling him or her to harm self or others | Understanding the nature of command hallucinations helps in determining the appropriate level of supervision needed |
| Minimize the patient's exposure to stimuli; keep environment calm, quiet, with little distraction; remove all hazardous items from the patient's environment | Limiting stimuli helps to prevent overwhelming the patient, which could lead to increased anxiety and agitation; removal of items reduces the risk of use if behavior escalates |
| Assist patient in identifying signs and symptoms of increasing anxiety and in using measures to reduce anxiety and agitation when they occur; suggest the use of physical activity, talking about feelings, or asking for medication | Being able to identify signs and symptoms promotes early intervention; using measures such as physical activity or talking provides an outlet for reducing anxiety without harming self or others |

*(cont.)*

**PLAN OF CARE 11-1: (*CONT.*)**
**THE PATIENT WITH SCHIZOPHRENIA SPECTRUM DISORDER**

| | |
|---|---|
| Work with patient to employ strategies such as behavior modification to control impulses associated with delusions and hallucinations | Using behavior modification reinforces a positive method of dealing with delusions and hallucinations |
| Ensure the development of a plan if behavior escalation occurs; ensure a unified approach to the patient | Having a plan is necessary to reduce the safety risk for all involved; employing a unified approach demonstrates control over the situation |
| Contract with the patient for no self-harm | Using a no-harm contract emphasizes expectations, fosters participation in care and feelings of control over the situation, and promotes safety |
| If behavior escalation occurs, place the patient in the least restrictive environment; move others away from the area of escalation | Using the least-restrictive environment is necessary to protect the patient's rights; moving others away protects their safety |

**NURSING DIAGNOSIS:** Impaired social interaction related to paranoia and delusional thinking; manifested by inability to trust others and sustain relationships

**OUTCOME IDENTIFICATION:** Patient will begin to interact with others

| INTERVENTION | RATIONALE |
|---|---|
| Institute measures, such as antipsychotic agents and psychotherapy to control delusions | Controlling disordered thinking is needed before the patient can begin to engage socially |
| Assist the patient in talking about feelings related to public- and self-stigma associated with disorder and delusions | Verbalizing feelings helps to provide insight into underlying problems interfering with social relationships |
| Work with the patient to understand the acceptable limits involved with relationships | Understanding the limits involved with relationships is necessary for the patient to engage in a successful interaction |
| Assist the patient in using social skills training; break skills down into small discrete steps; encourage the use of role playing, social modeling, and social reinforcement | Using social skills training gradually introduces the patient to appropriate methods for developing social relationships for eventual mastery of critical social skills |
| Encourage practice of skills, emphasizing patience; provide feedback about performance | Practicing promotes the likelihood of success with a skill that takes time to develop; providing feedback promotes learning and fosters positive feelings about success |

(cont.)

### PLAN OF CARE 11-1: (*CONT.*)
### THE PATIENT WITH SCHIZOPHRENIA SPECTRUM DISORDER

| | |
|---|---|
| Help the patient in developing an initial single social relationship, emphasizing the need for honesty and respect | Developing an initial single social relationship permits the patient to focus on one interaction at a time and prevents the patient from becoming overwhelmed; encouraging honesty and respect are necessary to facilitate trust |

*Nursing Diagnosis—Definitions and Classifications 2009–2011. Copyright © 2011 by NANDA International. Use by arrangement with Blackwell Publishing Limited, a company of John Wiley & Sons, Inc.*

### CONSUMER PERSPECTIVE 11-1:
### LIVING WITH SCHIZOPHRENIA

*Sandy Jeffs has lived with schizophrenia for 33 years. Here she tells how she battles to get through every day:*

EVERY day I wake up with a mantra: "Top myself or eat breakfast." So far I have been waking up and eating breakfast.

I was just 23 when diagnosed with schizophrenia. It was terrifying, like a death sentence. It was seen as a psychiatric cancer.

But being diagnosed meant treatment started and I was given medication and psychological help.

I was unravelling and very unwell. One night I left my friend's house and walked the streets feeling every light was on me and someone was after me with a knife. I ended up being committed to a hospital.

My main symptoms are voices. They are real and as loud as you and I are talking. They are powerful, relentless, and they persecute me. They have a life of their own; they are different genders and personalities. I hate them and they hate me.

I just hope one day I get to have the last word. In the past four years I have been unwell and I hear them most days. At night I hear them so I listen to Beethoven on my MP3.

They say terrible things like, "You are a whore, Satan's whore." Once they told me food and drink was the devil's food so I fasted for a week.

When you go into a psychotic episode the voices take over and your thinking is confused. Your delusions become reality. I haven't worked but have been on a disability pension.

I have published poetry books and I do a lot of public speaking about schizophrenia.

http://www.dailytelegraph.com.au/news/national/sandy-jeffs-on-what-its-like-to-live-with-schizophrenia/story

patient's self stigma when entering into a therapeutic relationship. Strategies for empowerment can be implemented to minimize the stigmatization for persons with SSD within the therapeutic relationship (Corrigan & Larson, 2008). These strategies include seeking collaboration rather than compliance, fostering decision-making capabilities, and approaching treatment as a peer endeavor with equal partners working together to understand the illness experience to arrive at a successful treatment plan.

### Rapport

Developing adequate rapport is essential for an effective assessment. Persons with SSD may be quite stressed and anxious during the assessment experience, especially if they are being admitted to an in-patient facility or are being admitted to treatment involuntarily. Because SSD is a chronic disease, unless it is the initial presentation, the patient is likely to have been through the process of assessment previously, and those experiences may influence their attitude in the current situation.

The goal is to begin the development of the therapeutic relationship during this assessment process. In this therapeutic encounter, the nurse communicates caring and acceptance of the patient as a worthy human being. This acceptance is the first step in developing trust. Throughout the interactions, the nurse should be consistent in communication and continue to provide support, building the relationship over time.

> *When assessing a patient with schizophrenia, nurses need to be self-aware and to establish rapport with the patient to prevent the stigma associated with this disorder from interfering with the assessment and development of the therapeutic relationship.*

### Environmental Management

When meeting with the patient, allow for adequate interpersonal space during the assessment process. Arranging space for safety, comfort, and privacy is important. Approach the person in a calm and reassuring manner. It may be desirable to break up the assessment process over several sessions depending on the person's ability to attend to the task. Mental health assessments often include questions that may be uncomfortable for persons with an acute psychosis, so priority setting is important. Brief, focused assessments may be necessary. In addition, be consistent and follow through on comments, suggestions, or promises, which will help foster a sense of trust. Be alert for signs of agitation or fear, which can impact the patient's safety.

### Health History and Examination

The priority during the first encounter with the patient is assessment for suicidal or homicidal ideation, command hallucinations, current medications, and/or physical health problems or injuries. Questions related to these issues are the most critical to ensure the patient's safety.

As appropriate, a detailed assessment is initiated. It should include a description of the presenting problem. Use a broad-opening statement such as "Tell me what brought you to the clinic" to elicit information. From there, obtain the following: a family history including mental illness diagnoses; a medical history and current treatments; use of legal and illegal substances; a psychiatric history including hospitalizations and treatment modalities; a personal history including information on education, employment, spiritual and cultural influences; interpersonal relationships; a history of trauma or abuse; and a legal history. In addition, assess for suicidal, homicidal, aggressive, or self-harm tendencies with each encounter in an out-patient setting and at least once a shift in an inpatient setting. Such detail is necessary to collaboratively formulate a uniquely personal treatment plan.

Assessment of the patient's current symptoms is important. Use a methodical, attentive approach to ensure that the information obtained is complete. SSD is a complex and chronic disorder with an extremely wide variation in the presentation of symptoms. Thus, be knowledgeable of the typical signs and symptoms and be alert for their appearance. Complete a mental status examination, making sure to assess mood, affect, speech, perceptual disturbances, thought process and content, sensorium, cognition, judgment, and insight. Throughout this examination, be alert for positive and negative symptoms of SSD (**Table 11-2**). Keep in mind that negative symptoms are blamed for much of the disability of SSD and are less amenable to standard treatment protocols such as pharmacotherapy.

There are no specific laboratory findings associated with SSD. At times, patients may experience associated medical syndromes. For example, persons with SSD are prone to ingest excessive amounts of fluids and may develop water intoxication, which causes electrolyte imbalances. Neuroleptic malignant syndrome (NMS), a complication of the use of antipsychotics, will cause elevations in creatinine phosphokinase (CPK). Thus laboratory testing may be used to address these problems.

> *The psychiatric-mental health nurse needs to use a broad opening statement to obtain information from the patient about his or her current status. Throughout the assessment, the nurse is vigilant in observing positive and negative symptoms of schizophrenia.*

Two other medical conditions often associated with SSD are metabolic syndrome and diabetic ketoacidosis. Interest in these two conditions increased as it became evident that second-generation antipsychotic drugs induced metabolic syndrome in many persons with SSD

**TABLE 11-2: POSITIVE AND NEGATIVE SYMPTOMS OF SSD EXAMPLES OF DISTURBED SPEECH**

| POSITIVE SYMPTOMS | DEFINITION/DESCRIPTION | EXAMPLES |
|---|---|---|
| Hallucinations | A sensory experience not caused by external stimuli. Can be auditory (most common), visual, olfactory, gustatory, or tactile | *Auditory:* Hearing voices, music, animal sounds, mechanical noises such as clock ticking<br>*Visual:* Seeing blood, people, or insects<br>*Olfactory:* Smelling feces or putrefaction<br>*Gustatory:* Metallic taste or blood<br>*Tactile:* Crawling insects or being beaten |
| Delusions | Firmly held false beliefs involving the self, interpersonal relationships, or the environment | *Grandiosity:* Woman believes she is pregnant with a messiah<br>*Persecution:* Man believes he is being targeted by mafia hit man<br>*Reference:* Woman believes story line on soap opera is about her<br>*Somatic:* Man believes his brain has dissolved<br>*Thought broadcasting:* Man believes coworkers know about his intrusive homosexual fantasies though he has not revealed them<br>*Control:* Woman believes dentist implanted a device in her mouth that directs her activities |
| Disorganized speech | The outward sign of disorganized thinking. Speech can be disorganized in a variety of ways. It can be oblique, incompletely related, or literally incomprehensible. Communication is impaired | *Tangential:* When asked his home address a man describes the bus route he took to the clinic, the people on the bus, and the stores near his home<br>*Loose association:* "Breakfast at eight. Eight sisters and all are married like Maryann, Sister Maryann teaching children penmanship…."<br>*Clanging:* "I slept, kept, swept…"<br>*Echolalia:* Nurse says "Time for vitals then dinner." Client answers "Vitals and dinner, dinner, dinner…" |
| Disorganized behavior | Behavior that is not goal directed, which leads to difficulties in activities of daily living. This also may include catatonic excitement, rigidity, or stupor | Client paces from one end of hall to the other, touching each doorknob<br>*Excitement:* Hyperactive, assaultive, driven<br>*Rigidity:* Sits straight up in chair with left hand planted firmly on top of head for hours<br>*Stupor:* Lying in bed, not responsive to surroundings |
| Disorganized thought | May be single most important symptom. Contributes to the burden of disability | Indecisive, poor problem solving, concrete thinking, thought blocking, difficulty planning and initiating activities |
| NEGATIVE SYMPTOMS | DEFINITION/DESCRIPTION | EXAMPLES |
| Affective flattening | Limited range of emotion and little interpersonal connectivity such as poor eye contact | Woman describes brutal rape with no emotion |
| Alogia | Sometimes referred to as poverty of speech and is characterized by brief, bland, minimalist replies | Man replies "OK" to all requests/statements and only with prompting during a 30-minute conversation about seeking a new apartment |
| Avolition | Limited ability to plan and organize goal-directed activities | Woman subsists on crackers and tea though she has sufficient resources and transportation to go to the supermarket |
| Anhedonia | Loss of interest in formerly pleasurable activities | Formerly artistic young woman stops her beloved jewelry making. Does little but smoke and stare out the window |

and diabetic ketoacidosis in a smaller but significant number. **Evidence-Based Practice 11-1** highlights a study addressing weight gain associated with metabolic syndrome and use of second-generation antipsychotic agents. Additionally, later studies have documented persons with SSD die up to 25 years earlier than the general population from preventable disorders hastened by unhealthy lifestyles and lack of access to primary care (Parks, Svedsen, Singer, & Foti, 2006). Nurses need to be aware of the possibility of associated medical problems to advocate for and ensure adequate care. Recent studies also demonstrate that nurses working as care managers make a significant difference in meeting the health care needs of the SSD population (Druss, von Esenwein, Compton, Rask, Zhao, & Parker, 2010). One recent study is highlighted in **Evidence-Based Practice 11-2**.

## Diagnosing and Planning Appropriate Interventions: Meeting the Patient's Focused Needs

Identifying and planning for needs for the person with SSD depends on multiple factors including the person's

---

### EVIDENCE-BASED PRACTICE 11-1: INTERVENTION FOR SCHIZOPHRENIA SPECTRUM DISORDERS

#### STUDY

Beebe, L.H., & Smith K. (2010). Feasibility of the walk, address, learn and cue (WALC) intervention for schizophrenia spectrum disorders. *Archives of Psychiatric Nursing, 24*(1), 54-62.

#### SUMMARY

The authors conducted a feasibility study involving a group of 17 individuals with SSD. A specific intervention, called the Walk, Address sensations, Learn about exercise, and Cue exercise behavior (WALC) intervention, which was designed to motivate exercise in the elderly, was adapted for the population being studied. Adaptations included low-intensity stretches, exercise education, and exercise cues. Approximately two-thirds of all groups were attended and nearly half of participants attended at least 75% of groups. The authors concluded that follow-up studies are needed to evaluate how this intervention may impact future exercise behavior in the hopes of identifying "evidence-based interventions to increase exercise in this group."

#### APPLICATION TO PRACTICE

This study is of particular interest for psychiatric-mental health nurses because it combines interventions deemed appropriate for persons with SSD. It promotes exercise, which may address the metabolic side effects of second-generation antipsychotics and may potentially combat feelings of depression common in persons with SSD. The intervention also addresses potential problems in executive functioning when planning a complex activity through the use of information, education, and cues. These interventions provide growing evidence about effective measures aimed at potentially combating weight gain and promoting quality of life in persons with SSD.

#### QUESTIONS TO PONDER

1. *Other than walking, what other types of exercise might a psychiatric-mental health nurse suggest to include as part of a similar exercise program?*
2. *How might a patient's delusions or hallucinations affect the implementation of such an exercise program?*

**EVIDENCE-BASED PRACTICE 11-2:**
**EFFECTS OF A PLANNED INTERVENTION ON INDIVIDUALS WITH SEVERE MENTAL ILLNESS**

### STUDY

Druss, B., von Esenwein, S., Compton, M., Rask, K., Zhao, L., & Parker, R. (2010). A randomized trial of medical care management for community mental health settings, The Primary Care Access, Referral, and Evaluation (PCARE) study. *American Journal of Psychiatry, 167* (2), 151-159.

### SUMMARY

The researchers conducted a quasi-experimental study involving 407 individuals with severe mental illness. The individuals were randomly assigned to one of two groups: a management intervention group and a usual care group. The individuals in the management intervention group received communication and advocacy with medical providers, health education, and support in navigating the system. Findings revealed that there were significant differences between the groups when evaluated after 12 months. The group receiving the management intervention showed significant improvement in the mental component of the evaluation. This group also received more services.

### APPLICATION TO PRACTICE

This study is important for psychiatric-mental health nurses because it shows that specific interventions can foster improvement in the functioning of individuals with severe mental illness. Poor quality of care contributes to excess morbidity and mortality among patients with severe mental illness. Psychiatric-mental health nurses, when applying the therapeutic use of self and the interpersonal process, play a key role in advocating for and teaching patients. This study helps to underscore the positive effects of such activities.

### QUESTIONS TO PONDER

1. *What other areas of the therapeutic nurse-patient relationship would be appropriate to use for further study and research?*
2. *This study addresses patients with severe mental illness. How would this study apply to patients with SSD?*

---

current status and the resources available. Persons with SSD comprise some of the most vulnerable populations in our society. An estimated one-third to one-half of persons who are homeless are mentally ill. Approximately one-half of that population suffers from SSD (McQuistion & Gillig, 2006). Priority needs often include safety, nourishment, shelter, and medical care. Cooperating or committing to active mental health treatment may be weeks or months down the road once the nurse is able to establish a therapeutic relationship with the patient with SSD.

Awareness of illness is another factor. While some persons with SSD are acutely aware that they have a problem, others may seem quite oblivious. That decreased awareness of illness, termed anosognosia, is actually a neurological symptom distinct from denial of illness. It complicates planning because the individual does not see a need to engage in the treatment process because they are "not sick" (Amador, 2003).

Community resources also must be considered. Psychiatric-mental health treatment systems in the United

States today typically are significantly underfunded. Psychiatric hospital bed space has decreased dramatically (Treatment Advocacy Center, 2008). Additionally, funding for community mental health treatment is actually decreasing in real dollars allocated (New Freedom Commission, 2003). Subsequently, due to this lack of funding for workforce training, many of the evidence-based practices for treating SSD are unavailable.

Recently, the push toward empowerment for persons with SSD has received increased support at the grass roots level. In addition, individuals with SSD are becoming more aware of themselves and their role in managing their illness in relation to their individual life goals. Recognizing, affirming, and collaborating with the personal strength and resilience exercised by persons with SSD is a critical part of the planning process (Deegan, 2010).

Due to the varying assessment findings noted and the wide range of problems faced by patients with SSD, several nursing diagnoses would apply. Examples of possible nursing diagnoses would include:

- Disturbed sensory perception related to disordered thinking, difficulty in cognitive processing of information, difficulty in maintaining focus of attention
- Impaired social interaction related to inability to trust, paranoia, delusional thinking
- Self-care deficit related to inability to manage routine daily activities, thought disturbances, inattention
- Social isolation related to lack of trust, impairment in processing interpersonal stimuli (e.g., maintaining eye contact), over-assessment of threat from others
- Risk for injury related to lack of impulse control, command hallucinations
- Risk for self- or other-directed violence related to lack of impulse control, command hallucinations, paranoia, lack of trust

These nursing diagnoses also will vary based on the acuity of the patient's illness, developmental stage, co-morbidities, current treatment regimen, and sources of support. For example, the person with SSD with acute psychosis may have disturbed sensory perception, self-care deficit, and risk for violence simultaneously. During periods of remission, nursing diagnoses such as diversional activity

> *Patients with schizophrenia often present with a wide range of symptoms. Therefore, nursing diagnoses appropriate for a patient must reflect this variation.*

deficit, loneliness, or chronic low self-esteem may be the priority areas to be addressed. However, nurses need to remember that disorders of thought or cognition are recognized as the most disabling aspect of the disorder and they persist through acute illness and interepisodic periods.

Based on the identified nursing diagnoses, the nurse and patient collaboratively would determine the outcomes to be achieved. For example, for the nursing diagnosis of impaired social interaction, the nurse would first develop a therapeutic interpersonal relationship with the patient. Gradually, as the patient becomes ready, the nurse would assist the patient to engage in interactions with others, such as other patients, family members, or other staff members.

## Implementing Effective Interventions: Timing and Pacing

When implementing interventions for patients suffering from a chronic disorder such as SSD, timing and pacing of effective interventions are critical. During an initial episode of psychosis or during a relapse, persons are often hospitalized in a community facility such as a psychiatric unit of a general hospital or a residential crisis facility. The initial interventions focus on promoting safety and establishing a therapeutic relationship as a means to reassure persons with SSD and their families. For example, constant monitoring of the patient is often indicated. This may mean that the patient would have to be placed in an environment in which the amount of stimuli is controlled, such as a secluded area, or it may require a one-to-one monitoring by a staff member. The priority safety needs reflect the assessment findings, such as evidence of command hallucinations or thoughts of harm to self or others. **How Would You Respond 11-1** provides an example of implementation for a patient with a thought disorder.

The nurse intervenes in positive symptoms through medication, communication, and environmental manipulation as needed. Immediately establishing communication with families is desirable. Expression of support and empathy as well as providing information for family members are primary tasks for nurses employed in inpatient and residential facilities. **Therapeutic Interaction 11-1** provides a sample interaction that applies the interpersonal process.

Patients receiving treatment involuntarily in the hospital or community setting require special attention. At times, patients may need coerced treatment of persons with SSD to ensure the safety of the person and the community. However, this may produce resentment and influence individuals to avoid treatment in the future.

Based on research, the perception of coercion can be reduced for persons with SSD who are subject to involuntary treatment by promoting the process of procedural justice (MacArthur Research Network, 2001). The elements of procedural justice are transparency (patient is kept apprised of situation), the belief that those involved in treatment have benevolent motives (nurses and other providers are interested in their well-being), and the opportunity for the patient to have a "voice" in the process (to be able to state their position and feelings) (MacArthur Research Network, 2001). Thus, the nurse

promotes active participation by the patient in the elements of his or her care, a key aspect of the therapeutic relationship and interpersonal process. Nurses are in a unique position, especially in the in-patient setting, where most involuntary treatment episodes are initiated, to promote procedural justice and thereby reduce the perception of coercion.

As patients become stable, nurses modify the interventions to focus on the patient's transition back to the community and out-patient treatment. Interventions at this juncture include collaboration in promoting treatment

### HOW WOULD YOU RESPOND? 11-1: A PATIENT WITH A THOUGHT DISORDER

Jerry Brown is a 30-year-old white male who was transferred from the county jail to an acute care psychiatric unit. Jerry was arrested outside his parents' home about 3 days ago after an attempt to break into the house at 2 a.m. about 3 days ago. When the nurse begins the admission process, Jerry confides that his parents are agents of the Demon Saboteur. Per Jerry, the Demon who has been living in his parents' home for the past year is now "transmigrating through the wires" to Jerry's apartment and is communicating threats to Jerry through the television. The reason Jerry was breaking into the house was to "cut the wires" to stop the Demon Saboteur's activities.

Jerry is dressed in a jail jumpsuit and appears fatigued with bags under his eyes and hollow cheeks. He admits that he has not been sleeping. He also appears not to have showered or brushed his teeth for several days. He is hypervigilant but accepts an offer of juice and crackers. Jerry answers questions noting he has never worked and is receiving government benefits. He lives alone in a small apartment

in the city. Jerry admits he does not take prescribed drugs as he feels he is not ill so he does not need medicine. He graduated from high school and attended a community college for one semester. His jail records indicate that he has had 4 arrests in the past 3 years for similar incidents involving his parents' home and once for possession of cannabis. He has also been hospitalized twice but was lost to treatment after discharge. Jerry allows you to notify his younger sister that he is in the hospital though he does not want to talk to her. In conversation with his sister you find that Jerry's parents love him but fear him when he is acutely ill. His sister is also very interested in his welfare but feels torn between her brother and her exasperated parents. She is relieved he is out of jail but wishes somehow this cycle could be stopped. Jerry is started on antipsychotic medication, specifically a second generation antipsychotic. After several days of therapy, Jerry begins to discuss his life outside the hospital. He discusses his solitary existence and loss of contact with people his own age.

### CRITICAL THINKING QUESTIONS

1. *How do Jerry's assessment findings correlate to the diagnostic criteria for schizophrenia, paranoid type?*
2. *What would be two priority nursing diagnoses for Jerry?*
3. *How would psychoeducation play a role in Jerry's treatment?*
4. *How would you respond to his sister's concern about her brother?*

**APPLYING THE CONCEPTS**

Jerry is demonstrating delusions involving paranoid thoughts that the Demon is out to get him. He also exhibits hypervigilance and has had difficulties with work and social functioning, as evidenced by his four arrests and living alone. Physically, he shows signs of inadequate sleep and hygiene. Priority nursing diagnoses would include disturbed sensory perception, impaired social interaction, deficient self care, and risk for violence.

With the start of antipsychotic therapy, Jerry would need to learn about the drug therapy, its actions, frequency, duration, and intended effects. Psychoeducation would also focus on monitoring for side effects, especially extrapyramidal symptoms and neuroleptic malignant syndrome. Since he is taking a second-generation agent, he would need to be cautioned about possible orthostatic hypotension and to be instructed in measures to reduce the risk of metabolic syndrome. Jerry and his family also need education about the disorder and possible relapse, especially if medication adherence is a problem.

The nurse would use therapeutic communication skills to elicit exactly what the sister's concerns are and then formulate a plan to address these concerns. The nurse would develop a therapeutic relationship with the sister to foster a sense of understanding about her brother's condition and how best to support him.

adherence and relapse prevention through actions such as psychoeducation, promoting organized behavior, setting realistic social, vocational, and personal goals, and making referrals to appropriate community resources for both the patient and family. Nurses play a major role in patient and family psychoeducation. **Patient and Family Education 11-1** provides suggestions for teaching.

Antipsychotic agents are commonly prescribed for patients to control their symptoms. However, patients often have difficulty adhering to the medication regimen. Nurses play a key role in working with patients to facilitate adherence to a prescribed medication regimen. Studies suggest that perhaps 75% of persons with SSD are non-adherent with oral medication. Such non-adherence contributes significantly to relapse (Lieberman, Stroup, McEvoy, Swartz, Rosenheck, & Perkins, 2005).

> *An important consideration when implementing care for a patient with schizophrenia is to ensure adherence to the prescribed medications. Patient and family psychoeducation is a key intervention.*

Research has identified three routes to increased adherence. Nurses can promote one or more of these

routes with the patient. The first is the use of long-acting antipsychotic medications. While the number of agents in this category is limited, this method simplifies the medication regimen for many patients. Nurses can advocate for a longer-acting medication if the patient and nurse determine that this is a valuable option. A second method that may be helpful in promoting adherence is to connect an effective medication regimen to meeting the patient's personal goals. For example, if the patient wishes to finish his or her education, it may be effective to discuss how medication may assist in eliminating or minimizing the disturbing experience of hallucinations, thereby allowing the patient to concentrate on studies. A third route to medication compliance may be tailoring adherence cues to the person's lifestyle. For example, encouraging the patient to place the medication bottle in a cup with his or her toothbrush may provide a reminder to take the medication before going to bed or when arising in the morning (Miller, 2005).

## Evaluation: Objective Critique of Interventions and Self-Reflection

Evaluation is a process that begins immediately after the initiation of each intervention and continues through each episode of care. The evaluation process in nursing is dictated by the collaborative goals and outcomes set in the planning phase of the nursing process. It is essential to gather the objective data regarding a patient's

### THERAPEUTIC INTERACTION 11-1:
### INITIAL INTERACTION WITH PATIENT WITH SCHIZOPHRENIA

Mr. P. is an 80-year-old man who was admitted to the inpatient psychiatric nursing unit last evening with a primary diagnosis of schizophrenia.

| | |
|---|---|
| **Nurse:** "Good morning, Mr. P. I am Nurse Jones and I am here to assist you today." | Introduces self in order to identify role and begin establishment of rapport |
| **Mr. P.:** "I do not need your help." (pacing around room). "I have all of the help I need from my parents; they are here with me." (referring to others who are not present) | Denying need for help; delusional about parents being in the room |
| **Nurse:** "Mr. P., I am here to help you. I would like to walk with you. Will you come with me to walk in the hallway?" | Continues to develop rapport; focuses on positive behavior of pacing as a means to channel anxiety and energy |
| **Mr. P.:** "You are just like my children, trying to control me." | Expresses distrust of others, specifically the nurse and his children |
| **Nurse:** (stays quietly with patient while he continues to pace in the room) | Building trust by not rejecting patient or his behavior |
| **Nurse:** "Mr. P., now it is time for breakfast. Will you come with me to the breakfast room?" | Continues to build trusting relationship with patient |
| **Mr. P.:** (walks out of room with nurse, but does not say anything to her; walks with her to breakfast room) | Display of beginning of relationship on which trust can be built |

status in each identified problem area such as self-care, communication, thought and perceptual alterations, role functioning, and interpersonal/family relationships. It is equally important to discuss the patient's perceptions of his or her response to treatment and to ascertain if the outcomes have been met. Coming to a mutual understanding about what has been most helpful or not helpful during this time is also desirable. When mental health professionals do not understand the patient's point of view, they run the risk of making assumptions about the acceptability of treatment options. In such circumstances, the opportunity for appropriate treatment negotiation may be lost and lead to relapse if the patient's concerns are not heard or not addressed during evaluation.

Self-reflection on the part of the mental health professional is an equally important part of the evaluation. As the interpersonal relationship develops, it will be important for the professional to acknowledge his/her own thoughts, associations, and feelings related to the patient. At times, the professional may need to "step back" from the encounter to reflect and develop awareness of the influence that he or she is having on the therapeutic relationship. Self-reflection is facilitated by consultation with professional colleagues in the mental health field.

## PATIENT AND FAMILY EDUCATION 11-1: LIVING WITH SCHIZOPHRENIA

- Know the signs and symptoms of a relapse (changes in mood, affect, speech, attention, memory, behavior), or the development of hallucinations or delusions. Call your health care provider as soon as you or your family notices any changes.

- Follow the instructions for taking the medication exactly as prescribed.

- Use a calendar, pill box, or another method to help you remember when to take the medications.

- If you experience dry mouth from the medication, try sips of water or sugarless candies or gum.

- Change positions gradually; wait a few minutes before standing up after lying down or sitting.

- Notify your prescriber if you develop tremors, restlessness, strange movements, or other unusual symptoms.

- Call your prescriber immediately if you develop severe muscle rigidity or a fever.

- Do not drink alcohol when taking medications; check with prescriber before taking any over-the-counter medications or herbal preparations.

- Set realistic goals for yourself.

- Use the coping strategies that you were taught, especially during times of stress or crisis, such as changing the environment, reducing stimuli, and maintaining social support.

- Keep appointments for scheduled therapies.

- Obtain support from local community agencies.

## SUMMARY POINTS

- Thought disorders involve disturbances in thinking, reality orientation, and social involvement. Schizophrenia Spectrum Disorders (SSD) are thought disorders of which schizophrenia is a specific diagnostic category.

- Thought disorders include schizophrenia and its five subtypes: schizophreniform disorder, schizoaffective disorder, delusional disorder, brief psychotic disorder, and shared psychotic disorder.

- A patient with schizophrenia typically exhibits positive and negative symptoms. Positive symptoms include: delusions, hallucinations, disorganized speech, and disorganized behavior. Negative symptoms include: affective flattening, alogia, avolition, ambivalence, and anhedonia.

- The etiology of SSD is unknown. The greatest known risk factor is genetics; however,

environmental factors such as maternal stress and intrauterine infection may also play a role. Psychosocial factors contribute to exacerbations of the disorder in genetically vulnerable individuals.

- Evidence-based practice treatment strategies most applicable to persons with SSD include psychotropic medication, cognitive behavioral therapy (CBT), family psycho-education, assertive community treatment (ACT), integrated dual diagnosis treatment (IDDT), illness self-management training, assertive community treatment, and supported employment.

- Pharmacological therapy involves the use of antipsychotic agents, typically classified as first- or second-generation antipsychotics. These agents do not cure the disorder but they are effective in managing the symptoms of the disorder. Patient

(cont.)

## SUMMARY POINTS (*CONT.*)

adherence to the medication regimen is essential to ensure the effectiveness of therapy.

- There is an intense stigma associated with all mental illness but especially SSD. To work effectively with persons with SSD, psychiatric-mental health nurses must recognize their reactions to the population

and how these reactions could influence the therapeutic relationship.

- Integration of the interpersonal process throughout the nursing process helps to promote positive patient outcomes. Effective prioritized interventions in acute illness are critical. Families also require significant education and support.

## NCLEX-PREP*

1. A patient is brought to the emergency department by an emergency medical team because the patient was behaving violently. When talking with the patient, the nurse notices that he suddenly shifts the conversation from one topic to another but the topics are completely unrelated. The nurse would document this finding as which of the following?

   a. Delusion
   b. Hallucination
   c. Neologism
   d. Loose association

2. The nurse is conducting an interview with a patient diagnosed with schizophrenia. Throughout the conversation, the patient responds to questions and statements with, "okay." The nurse interprets this as reflecting which of the following?

   a. Affective flattening
   b. Alogia
   c. Avolition
   d. Anhedonia

3. After reviewing information related to the symptoms of schizophrenia, a group of nursing students indicate the need for additional review when they identify

which of the following as a positive symptom?

   a. Delusion
   b. Hallucination
   c. Affective flattening
   d. Echolalia

4. A patient is diagnosed with schizophrenia, catatonic type. Which of the following would the nurse expect to assess? Select all that apply.

   a. Stereotyped movements
   b. Mutism
   c. Absence of delusions
   d. Echopraxia
   e. Odd beliefs

5. The nurse is preparing to assess a patient with acute psychosis for the first time. Which of the following would be a priority?

   a. Providing a gentle touch to calm the patient
   b. Taking as long as necessary to gather all the information
   c. Focusing on the type of delusions the patient is experiencing
   d. Assessing for indications of suicidal ideation

(*cont.*)

## NCLEX-PREP* (*CONT.*)

6. A patient is receiving a second-generation antipsychotic agent. Which of the following might this be?

    a. Chlorpromazine
    b. Haloperidol
    c. Fluphenazine
    d. Aripiprazole

7. A patient with schizophrenia is about to start medication therapy with clozapine.

Which of the following would be most important for the nurse to do?

    a. Obtain a baseline white blood cell count
    b. Monitor the patient for high fever
    c. Suggest the use of hard candy to alleviate dry mouth
    d. Assess for cogwheel rigidity

*Answers to these questions appear on page 639.

## REFERENCES

Amador, X. (1998). *Insight and Psychosis.* NY: Oxford University Press.

American Psychiatric Association. (2004). Practice guideline for the treatment of patients with schizophrenia. 2nd Edition, Arlington, VA.

American Psychiatric Association. (2000). *Diagnostic and Statistical Manual of Mental Disorders,* 4th edition, Text Revision. Washington, DC: Author.

Arey, B., & Marder, S. (2008). Other medications. In K. Mueser & D. Jeste (Eds.), *Clinical handbook of schizophrenia* (pp. 186–195) NY: Guilford Press.

Auslander, L., & Jeste, D. (2004). Sustained remission of schizophrenia among community-dwelling older outpatients. *American Journal of Psychiatry, 161*(8), 1490–1493.

Beebe, L.H., & Smith K. (2010). Feasibility of the walk, address, learn and cue (WALC) intervention for schizophrenia spectrum disorders. *Archives of Psychiatric Nursing, 24*(1), 54–62.

Bellack, A. (2006). Scientific and consumer models of recovery in schizophrenia: Concordance, contrasts, and implications. *Schizophrenia Bulletin, 32,* 432–442.

Boyle, P., Delos Reyes, C., & Kruszynski, R. (2005) Integrated dual disorder treatment. In R. Drake, M. Merrens, & W. Lynde (Eds.). Evidence-based mental health practice (pp. 349–366). New York: W. W Norton Company.

Castle, D., & Morgan, V. Epidemiology. In K. Mueser & D. Jeste (Eds), *Clinical handbook of schizophrenia* (pp. 15–23) NY: Guilford Press.

Copeland, M. (1999). *Wellness Recovery Action Plan.* West Dummerston, VT: Peach Press.

Corrigan, P., & Larson, J. (2008). Stigma. In K. Mueser, & Jeste, D. (Eds), *Clinical handbook of schizophrenia* (pp. 533–540) NY: Guilford Press.

Deegan, P. Conspiracy of hope. Retrieved May 8, 2010 from http://www.patdeegan.com/aboutus.html

Doegenes, M., Moorhouse, M., & Murr, A. (2010). *Nursing diagnosis manual: Planning, individualizing, and documenting client care.* Philadelphia: F.A. Davis.

Downar, J., & Kapur, S. (2008). Biological Theories. In K. Mueser, & D. Jeste (Eds.), *Clinical handbook of schizophrenia* (pp. 25–34) NY: Guilford Press.

Druss, B., von Esenwein, S., Compton, M., Rask, K., Zhao, L., & Parker, R. (2010). A randomized trial of medical care management for community mental health settings, The Primary Care Access, Referral, and Evaluation (PCARE) study. *American Journal of Psychiatry, 167*(2), 151–159.

Evans, F.B. (1996). *Harry Stack Sullivan: Interpersonal theory and psychotherapy.* NY: Routledge.

Ferriera, A. (1961). The etiology of schizophrenia: a review. *California Medicine, 94*(6), 369–377.

Gerber, G., & Prince, P. (1999). Measuring client satisfaction with assertive community treatment. *Psychiatric Services, 50,* 546–550.

Gingerich, S., & Mueser, K. (2005). Illness management and recovery. In R. Drake, M. Merrens, & W. Lynde (Eds.), *Evidence-based mental health practice* (pp. 395–424). NY: W. W. Norton.

Kuipers, E., Bebbington, P., Dunn, G., Fowler, D., Freeman, D., & Watson P. (2006). Influence of career expressed emotion and affect in nonaffective psychosis. *British Journal of Psychiatry, 188,* 173–179.

Lavretsky, H. (2008). History of schizophrenias a psychiatric disorder. In K. Mueser, & D. Jeste (Eds), *Clinical handbook of schizophrenia* (pp. 3–13) NY: Guilford Press.

Lieberman, J. T., Stroup, S., McEvoy, J., Swartz, M., Rosenheck, R., Perkins, D., Keefe, R., Davis, S., Davis, C., Lebowitz, B., Severe, M., & Hsiao, J. (2005). Effectiveness of antipsychotic drugs in patients with chronic schizophrenia. *NEJM , 253*(12), 1209–1223.

MacArthur Research Network on Mental Health and the Law. (2001). MacArthur Coercion Study. Retrieved May 7, 2010 from http://www.macarthur.virginia.edu/coercion.html

Marwaha, S., & Johnson, S. (2004). Schizophrenia and employment: A review. *Social Psychology and Psychiatric Epidemiology, 39,* 337–349.

McClintock, S., Ranginwala, N., & Husain, M. (2008). Biological Electroconvulsive Therapy. In K. Mueser, & D. Jeste (Eds.), *Clinical handbook of schizophrenia* (pp. 196–203) NY: Guilford.

McDonald, M., Hertz, R., Lustik, M., & Unger, A. (2005). Health care spending among community dwelling adults with schizophrenia. American Journal of Managed Care, *11*(8), 242–47.

McGurk, S., & Mueser, K. (2004). Cognitive functioning, symptoms, and work in supported employment: A review and heuristic model. *Schizophrenia Research, 70,* 147–73.

McGrath, J., Saha, S., Chant, D., & Welham, J. (2008). Schizophrenia: a concise overview of incidence, prevalence, and mortality. *Epidemiologic Reviews, 30,* 87–76.

McQuistion, H., & Gillig P. (2006). Mental illness and homelessness: An introduction. In P. Gillig & H. McQuistion (Eds.), *The mentally ill homeless person* (pp. 1–8). Washington DC: American Psychiatric Publishing.

Miller, A. (2005). Medications. In R. Drake, M. Merrens, & D. Lynde (Eds.), In *Evidence-based mental health practice: A textbook* (pp. 453–477). NY: W. W. Norton.

Morrison, A.P. (2005). Trauma and psychosis: Theoretical and clinical implications. *Acta Psychiatic Sandinavia 112,* 327–329.

Murray, C., & Lopez, A. (1996). The global burden of disease: A comprehensive assessment of mortality and disability from diseases, injuries, and risk factors in 1990 and projected to 2010. Cambridge: *Harvard University Press.*

Murray-Swank, A., & Dixon, L. (2005). Evidenced-based practices for families of individuals with severe mental illness. In R. Drake, M. Merrens, & D. Lynde (Eds.), *Evidence-based mental health practice: A textbook* (pp. 425–452). NY: W.W. Norton.

Munich, R.L. (1997). Contemporary treatment of schizophrenia. *Bulletin of the Menninger Clinic, 61,* 189–221.

New Freedom Commission on Mental Health. (2003). *Achieving the promise: Transforming mental health in America.* (DHHS Publication No. SMA-O3–383). Rockville, MD: Department of Health and Human Services.

Palmer, B., & Heaton, R. (2000). Executive dysfunction in schizophrenia. In T. Sharma and P. Harvey (Eds.), *Cognition in schizophrenia: Impairment, importance and treatment strategies* (pp. 51–72). NY: Oxford University Press.

Parks, J., Svedsen, D., Singer, P., & Foti, M. (2006). Morbidity and mortality in people with serious mental illness. Thirteenth Annual Technical Report, National Association of State Mental Health Program Directors, Alexandria, VA.

Resnik, S., Fontana, A., Lehman, A., & Rosenheck, R. (2005). An empirical conceptualization of the recovery orientation. *Schizophrenia Research, 75,* 119–126.

Ridgeway, P. (2008). Supported housing. In K. Mueser & D. Jeste (Eds.), *Clinical handbook of schizophrenia* (pp. 287–297). NY: Guilford Press.

Stein. L., & Santos, A. (1998). *Assertive community treatment of persons with severe mental illness.* NY: W W. Norton.

Sullivan, P., Kendler, K., & Neale, M. (2003). Schizophrenia as a complex trait: Evidence from a meta-analysis of twin studies. *Archives of General Psychiatry, 60,* 1187–1192.

Tenhula, W., & Bellack, A. (2008). Social skills training. In K. Mueser & D, Jeste (Eds.), *Clinical handbook of schizophrenia* (pp. 287–297). NY: Guilford Press.

Thelander, B. (1997). The psychotherapy of Hildegard Peplau in the treatment of people with serious mental illness. *Perspectives in Psychiatric Care. 33*(3), 24–32.

Treatment Advocacy Center, Severe shortage of psychiatric beds sounds national alarm bell. Retrieved May 7, 2010 from http://www.treatmentadvocacycenter.org/index.php?option=com_content&task=view&id=81&Itemid=247

Torrey, E.F. (1980). *Schizophrenia and civilization.* NY: Aronson.

Torrey, E.F. (2006). *Surviving schizophrenia.* NY: Harper.

Velligan, D., & Bow-Thomas, C. (2000). Two cases of cognitive adaptation training for outpatients with schizophrenia. *Psychiatric Services, 51,* 25–29.

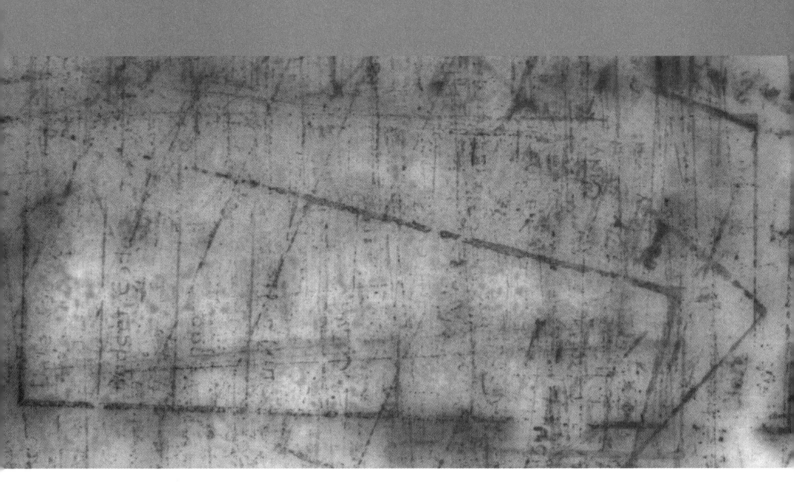

## CHAPTER CONTENTS

## EXPECTED LEARNING OUTCOMES

**After completing this chapter, the student will be able to:**

1. Define affective disorders.
2. Identify the disorders classified as affective disorders.
3. Discuss the history and epidemiology of affective disorders.
4. Analyze current theories related to the etiology of affective disorders, including relevant neurobiological and psychodynamic theories.
5. Distinguish among the *Diagnostic and Statistical Manual of Mental Disorders, 4th edition, Text Revision (DSM-IV-TR)* diagnostic criteria for affective disorders.

6. Discuss suicide and how it is related to affective disorders.

7. Describe common assessment strategies for individuals with affective disorders.

8. Demonstrate effective therapeutic use of self when communicating with a person diagnosed with an affective disorder or experiencing suicidal thoughts.

9. Explain various treatment modalities including those that are evidence-based practice (EBP) for the person demonstrating signs and symptoms of an affective disorder and/or is suicidal.

10. Apply the nursing process from an interpersonal perspective to the care of patients with affective disorders or who are experiencing suicidal thoughts.

## KEY TERMS

Affective disorder

Ambivalence

Hypomania

Mania

Melancholia

Mood

Serotonin syndrome

Suicidal Ideation

Suicide

Most people experience transient periods of depressed moods in their life. Fluctuations in MOOD (a person's overall emotional status), especially during times of loss, change, and other social stressors are normal as one's mood is not static. However, fluctuations occurring for a sustained period of time are suggestive of an AFFECTIVE DISORDER. An affective disorder, a term frequently used interchangeably with depressive or mood disorders, predominantly involves a persistent disturbance in mood. Affective disorders also influence a person thoughts, emotions, and behavior. The affective disorders include: major depressive disorder, dysthymic disorder, bipolar disorder types I and II, and cyclothymic disorder. Another affective disorder, called seasonal affective disorder (SAD), deals with periods of depression during winter months or that which occurs in parts of the world that experience decreased light and sun. It is not presently listed as a disorder in the *DSM IV-TR* but there is some discussion of including it in the next edition. Psychiatric-mental health nurses need to be able to identify and differentiate the different types of affective disorders.

This chapter addresses the historical perspectives and epidemiology of affective disorders as defined in the *Diagnostic and Statistical Manual, 4th edition, Text Revision* (*DSM-IV-TR*, 2000). Suicide, often a sequela of affective disorders is also addressed. Current psychosocial and biological etiological influences of affective disorders are addressed along with current treatment modalities. Application of the nursing process from an interpersonal perspective is presented, including a nursing plan of care for a patient with an affective disorder who is suicidal.

## HISTORICAL PERSPECTIVES

Affective disorders were described as early as 4th century B.C. in Greek medical literature. Hippocrates used the term MELANCHOLIA (black bile) to describe sad or dark moods noted in patients with depression and the term MANIA to describe mental disturbances such as elevated mood, grandiosity, difficulty with attention span, and sometimes psychosis in some patients.

During the 17th and through the 18th centuries, Europeans continued to use the term melancholia for a range of mental illnesses. The depressed were less burdensome to the community, especially in large crowded cities, and were usually ignored. Thus they suffered alone with no hope of a cure. However, manic and psychotic persons were more likely to be locked up in "insane or lunatic asylums." Conversely, the wealthy frequented the famous European spa towns to "take the waters"

in the hopes that these experimental treatments would relieve their symptoms. There is little evidence proving the effectiveness of this treatment especially on a long-term basis.

By the end of the 19th century, practitioners had begun to experiment with hypnosis as a treatment for "nervous" complaints. Influenced by this method, Sigmund Freud believed buried childhood memories were the cause of depression in adult life. So he used hypnosis to assist the patient to unlock these buried or suppressed memories in order to deal with the effects of the past experience on their present life. Hypnosis as a treatment remained popular in Europe and the United States during and after World War II. By 1938, electroconvulsive therapy (ECT) was being used because it was found to lessen depressive symptoms. It is still used today although the method of delivery has changed drastically. During the 1950s, psychopharmacology became prominent with the discovery of antidepressants. Tricyclic antidepressants were first, followed by the monoamine oxidase inhibitors (MAOIs). In the 1970s, serotonin reuptake inhibiters (SSRIs) were discovered. Newer medications targeting various other neurotransmitters are constantly being tested and approved for use in treatment of affective disorders, such as the serotonin/norepineherine reuptake inhibitors (SNRIs). Talk therapies, like cognitive behavioral therapy (CBT) are frequently used to treat affective disorders. Research studies have indicated the most effective treatment for affective disorders is a combination of psychopharmacology and talk therapy (emental-health.com, 2010; Andreasen & Black, 2001).

> During the 1940s, electroconvulsive therapy was used to treat depression. The use of medications to treat affective disorders arose during the 1950s and continues through today.

## EPIDEMIOLOGY

Statistics and prevalence for affective disorders according to the National Institute of Mental Health's web site, ([NIMH], 2010) and derived from the 2004 U.S. census reveal that approximately 20.9 million American adults, or about 9.5 percent of the population of the United States age 18 and older in a given year, have a mood disorder, with an average age of onset of 30 years. Statistics related to specific affective disorders show the following:

- Depressive disorders often co-occur with anxiety disorders and substance abuse disorders.
- Major Depressive Disorder is the leading cause of disability in the United States for individuals between the ages of 15 to 44 years, affecting approximately 14.8 million American adults, or about 6.7 percent of the U.S. population age 18 and older in a given year.
  - While major depressive disorder can develop at any age, the median age at onset is 32 years.
  - Major depressive disorder is more prevalent in women than in men.
  - Dysthymic disorder affects approximately 1.5 percent of the United States population age 18 years or older, or approximately 3.3 million American adults, with an average age of onset of 31 years.
- Bipolar disorder affects approximately 5.7 million American adults, or about 2.6 percent of the United States population age 18 years and older in a given year, with a median age of onset of 25 years.
- Approximately 33,300 (about 11 per 100,000) people died by suicide in the United States in 2006.
  - More than 90 percent of people who kill themselves have a diagnosable mental disorder, most commonly a depressive disorder or a substance abuse disorder.
  - The highest suicide rates in the United States are found in white men over age 85.
  - Four times as many men as women die by suicide; however, women attempt suicide two to three times as often as men (NIMH, 2010).

> *Major depressive disorder is a leading cause of disability in the United States, affecting greater numbers of women than men.*

## DIAGNOSTIC CRITERIA

Affective disorders include the following: major depressive disorder; dysthymic disorder; Bipolar I disorder; Bipolar II disorder; and cyclothymic disorder. Each disorder has specific set of diagnostic criteria that a patient must meet for diagnosis. **Box 12-1** highlights the major diagnostic criteria as identified by the *DSM-IV-TR* (American Psychological Association, 2000).

## Major Depressive Disorder

A patient with major depressive disorder has experienced a change from previous functioning with evidence of a depressed mood or decreased interest or pleasure in his or her usual activities. This change in mood lasts most of the day for over two weeks. The patient can report this mood change or it can be observed by others. The patient also must exhibit other symptoms as listed in Box 12-1.

Major depressive disorder can be further classified by the current status as:

- Single or recurrent episode
- Mild, moderate, or severe
- With or without psychotic features (such as hallucinations or delusions)
- With catatonic features (psychomotor disturbances such as excessive motor activity, waxy flexibility or stupor, mutism, extreme negativism echolalia, or echopraxia)
- With melancholic features (lack of reactivity to usually pleasurable activities, loss of pleasure in all or almost activities, distinct depression, depression usually worse in the morning, marked psychomotor retardation or agitation, significant anorexia or weight loss, or escessive or inappropriate guilt)
- Chronic
- With seasonal pattern (recurrence associated with a specific time of the year)
- With postpartum onset (within four weeks after birth [APA, 2000])

> *The diagnosis of major depressive disorder must include depressed mood or loss of interest or pleasure in conjunction with at least four other symptoms: significant weight loss; hypersomnia or insomnia; psychomotor agitation or slowness; fatigue or energy loss; difficulty concentrating or indecisiveness; or recurrent thoughts of death.*

## Dysthymic Disorder

Dysthymic disorder involves depressive symptoms that are chronic and must be present for at least two years for adults or one year for children and adolescents. Dysthmia is

### BOX 12-1: DIAGNOSTIC CRITERIA

#### MAJOR DEPRESSIVE DISORDER

In addition to the depressed mood or loss of interest or pleasure in usual activities, at least four of the following must be present:

- Significant weight loss without dieting or weight gain or markedly decreased or increased appetite
- Hypersomnia or insomnia
- Psychomotor agitation or slowness
- Fatigue or energy loss
- Feelings of worthlessness or guilt
- Difficulty concentrating or indecisiveness
- Recurrent thoughts of death, either with or without suicide ideation
- Symptoms cause significant distress or impair social, occupational, educational, or other functioning
- Symptoms are not caused by a substance or a general medical condition

#### DYSTHYMIC DISORDER

In addition to the individual's chronic depressive symptoms, the individual has never been without at least two of the following symptoms for more than two months:

- Poor appetite or overeating
- Hypersomnia or insomnia
- Fatigue or energy loss
- Feelings of hopelessness or helplessness
- Low self-esteem
- Difficulty concentrating or indecisiveness

Additionally, the person has:

- Never been diagnosed with a major depressive disorder
- Never been diagnosed with a manic, mixed, or hypomanic episode, and does not meet the criteria for cyclothymic disorder

Also, the symptoms:

- Are not caused by a substance, medication or general medical condition.
- Cause the patient significant distress or impair social, occupational, educational, or important functioning

#### BIPOLAR I DISORDER

*Manic Episode*
- Abnormally persistently elevated and expansive or irritable mood for at least one week.
- Presence of at least three or more of the following:
  - Excessive participation in pleasurable and often high-risk activities
  - Decreased need for sleep
  - Inflated self-esteem or grandiosity
  - Easy distractibility
  - Excessive speech or pressure to keep talking
  - Flight of ideas or racing thoughts
  - Increase goal-oriented activity or psychomotor agitation
  - Markedly impaired functioning in more than one area (occupational and/or social)
- Symptoms not due to effects of a substance or general medical condition

*(cont.)*

## BOX 12-1: DIAGNOSTIC CRITERIA (*CONT.*)

*Major Depressive Episode*

- During the same two-week period, presence of five or more of the following symptoms:
  - Depressed mood most of the day, nearly every day, as indicated by either subjective report or observation. In children and adolescents, can be irritable mood.
  - Decreased interest in nearly all normally pleasurable activities is present
  - Significant weight gain or weight loss
  - Significant decrease or increase in appetite
  - Experiences fatigue or energy loss
  - Psychomotor retardation or agitation
  - Hypersomnia or insomnia
  - Difficulty with concentration, decreased thought, or indecisiveness
  - Feelings of worthlessness or excessive guilt
  - Thoughts of death with or without suicidal ideation are recurrent

*Mixed Episode*

- For one week or longer, criteria met for both manic and major depression episodes nearly every day.
- Marked decreased ability to function occupationally, educationally, or socially.
- Symptoms are not a result of general medication condition or medication effects or drug abuse.

### BIPOLAR II DISORDER

- Recurring major depressive episode and at least one hypomanic episode

**HYPOMANIA**

- For at least four days, experience of an elevated, expansive or irritated mood clearly different from normal mood
- At least three of the following present:
  - Inflated self-esteem or grandiosity
  - Decreased need for sleep
  - More talkative or pressured speech
  - Subjective experience that thoughts are racing
  - Distractibility
  - Increase in goal directive activities
  - Excessive involvement in pleasurable activities that have a high potential for painful consequences
- Symptoms causing a decrease ability to function in social, occupational, or educational situations, and causing patient emotional distress; episode not severe enough to cause marked impairment in social or occupational functioning, or to necessitate hospitalization; psychotic features absent
- Symptoms not a result of general medication condition or medication effects or drug abuse.

### CYCLOTHYMIC DISORDER

- For at least two years, evidence of numerous periods of hypomania and depressive symptoms without meeting criteria for major depressive disorder
- Symptoms never absent during the 2-year period
- No evidence of major depressive episode, manic episode or mixed episode
- Symptoms not due to effects of a substance, or general medical condition
- Significant distress or impairment in social, occupational, or other important areas of functioning

*From the Diagnostic and Statistical Manual of Mental Disorders, Fourth Edition, Text Revision, (Copyright © 2000). American Psychiatric Association.*

considered a milder form of depression. The patient experiences a depressed mood which can be self-reported, such as "feeling sad or down in the dumps" or observed. The patient also must exhibit other symptoms as listed in Box 12-1.

## Bipolar I Disorder

Bipolar I disorder is characterized by the occurrence of one or more manic episodes or mixed episodes (mania and major depression), and often one or more major depressive episodes (see Box 12-1). Substance-induced mood disorders either due to medication or drug of abuse are excluded as well as mood disorder due to a general medical condition. Mixed episodes may present as extreme irritability and/or agitation at times. A patient experiencing a mixed episode also may be experiencing psychotic features and will most likely require hospitalization to prevent harm to self or others.

## Bipolar II Disorder

Bipolar II disorder is characterized by recurring major depressive episode (see previous sections) either currently or in the past, and at least one hypomanic episode. The patient has never experienced symptoms that meet the criteria for a manic or mixed episode.

## Cyclothymic Disorder

Cyclothymic disorder is defined by chronic fluctuations of mood from numerous periods of both depressive symptoms and hypomania. A diagnosis is not made unless the patient has been free of major depression, manic, or mixed episodes for at least two years. Additionally, other psychiatric disorders must be ruled out along with general medical conditions, or substance abuse or medication (APA, 2000).

## Suicide

The *DSM-IV-TR* does not include diagnostic criteria for SUICIDE or suicidal behavior. Additionally, suicide is not considered a disorder. However it is a behavior often

*Suicide is considered a behavior and not a disorder. The DSM-IV-TR does not identify diagnostic criteria for this behavior. Ambivalence is frequently the underlying theme involved with suicide.*

resulting from an affective disorder. Suicide is frequently described as an act of AMBIVALENCE (conflicting or opposing ideas, attitudes or emotions)

## ETIOLOGY OF AFFECTIVE DISORDERS

At this time in history there is no single scientific theory that explains the cause of affective disorders. Many theorists suggest multiple causes as an explanation for the development of affective disorders.

## Psychosocial Theories

A number of psychosocial/psychological theories suggest psychodynamic influences play a role in causing affective disorders. For example, learned helplessness theory is based on studies performed Seligman (1992) dealing with dogs and avoidable shock (see Chapter 10 for an expanded discussion of Seligman's work). Cognitive theory (Beck, et. al., 1979) is based on the premise that negative and faulty thoughts lead to negative feelings and behaviors. Freud and other therapist have posited that anger turned inward can lead to depression. He believed that a loss of a love object, either real such as through death or perceived such as by rejection or loss of value to the person led to melancholia. Childhood temperament is thought to be a factor. Stress for prolonged periods of time has been studied as a factor leading to affective disorders. Several of these theories are summarized in **Table 12-1**.

## Biological Theories

There are numerous theories suggestive of a biological basis for depression and bipolar. While none of them have been fully accepted as a definitive or exact cause, research continues to provide us with new knowledge about these illnesses and some are discussed in the following section.

### Neurobiological influences

The most common theories addressing neurobiological influences involve the neurotransmitters serotonin, dopamine, and norepinephrine. It is believed that patients who are experiencing affective disorders, especially the

*Neurotransmitters, such as serotonin, dopamine, and norepinephrine, have been identified as playing a role in affective disorders.*

**TABLE 12-1: SELECTED PSYCHODYNAMIC INFLUENCES ASSOCIATED WITH AFFECTIVE DISORDERS**

| THEORY | DESCRIPTION |
|---|---|
| Learned Helplessness (M. Seligman) | Harnessed canines exposed to a sustained electrical shock could not escape; additional experiments followed with the same dogs, unharnessed and exposed to the electrical shock; canines despite being free to escape or avoid the shock did not |
| | Adaptation of experiments to humans: added the human dimension of attribution of meaning (cognitive explanations) to negative events in a person's life using an optimistic vs. pessimistic lens (self-explanation) |
| | Proposed that prior inescapable negative events, negative cognition, and locus of control are important contributors to depression in humans |
| Cognitive theory (A. Beck, et al.) | Cognitive distortions (negative expectations of environment, self, and future) as the underlying mechanism leading to negative, defeatist attitudes |
| | Distortions develop because of a defect in the development of cognition leaving the person to feel inadequate and worthless |
| | Pessimistic and hopeless attitude for the future |
| Psychoanalytical theory (S. Freud) | Melancholia developing after loss of an identified love object leaving person feeling ambivalent |
| | Rage resulting from the loss directed inward resulting in depression |

depressive symptoms, have an altered level of these neurotransmitters or dysfunction at the receptor sites. However, the exact role of the neurotransmitters is not known. Treatment with medications that block the reuptake of various neurotransmitters have shown positive outcomes for patients (emental-health.com, 2010; Andreasen & Black, 2001).

## Genetics

Most researchers agree there seems to be a genetic predisposition for developing affective disorders. Affective disorders tend to "run in families," and a definite association has been scientifically established (Andreasen & Black, 2001). Much research has been conducted regarding genetics. Numerous investigators have documented that susceptibility to a depressive disorder is twofold to fourfold greater among the first-degree relatives of patients with mood disorder than among other people. The risk among first-degree relatives of people with bipolar disorder is about six to eight times greater. Some evidence indicates that first-degree relatives of people with mood disorders are also more susceptible than other people to anxiety and substance abuse disorders (Tsuang & Faraone, 1990). Genetics continues to be an explosive field for research.

## TREATMENT OPTIONS

An interdisciplinary team approach is used to treat patients with affective disorders regardless of the setting. Nurses' role in the treatment team is of major importance as they are often the professional who spends the most time with the patient. Advanced practice nurses may treat patients in hospitals, clinics, or private practice settings.

Various treatment options are available for patients who are diagnosed with affective disorder or having suicidal thoughts. They include but are not limited to: face-to-face or Internet individual therapy, family therapy, cognitive behavioral therapy, face to face or Internet-based self-help groups, and pharmacological therapy. **Evidence-Based Practice 12–1** highlights a comparison of face-to-face and Internet therapy related to self-disclosure. Research has indicated that while all options are viable depending on the severity of the illness, a combination of psychotherapy or "talk therapy" and medication usually results in the best outcomes (NIMH, 2009).

## Psychopharmacology

Psychopharmacology is a treatment option usually reserved for patients suffering moderate to severe depression, and/or bipolar I or II disorder. Medications used to treat patients with affective disorders include antidepressants and mood stabilizers:

- Tricyclic antidepressants such as amytriptyline, imipramine, amoxapine, and doxepin
- Selective serotonin reuptake inhibitors (SSRIs) such as fluoxetine, paroxetine, sertraline, and escitaloprpram
- Serotonin/norepienephrine reuptake inhibitors (SNRIs) such as duloxetine and venlafaxine
- Selective reuptake inhibitors (also known as serotonin 2 antagonist reuptake inhibitors [SARIs]) such as trazodone
- Selective atypical antidepressantss such as bupropion and mirtazapine

---

**EVIDENCE-BASED PRACTICE 12-1:**
**INTERNET THERAPY**

### STUDY

Rogers, V., Quinn Griffin, M., Wykle, M., & Fitzpatrick, J., (2009) Internet versus face-to-face therapy: Emotional self-disclosure issues for young adults. *Issues in Mental Health Nursing, 30:* 596–602.

### SUMMARY

With the emerging use of the Internet for therapy treatment options, the researchers conducted a study about young adults. A convenience sample of 328 young adult Internet users was recruited from Facebook to complete an online survey. They were asked their preference for face-to-face therapy (F2FT) or Internet therapy (IT). The F2FT group consisted of 263 young adults; the IT group had 65 members. There were no significant differences between the groups on the background characteristics of age, gender, marital status, ethnicity, level of education, income, location, frequency of logging onto the Internet, and therapy history. The Emotional Self-Disclosure Scale (ESDS) was used to assess the eight emotional self-disclosure subscales. Findings revealed significant differences between the two groups on four of the eight subscales (depression, jealousy, anxiety, and fear) indicating that the F2FT group would disclose these emotions to a therapist more frequently than the IT group would. Additionally, 80% of the participants reported a preference for F2FT over IT. An important finding was that 60% of the participants reported a history of F2FT in their past.

### APPLICATION TO PRACTICE

This study was one of the first to explore preferences for treatment for young adults. Additionally, the study provided information about young adult's willingness to disclose emotional issues with their therapist in both formats, with face-to-face therapy participants demonstrating an increase in self-disclosure. This ability for self-disclosure has been linked with positive outcomes in therapy.

### QUESTIONS TO PONDER

1. *Which of the two methods would you prefer and why?*
2. *What consequences might occur with the use of IT?*

---

- Monoamine oxidase inhibitors (MAOIs) such as tranylcypromine, phenelzine, and isocarboxazid
- Mood stabilizers such as lithium and anticonvulsants (carbamazepine, divalproex sodium, and lamotrigine)

**Drug Summary 12–1** highlights the major drugs and associated implications for the interpersonal process.

Antidepressants are the medication of choice for treatment of depression. However, they must be used cautiously in patients with bipolar disorders because they can promote the development of a manic episode. In addition, it often takes time and requires trial and error to find the "right" antidepressant. Although some antidepressants such as selective serotonin reuptake inhibitors may exert their therapeutic effects within a week or so, complete effectiveness may not be achieved for several weeks.

Each group of drugs is associated with side effects. For example, tricyclic antidepressants often cause sedation, orthostatic hypotension, and anticholinergic effects such as dry mouth, blurred vision, constipation, and urinary retention. The anticholinergic effects of this group is often cited as a reason for stopping the medication. Another group of antidepressants, selective serotonin reuptake inhibitors (SSRIs), are associated with sedation, nausea, and sexual dysfunction including decreased libido and erectile dysfunction. In addition, SSRIs interact with numerous medications placing the patient at risk for serotonin intoxication or SEROTONIN SYNDROME due to an overactivity of serotonin or disruption in the neurotransmitter's metabolism. This is a life-threatening situation that requires discontinuation of the SSRI. A patient taking a monamine oxidase inhibitor (MAOI) is at risk for developing a hypertensive crisis if he or she ingests foods that are high in the dietary amine tyramine (Box 12-2) or takes medications whose action mimics the sympathetic nervous system, such as albuterol or amphetamines.

Mood stabilizers including lithium, and anticonvulsants are commonly prescribed for patients with bipolar disorders (see Drug Summary Table 12–1). Lithium is considered the gold standard for treatment of bipolar disorder. However, the margin of safety between therapeutic effectiveness and toxicity is narrow. Therapeutic drug levels range from 0.5 mEq/L to 1.2 mEq/L. Toxicity occurs when drug levels are greater than 1.5 mEq/L. The risk of toxicity also is increased if the patient reduces his or her salt intake or experiences significant diaphoresis or increased

## DRUG SUMMARY 12-1:
## COMMON ANTIDEPRESSANTS USED TO TREAT AFFECTIVE DISORDERS

| DRUG | IMPLICATIONS FOR NURSING CARE |
|---|---|
| **TRICYCLIC ANTIDEPRESSANTS (TCAS)** | |
| amitriptyline (Elavil)<br>amoxapine (Asendin)<br>clomipramine (Anafranil)<br>desipramine (Norpramin)<br>doxepin (Sinequan)<br>imipramine (Tofranil)<br>maprotiline (Ludiomil)<br>nortriptyline (Aventy, Pamelor) | • Urge the patient to take the prescribed drug at bedtime to reduce the risk of injury related to sedation<br>• Offer suggestions for the patient to combat anticholinergic effects, such as dry mouth (using sugarless hard candy or gum), constipation (high fiber intake, moderate physical activity)<br>• Advise patient to change positions slowly to minimize the effects of orthostatic hypotension<br>• Discuss with patient the time to achieve effectiveness and that it may take from 2-4 weeks before symptoms resolve<br>• Emphasize the need for adherence to therapy and to not stop taking the drug abruptly to prevent withdrawal symptoms<br>• Monitor the patient for therapeutic effectiveness of the drug. Anticipate the need to advocate for a change in drug if not effective<br>• Assess the patient for evidence of suicidal thoughts, especially as depression lessens |
| **SELECTIVE SEROTONIN REUPTAKE INHIBITORS (SSRIs)** | |
| fluoxetine (Prozac)<br>paroxetine (Paxil)<br>sertraline (Zoloft)<br>fluvoxamine maleate (Luvox) | • Advise the patient to take the drug in the morning; if sedation occurs, encourage the patient to take the drug at bedtime<br>• Monitor the patient for signs of serotonin syndrome such as fever, sweating, agitation, tachycardia, hypotension, and hyperreflexia |

*(cont.)*

**DRUG SUMMARY 12-1: (CONT.)**
**COMMON ANTIDEPRESSANTS USED TO TREAT AFFECTIVE DISORDERS**

| DRUG | IMPLICATIONS FOR NURSING CARE |
|---|---|
| **SELECTIVE SEROTONIN REUPTAKE INHIBITORS (SSRIs) (CONT.)** | |
| citalopram (Celexa)<br>escitalopram (Lexapro) | • Inform the patient about possible sexual dysfunction with the drug; if this occurs and causes the patient distress, advocate for a change in the drug<br>• Discuss with patient the time to achieve effectiveness and that it may take from 2–4 weeks before symptoms resolve<br>• Emphasize the need for adherence to therapy and to not stop taking the drug abruptly to prevent withdrawal symptoms<br>• Assess the patient for evidence of suicidal thoughts, especially as depression lessens |
| **SEROTONIN/NOREPINEPHRINE REUPTAKE INHIBITORS (SNRIs)** | |
| desvenlafaxine (Pristiq)<br>duloxetine (Cymbalta)<br>venlafaxine (Effexor and Effexor XR) | • Advise the patient taking desvenlafaxine or duloxetine to have his blood pressure monitored because the drug may increase blood pressure<br>• Instruct patient taking venlafaxine to take the drug with food and a full glass of water; if the patient has difficulty swallowing capsules, suggest the patient open the capsule and sprinkle contents on an spoonful of applesauce and take immediately; reinforce the need to follow the capsule with a full glass of water<br>• Encourage the patient to check with his prescriber before taking any other prescription or over-the-counter drugs<br>• Warn patient of possible sedation and dizziness and the need to avoid hazardous activities until the drug's effects are known<br>• Emphasize the need for adherence to therapy and to not stop taking the drug abruptly to prevent withdrawal symptoms<br>• Assess the patient for evidence of suicidal thoughts, especially as depression lessens |
| **SELECTIVE REUPTAKE INHIBITORS (SARIs)** | |
| nefazodone (Serzone)<br>trazodone (Desyrel) | • Work with the patient to develop a schedule that minimizes the risk for dizziness; suggest taking drug after meals or light snack to promote absorption and decrease risk of dizziness<br>• Inform the male patient taking trazodone to report a persistent painful erection immediately<br>• Encourage the patient to check with his prescriber before taking any other prescription or over-the-counter drugs |

(cont.)

**DRUG SUMMARY 12-1: (*CONT.*)**
**COMMON ANTIDEPRESSANTS USED TO TREAT AFFECTIVE DISORDERS**

| DRUG | IMPLICATIONS FOR NURSING CARE |
|---|---|
| **SELECTIVE REUPTAKE INHIBITORS (SARIs) (*CONT.*)** | |
| | • Warn patient of possible sedation and dizziness and the need to avoid hazardous activities until the drug's effects are known<br>• Emphasize the need for adherence to therapy<br>• Assess the patient for evidence of suicidal thoughts, especially as depression lessens |
| **SELECTIVE ATYPICAL ANTIDEPRESSANTS** | |
| buropion (Wellbutrin and Wellbutrin XR)<br><br>mirtazapine (Remeron) | • Inform patient that he or she may experience possible increased restlessness, agitation, insomnia, and anxiety at the start of therapy<br>• Advise patient taking mirtazapine to watch for signs of infection such as fever, sore throat, and to report immediately if they occur<br>• Discuss with patient the time to achieve effectiveness and that it may take up to 4 weeks before symptoms resolve<br>• Encourage the patient to check with his prescriber before taking any other prescription or over-the-counter drugs<br>• Warn patient of possible sedation and dizziness and the need to avoid hazardous activities until the drug's effects are known<br>• Emphasize the need for adherence to therapy<br>• Assess the patient for evidence of suicidal thoughts, especially as depression lessens |
| **MONOAMINE OXIDASE INHIBITORS (MAOIs)** | |
| tranylcypromine (Parnate)<br><br>phenelzine sulfate (Nardil)<br><br>isocarboxazid (Marplan) | • Instruct patient to avoid foods containing tyramine to prevent hypertensive crisis; assist patient in identifying foods to avoid<br>• Remind patient that he or she must avoid tyramine foods for 2 weeks after MAOI therapy is discontinued<br>• Review potential drugs that may interact with MAOIs and encourage patient to avoid these<br>• Teach patient about signs and symptoms of hypertensive crisis such as headache, stiff neck, sweating, nausea, and vomiting; emphasize the need to seek medical attention immediately if any occur<br>• Discuss with patient the time to achieve effectiveness and that it may take from 2-4 weeks before symptoms resolve<br>• Emphasize the need for adherence to therapy and to not stop taking the drug abruptly to prevent withdrawal symptoms |

*(cont.)*

### DRUG SUMMARY 12-1: (*CONT.*)
### COMMON ANTIDEPRESSANTS USED TO TREAT AFFECTIVE DISORDERS

| DRUG | IMPLICATIONS FOR NURSING CARE |
|---|---|
| **MONOAMINE OXIDASE INHIBITORS (MAOIs) (*CONT.*)** | |
| | • Develop a plan with the patient for scheduling the drug doses; advise patient to take the last dose of the day earlier in the day than at bedtime to reduce the risk of insomnia. |
| | • Offer suggestions to combat dry mouth |
| | • Assess the patient for evidence of suicidal thoughts, especially as depression lessens |
| **MONOAMINE OXIDASE INHIBITORS (MAOIs)** | |
| tranylcypromine (Parnate)<br><br>phenelzine sulfate (Nardil)<br><br>isocarboxazid (Marplan) | • Instruct patient to avoid foods containing tyramine to prevent hypertensive crisis; assist patient in identifying foods to avoid<br><br>• Remind patient that he or she must avoid tyramine foods for 2 weeks after MAOI therapy is discontinued<br><br>• Review potential drugs that may interact with MAOIs and encourage patient to avoid these<br><br>• Teach patient about signs and symptoms of hypertensive crisis such as headache, stiff neck, sweating, nausea, and vomiting; emphasize the need to seek medical attention immediately if any occur<br><br>• Discuss with patient the time to achieve effectiveness and that it may take from 2-4 weeks before symptoms resolve<br><br>• Emphasize the need for adherence to therapy and to not stop taking the drug abruptly to prevent withdrawal symptoms<br><br>• Develop a plan with the patient for scheduling the drug doses; advise patient to take the last dose of the day earlier in the day than at bedtime to reduce the risk of insomnia.<br><br>• Offer suggestions to combat dry mouth<br><br>• Assess the patient for evidence of suicidal thoughts, especially as depression lessens |
| **MOOD STABILIZERS** | |
| lithium carbonate (Lithobid, Lithotabs, Lithonate)<br><br>carbamazepine (Tegretol)<br><br>divalproex sodium (Depakote) | • Work with the patient to develop a schedule for laboratory testing of drug levels to promote compliance; remind patient that the level must be obtained 12 hours after the last dose has been taken<br><br>• Discuss with the patient the signs and symptoms of lithium toxicity:<br>-Levels 1.5 to 2.0 mEq/L: blurred vision, ataxia, tinnitus, persistent nausea and vomiting, severe diarrhea |

*(cont.)*

**DRUG SUMMARY 12-1: (*CONT.*)**
**COMMON ANTIDEPRESSANTS USED TO TREAT AFFECTIVE DISORDERS**

| DRUG | IMPLICATIONS FOR NURSING CARE |
|---|---|
| **MOOD STABILIZERS (*CONT.*)** | |
| oxcarbazepine (Trileptal) <br> lamotrigine (Lamictal) <br> tiagabine HCL (Gabitril) | -Levels 2.0 to 3.5 mEq/L: excessive dilute urine output, increasing tremors, muscle irritability, psychomotor retardation, mental confusion <br><br> -Levels over 3.5 mEq/L: impaired level of consciousness, nystagmus, seizures, coma, oliguria or anuria, arrhythmias, cardiovascular collapse <br><br> • Collaborate with patient how to ensure adequate sodium intake; reinforce the need for 6 to 8 large glasses of fluid each day; urge the patient to avoid caffeine beverages which increase urine output <br><br> • Advise patient to increase fluid intake if sweating, fever, or dieresis occurs <br><br> • Suggest the patient take the drug with food if gastrointestinal upset occurs <br><br> • Collaborate with the patient to develop a schedule for blood level testing to promote adherence <br><br> • Institute safety measures to reduce the risk of falling secondary to drowsiness or dizziness <br><br> • Emphasize the need for adherence to therapy and to not stop taking the drug abruptly to prevent withdrawal symptoms <br><br> • Assess the patient for evidence of suicidal thoughts, especially as depression lessens |

**BOX 12-2: FOODS HIGH IN TYRAMINE**

- Aged cheeses including dishes made with aged cheese (except cottage cheese, cream cheese, ricotta cheese, or processed cheese)
- Aged or fermented meats such as pepperoni, salami, summer sausage, beef logs
- Fava bean pods
- Tofu (bean curd)
- Overripe fruit; ripe avocados or figs
- Tap or microbrewery beer; sherry or chianti
- Sauerkraut
- Pickled herring
- Soy sauce or soybean condiments
- Yogurt
- Sour cream
- Brewer's yeast; yeast extract
- Monosodium glutamate

urinary output without adequate replacement. The normal sodium balance is upset, leading to increased reabsorption of lithium by the kidneys, thus increasing drug levels.

*Psychopharmacologic agents used to treat patients with affective disorders include antidepressants and mood stabilizers. Antidepressant agents target neurotransmitters to achieve their therapeutic effect. These neurotransmitters include dopamine, norepinephrine, and serotonin.*

Patient and family education is needed for those patients starting antidepressant therapy. For example, if the patient is prescribed a MAOI, dietary restrictions about foods high in tyramine need to be addressed. For the patient taking lithium, he or she needs instruction about maintaining an adequate salt and fluid intake as well as frequent monitoring of blood levels. Successful education requires that patients be compliant, nonsuicidal, and willing to learn. **Patient and Family Education 12-1** highlights important information for patients taking antidepressants and their families.

> *Patients taking lithium need to have their drug levels monitored closely to reduce the risk of toxicity.*

## ElectroconvulsiveTherapy

Electroconvulsive therapy (ECT) is another treatment option usually reserved for patients who have not responded to medications and other treatment modalities. Before ECT is administered, a patient is given a muscle relaxant and receives short-acting anesthetic. Electrodes are placed on one or both temporal areas for delivery of the electrical impulse. The electrical impulse induces seizure activity. The patient does not consciously feel the electrical impulse administered in ECT. After ECT, the patient may experience transient confusion and disorientation. Memory loss also may occur but this is only temporary.

A patient typically will undergo ECT several times a week, and often will need to take an antidepressant or mood stabilizer to supplement the ECT treatments and prevent relapse. Although some patients will need only a few courses of ECT, others may need maintenance ECT, usually once a week at first, then gradually decreasing to monthly treatments for up to one year. Some patients have been able to receive outpatient maintenance ECT early in the morning, and go to work in the afternoon. Research has indicated that after one year of ECT treatments, patients showed no adverse cognitive effects (NIMH, 2010).

## Cognitive Behavioral Therapy

Cognitive behavioral therapy (CBT) is a form of psychotherapy or "talk therapy" which has been used successfully in depression. CBT is based on the assumptions that the way an individual perceives a situation influences their thoughts, emotions, and behaviors. In addition, persons may be influenced by core beliefs that result from life experiences. CBT helps patients restructure their perceptions thereby resulting in changes in the patient's behavior and

---

**PATIENT AND FAMILY EDUCATION 12-1: TAKING ANTIDEPRESSANTS**

- Avoid use of alcohol and illegal substances as they can interact with your medication and cause a relapse.

- Take the medication exactly as your doctor has prescribed it.

- Be aware that it might take several weeks before you notice any changes in your symptoms. Continue to take the medication even if your symptoms do not subside.

- If you miss a dose, do not double up on the next dose.

- Do not stop the drug suddenly because you might experience withdrawal symptoms.

- Use sugarless hard candy or gum or frequent sips of water you if experience dry mouth.

- Avoid activities that require you to be alert, such as driving, because you may experience drowsiness or dizziness.

- Check with your physician before taking any other medications, including over-the-counter medications and herbal preparations.

- Be alert for signs of worsening depression, mania, or suicide. Call your prescriber immediately if you experience any of these.

- Keep appointments for follow-up care and any lab testing that is scheduled.

- Be aware of national and local support groups for patients and family members.

emotions. It emphasizes a focus on the present, structures sessions through the use of homework and exercises, and is time limited.

## APPLYING THE NURSING PROCESS FROM AN INTERPERSONAL PERSPECTIVE

Patients with affective disorders may be seen in a variety of settings such as acute care settings, day hospitalization programs, community and out-patient centers, and long-term care facilities. Patients who are suicidal, homicidal, or experiencing psychotic symptoms require the highest level of care such as the close supervision in an acute care setting. Many individuals who have co-morbidities such as substance abuse, diabetes, cardiovascular, or respiratory disorders may develop an affective disorder such as major depression. As a result, patients often can be encountered in general medical facilities, emergency rooms, and specialty clinics. Therefore, nurses need a firm understanding of the nursing process that integrates the interpersonal process when caring for patients with affective disorders. **Plan of Care 12-1** provides an example for a patient with major depressive disorder experiencing suicidal thoughts.

### Strategies for Optimal Assessment: Therapeutic Use of Self

Part of learning how to apply therapeutic use of self for the nurse generalist is to spend time evaluating one's own self-perceptions, values, and beliefs. Nursing faculty may have students participate in values clarification exercises to facilitate this introspective journey. Therapeutic use of self, while different than those skills learned from a psychomotor standpoint such as inserting a foley catheter or changing a wound dressing, is nonetheless a valuable nursing tool and skill. Many feel this skill is the cornerstone or foundation of nursing and is most certainly true when talking about the interpersonal process and therapeutic relationship. Recall from Chapter 2 that Peplau (1991) identified six roles of the nurse: stranger, teacher, resource manager, counselor, surrogate, and leader. During nurse-patient relationship, the nurse commonly assumes many if not all of these roles.

As the nurse begins the nurse-patient relationship and meets the patient for the first time, he or she is a stranger to the patient. The nurse can also be viewed as an authority figure for the patient. The nurse is responsible for beginning to establish trust and rapport with the patient. This can be done by showing concern, empathy, and honesty. Pay attention to verbal and nonverbal cues and use therapeutic verbal techniques. Be alert to the possible stigma associated with patients experiencing an affective disorder.

**Consumer Perspective 12-1** provides insight from a patient on what it is like to have Bipolar II disorder.

Conduct the assessment in a safe and quiet place where the patient can feel comfortable and safe. Be sure to include a past medical history, including both physical and psychological details. Any underlying physical cause for the mood disorder needs to be ruled out. When assessing the patient with an affective disorder, also include subjective and objective data related to mood, affect, psychomotor functioning, sleeping patterns, appetite, self-care abilities, cognitive functioning, cultural, ethnic, spiritual factors, and any recent stressors precipitating the episode. Assessment findings may include disturbances in any or all of the above areas. Also, assess for history of past violence, either self-directed and/or other-directed. This information is vital because it can help predict possible similar behaviors by the patient, especially if hospitalized.

Another key area to assess during the initial encounter on admission is SUICIDAL IDEATION (intruding thoughts of harming one's self) or evidence of a suicide plan. This assessment continues as the therapeutic relationship evolves. The nurse needs to ask the patient directly about any thoughts of suicide and if they have a past history of suicide attempt. **Therapeutic Interaction 12-1** illustrates an interaction between a patient and nurse to evaluate for suicidal ideation.

Regardless of how much rapport has been established, assessing for information related to suicide may be uncomfortable and anxiety producing. A common myth is that if one brings up the subject, the patient will be more inclined to commit suicide. However, this is inaccurate and just the opposite is true. Patients who commit suicide because of their ambivalence can often be assisted by nurses to see an alternative to this desperate act.

Most patients give verbal and nonverbal clues about their intent to commit suicide. Verbal warnings could be statements like: "you won't have to worry about me soon" or "everything is going to be OK soon." Nonverbal acts are frequently manifested by giving away prized possessions, getting affairs in order such as making wills or closing out checking accounts. **How Would You Respond?** 12-1 provides an example of a patient with an affective disorder who is exhibiting suicidal thoughts.

> *The nurse needs to assess a patient for suicidal ideation by asking direct questions about suicidal thoughts and any previous attempts at suicide.*

## PLAN OF CARE 12-1:
## THE PATIENT WITH MAJOR DEPRESSION AND SUICIDAL IDEATION

**NURSING DIAGNOSIS:** Risk for suicide; related to impaired judgment, feelings of hopelessness and despair Risk for self-directed violence; related to self-harm ideation.

**OUTCOME IDENTIFICATION:** Patient will demonstrate control of behavior without harm to self.

| INTERVENTION | RATIONALE |
|---|---|
| Approach the patient calmly and non-judgmentally; demonstrate an accepting attitude | Using a calm, nonjudgmental, accepting approach promotes trust and the development of the nurse-patient relationship and fosters feelings of the patient's self-worth |
| Assess patient for thoughts of suicidal ideations (with or without plan) at each shift while awake, and periodically throughout the day; ask patient directly about thoughts of or plan for suicide | Assessing provides a baseline from which to individualize a plan; frequent assessment is needed to ensure the patient's safety; direct questioning is required to identify risk |
| Assess the patient for indicators suggesting potential for harm to self such as increasing withdrawal, tearfulness, excessive rumination; ensure the safety of the patient | Identifying indicators of potential harm allows for early intervention |
| Contract with the patient for no-self harm; assess if patient can verbally agree to notify staff if feeling unsafe. If unable, institute suicide precautions including one-to-one supervision | Contracting for a no-harm contract emphasizes expectations, fosters participation in care and feelings of control over the situation, and promotes safety; suicide precautions promote safety |
| Minimize the patient's exposure to stimuli; keep environment calm, quiet with little distraction; remove all hazardous items from the patient's environment | Limiting stimuli helps to prevent overwhelming the patient, which could lead to increased depression, hopelessness, and powerlessness; removing items reduces the risk and the "means" of use if suicidal thoughts occur |
| Administer antidepressant medications as ordered; ensure that patient has swallowed medication | Using antidepressant agents assists in addressing signs and symptoms associated with depression and suicidal ideation; ensuring that patient has swallowed medication prevents possible hoarding for overdose |
| Be alert for changes in patient's behavior as antidepressant therapy begins to exert effect and reassess for possible suicidal ideation | Reassessing for suicidal ideation when antidepressant therapy becomes effective is important because the patient now potentially has the energy to complete the act |

*(cont.)*

**PLAN OF CARE 12-1: (*CONT.*)**
**THE PATIENT WITH MAJOR DEPRESSION AND SUICIDAL IDEATION**

| | |
|---|---|
| Educate and evaluate for possible medication side effects; assist patient in advocating for medication changes due to potential side effects | Evaluating and educating about side effects is important to ensure compliance with therapy and to prevent untoward reactions |
| Encourage patient to verbalize feelings related to situation and discuss problem causing distress; point out maladaptive thinking: provide patient with a realistic appraisal of the situation | Encouraging verbalization of feelings helps the patient identify underlying feelings related to self-harm; discussing the problem causing the distress brings the issue into the forefront to promote a realistic reframing of the problem |

**NURSING DIAGNOSIS:** Powerlessness; related to perceived lack of control of life circumstances; manifested by indecisiveness and dependency on others in decision making.

Hopelessness; related to intense feelings of negativity about self and circumstances; manifested by no sense of future orientation and loss of pleasure in life.

**OUTCOME IDENTIFICATION:** Patient will verbalize the beginning of feeling in control of the situation. Patient will begin participation in own care and decision making

| INTERVENTION | RATIONALE |
|---|---|
| Assist patient in identifying the underlying reasons for feeling hopeless and powerless; encourage patient to discuss feelings; listen actively in an accepting nonjudgmental manner | Expressing feelings help to identify patient's view of the situation and plan appropriate interventions; actively listening provides opportunities for validation and clarification and helps promote trust and the nurse-patient relationship |
| Help patient identify more realistic means for addressing the underlying situation; point out strengths and positive aspects about the patient | Identifying more realistic interpretations or ways to address the situation promotes feelings of control and self-confidence; pointing out strengths promotes feelings of self-worth |
| Work with patient to identify situations that can precipitate feelings of helplessness and lack of control; assist patient in interpreting situations objectively | Identifying precipitating situations can facilitate the patient's ability to control them; objectively interpreting situations fosters control over them |
| Assess patient's usual methods for problem solving and decision making; help patient identify problematic or maladaptive methods; offer suggestions for more adaptive methods; encourage patient participation in care and decision making, addressing one item or issue at a time | Helping the patient change maladaptive methods to adaptive ones promotes feelings of success and control; encouraging patient participation provides the patient with a "voice" and fosters feelings of control; focusing on one item-issue prevents overwhelming the patient and enhances chances of success |

*(cont.)*

↺ **PLAN OF CARE 12-1:** (*CONT.*)
**THE PATIENT WITH MAJOR DEPRESSION AND SUICIDAL IDEATION**

**NURSING DIAGNOSIS:** Bathing self-care deficit; related to depressed mood and emotional fatigue; manifested by lack of interest in bathing for over a week.

**OUTCOME IDENTIFICATION:** Patient will participate in self-care activities, gradually increasing participation until independent

| INTERVENTION | RATIONALE |
|---|---|
| Determine patient's level of ability in providing self-care | Determining ability to perform self-care provides a baseline for individualized interventions and future evaluation |
| Provide assistance with care as necessary, checking with patient first before giving assistance; break care steps up into steps as appropriate and provide for short rest periods; if necessary, provide clear concrete demonstration of activity | Asking for patient's permission before providing assistance promotes patient control of situation; breaking care into steps, providing demonstration, and providing rest periods reduces the risk of fatigue interfering with patient's ability to provide care |
| Work with the patient to establish a routine for care including the time frame for completing the activities; provide the patient with personal supplies | Establishing a routine lessens the energy needed for decision making related to care; providing personal items for care reduces fears and anxieties. |
| Provide patient with positive reinforcement and recognition for completing activities | Providing positive reinforcement promotes feelings of self-worth and enhances the chances for continued participation, compliance, and success |

*Nursing Diagnosis: Definitions and Classifications 2009–2011. Copyright © 2011 by NANDA International. Use by arrangement with Blackwell Publishing Limited, a company of John Wiley & Sons, Inc.*

If assessment reveals suicidal ideation, safety is paramount. When a patient cannot commit to safety on the unit, the nurse must obtain orders for one-to-one observation, which means a staff member will be present with the patient at all times. The need for this intervention is assessed continuously and the safety of the patient remains the number one priority.

## Diagnosing and Planning Appropriate Interventions: Meeting the Patient's Focused Needs

Once a full assessment is completed, the nurse and the patient, as long as they are cognitively able, proceed to develop a plan of care with mutual goals and expectations for outcomes. If the patient is unable to do this on admission, the nurse assumes the role of leader or surrogate and makes the plan. Once the patient is stable enough to participate in their plan of care, the nurse then collaborates with the patient. The nurse can help the patient identify their needs and specific problems and begin a plan for recovery (Peplau, 1991).

Due to the wide range of assessment findings noted in and multiple problems faced by patients with affective disorders, numerous nursing diagnoses would apply. Examples of possible nursing diagnoses would include:

• Hopelessness related to intense feelings of guilt, worthlessness, loss of pleasure

### CONSUMER PERSPECTIVE 12-1: A PATIENT WITH BIPOLAR II DISORDER

There's an undeniable stigma associated with a psychiatric illness. It's never easy for someone with such a diagnosis to admit it or talk about it, but I feel that the only way health care professionals can truly understand and treat people with psychiatric illnesses is to hear from people like me directly. I have type II bipolar disorder and have been in treatment for twenty years. In that time, I've been on several medication regimens and have been both well-controlled and not so well-controlled. For the last ten years, I've been on one medication that keeps my bipolarity well-controlled. This medication, coupled with therapy, has allowed me to live as normal a life as someone with my diagnosis can. Over the past few years I've become quite comfortable discussing my illness and how I treat it. It's human nature to be curious, so I want to share my experiences to help you understand how I live with bipolar disorder. I like to think that I live a relatively normal life. I'm married, in school, and worked as a paramedic for ten years. When I've told friends about being bipolar, they've always acted surprised. I remember one specific reaction where a fellow medic told me "But you seem so normal!" She wasn't the only person who reacted this way to my disclosure.

Receiving a psychiatric diagnosis can seem like a death sentence. When I was finally diagnosed, it felt like my life was coming to an end. There is an unspoken terror that grips you; a fear that you'll always be labeled as "crazy." Thankfully, I've been able to live my life well, albeit making some modifications to accommodate my diagnosis. I have a very understanding wife (a doctoral candidate in psychology no less) who lets me know when I'm slipping back into old habits. She's the only person I can really listen to when I'm hypo manic or depressive. I trust her judgment and when she tells me she's taking me to the psychiatrist, I go without hesitation. I've taken myself off of medication twice in my life, and both times were disastrous. My backslides into bipolarity sans medication were more insidious than I could have imagined. I became the person I always feared I would and pushed those I cared about away from me. Thankfully, my wife convinced me to restart my regimen and got me back on track. I know that I'll never be able to be off my medication and I've come to terms with it. In order for me to live the life I want to, I have learned to make compromises.

As for my day to day, there are many days when I don't even think about being bipolar. It is possible for me to go whole weeks without actively thinking about my diagnosis. I do have a strictly regimented medication schedule, however, and I have to follow it to the letter. It's a small price to pay for my peace of mind (literally). It is possible for those with psychiatric illness to live well; I have firsthand experience.

- Powerlessness related to feelings of helplessness, lack of control, dependency on others
- Risk for suicide related to depressed mood, feelings of worthlessness, suicidal ideation
- Self-care deficit (bathing, dressing) related to depressed mood, lack of interest in self or activities
- Risk for self-directed or other-directed violence related to impulsivity and impaired judgment, risk-taking behaviors
- Ineffective role performance related to depressed mood, lack of interest in self
- Situational low or chronic low self-esteem related to persistent depressed mood, feelings of helplessness, guilt, shame

These nursing diagnoses also will vary based on the acuity of the patient's illness, developmental stage, co-morbidities, current treatment regimen, and sources of support. For example, the acutely ill person with major depressive disorder may have situational low self-esteem, hopelessness, powerlessness, self-care deficit, and risk for violence simultaneously. During periods of remission, nursing diagnoses such as knowledge deficit or chronic low self-esteem may be the priority areas to be addressed.

Based on the identified nursing diagnoses, the nurse and patient collaboratively would determine the outcomes to be achieved. For example, the patient no longer has suicidal thoughts and expresses they feel hopeful about their future.

> **THERAPEUTIC INTERACTION 12-1:**
> **A PATIENT EXPERIENCING SUICIDAL IDEATION**

M. is a young adult male who has been diagnosed with major depression. He is admitted to the acute care unit of the psychiatric facility. The nurse is interacting with him to establish his risk for self harm.

| | |
|---|---|
| **Nurse:** "Are you having thoughts of suicide or harming yourself?" | Acting direct assessment question. |
| **M.:** "Yes, I think about it all the time." | |
| **Nurse:** "It must be scary to have these thoughts." | Empathizing with patient and exploring underlying feelings behind statement. |
| **M.:** "Yes, these thoughts scare me and are the reason my doctors suggested I come here." | |
| **Nurse:** "Do you have a plan to harm yourself or a method to harm yourself?" | Further assessing for plan and if present, lethality of plan |
| **M.:** "I don't want to kill myself. I don't have a plan I just think about being dead so I don't hurt anymore. I just feel hopeless." | |
| **Nurse:** "Feeling hopeless is often a symptom of depression. Part of your treatment here will be taking an anti depressant medication along with individual and group therapy." | Educating and explaining what to expect while hospitalized. |
| **M.:** "I know I can't continue to go on like this so I am willing to try anything." | |
| **Nurse:** "So, can I trust that you can and will tell the staff if your thoughts become unmanageable so we can make sure you are safe?" | Validating that the nurse heard patient and working to develop trust with patient. Also, clarifying if patient can tell staff if his thoughts of harm become unmanageable. |
| **M.:** "Yes, I will tell the staff if I don't feel safe while here. I don't really want to die. I want to get better." | |

## Implementing Effective Interventions: Timing and Pacing

After problems are identified and outcomes and goals have been set, the nurse works with the patient implementing interventions. These interventions will vary depending on the actual diagnosis; for example, if a patient has low self-esteem the nurse can work with the patient to develop a more healthy sense of self. As described in Chapter 4, nurses need to be mindful of their boundaries and maintain professionalism at all times. The patient may begin to test the nurse during this phase. It is essential to establish

### HOW WOULD YOU RESPOND? 12-1:
### A PATIENT WITH DEPRESSION AND SUICIDAL THOUGHTS

Carol is a 24-year-old female being admitted to the acute care psychiatric unit. She has been diagnosed with Bipolar I disorder. Carol has no medical conditions or illnesses. During the nursing assessment, Carol states she was treated for Bipolar I disorder when she was 18 but did not require hospitalization. Carol was prescribed lithium but stopped taking it about a year ago. She reports that she recently moved to the city to teach secondary school, has a limited support system, and lives alone. Approximately three weeks ago, she experienced a burst of energy and wasn't able to sleep for several days.

She states she then started feeling sad, worthless, hopeless, lonely, and guilt about leaving her parent's home. Carol has a blunted affect, unkempt, and her clothes are dirty. She frequently bursts into tears during her intake. Carol has lost 11 pounds over the past two weeks, has no appetite, and difficulty sleeping. She has missed several days of work this past week due to her not having the "energy to get out of bed." Carol admits to recurrent thoughts of hanging herself but is afraid if she commits suicide she will "go to hell." You are assigned to provide care to Carol.

### CRITICAL THINKING QUESTIONS

1. *How would you describe what Carol is experiencing?*

2. *Does Carol meet the diagnostic criteria for Bipolar I disorder? Explain your answer.*

3. *What would you identify as a priority for Carol at this time?*

### APPLYING THE CONCEPTS

Based on the findings from the assessment, Carol appears to be experiencing a depressive episode that followed what appeared to be a manic episode as evidenced by not sleeping, burst of energy, then her crying, loss of weight and appetite, difficulty sleeping, and missing work. Her statement about having no energy provides further evidence of depression. In addition, Carol is verbalizing thoughts of suicide. The assessment findings revealed her recurrent thoughts of "hanging herself," statements of feeling lonely, hopeless, and worthless, and her unkempt appearance suggesting a lack of interest in herself all help to support the diagnostic criteria for Bipolar I, depressive disorder.

The priority for Carol at this time is addressing her suicidal thoughts and ensuring her safety because she is at risk for self-directed violence.

appropriate limits if necessary and point out inappropriate behaviors in a nonjudgmental and nonthreatening manner. Explain calmly to the patient what behavior is expected and what the consequences are for not adhering to the expectations. Never use punishment as a threat for noncompliance. Continue to work with the patient to meet the stated outcomes or goals (Peplau, 1991).

When providing care to a patient with suicidal behavior, remember that suicide most frequently occurs as a patient is going into a depression or coming out of a depression. When a patient is placed on antidepressants, the medication works first on energy level, then on thought processes and lastly on lifting the mood. Thus, the patient who previously did not have the energy to follow through with suicidal actions, now has an increased energy level to accomplish the act. An important time for hypervigilance by health care providers and families is once the patient is started on medications. Patients also need to be educated about this fact.

> *Nurses need to vigilantly monitor patients with suicidal thoughts for suicidal behavior as antidepressant medications begin to exert their effect, providing the patient with the necessary energy to follow through with the task.*

## Evaluating: Objective Critique of Interventions and Self-Reflection

The nurse evaluates how much progress has been made toward achieving expected outcomes. For any goals not met, the nurse needs to self-reflect on anything he or she may have done differently while providing nursing care. Evaluating how the patient presented upon admission and where they are as discharge approaches is important. During this phase of the nurse-patient relationship, the nurse and the patient should reflect on progress made toward reaching the patient goals. Point out positives to the patient and include a plan for aftercare as appropriate.

This phase is also part of the termination of the patient-patient relationship. Many times a patient will have a setback due to their feeling of loss of this relationship. The nurse's role is to help them explore their feelings and ease this transition while maintaining boundaries (Peplau, 1991).

## SUMMARY POINTS

- Everyone experiences transient periods of depressed or elated mood at different times of their lives. Affective disorders involve a persistent or sustained disturbance in mood.

- Affective disorders include major depressive disorder, dysthymic disorder, bipolar I and II disorders, and cyclothymic disorder.

- Major depressive disorder is a leading cause of disability in the United States for persons between the ages of 15 to 44 years. It occurs more commonly in women than in men.

- For major depressive disorder to be diagnosed, the individual must experience a change from previous functioning with evidence of a depressed mood or decreased interest or pleasure in usual activities that lasts most of the day for over two weeks.

- Dysthmic disorder is a milder form of depression in which the individual often reports "feeling sad or down."

- Bipolar I disorder involves the occurrence of one or more manic episodes, mixed episodes (mania and major depression), and often one or more major depressive episodes. Manic episodes are characterized by a persistently elevated and expansive or irritable mood.

- Suicide is a behavior, not a disorder. It is an act of ambivalence that can often result from an affective disorder.

- The exact cause of affective disorders is not known.

- Psychological theories have attempted to explain the cause of affective disorders. These theories involve learned helplessness, cognitive theory, anger turned inward, child temperament, and prolonged stress.

- Neurobiological theories focus on the neurotransmitters dopamine, norepinephrine, and serotonine.

- The nurse employs the therapeutic use of self throughout the nursing process

*(cont.)*

## SUMMARY POINTS (*CONT.*)

for a patient with an affective disorder. Developing trust and rapport and ensuring the patient's safety are crucial during assessment. The nurse also assesses the patient for suicidal ideation and past and current attempts verbally through direct questions and observation of nonverbal actions.

- Implementing effective interventions requires appropriate timing and pacing, maintenance of professional boundaries, and continual reassessment for suicidal behavior, especially when the patient is going into a depression or coming out of one.

- Evaluation may lead to feelings of loss by the patient as the relationship draws to a close. The nurse needs to help the patient explore his or her feelings and ease the

transition while maintaining appropriate boundaries.

- Research has indicated that psychotherapy and medication typically result in the best outcomes for patients with affective disorders.

- Psychopharmacology involves the use of antidepressants and mood stabilizers. Patients receiving MAOIs need to avoid foods containing tyramine to prevent the development of a hypertensive crisis. Lithium has a narrow therapeutic margin of safety. Drugs levels need to be monitored closely.

- Electroconvulsive therapy is used to treat patients who have not responded to other treatment modalities. Patients may experience transient confusion, disorientation, and memory loss after this therapy.

## NCLEX-PREP*

1. Which statement by a patient with bipolar disorder would indicate the need for additional education about his prescribed lithium carbonate therapy? "I will:
   a. drink about 2 liters of liquids daily."
   b. restrict my intake of salt."
   c. take my medications with food."
   d. have my blood drawn like the doctor ordered."

2. A patient has been severely depressed and expressing suicidal thoughts. She was started on antidepressant medication four days ago. She is now more energized and communicative. Which of the following would be most important for the nurse to do?
   a. Allow the patient to have unsupervised passes to her home.

   b. Encourage the patient to participate in group activities.
   c. Increase vigilance with the patient's suicidal precautions.
   d. Recognize that the patient's suicidal potential has decreased.

3. A group of nurses in the emergency department (ED) are discussing a patient who has been admitted almost every holiday with suicide ideation. One of the nurses stated that the patient is not serious about hurting himself and should not be admitted the next time he comes in. Which response by the charge nurse would be most appropriate?
   a. "Telling him we cannot see him may be the answer to stop this behavior."

(*cont.*)

NCLEX-PREP* (CONT.)

b. "Each episode must be individually evaluated and all options explored."

c. "He obviously needs support that he is not getting elsewhere."

d. "We should avoid showing any emotion to him the next time he comes in."

4. A group of nursing students are reviewing the different classes of antidepressants. The students demonstrate understanding of the information when they identify sertraline as exerting its action on which neurotransmitter?

   a. Serotonin
   b. Dopamine
   c. Gamma-aminobutyric acid (GABA)
   d. Norepinephrine

5. Which statement would the nurse expect a newly admitted married patient with mania to make? "I can:

   a. not do anything right anymore."
   b. manage our finances better than any accountant."
   c. understand why my spouse is so upset that I spend so much money."
   d. not understand where all our money goes."

6. When developing the plan of care for a patient who has attempted suicide, an understanding of which of the following would be most critical for the nurse to integrate into the plan?

   a. Patients who attempt suicide and fail will not try again.
   b. The more specific the plan, the greater the risk of suicide.
   c. People who talk about suicide rarely go ahead and attempt it.

d. People who attempt suicide and fail do not really want to die.

7. In planning care for a patient newly admitted with severe major depressive disorder, the primary nursing intervention would be to:

   a. Avoid a stressful situation by asking for the patient's participation in the plan.
   b. Teach the patient about relapse and the signs and symptoms of mania.
   c. Assess if the patient has more than two weeks worth of medication.
   d. Evaluate the patient's cognitive functioning and ability to participate in planning care.

8. The most important reason why a full physical health assessment is warranted for patients with depressive symptoms is that:

   a. they are less likely to complain about their physical health and may have an undiagnosed medical problem.
   b. physical health complications are likely to arise from antidepressant therapy.
   c. the attention afforded to the patient during the assessment is beneficial in decreasing social isolation.
   d. physiological changes may be the underlying cause of depression, and, if present, must be addressed.

9. The psychiatric nurse understands that dysthymia differs from a major depression episode in that dysthymia:

   a. Typically has an acute onset.
   b. Involves delusional thinking.
   c. Is a chronic low-level depression.
   d. Does not include suicidal ideation.

*Answers to these questions appear on page 639.

## REFERENCES

American Psychiatric Association. (2000). *Diagnostic and statistical manual of mental disorders* (4th ed., text rev.). Washington, DC: Author.

Andreasen, N. C., & Black, D. W. (2001). *Introductory textbook of psychiatry*. Washington, DC. American Psychiatric Publishing, Inc.

Beck, A.T., Rush, A.J., Shaw, B.F., & Emery, G. (1979). Cognitive Theory of depression. New York: Guilford Press.

Emental-health.com. (2010). Historical perspectives of depression. Retrieved May 31, 2010 from http://emental-health.com/depr_history.htm

Freud, S. (1920). *An introduction to psychotherapy*. NY: Horace Liveright.

National Institute for Mental Illness (NIMH) (2009). *How is depression detected and treated?* Retrieved May 31, 2010 from http://www.nimh.nih.gov/health/publications/depression/how-is-depression-detected-and-treated.shtml

National Institute for Mental Illness (NIMH) (2010).*The numbers count: Mental disorders in American.* Retrieved May 31, 2010 from http://www.nimh.nih.gov/health/publications/the-numbers-count-mental-disorders-in-america/index.shtml#Mood

Peplau, H. E. (1991). *Interpersonal relations in nursing: A conceptual frame of reference for psychodynamic nursing.* New York: Springer Publishing Company.

Rogers, V, Quinn Griffin, M., Wykle, M., & Fitzpatrick, J., (2009) Internet versus face-to-face therapy: Emotional self-disclosure issues for young adults. *Issues in Mental Health Nursing.* 30: 596–602.

Seligman, M.E. (1992). *Helplessness.* New York, NY: Freeman,

Tsuang, M.T., Faraone, S.V. (1990). *The genetics of mood disorders.* Baltimore: The Johns Hopkins University Press.

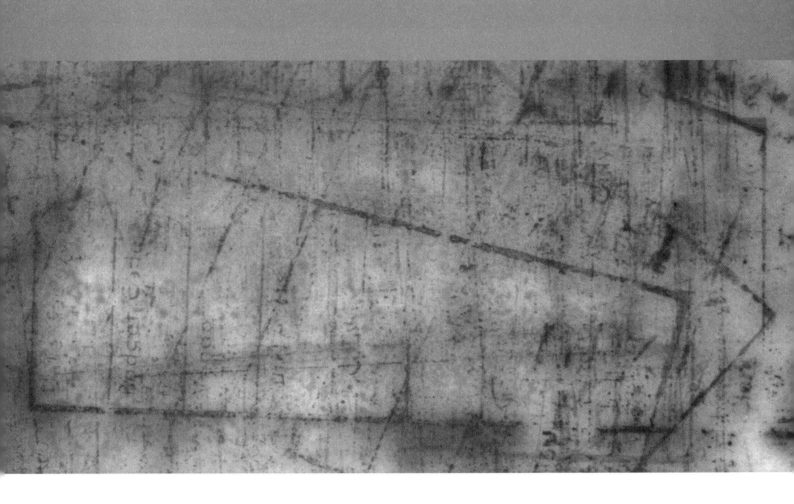

## CHAPTER CONTENTS

## EXPECTED LEARNING OUTCOMES

**After completing this chapter, the student will be
able to:**

1. Define anxiety.
2. Identify the disorders classified as anxiety disorders.
3. Describe the historical perspectives and epidemiology
   associated with anxiety disorders.
4. Discuss current scientific theories related to the
   etiology of anxiety disorders, including relevant
   psychodynamic and neurobiological influences.
5. Distinguish among the diagnostic criteria for anxiety
   disorders as outlined in the *Diagnostic and Statistical
   Manual of Mental Disorders, 4th edition, Text Revision
   (DSM-IV-TR)*.

# CHAPTER 13
# ANXIETY DISORDERS

Marianne Goldyn

6. Explain the various treatment options available for anxiety disorders.
7. Apply the nursing process from an interpersonal perspective to the care of patients with anxiety disorders.

## KEY TERMS

Agoraphobia

Anxiety

Biofeedback

Compulsions

Fear

Flooding

Hysteria

Obsessions

Panic disorder

Phobia

Systematic desensitization

Worry

ANXIETY is a common human emotion that is often difficult to define. Words used to describe anxiety reflect one's inner experience and, subsequently, can be quite subjective. Typically, anxiety refers to a vague feeling involving some dread, apprehension, or other unknown tension. Life experiences teach us that anxiety can be a normal emotional response to a stressor. As a healthy response, anxiety is a catalyst to achieve, to stay focused, and to cope in threatening situations. Anxiety becomes a symptom of a disorder or pathological when it interferes with one's ability to function. Anxiety disorders include: panic disorder; obsessive-compulsive disorder (OCD); posttraumatic stress disorder (PTSD); acute stress disorder; generalized anxiety disorder (GAD); and phobias, such as social phobia, agoraphobia, and specific phobia.

Persons who feel anxiety often experience somatic symptoms such as muscle pain, blurred vision, tachycardia, dyspnea, difficulty swallowing, loss of appetite, increased sweating, loss of libido, or dry mouth. Cognitive symptoms also can be manifested, especially with anxiety disorders. These include: poor memory, confusion, difficulty concentrating, distorted thinking, unrealistic fears, repetitive fearful ideation, or hypervigilence. In addition, some people with anxiety disorders perform certain rituals such as handwashing, counting, or avoiding certain situations such as large crowded areas, bridges, and elevators in order to cope with their symptoms.

> *Anxiety is a vague feeling of discomfort. It can be a healthy response leading an individual to become more focused and able to cope with threatening situations, or it can become pathological and interfere with a person's ability to function.*

Much has been written about the similarities and differences between FEAR, WORRY, and anxiety. For the purpose of this chapter, fear and anxiety are viewed as the two core symptom clusters of anxiety. Fear in this context refers to feelings consistent with panic and phobias. Anxiety, as stated earlier, is a vague, uncertain feeling of dread, while worry is more indicative of symptoms such as anxious misery, apprehensive expectations, and obsessions. All of the anxiety disorders maintain some form of anxiety or fear coupled with some form of worry. However, what triggers them differs (Stahl, 2008).

This chapter addresses the historical perspectives and epidemiology of anxiety disorders followed by a detailed description of the anxiety disorders as defined in the *Diagnostic and Statistical Manual, 4th edition, Text Revision* ([*DSM-IV-TR*], 2000). Specific scientific theories focusing on psychodynamic, behavioral, and neurobiological influences are described plus common treatment options, including pharmacotherapy and nonpharmacotherapy strategies. Application of the nursing process from an interpersonal perspective is presented, including a plan of care for a patient with an anxiety disorder.

## HISTORICAL PERSPECTIVES

The American Psychiatric Association (APA) did not officially recognize anxiety disorders until 1980. However, anxiety and anxiety disorders have played substantial roles in human history. The earliest interpretations of anxiety disorders appear to be mostly spiritual, with many early spiritual treatments resembling some aspects of modern psychotherapy. For example, in early Christian thought, logismoi were distressing, obsessive thoughts that were unhealthy and believed to lead people away from God. The spiritual leaders took on roles as confessors or counselors by employing healing dialogue to lessen these obsessions. Often the treatment for logismoi was to redirect and replace unhealthy thoughts with realistic ones, which is similar to modern-day techniques of cognitive behavioral therapy. In addition, the ancient preparation and use of natural substances have similarities to modern pharmaceuticals (Anderson, 2007).

Medical interpretations of anxiety disorders are not entirely new, reaching as far back as classical Greek civilization. Greeks coined the word "agoraphobic," which was initially given to people who were afraid to go outside to the market. Today this term refers to people who suffer from an anxiety disorder.

During the 17th and 18th centuries, in Germany, France, England, and North America, the term HYSTERIA (which is Greek for uterus) was used to describe anxiety and anxiety-related disorders specifically in women. During the 1800s, French psychiatrist Jean Martin Charcot spent a great deal of energy studying hysteria and concluded that it derived from a particular hereditary disposition and was unleashed by an environmental stimulus. He postulated that certain people are genetically predisposed to develop hysteria just as today we know that there is a genetic predisposition to diseases such as cancer. Charcot observed numerous cases of hysterical symptoms arising in both men and women, including headaches, heart palpitations, chest pain, irregular pulse rate, constipation, dizziness, fainting spells, trembling of the hands and neck, emotional and sleep disorders, and mental disorientation. While the symptoms between men and women were similar, he believed that symptoms in men were triggered by traumatic events, such as workplace accidents and train crashes. In women, on the other hand, Charcot believed that hysterical attacks were triggered by emotions or passions; jilted lovers; and weepy, romantic girls (Porter, 1997).

In 1895, Sigmund Freud's earliest descriptions of anxiety were documented using the term "anxiety neurosis." Initially, Freud described anxiety neurosis as anxiety that resulted from a repressed libido. Later he expanded the concept of anxiety neurosis to include a diffuse sense of worry or dread that originates in a repressed thought or wish and not just in the repression of sexual energy. According to Freud, anxiety neurosis resulted in hysteria, obsessions, phobias, and somatic symptoms such as fatigue and dizziness (Sadock & Sadock, 2007).

Much of the current understanding of anxiety and anxiety-related disorders can be traced back primarily to times of war. For example, in the mid-1800s, Otto Domrich became the first in the field of medical psychology to write about "anxiety attacks." This term replaced earlier notions of "neurocirculatory neurasthenia," "soldier's heart," and "hyperventilation syndrome" that dated back to the French Revolution. These terms depicted the state of combined anxiety and cardiopulmonary symptoms that might be induced by the terrors of the battlefield (Stone, 1997).

During World War I, the number of psychiatric casualties dramatically increased such that hospitals were quickly opened to house them. According to one estimate, mental breakdowns represented 40% of British battle casualties. Military authorities attempted to hide reports of these psychiatric casualties because of their demoralizing effect on the public. Initially, the symptoms of mental breakdown were attributed to a physical cause. The British psychologist Charles Myers examined some of the first cases and attributed their symptoms to the concussive effects of exploding shells. Myers called the resulting nervous disorder "shell shock." The name stuck, even though it soon became clear that the syndrome could be found in soldiers who had not been exposed to any physical trauma. Gradually, military psychiatrists were forced to acknowledge that the symptoms of shell shock were due to psychological trauma (Herman, 1997).

During World War II, psychiatric collapse accounted for the loss of 504,000 men from the American fighting forces. In every one of America's wars in the 20th century, the rates of psychiatric collapse among soldiers exceeded the numbers killed in action. Psychiatric casualties constituted the single largest category of disability discharges in World War II (Gabriel, 1987).

No precise data on the number of soldiers suffering from posttraumatic stress disorder (PTSD) after the Vietnam War exist. Figures range from 500,000 to 1,500,000 PTSD cases, indicating that at least 18% and possibly as many as 54% of the armed forces suffered psychiatric symptoms. The chances that a soldier would become a psychiatric casualty in Vietnam were about the same as his or her chances of being killed in action (Gabriel, 1987). Veterans of the Gulf War, Operation Desert Shield, and Desert Storm exhibit rates of PTSD, generalized anxiety disorder, and panic disorders that are nearly twice that of non-deployed military personnel (Black et al., 2004). More recent studies have indicated that one in three Iraqi combat veterans have been diagnosed with PTSD, generalized anxiety disorder, or a panic disorder and one in six from Afghanistan have been diagnosed with an anxiety disorder (Milliken et al. 2007).

> *Historically, terms such as hysteria, anxiety neurosis, and shell shock were used to identify anxiety disorders.*

## EPIDEMIOLOGY

Anxiety disorders are the most common psychiatric diagnoses and the most costly psychiatric illnesses in the United States. It is estimated that three out of ten people will suffer from an anxiety disorder in their lifetime (Kessler, Berglund, Demler, Jin, Merikangas, & Walters, 2005). Approximately 40 million American adults ages 18 and older, or about 18.1% of people in this age group in a given year, have an anxiety disorder. Disability common to these disorders exceeds that associated with other psychiatric conditions and most medical conditions including cardiovascular disease, pulmonary disease, gastrointestinal diseases, and cancer (Merikangas, Ames, Cui, Stang, Ustun, Von Korff, & Kessler, 2007). Despite the high prevalence rates of anxiety disorders as well as their economic burden, they often go unrecognized and untreated.

Anxiety disorders frequently co-occur with depressive disorders or substance abuse disorders (Kessler, Chiu, Demler, & Walters, 2005). Most people with one anxiety disorder also have another anxiety disorder. Nearly three-fourths of those with an anxiety disorder will have their first episode by age 21.5 years (Kessler, Berglund, et al., 2005). The presence of any anxiety disorder is associated with a 21.9% prevalence of self-medication with drugs and alcohol. For example, persons with generalized anxiety disorder (GAD) show the highest self-medication rate of 35.6% while persons with bipolar I disorder show the lowest self-medication rate of 12.6%. Caucasians are more likely to self-medicate than any other race (84.5%) and men (55.4%) are more likely to self-medicate than women (44.6%) (Bolton, Cox, Clara, & Sareen, 2006).

> *Anxiety disorders, the most common and most costly psychiatric diagnosis in the United States, commonly occur with other conditions such as substance abuse and depression.*

## Incidence

Statistics related to specific anxiety disorders reflect:

- *Approximately 6 million adults, ages 18 and older, or about 2.7% of people in this age group have panic disorder in a given year* (Kessler, Chiu et al., 2005).
  - It typically develops in early adulthood, with a median age of onset of 24 years, but can extend throughout adulthood (Kessler, Bergland et al., 2005).
  - About one in three people with panic disorder develops **AGORAPHOBIA**, a condition in which the individual becomes afraid of being in a place or situation where escape might be difficult or help unavailable in the event of a panic attack (Robins & Regier, 1991).
- *Approximately 2.2 million American adults, age 18 or older, or about 1.0% of people in this age group, have obsessive-compulsive disorder (OCD) in a given year* (Kessler, Chiu et al., 2005).
  - The first symptoms of OCD often begin during childhood or adolescence.
  - The age of onset is 19 years (Kessler, Berglund, et al., 2005).
- *Approximately 7.7 million American adults age 18 and older, or about 3.5% of people in this age group, have a diagnosis of posttraumatic stress disorder (PTSD) in a given year* (Kessler, Chiu et al., 2005).
  - It can develop at any age, including childhood, but research shows that the median age of onset is 23 years (Kessler, Berglund, et al., 2005).

- About 19% of Vietnam veterans experienced PTSD at some point after the war (Dohrenwend, Turner, Turse, Adams, Koen, & Marshall, 2006).
- The disorder also frequently occurs after violent personal assaults such as rape, mugging, domestic violence, terrorism, natural or human-caused disasters, and accidents.
- *Approximately 6.8 million American adults, or about 3.1% of people age 18 and over, have a diagnosis of generalized anxiety disorder (GAD) in a given year* (Kessler, Chiu, et al., 2005), beginning across the life cycle with a median age of onset of 31 years (Kessler, Berglund, et al., 2005).
- *Approximately 15 million American adults age 18 and over, or about 6.8% of people in this age group have social phobia in a given year* (Kessler, Chiu, et al., 2005), typically beginning in childhood or adolescence, usually around 13 years of age (Kessler, Berglund, et al., 2005).
- *Approximately 1.8 million American adults age 18 and over, or about 0.8% of people in this age group, have agoraphobia without a history of panic disorder in a given year*, with a median age of onset of 20 years (Kessler, Chiu, et al., 2005).
- *Approximately 19.2 million American adults age 18 and over, or about 8.7% of people in this age group, have some type of **SPECIFIC PHOBIA** (marked and persistent fear and avoidance of a specific object or situation) in a given year* (Kessler, Chiu, et al., 2005), typically beginning in childhood with a median age of onset of 7 years (Kessler, Berglund, et al., 2005).

## Morbidity and Mortality

Anxiety disorders, through effects of the neurologic, endocrine, and immune mechanisms or direct neural stimulation that result in conditions such as hypertension or cardiac arrhythmia, can contribute to morbidity and mortality. In addition, severe anxiety disorders may be complicated by suicide, with or without secondary mood disorders (e.g., depression). Anxiety disorders have high rates of comorbidity with major depression and alcohol and drug abuse. Some of the increased morbidity and mortality associated with anxiety disorders may be related to this high rate of comorbidity.

Between 1980 and 1985, the National Institute of Mental Health (NIMH) funded the Epidemiologic Catchment Area (ECA) program of research. This program was designed to determine prevalence and incidence of mental disorders and the use of and need for services by the mentally ill. One of its findings revealed that panic disorder was associated with suicide attempts 18 times higher than populations without psychiatric disorders. The ECA study also found no difference in rates of panic disorder among White, African American, or Hispanic populations in the United States. However, some studies have found higher rates of PTSD in minority populations, which may be due to higher rates of specific traumatic events, such as assault.

The female-to-male ratio for any lifetime anxiety disorder is 3:2. It is not clear why females have higher rates of most anxiety disorders than males do. Some theories suggest that the gonadal steroids may play a role. Other research on women's responses to stress also suggests that women experience a wider range of life events (e.g., those happening to friends) as stressful as compared with men, who react to a more limited range of stressful events, specifically only those affecting themselves or close family members (Yates, 2009).

> *Anxiety disorders occur more commonly in women than in men and can contribute to illness and death through effects on the endocrine, immune, and nervous system.*

## DIAGNOSTIC CRITERIA

Anxiety disorders include the following: panic disorder, obsessive-compulsive disorder (OCD), posttraumatic stress disorder (PTSD), generalized anxiety disorder (GAD), and phobias. Each disorder has a specific set of diagnostic criteria that a patient must meet for diagnosis. **Box 13-1** highlights the major diagnostic criteria as identified by the *DSM-IV-TR* (APA, 2000).

### Panic Disorder

**PANIC DISORDER** involves sudden, intense, and unprovoked feelings of terror and dread. People who suffer from this disorder generally develop strong fears about when and where their next panic attack will occur, and subsequently, often restrict their activities. Panic disorder usually occurs after frightening experiences or prolonged stress, but it can also occur spontaneously. A panic attack may lead an individual to be acutely aware of any change in normal body function, interpreting it as a life-threatening illness. In addition, panic attacks lead a sufferer to expect future attacks, which may cause drastic behavioral changes in order to avoid these attacks.

### Obsessive-Compulsive Disorder (OCD)

Obsessive-compulsive disorder (OCD) is an anxiety disorder characterized by thoughts or actions that are repetitive, distressing, and intrusive. OCD sufferers usually know that their compulsions are unreasonable or irrational, but they serve to alleviate their anxiety. Often, the logic of someone with OCD will appear superstitious, such as an insistence to walk in a certain pattern. OCD sufferers may obsessively clean personal items or hands or constantly check locks, light switches, etc.

### Posttraumatic Stress Disorder (PTSD)

Posttraumatic stress disorder (PTSD) is an anxiety disorder that results from previous trauma such as military combat, rape, hostage situations, or a serious accident. PTSD often leads to flashbacks and behavioral changes in order to avoid certain stimuli. Thoughts, feelings, and behavior patterns become seriously affected by reminders of the event, sometimes months or even years after the traumatic experience.

### Generalized Anxiety Disorder (GAD)

Generalized anxiety disorder (GAD) is a chronic disorder characterized by excessive, long-lasting anxiety and worry about nonspecific life events, objects, and situations. GAD sufferers often feel afraid and worry about health, money, family, work, or school, but have trouble both identifying the specific fear and controlling the worries. Their fear is usually unrealistic or out of proportion with what may be expected in their situation. Sufferers expect failure and disaster to the point that it interferes with daily functions like work, school, social activities, and relationships. People with GAD have recurring fears or worries, such as about health or finances, and they often have a persistent sense that something bad is about to happen. The reason

> *Although panic disorder can occur spontaneously, it typically results after frightening experiences or prolonged stress. Patients with OCD use obsessions and compulsions to relieve anxiety. Patients with PTSD experience flashbacks and change behavior in an effort to avoid stimuli associated with a previous trauma.*

### BOX 13-1: DIAGNOSTIC CRITERIA

#### PANIC DISORDER

A. Evidence of recurrent unexpected panic attacks with at least one of the attacks being followed by 1 month (or more) of one (or more) of the following:
- Persistent concern about having additional attacks
- Worry about the implications of the attack or its consequences (e.g., losing control, having a heart attack, "going crazy")
- Significant change in behavior related to the attacks

B. The presence (or absence) of agoraphobia

C. The panic attacks are not due to the direct physiological effects of a substance or a general medical condition

D. The panic attacks are not better accounted for by another mental disorder, such as social phobia, OCD, PTSD, or separation anxiety disorder

#### OBSESSIVE-COMPULSIVE DISORDER (OCD)

A. Evidence of either obsessions or compulsions:
- **OBSESSIONS** as defined by:
  - Recurrent and persistent thoughts, impulses, or images experienced at some time during the disturbance are intrusive and inappropriate, causing marked anxiety or distress
  - The thoughts, impulses, or images are not simply excessive worries about real-life problems
  - Attempts to ignore or suppress such thoughts, impulses, or images, or to neutralize them with some other thought or action by the person
  - Recognition that the obsessive thoughts, impulses, or images result from his or her own mind (not imposed from without as in thought insertion)
- **COMPULSIONS** as defined by:
  - Repetitive behaviors (e.g., hand washing, ordering, checking) or mental acts (e.g., praying, counting, repeating words silently) that the person feels driven to perform in response to an obsession or according to rules that must be applied rigidly
  - The behaviors or mental acts are aimed at preventing or reducing distress or preventing some dreaded event or situation; however, there is no realistic connection of behaviors or mental acts with what they are designed to neutralize

B. Recognition that obsessions or compulsions are excessive or unreasonable at some point during the course of the disorder

C. The obsessions or compulsions causing marked distress are time consuming (take more than 1 hour a day), or significantly interfere with the person's normal routine, occupational (or academic) functioning, or usual activities or relationships

D. If another Axis I disorder is present, the content of the obsessions or compulsions is not restricted to another Axis I disorder, if present

E. The disturbance is not due to the direct physiological effects of a substance or a general medical condition

#### POSTTRAUMATIC STRESS DISORDER (PTSD)

A. Exposure to a traumatic event in which both of the following have been present:
- Person experienced, witnessed, or was confronted with an event or events that involved actual or threatened death or serious injury, or a threat to the physical integrity of self or others
- Person's response involved intense fear, helplessness, or horror. (*Note*: In children, this may be expressed instead by disorganized or agitated behavior.)

*(cont.)*

## BOX 13-1: DIAGNOSTIC CRITERIA (*CONT.*)

B. The traumatic event is persistently re-experienced in one (or more) of the following ways:
- Recurrent and intrusive distressing recollections of the event, including images, thoughts, or perceptions. (*Note*: In young children, repetitive play may occur in which themes or aspects of the trauma are expressed.)
- Recurrent distressing dreams of the event. (*Note*: In children, there may be frightening dreams without recognizable content.)
- Acting or feeling as if the traumatic event were recurring; includes a sense of reliving the experience, illusions, hallucinations, and dissociative flashback episodes, including those that occur upon awakening or when intoxicated. (*Note*: In young children, trauma-specific reenactment may occur.)
- Intense psychological distress at exposure to internal or external cues that symbolize or resemble an aspect of the traumatic event
- Physiological reactivity on exposure to internal or external cues that symbolize or resemble an aspect of the traumatic event

C. Persistent avoidance of stimuli associated with the trauma and numbing of general responsiveness (not present before the trauma), as indicated by three (or more) of the following:
- Efforts to avoid thoughts, feelings, or conversations associated with the trauma
- Efforts to avoid activities, places, or people that arouse recollections of the trauma
- Inability to recall an important aspect of the trauma
- Markedly diminished interest or participation in significant activities
- Feeling of detachment or estrangement from others
- Restricted range of affect (e.g., unable to have loving feelings)
- Sense of a foreshortened future (e.g., does not expect to have a career, marriage, children, or a normal life span)

D. Persistent symptoms of increased arousal (not present before the trauma), as indicated by two (or more) of the following:
- Difficulty falling or staying asleep
- Irritability or outbursts of anger
- Difficulty concentrating
- Hypervigilance
- Exaggerated startle response

E. Duration of the disturbance more than 1 month.

F. Clinically significant distress or impairment in social, occupational, or other important areas of functioning. Further specified as: acute ( if duration of symptoms is less than 3 months); chronic (if duration 3 months or more); or with delayed onset (if symptoms develop at least 6 months after the stressor).

### GENERALIZED ANXIETY DISORDER (GAD)

A. Excessive anxiety and worry (apprehensive expectation), occurring more days than not for at least 6 months, about a number of events or activities (such as work or school performance)
- Difficulty controlling the worry
- The anxiety and worry associated with three (or more) of the following six symptoms, with at least some symptoms present for more days than not for the past 6 months. (*Note*: Only one item is required in children.)

*(cont.)*

**Q**   **BOX 13-1: DIAGNOSTIC CRITERIA (*CONT.*)**

GENERALIZED ANXIETY DISORDER (GAD) (*CONT.*)

- Restlessness or feeling keyed up or on edge
- Being easily fatigued
- Irritability
- Muscle tension
- Difficulty falling or staying asleep, or restless unsatisfying sleep
- Difficulty concentrating or the mind going blank
- Symptoms can also include nausea, vomiting, and chronic stomachaches.

SPECIFIC PHOBIA

A. Marked and persistent fear that is excessive or unreasonable, initiated by a stimulus (the presence or anticipation of a specific object or situation, such as flying, heights, animals, receiving an injection, or seeing blood)

B. Almost invariably immediate anxiety response with exposure to the phobic stimulus, possibly taking the form of a situationally bound or situationally predisposed panic attack

C. Recognition by the person that the fear is excessive or unreasonable

D. Avoidance of or endurance with intense anxiety or distress of the  phobic situation(s)

E. Significant interference with the person's normal routine; occupational (or academic) functioning, social activities or relationships, or marked distress about having the phobia with the avoidance; anxious anticipation; or distress in the feared situation(s)

F. Duration of at least 6 months in individuals under age 18 years

G. The anxiety, panic attacks, or phobic avoidance associated with the specific object or situation, not better accounted for by another mental disorder

SOCIAL PHOBIA

A. A marked and persistent fear of one or more social or performance situations in which the person is exposed to unfamiliar people or to possible scrutiny by others; fear that he or she will act in a way (or show anxiety symptoms) that will be humiliating or embarrassing

B. Anxiety almost invariably on exposure to the feared social possibly taking the form of a situationally bound or situationally predisposed panic attack

C. Recognition that fear is excessive or unreasonable

D. Avoidance of, or endurance of with intense anxiety or distress, the feared social or performance situation

E. Significant interference with the person's normal routine; occupational (academic) functioning; or social activities or relationships; or marked distress related to the avoidance, anxious anticipation, or distress in the feared social or performance situation(s)

F. Duration of at least 6 months in individuals under age 18 years

G. The fear or avoidance is not due to the direct physiological effects of a substance or a general medical condition and is not better accounted for by another mental disorder

*(cont.)*

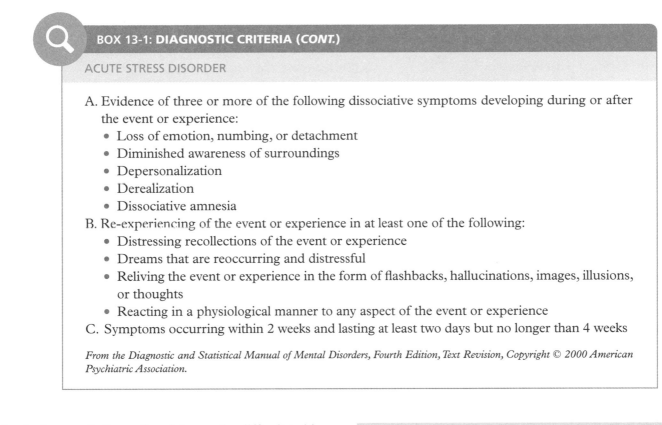

BOX 13-1: DIAGNOSTIC CRITERIA (*CONT.*)

ACUTE STRESS DISORDER

A. Evidence of three or more of the following dissociative symptoms developing during or after the event or experience:
- Loss of emotion, numbing, or detachment
- Diminished awareness of surroundings
- Depersonalization
- Derealization
- Dissociative amnesia

B. Re-experiencing of the event or experience in at least one of the following:
- Distressing recollections of the event or experience
- Dreams that are reoccurring and distressful
- Reliving the event or experience in the form of flashbacks, hallucinations, images, illusions, or thoughts
- Reacting in a physiological manner to any aspect of the event or experience

C. Symptoms occurring within 2 weeks and lasting at least two days but no longer than 4 weeks

*From the Diagnostic and Statistical Manual of Mental Disorders, Fourth Edition, Text Revision, Copyright © 2000 American Psychiatric Association.*

for the intense feelings of anxiety may be difficult to identify. However, the fears and worries are very real and often keep individuals from concentrating on daily tasks.

## Specific Phobia

PHOBIAS are intense fears about certain objects or situations. Specific phobias may involve things such as encountering certain animals or flying in airplanes. One example is agoraphobia. Agoraphobia involves intense fear and anxiety of any place or situation where escape might be difficult, leading to avoidance of situations such as being alone outside of the home; traveling in a car, bus, or airplane; or being in a crowded area (Kessler, Berglund, et al., 2005). Individuals will situate themselves so that escape will not be difficult or embarrassing. Additionally, they will change their behavior to reduce anxiety about being able to escape.

## Social Phobia

Social phobia is a type of phobia characterized by a fear of being negatively judged by others or a fear of public embarrassment due to impulsive actions. This includes feelings such as stage fright, a fear of intimacy, and a fear of humiliation. This disorder can cause people to avoid public situations and human contact to the point that normal life is rendered impossible.

## Acute Stress Disorder

Acute stress disorder occurs when a person has been exposed to a traumatic event or experience involving intense fear, horror, or helplessness. It is labeled acute because it refers to the anxiety and behavioral disturbances that develop and are alleviated within the first month after exposure to an extreme trauma The event or experience must involve a threat of death, serious injury, or physical integrity. The event or experience may be to the person themselves or to others around them.*

## ETIOLOGY

The exact etiology of anxiety disorders is not known. Numerous research studies have attempted to address the underlying causes of anxiety, but without success.

### Psychosocial Theories

Two psychosocial influences dominate the thinking related to the development of anxiety disorders. These are the psychodynamic influences of theorists such as Sigmund

---

*From the *Diagnostic and Statistical Manual of Mental Disorders, 4th Edition, Text Revision*. Copyright © 2000 American Psychiatric Association.

Freud, Harry Sullivan, and Hildegard Peplau, and behavioral and learning theories.

## Psychodynamic Influences

In 1894, Sigmund Freud first published his writings on the psychodynamic nature of anxiety. His last publication on the topic was in 1926. According to Freud, the conflicting demands between the id, ego, and superego produce anxiety. He described anxiety as a signal to the ego that an unacceptable drive was pressing for conscious representation or discharge. For example, when the ego blocks the pleasurable desires of the id, anxiety is felt. This diffuse, distressed state develops when the ego senses that the id is going to cause harm to the individual. Freud identified three types of anxiety:

- *Reality anxiety*: The most basic form, rooted in reality such as fear of a bee sting or fear felt just prior to an accident; also referred to as ego-based anxiety.
- *Neurotic anxiety*: Arising from an unconscious fear that the libidinal impulses of the id will take control at an inopportune time; driven by a fear of punishment that will result from expressing the id's desires without proper sublimation.
- *Moral anxiety*: Resulting from fear of violating moral or societal codes; appearing as guilt or shame.

Freud believed that when anxiety is present, it alerts the ego to resolve the conflict by means of defense mechanisms. (See Chapter 10 for a more in-depth discussion of defense mechanisms.) Of all the defense mechanisms, Freud believed that repression is the most powerful and pervasive defense mechanism working to push unacceptable id impulses out of awareness and back into the unconscious mind. Repression is the foundation from which all other defense mechanisms work. The goal of every defense mechanism is to repress, or push threatening impulses out of awareness. Freud said that our early childhood experiences, many of which he believed are sexually laden, are too threatening and stressful for us to deal with consciously. Individuals then reduce the anxiety of this conflict through the defense mechanism of repression (Freud, 1938).

Freud's pupil and later critic Otto Rank separated from Freud by describing anxiety as a result of birth trauma. According to Rank, the anxiety experienced during birth was the model for all anxiety experienced afterward. While he viewed anxiety as trauma from birth, another theorist, Harry Stack Sullivan, believed anxiety stemmed from the early relationship between the mother and the child and the transmission of the mother's anxiety to the infant.

Sullivan called his approach an interpersonal theory of psychiatry because he believed psychiatry is the study of what goes on between people. This is in contrast to Freud's paradigm that focused on what goes on inside people. Freud's is a drive model whereas Sullivan's is an interpersonal model.

For Sullivan, relationships are primary. Personality is a hypothetical entity that cannot be observed or studied apart from interpersonal situations. The only way personality can be known is through the medium of interpersonal interactions. Therefore, what is to be studied is not the individual person, but the interpersonal situation.

Like Sullivan, Hildegard Peplau (1991) also believed that relationships are primary. She applied psychodynamic theories not only to individuals but also to the nursing process. She clearly illustrated in her writings and teaching that she felt nursing was a significant and therapeutic, interpersonal process. Peplau wrote extensively about unexplained discomfort and within these writings described four types of anxiety:

- *Mild anxiety*: This anxiety motivates individuals every day; considered "normal anxiety" and viewed as a positive motivator for personal growth and success.
- *Moderate anxiety*: The individual begins to hear, see, and grasp less due to a narrowing of their perceptual field; decreased awareness of the environment and decreased focus, noticing only those things that are brought to their attention.
- *Severe anxiety*: The individual's thoughts become scattered, focusing on small details; inability to problem solve or use the learning process to make decisions.
- *Panic*: The individual experiences intense fear accompanied by physical symptoms such as chest pain, heart palpitations, dizziness, shortness of breath, and abdominal distress; possible inability to cooperate or collaborate with the nurse.

Peplau believed that clearly identifying and understanding the type of anxiety an individual is experiencing is pivotal for good nursing care. She believed that nursing interventions were not required during mild episodes of anxiety. For moderate levels of anxiety, Peplau believed many useful nursing interventions could take place such as problem solving/talk therapy, cognitive reframing, and teaching anxiety reduction techniques such as relaxation training, meditation, counting, and deep breathing. During periods of severe anxiety, Peplau suggested that individuals cannot effectively problem solve or make connections because they are self absorbed, feeling an impending sense of doom and experiencing physiological symptoms such as hyperventilation and tachycardia. Nursing interventions during this time focus on providing short, firm concrete directions to assist the person to remain calm, to protect the person from self-injury, either intentional or related to inattention or poor reality testing, and to protect the milieu from disruption and injury.

Peplau postulated that persons with panic levels of anxiety were unable to focus on even one detail within the environment. She believed that terror, emotional paralysis, hallucinations, or delusions might occur during panic. Individuals can become mute, extremely agitated, irrational, hypervigilant, and hyperactive. When a person experiences panic, Peplau suggested the nurse remains with the individual until the panic subsides. This action provides a certain amount of security, or "thereness" of the nurse.

> *Peplau identified four categories of anxiety: mild, moderate, severe, and panic.*

## Behavioral Influences

Prior to more recent biologic and pharmacologic studies about anxiety, the widely accepted theory of anxiety disorders fell within behavioral or learning theories. While Freud was working on the psychodynamics of anxiety, a radically different view of anxiety and fear greatly influenced by Pavlov's theory of classical condition (1927) was emerging through the work of John B. Watson and J.J.B. Morgan (1917). They argued that anxiety was a conditioned response to an unpleasant stimulus. This theory, also known as respondent conditioning, was disregarded by many. However, it laid the groundwork for cognitive and social learning theories of anxiety and has undergone considerable transformation. These theories primarily focused on simple phobias and fears. Thus, the concepts of classical conditioning were not adequate to explain more complex anxiety states. Most learning and behavioral theorists now embrace interactive models that attempt to explain the multifaceted nature of anxiety disorders. These models take into account how individual risk factors interact with environmental factors to produce anxiety states or disorders. For example, an interactive model of anxiety would suggest that individuals with controlling, time conscious, and impatient personality (type A) would be more prone to anxiety in a highly chaotic or stressful work environment (Taylor & Arnow, 1988).

## Biological Theories

Biological theories focus primarily on neurostructural and neurochemical influences. Genetics also is associated with influencing the development of anxiety disorders.

## Neurobiological Influences

The anxiety disorder spectrum is so broad that the neurobiology that seems most relevant in one anxiety disorder may have little to do with other anxiety disorders. As stated earlier, all of these disorders seem to have the core feature of fear and/or worry. More than ever, the past decade has produced more scientific evidence regarding the neurocircuitry and neurochemistry associated with fear and worry.

Symptoms of anxiety or fear are associated with the malfunctioning of amygdala-centered circuits. The amygdala is an almond-shaped structure in the brain located near the hippocampus. It has anatomical connections that allow it to integrate sensory and cognitive information and then determine whether there will be a fear response. In contrast to fear, symptoms of worry such as anxious misery, apprehension, catastrophic thinking, and obsessions are linked to the cortico-striatal-thalamic-cortical (CSTC) loop circuitry. Both the amygdala and the cortico-striatal-thalamic-cortical loop contain gamma-amino-butyric acid (GABA), norepinephrine, and serotonin as the main neurotransmitters. Other neurotransmitters and peptides, such as dopamine, glutamate (a precursor to GABA), and corticotrophin releasing factor (CRF) have also been studied as playing a role in the development of anxiety symptoms. In addition, voltage-gated ion channels are involved in neurotransmission within these circuits (Stahl, 2008).

GABA is the main neurotransmitter involved in anxiety responses and in the anxiolytic action of many of the medications used to treat anxiety disorders. It directly influences an individual's personality and ability to handle stress. GABA is an inhibitory neurotransmitter that plays a regulatory role in reducing the activity of many neurons, including those in the amygdala and the CSTC loop, which affects one's sense of worry. It acts as the primary calming, or "peacemaker" chemical, inducing relaxation, reducing stress and anxiety, and increasing alertness. Overactivation or malfunction of the amygdala circuits leads to pathological anxiety or fear. GABA-ergic agents such as benzodiazepines act at postsynaptic GABA receptors to enhance the inhibitory action of GABA, thus decreasing the fear or anxiety symptoms.

As stated previously, anxiety disorders frequently co-occur with depressive disorders. Anxiety and depressive disorders also share symptoms, brain circuits, and neurotransmitters. Recall from Chapter 12 that altered levels of the neurotransmitter, serotonin, have been implicated in depressive disorders. It also has been postulated that serotonin works to decrease anxiety symptoms because it works in the amygdala to regulate the vulnerability of fear circuits (Stahl, 2008). Studies show that certain antidepressants increase the amount of available serotonin by blocking its reuptake. These medications have proven efficacious for anxiety disorders as well.

Norepinephrine, the neurotransmitter often associated with the "fight or flight" response to stress, also has regulatory input to the amygdala. This neurotransmitter is strongly linked to physical responses and reactions, including increasing heart rate and blood pressure as well as creating a sense of panic and overwhelming fear or dread. Excessive output of norepinephrine from the locus coeruleus results not only in autonomic overdrive but also can trigger symptoms of anxiety and fear, nightmares, hyperarousal states, flashbacks, and panic attacks. Blocking alpha-1- and beta-1-adrenergic receptors within the amygdala leads to a lessening of these symptoms. This is why beta blockers such as propranolol and, more recently, alpha-1-adrenergic blockers such as prazosin (Minipress) have been used to treat anxiety symptoms (Stahl, 2008).

> *Specific brain structures such as the amygdala and neurotransmitters such as GABA, norepinephrine, and serotonin have been associated with anxiety disorders. GABA is the primary neurotransmitter involved.*

### Genetic Vulnerability

The study of genetic vulnerability or the idea that a person may have a biological predisposition to develop a disorder when certain environmental factors present themselves has been gaining attention within the psychiatric arena. Of the known risk factors for anxiety disorders, the most validated is family history. Smoller and Farone (2008) reported that genetic epidemiologic studies have clearly shown that all of the anxiety disorders aggregate in families and that familiality is primarily due to genetic factors (Smoller & Farone, 2008). Interestingly, studies of temperament since the 1950s have concluded that temperamental differences in individuals have a biological or genetic basis, particularly in regard to fear and stress reactions.

For example, psychologist Jerome Kagan has demonstrated that people born with a certain brain circuitry also have a "hyperreactive amygdala." He reports that infants born with this vulnerability have a "high reactivity" when exposed to new stimuli and later become inhibited, shy, and anxious adults (Henig, 2009). Another psychiatrist, Stephen Stahl (2008), discussed the idea that there are vulnerable circuits in the brain that are created by certain genes. These circuits, when stressed by environmental factors, such as childhood sexual abuse, can lead to anxiety disorders later in life.

Most recently, in March of 2011, at the Anxiety Disorders of America 31st Annual Conference, investigators presented an abstract representing the first longitudinal imaging and genetic study of tempermental and neurobiological risk factors for anxiety. In this study, a specific gene, the *RTN4* gene, was associated with intermediate phenotypes (physical characteristics) of anxiety disorders. This gene may be associated with temperament and reactivity of the amygdala, which is one of the strongest functional magnetic resonance imaging correlates of temperament (Helwick, 2011). This research helps to further underscore the need that more effective strategies for the treatment and prevention of anxiety disorders require a better understanding of the etiology of these disorders. Much of this understanding appears to be in the area of genetic vulnerability.

## TREATMENT OPTIONS

Various treatment options are available for anxiety disorders. Anxiety disorders will most likely require concomitant use of nonpharmacological and pharmacological strategies. Studies show that for many patients, a combination of both is more efficacious than any monotherapuetic strategy (Bandelow, Seidler-Brandler, Becker, Wedekind, & Ruther, 2007).

### Pharmacological Therapy

Pharmacological therapy for anxiety disorders is similar to that for depression. Specifically, selective serotonin reuptake inhibitors (SSRIs) and selective norepinephrine reuptake inhibitors (SNRIs) are the drugs of choice for treating both depressive disorders and anxiety disorders. Patients need to understand that the therapeutic anxiolytic effects of SSRIs and SNRIs range from approximately two to eight weeks, but more commonly, six to eight weeks. This time frame is typically longer than what is seen when used to treat depression. Also, higher doses of SSRIs are required to treat anxiety symptoms when compared to depression symptoms. **Drug Summary 13-1** highlights the major medications commonly used to treat anxiety disorders. Different combinations of pharmacologic agents may be used depending on the specific anxiety disorder.

## Generalized Anxiety Disorder (GAD)

Both serotonin selective reuptake inhibitors (SSRIs), generally prescribed in higher doses, and selective norepinephrine reuptake inhibitors (SNRIs), typically prescribed in usual doses, are considered first line treatment for GAD. However, due to the serotonergic properties of SSRIs and SNRIs, some individuals report feeling more anxious and excited instead of calm. Because these agents have a delayed onset of action, benzodiazepines are often prescribed concurrently when initiating treatment. Benzodiazepines are also used when there is only a partial response to an SSRI or SNRI or for intermittent use when anxiety symptoms worsen and quick relief is required (Stahl, 2008). Another first line agent for treating GAD is buspirone (Buspar), used alone or as an adjunct to SSRIs or SNRIs. (See Chapter 12 for an expanded discussion of SSRIs and SNRIs.)

If a patient does not respond to initial treatment choices, switching to an agent within the same class is often considered. When a patient fails to respond to any first-line treatment, trials of mirtazapine (Remeron), trazodone (Desyrel), tricyclic antidepressants or sedating antihistamines such as hydroxyzine (Vistaril) may be used. Other second-line agents may include the novel alpha-2 delta ligands, gabapentin (Neurontin), or pregabalin (Lyrica). These drugs are approved for seizures, neuropathic pain, and fibromyalgia. Currently, they are being tested as treatment for anxiety disorders (Stahl, 2008). Atypical antipsychotics are often used as adjunct treatment in patients that have severe, refractory, and disabling symptoms that are unremitting. (See Chapter 12 for a more detailed discussion of tricyclic antidepressants; see Chapter 11 for a more detailed discussion of antipsychotics.)

## Panic Disorders

Treatment for panic disorders is similar to that for GAD. SSRIs generally prescribed in doses higher than for treating depression and SNRIs prescribed in usual doses are considered first-line treatment. Benzodiazepines are used when there is only partial response to an SSRI or SNRI or for intermittent use. They also are used alone as first-line treatment when symptoms are acute, severe, and disabling.

Second-line treatment may include the novel alpha-2 delta ligands, gabapentin or pregabalin. Occasionally, mirtazapine and trazodone are used alone or to augment therapy with SSRIs and/or SNRIs. Often, tricyclic antidepressants (TCAs) are used and the MAOIs, while commonly avoided due to their unfavorable side effect profile, are particularly efficacious in the treatment of panic disorders (Stahl, 2008). Other adjunctive treatments include the use of atypical antipsychotics such as quetiepine (Seroquel) and olanzapine (Zyprexa) and anticonvulsants such as lamotrigine (Lamictal) and topiramate (Topamax). (See Chapter 12 for a more in-depth discussion of MAOIs.)

## Obsessive-Compulsive Disorder (OCD)

High doses of SSRIs are considered first-line treatment for OCD. Commonly, two or three different SSRIs at high doses are tried if the first SSRI is not effective. Second-line agents include clomipramine (Anafranil) and SNRIs, particularly venlafaxine (Effexor) (Dell'Osso, Nestadt, Allen, & Hollander, 2006) and MAOIs. If a patient responds only partially or does not respond to SSRI therapy, atypical antipsychotics may be used for augmentation. Risperidone (Risperdal) is considered a first-line agent for such augmentation (Fineberg & Gale, 2005). Additionally, atypical antipsychotic agents are the only established agents for treating SSRI-refractory OCD (Keuneman, Pokos, Weerasundera, & Castle, 2005). Other pharmacological options for refractory OCD based on limited research data include intravenous clomipramine and citalopram (Celexa), as well as combined SSRI-clomipramine treatment.

Many other drugs have been studied in OCD treatment. Opioid agonists such as tramadol hydrochloride (Ultram) and morphine have shown encouraging results. These drugs inhibit glutamate release in cerebral cortex, disinhibit serotonergic neurons in dorsal raphe, and increase dopamine transmission in the striatum leading to a decrease in distressing, obsessional thoughts, and a reduction in compulsive actions. In addition, glutamate (MSG) has been cited as a novel treatment target. Drugs, such as riluzole (Rilutek), memantine (Namenda), and N-acetylcysteine that lessen glutamatergic transmission have shown encouraging results. However, more research is needed (Lafleur, Pittenga, Kelmendi, et al. 2006).

## Posttraumatic Stress Disorder (PTSD)

SSRIs and SNRIs are considered first-line agents for treating PTSD. Second-line agents include the novel alpha-2 delta ligands, gabapentin or pregabalin, tricyclic antidepressants, and MAOIs. Due to the wide variation of symptoms that comprise PTSD, pharmacologic agents often leave patients with residual symptoms, such as insomnia, because one medication usually cannot manage all of the symptoms. Therefore most patients diagnosed with PTSD do not respond to monotherapy (Stahl, 2008). Research has shown that prazosin, an alpha-1 blocker, is effective for patients in which trauma-related nightmares and insomnia are prominent complaints. In addition, strong evidence supports it as an alternative treatment of PTSD, particularly for augmentation (Berger, Mendlowicz, Marques-Portella, Kinrys, Fontenelle, Marmar, & Figueira, 2009). Other medications that may be used as adjunctive treatment

## DRUG SUMMARY 13-1:
## AGENTS USED FOR ANXIETY DISORDERS

| DRUG | IMPLICATIONS FOR NURSING CARE |
|---|---|
| **BENZODIAZAPINES** | |
| aprazolam (Xanax) <br> clonazepam (Klonopin) <br> diazepam (Valium) <br> lorazepam (Ativan) | • Institute safety precautions to prevent injury secondary to sedative effects of the drug; warn the patient of these effects including decreased response time, slowed reflexes <br><br> • Encourage the patient to change positions slowly to minimize the effect of orthostatic hypotension <br><br> • Teach the patient that the full effects of the drug may not be noted for several weeks. Work with the patient to use other methods such as guided imagery and progressive relaxation to assist in relieving anxiety until drug reaches its therapeutic effectiveness <br><br> • Counsel the patient that one or more agents may need to be tried to determine the most effective drug <br><br> • Allow the patient to verbalize feelings and issues related to drug therapy; work with the patient and family to develop a method for adhering to drug therapy <br><br> • Urge the patient not to stop taking the drug abruptly because of possible withdrawal symptoms such as insomnia, increased anxiety, abdominal and muscle cramps, tremors, vomiting, sweating, and delirium <br><br> • Monitor the patient for compliance with therapy; be aware that physical and psychological dependence can occur <br><br> • Assess the patient for possible suicidal ideation, especially if the patient also has a concurrent depressive disorder <br><br> • Urge the patient to avoid consuming alcohol |
| **ANTICONVULSANTS** | |
| lamotrigine (Lamictal) <br> topiramate (Topomax) | • Institute safety precautions to prevent injury secondary to sedative effects of the drug; warn the patient of these effects including decreased response time, slowed reflexes <br><br> • Instruct female patients to notify the prescriber if starting or stopping oral contraceptives or other hormone preparations, if they become pregnant, or experience changes in their menstrual pattern <br><br> • Advise the patient not to discontinue abruptly or restart without notifying the prescriber <br><br> • Educate the patient that lamotrigine may cause a serious rash. Urge the patient to contact the prescriber immediately if a rash or symptoms of hypersensitivity occur |

*(cont.)*

**DRUG SUMMARY 13-1: (CONT.)**
**AGENTS USED FOR ANXIETY DISORDERS**

| DRUG | IMPLICATIONS FOR NURSING CARE |
|---|---|
| **ANTICONVULSANTS (*CONT.*)** | |
| lamotrigine (Lamictal)<br>topiramate (Topomax) | • Educate the patient that there may be a possible worsening of depressive symptoms or suicidal ideation, especially if the patient also has a concurrent depressive disorder |
| **PARTIAL SEROTONIN AGONIST** | |
| buspirone (BuSpar) | • Institute safety precautions to prevent injury secondary to dizziness, drowsiness<br>• Monitor the patient closely for withdrawal when switching from benzodiazepines to this agent<br>• Teach the patient that the full effects of the drug may not be noted for 1 to 2 weeks. Work with patient to use other methods such as guided imagery, progressive relaxation to assist in relieving anxiety until drug reaches its therapeutic effectiveness<br>• Educate the patient not to take with grapefruit juice |
| **BETA BLOCKERS** | |
| propranolol (Inderal) | • Counsel the patient not to stop the drug abruptly<br>• Monitor apical pulse and blood pressure closely for changes; if hypotension occurs or pulse rate varies widely, withhold the drug<br>• Administer the drug with food to promote absorption<br>• Institute safety precautions to prevent injury<br>• Educate the patient that this drug may mask signs of thyrotoxicosis and hypoglycemia |
| **ALPHA-1 BLOCKERS** | |
| prazosin (Minipress) | • Counsel the patient not to stop the drug abruptly<br>• Institute safety precautions to minimize the risk of injury from orthostatic hypotension; counsel the patient to change positions slowly<br>• Explain that drug may cause sexual dysfunction; encourage the patient to verbalize feelings related to this condition<br>• Educate patients that they should avoid exercising in hot weather while taking this medication<br>• Counsel patients to avoid consuming alcohol with this medication |

*(cont.)*

## DRUG SUMMARY 13-1: (*CONT.*)
## AGENTS USED FOR ANXIETY DISORDERS

### ALPHA-2 DELTA LIGANDS

| | |
|---|---|
| gabapentin (Neurontin)<br>pregabalin (Lyrica) | • Institute safety precautions to prevent injury secondary to sedative effects of the drug; warn the patient of these effects including decreased response time, slowed reflexes<br><br>• Counsel patients to avoid consuming alcohol with this medication<br><br>• Educate the patient regarding the signs and symptoms of angioedema<br><br>• Urge the patient not to abruptly discontinue this medication. It should be tapered off over one week<br><br>• Educate the patient that there may be a possible worsening of depressive symptoms or suicidal ideation, especially if the patient also has a concurrent depressive disorder<br><br>• *For gabapentin*: Counsel patients that if they are taking antacids such as Maalox, they should separate dosing by two hours |

*See Chapter 11 for a discussion of antipsychotic agents; see Chapter 12 for a discussion of antidepressants.*

include the antidepressant mirtazapine and naltrexone (ReVia) and acamprosate (Campral), which are used for alcohol dependence and abuse. The anticonvulsants such as lamotrigine and topiramate also may be used.

### Social Phobia

SSRIs and SNRIs are considered first-line agents for treating social phobia. However, the use of benzodiazepines as monotherapy is not well supported (Stahl, 2008). Tricyclic antidepressants and antidepressants such as mirtazapine and trazodone are not typically effective. MAOIs have shown some benefit, as have the novel alpha-2-delta ligands, gabapentin, or pregabalin. For patients with specific types of social phobia, such as performance anxiety, beta-blockers that are most notably used to treat hypertension can be useful. Like PTSD, adjunctive treatments include naltrexone and acamprosate and the anticonvulsants such as lamotrigine and topiramate.

> *Various groups of medications can be used to treat anxiety disorders. SSRIs and SNRIs are the primary agents used. Benzodiazepines also may be used in conjunction with these agents.*

### Pre-emptive or Prophylactic Treatments

A newly emerging concept for the treatment of anxiety disorders is called pre-emptive or prophylactic treatment. This concept is based on blocking the formation of fear conditioning by suppressing the presynaptic changes in the brain. This is accomplished with the use of "early fear extinction learning paradigms" or with medications. Some research supports the administration of beta blockers such as propranolol (Inderal) alone or with cortisol immediately following trauma exposure to block fear conditioning before it occurs (Tollenaar, Elzinga, Spionhovan, & Everaerd, 2009).

### Herbal Preparations

The use of herbal preparations as alternative therapies for anxiety is common practice. Attitudes that herbal remedies are "natural," have fewer side effects, and are readily available contribute to their appeal. Two herbal products commonly used to self-medicate symptoms of anxiety are valerian and kava kava.

The efficacy of kava kava (*Piper methysticum*) has been the subject of research. One meta-analysis documented greater efficacy of kava kava versus placebo for anxiety symptoms across several studies (Pittler & Ernst, 2000). One of the most extensive randomized, placebo-controlled studies evaluated the effects of kava kava in 100 patients diagnosed with agoraphobia, specific phobia, GAD, and adjustment disorder with anxiety (Volz & Kieser, 1997). Patients treated with 70 mg of kavalactones (the agent responsible for kava kava's psychotropic properties) three times daily showed significant improvement after eight weeks of treatment, with continued benefit at 24 weeks.

Kava kava is associated with several side effects including morning fatigue and mild gastrointestinal disturbances (Pepping, 1999). Toxic doses (greater than 300 g) may, however, cause progressive ataxia, muscle weakness, ascending paralysis, and scaling of skin on the extremities (Singh & Blumenthal, 1997). Reports of hepatotoxicity are currently being investigated by the Food and Drug Administration (FDA). Additionally, kava kava can potentiate the effects of central nervous system depressants, including ethanol, barbiturates, and benzodiazepines. Therefore, concomitant use should be avoided. Finally, kava kava should be avoided during pregnancy due to the potential for loss of uterine tone (Brinker, 1998). While kava kava may be an effective and well-tolerated anxiolytic agent for many patients, no evidence exists to suggest it is more effective than antidepressants or benzodiazepines.

Another herbal preparation is valerian (*Valeriana officinale*). Valerian has been studied using multiple dosages and preparations mostly as an herbal sleep remedy. Valerian has also been used in persons with mild anxiety, but the data supporting this indication are limited.

In one randomized, double-blind, placebo-controlled trial, researchers compared valerian with propranolol, a valerian-propranolol combination, and placebo in an experimental stress situation in 48 healthy adults. Unlike propranolol, valerian had no effect on physiologic arousal such as increased respiratory rate and increased heart rate, but significantly decreased subjective feelings of anxiety (Kohnen & Oswald, 1988).

In another preliminary, randomized, double-blind, placebo-controlled trial, 36 individuals with a diagnosis of generalized anxiety disorder were treated with placebo, diazepam, in a dosage of 2.5 mg three times daily, or valerian extract in a dosage of 50 mg three times daily for four weeks. Dosage was regulated at one week if an interviewing psychiatrist deemed an increase or decrease necessary. Although the study was limited by a small sample size, relatively low dosages of the active agents, and a short duration of treatment, the researcher found a significant reduction in the psychic factor of the Hamilton Anxiety Scale with diazepam and valerian (Andreatini, Sartori, Seabra & Leite, 2002).

A third randomized, double-blind, placebo-controlled trial compared 120 mg of kava, 600 mg of valerian, and placebo taken daily for seven days in relieving physiologic measures of stress induced under laboratory conditions in 54 healthy volunteers. Valerian and kava were found to significantly decrease systolic blood pressure, heart rate, and self-reported stress (Cropley, Cave, Ellis, & Middleton, 2002).

Side effects associated with valerian include sedation and withdrawal symptoms similar to those of benzodiazepine withdrawal following abrupt discontinuation. Although adverse effects and toxicity have not been adequately studied, four cases of hepatotoxicity associated with valerian use have been reported (Plushner, 2000). Additional studies are required to determine if valerian has any significant and sustained anxiolytic properties.

> *Two herbal preparations are commonly used for self-medication with anxiety disorders. These include kava kava and valerian. Further research is needed to determine their effectiveness.*

Some patients may use Ayurvedic herbal preparations such as *Bacopa monnieri* and *Centella asiatica*. Ayurveda is an advanced, highly integrated system of medicine that employs diverse herbal, mind-body, and energetic treatment modalities. These herbal preparations have been used for thousands of years to treat symptom patterns that resemble generalized anxiety. Double-blind controlled trials suggest that both herbs effectively reduce general anxiety symptoms (Stough, Lloyd, & Clarke, 2001). Some studies suggest that an Ayurvedic herbal compound formula "Geriforte" may also alleviate symptoms of generalized anxiety (Shah, Nayak, & Sethi, 1993). Although no serious adverse effects have been reported when these preparations are used at recommended dosages, patients who use Ayurvedic herbal preparations should be supervised by a trained Ayurvedic physician.

## Individual Psychotherapy

Psychotherapy when used to treat most of the anxiety disorders is typically oriented toward combating the patient's low-level, ever-present anxiety. Poor planning skills, high stress levels, and difficulty in relaxing often accompany such anxiety. According to the American Psychiatric Association (APA) Practice Guidelines (2006), psychodynamic therapy (a form of psychotherapy) has, from its beginnings, been concerned with responses to traumatic events and therefore is particularly useful for patients diagnosed with PTSD. Psychodynamic psychotherapists employ a mixture of supportive and insight-oriented interventions based on an assessment of the patient's symptoms, developmental history, personality, and available social supports. An ongoing assessment of the patient's ability to tolerate exploration of the trauma also is addressed (APA Practice Guidelines, 2006).

## Eye Movement Desensitization and Reprocessing

Eye movement desensitization and reprocessing (EMDR) is a fairly new type of psychotherapy. It is growing in popularity, particularly for treating posttraumatic stress disorder. EMDR is a unique approach to psychological issues. It does not rely on talk therapy or medications. Instead, EMDR uses a patient's own rapid, rhythmic eye movements to dampen the power of emotionally charged memories of past traumatic events. It is believed that these past events have set the groundwork for the current situations that trigger dysfunctional emotions, beliefs and sensations, and the positive experience needed to enhance future adaptive behaviors and mental health. Many EMDR patients also receive medications

During treatment, various procedures and protocols are used to address the entire clinical picture. One of the procedural elements is "dual stimulation" using bilateral eye movements, tones, or taps. During the reprocessing phases, the patient momentarily attends to past memories, present triggers, or anticipated future experiences while simultaneously focusing on a set of external stimulus. During that time, patients generally experience the emergence of insight, changes in memories, or new associations (Hamblen, et al., 2009).

While still considered controversial by some, the American Psychological Association has noted that EMDR is effective for treating symptoms of acute and chronic PTSD. It may be particularly useful for people who have trouble talking about the traumatic events they've experienced. The Department of Veterans Affairs and the Department of Defense (2010) have jointly issued clinical practice guidelines. These guidelines "strongly recommend" EDMR for the treatment of PTSD in both military and non-military populations. They also note that this approach has been as effective as other psychological treatments in some studies, and less effective in others.

## Biofeedback

BIOFEEDBACK, also referred to as *applied psychophysiological feedback,* is the process of displaying involuntary or subthreshold physiological processes, usually by electronic instrumentation, and learning to voluntarily influence those processes by making changes in cognition. It provides a visible and experiential demonstration of the mind-body connection. Biofeedback is also a therapeutic tool to facilitate learning how to self-regulate autonomic functions, such as heart rate and respiration for improving health (Stress Management Health Center, 2007). Although uncommon today, in part due to cost, health care professionals can be specifically trained and certified to assist patients to decrease stress and anxiety through biofeedback.

## Functional Neurosurgery

Neurosurgery as a form of treatment for psychiatric issues has historically been controversial. This history is marred by misguided applications of erroneous or overly simplistic approaches to psychiatric disease, often resulting in significant negative outcomes including morbidity. The earliest form of neurosurgery for psychiatric conditions or "psychosurgery" were prefrontal and transorbital lobotomies. These were crude procedures, that if not resulting in death, caused irreversible personality changes and cognitive impairment. Today, due to the level of precision available with modern neurosurgical procedures, advances in neuroimaging, and ethical considerations, there has been a cautious resurgence of surgical techniques used to treat psychiatric disorders. These techniques are referred to as neurosurgical lesioning because they ablate a biological function within a certain part of the brain.

Currently four lesioning neurosurgical procedures are used for the treatment of OCD and major depressive disorder: cingulotomy (lesioning the anterior portion of the cingulate gyrus, interrupting tracts between the cingulate gyrus and the frontal lobes), capsulotomy (lesioning in the anterior limb of the internal capsule, which serves as a relay route between cortical structures and the thalamus), subcaudate tractotomy (interrupting the relay between the cortex and thalamus via the striatum), and limbic leucotomy (essentially a combination of subcaudate tractotomy and cingulotomy). Research on the procedures has shown positive outcomes as evidenced by a decrease in objective measures of symptom report as well as increases in subjective reports of well being (Shah, Pesiridou, Gordon, Baltuch, Malone, & O'Reardon, 2008). Strides in neuroimaging and a greater understanding of neural circuitry have increased understanding of the neurobiological basis of psychiatric disorders. Based on this understanding, deep brain stimulation (DBS) has emerged as a potential neurosurgical treatment intervention that is performed without producing an irreversible lesion.

In 1987, deep brain stimulation was first performed in the thalamic region of the brain for successful treatment of Parkinson's tremor. Later it was performed in the subthalamic nucleus to treat Parkinson's disease and essential tremor (Hardesty & Sackeim 2007). Over the past decade, it has been studied as treatment for very severe, debilitating, treatment-resistant OCD with promising results. One study in particular suggested that stimulation of the subthalamic nucleus in individuals with severe forms of OCD may reduce symptoms but is associated with substantial risk of serious adverse events. Out of a total of 17 patients in whom stimulators were implanted, 11 had serious adverse events (Mallet et al., 2008). Based on this study, the FDA, on February 19, 2009, approved the use of an implanted brain device for patients with severe OCD. The FDA's "humanitarian device exemption" permits use of the device only on the most severely ill people with OCD. Fewer than 4,000 patients have such drastic, treatment-resistant OCD.

> *Although neurosurgery may be performed to treat OCD, deep brain stimulation (DBS), initially used for treating Parkinson's disease, is showing positive results for treating severe OCD.*

## Cognitive Behavioral Therapy

Cognitive behavioral therapy (CBT) incorporates a range of psychotherapeutic theories and practices including behavior therapy, behavior modification, and cognitive therapy. A large number of well-constructed studies have shown CBT to be highly useful in treating depression and anxiety disorders. Therefore, CBT is considered a first-line treatment option depending on the presenting symptoms and severity of anxiety (Carr & McNulty, 2006). **Evidence-Based Practice 13-1** highlights a study comparing CBT and psychodynamic therapy.

The hallmark of CBT is an intense focus on thought processes and belief systems. Patients learn to identify problematic beliefs and thought patterns, which are often irrational or unrealistic, and replace them with a more rational and realistic view. This is generally accomplished in a supportive environment where the treatment professional assigns homework, highlights concepts, and assists the patient through a path of self-discovery and change.

CBT focuses on the present rather than the past, and involves working collaboratively with patients, teaching them cognitive and behavioral skills. While there are a variety of CBT components, some of the more common techniques are presented here.

### Informational Interventions

Providing education is one of the most basic yet highly effective strategies used by psychiatric-mental health care professionals. This intervention is particularly useful with clients diagnosed with generalized anxiety disorder (GAD). Offering explanations about the nature of the disorder often demystifies the somatic sensations that patients experience. In addition, providing information helps to identify maladaptive thought processes and worrying as primary causes of anxiety. These interventions clarify for the patient the anxious nature of their thoughts and avoidance patterns in phobias and give them the opportunity to understand their symptoms. For patients diagnosed with posttraumatic stress disorder, simply having a discussion of dissociation and flashbacks helps to normalize and decrease the fear triggered by these symptoms.

### Self-Monitoring and Symptom Diary

One of the most effective tools for patients diagnosed with panic attacks is a diary or protocol of panic attacks. To monitor the occurrence of anxiety symptoms, the ability to identify anxious thoughts and the subsequent behaviors, such as avoidance, is essential to provide a rational description of the actual problem and to evaluate the treatment process. Patients are informed that this will help in the assessment of the frequency and nature of their panic attacks and provide information about the relationship of panic symptoms to internal stimuli such as emotions and images and to external stimuli, such as the situation, behavior, and substances.

### Cognitive Restructuring

Cognitive restructuring techniques are used to identify beliefs about the meaning and the consequences of

> *Cognitive behavioral therapy requires that a patient focuses on the present and examines problem beliefs and thought patterns. The patient then learns through education, self-monitoring, and cognitive restructuring how to replace these problematic thought patterns with more rational and realistic views.*

**EVIDENCE-BASED PRACTICE 13-1:**
**CBT VERSUS PSYCHODYNAMIC THERAPY**

STUDY

Leichsenring, F., Salzer, S., Jaeger, U., Kächele, H., Kreische, R., & Leweke, F. (2009). Short-term psychodynamic psychotherapy and cognitive behavioral therapy in generalized anxiety disorder: A randomized, controlled trial. *American Journal of Psychiatry, 166*(8), 875-881.

SUMMARY

This study compared the outcome of short-term psychodynamic psychotherapy with CBT in patients diagnosed with GAD. Patients with GAD were randomly assigned to receive either CBT (N = 29) or short-term psychodynamic psychotherapy (N = 28). Treatment included up to thirty weekly sessions. The primary outcome measure was the Hamilton Anxiety Rating Scale. Assessments were done at the completion of treatment and after six months. The study revealed that both therapies provided large, statistically significant improvements in anxiety symptoms. There were no significant differences in the Hamilton Anxiety Rating Scale between therapies or by two self-reported measures of anxiety. However, CBT was found to be superior in measures specific to trait anxiety, worry, and depressive symptoms.

APPLICATION TO PRACTICE

This study is helpful to provide evidence that CBT and individual psychodynamic therapy are effective treatment strategies. Although nurse generalists are not directly involved in these therapies, they play a major role in reinforcing the skills and techniques used with and learned from them. This study also impacts advanced nursing practice, since nurses trained at an advanced levels are able to provide both CBT and short-term psychodynamic psychotherapy.

QUESTIONS TO PONDER

1. *The study focused on patients with GAD. How might another anxiety disorder, such as OCD, impact the use of these two therapies and the results of the study?*
2. *Imagine that you had an anxiety disorder. Which of these two techniques do you think you would prefer and why?*

somatic symptoms. Catastrophic misinterpretations distort the meaning of somatic symptoms or overestimate the probability or the severity of feared outcomes. Patients are encouraged to consider the evidence and to think of alternative possible outcomes following the experience of the bodily sensation. Part of this process involves identifying the likely origin of the feared sensations and/or any misinformation about the meaning of the sensations (APA Practice Guidelines, 2006).

## Exposure Therapies

Exposure treatment involves presenting a patient with anxiety-producing stimuli for a long enough time to decrease the intensity of his or her emotional reaction. As a result, the feared situation or item no longer makes the patient anxious. Exposure treatment should be carried out in real situations whenever possible, called in vivo exposure. Alternatively, it can be done through imagination, which is called imaginal exposure. **SYSTEMATIC DESENSITIZATION** is a type of imaginal exposure where the patient is asked to imagine certain aspects of the feared object or situation combined with relaxation. Graduated exposure refers to exposing the patient to the feared situation in a gradual manner. **FLOODING** is a technique that exposes the patient to the anxiety-provoking or feared situation all at once. The patient is exposed to the stimuli until the anxiety and fear subside. Flooding, also called implosion therapy, is potentially dangerous, and should only be undertaken after careful consultation with a qualified practitioner.

Currently, the military is looking at a type of therapy that recreates the sights, smells, sounds and feel of combat using a "virtual reality helmet." This would provide a tool for veterans suffering with PTSD to vividly and safely confront their war experiences and allow reintegration of the parts of the self that were unable to tolerate the trauma when it originally occurred (Young, 2007).

*Exposure therapy can occur in real situations (in vivo exposure) or through the imagination (imaginal exposure).*

## Abdominal Breathing

When people are anxious, they tend to take rapid, shallow breaths that come directly from the chest. This type of breathing is called thoracic or chest breathing. Chest breathing disrupts the oxygen and carbon dioxide levels in the body, resulting in increased heart rate, dizziness, muscle tension, and other physical sensations. Blood is not being properly oxygenated and this may signal a stress response that contributes to anxiety and panic attacks. Teaching the patient how to perform abdominal or diaphragmatic breathing in which breaths are deep and even, is a simple and effective way to decrease anxious symptoms.

## Progressive Muscle Relaxation

Progressive muscle relaxation is a tension-reducing technique that involves the systematic tension and relaxation of specific muscle groups. Starting with the muscles in the face, the participant completely tenses all muscles and holds the tension for several seconds (usually to the count of ten). Next, the person completely relaxes for the same period of time, then repeats the process with the next set of muscles, such as the neck, the shoulders, and so on until every area

of the body has been relaxed. With practice, the participant learns to relax the body completely within seconds.

## Exercise

Patients who are anxious frequently engage in strenuous physical activity to alleviate symptoms. Open studies suggest that regular aerobic exercise of at least 20 to 30 minutes per day or strength training reduces anxiety (Paluska & Schwenk, 2000). Findings of a prospective, 10-week study of exercise in persons who experience panic episodes suggest that regular walking or jogging (4 miles, 3 times per week) reduces the severity and frequency of panic episodes (Stevinson, 1999).

## Guided Imagery

Guided imagery is a mind-body exercise based on prompting individuals to formulate meaningful mental pictures to achieve relaxation and reduce anxiety. Guided imagery has been shown to reduce anxiety, decrease the use of anxiolytics, and improve patient satisfaction in a variety of medical settings (Miller, 2003). Many guided imagery scripts include common elements such as asking the patient to sit or lie in a comfortable position, quieting the mind, removing negative thoughts and images, and calling to mind a vivid image or scenario that is calming and relaxing (a "safe place"). The content of a guided imagery script can include quiet and peaceful music with focus on a safe place where one feels secure and relaxed, or it may involve more active, physical sensations such as playing and winning a tennis match. For example, language used in a guided imagery exercise may be as follows:

> *"Position yourself as comfortably as you can, shifting your weight so that you're allowing your body to be fully supported by your chair or couch.... Take a deep, full, cleansing breath... inhaling as fully as you can... breathing deep into the belly if you can... and breathing all the way out.... Imagine a place where you feel safe and peaceful and easy... a place either make-believe or real...."*

## Music

Music and sound are used in many cultures and healing traditions for anxiety-reducing benefits. Studies have shown that music alters a person's psychophysiology (Kerr, Walsh, & Marshall, 2001). Soothing music has been shown to produce a hypometabolic response characteristic of relaxation in which autonomic, immune, endocrine, and neuropeptide systems are altered. Similarly, music therapy can produce desired psychological responses such as a reduction of anxiety and fear (Harris, 2009).

## Dietary Changes

Symptoms of generalized anxiety are frequently associated with a common condition known as reactive hypoglycemia, in which blood glucose drops to abnormally low levels following a glucose challenge. Patients who experience anxiety related to this condition benefit from dietary changes such as a low carbohydrate and high protein intake, consumption of foods with different glycemic indices, and avoidance of caffeine (Bell & Forse, 1999).

In addition, caffeine use is associated with an increased risk of anxiety. Caffeine consumption increases serum epinephrine, norepinephrine, and cortisol levels, and can result in feelings of "nervousness" in healthy adults or, in persons who are predisposed, increased feelings of generalized anxiety or panic episodes (Uhde, Boulenger, Jimerson, & Post, 1984). Patients who have chronic anxiety report that symptoms diminish when they abstain from caffeine (Bruce & Lader, 1989).

Moreover, a dietary deficiency of the amino acid tryptophan leads to reductions in brain serotonin levels. Persons who experience generalized anxiety or panic episodes reported more severe symptoms when they were being treated with an amino acid formula that did not include tryptophan (Klaassen, Klumperbeek, & Deutz, 1998).

Chronic stress and anxiety also can deplete the body's stores of vital nutrients. Many patients who suffer from agoraphobia are deficient in certain B-complex vitamins. This also may be a factor in other anxiety-related disorders. Vitamin B8 or inositol has been studied in patients suffering from panic disorder and agoraphobia. Results show that those taking inositol achieved a significant reduction in both severity and frequency of panic attacks and agoraphobia symptoms compared to the placebo group. Inositol also has been the focus of renewed research interest because of its role as a precursor of phosphatidylinositol, an important second messenger in the brain and an integral part of serotonin, norepinephrine, and other neurotransmitter receptors. Findings from several double-blind studies suggest that high doses of inositol reduce

> *Patients with anxiety disorders can learn techniques such as abdominal breathing, progressive muscle relaxation, and guided imagery and can use exercise, music, and diet to assist in reducing anxiety.*

many anxiety symptoms that respond to SSRIs, including panic episodes, agoraphobia, obsessions, and compulsions (Belmaker, Levine, & Kofman, 1998).

## APPLYING THE NURSING PROCESS FROM AN INTERPERSONAL PERSPECTIVE

Patients with anxiety disorders may be seen in a variety of settings such as acute care settings, day hospitalization programs, community and out-patient centers, and long-term care facilities. Many individuals may have co-morbidities such as substance abuse, diabetes, cardiovascular, or respiratory disorders. As a result, patients often can be encountered in general medical facilities, emergency departments, and specialty clinics. Therefore, nurses need a firm understanding of the nursing process that integrates the interpersonal process when caring for patients with anxiety disorders. **Plan of Care 13-1** provides an example for a patient with an anxiety disorder.

## Strategies for Optimal Assessment: Therapeutic Use of Self

According to Peplau (1991), the nursing process is therapeutic when the nurse and the patient can come to know and to respect what is the same and what is different in one another, thereby coming together to share in the solution of a problem. When working with patients experiencing anxiety disorders, unique challenges can occur. Symptoms may be vague or, if they are not physiologically based, may not be visible. Emotional problems can also manifest as different symptoms, arising from numerous causes. Similarly, past events may lead to very different types of presenting behaviors or symptoms. Many patients are unable to describe their problems. They may be highly withdrawn, highly anxious, or out of touch with reality. Their ability to participate in the problem-solving process may also be limited if they see themselves as powerless.

### Self-Assessment

Prior to and in order to respectfully and objectively work with a patient, nurses must complete a personal self-assessment through the process of reflection. Reflecting and examining oneself develop both insight and self-awareness (Gustafsson & Fagerberg, 2004) and is an essential component within nursing if satisfactory levels of care are to be maintained at a professional standard (Kuokkanen & Leino-Kilpi, 2000). Reflecting on one's own attitudes, values, and prejudices is a critical component of being able to

**PLAN OF CARE 13-1:**
**THE PATIENT WITH AN ANXIETY DISORDER (WITH PANIC) AND**
**OBSESSIVE-COMPULSIVE DISORDER**

**NURSING DIAGNOSIS:** Anxiety (*severe*); related to exposure to traumatic event; manifested by perceived threats and recurrent panic attacks. Ineffective coping; related to anxiety of perceived need to check and re-check things; manifested by participation in repeated ritualistic behavior to reduce anxiety.

**OUTCOME IDENTIFICATION:** Patient will demonstrate participation in fewer ritualistic behaviors with an improved level of independent function.

| INTERVENTION | RATIONALE |
|---|---|
| Assess the level of the patient's anxiety; stay with the patient and provide for safety and security | Determining the level of the patient's anxiety provides a baseline from which to intervene |
| Maintain a calm, reassuring approach; keep verbal exchanges short and direct | Maintaining a calm, reassuring approach prevents adding to the patient's anxiety Keeping exchanges short and direct reducing the risk of overwhelming an already overwhelmed patient; a patient experiencing significant anxiety has difficulty focusing and concentrating |
| Administer prescribed antianxiety agents if indicated | Administering antianxiety agents helps to reduce or control feelings of anxiety |
| Encourage the use of appropriate defense mechanisms | Using appropriate defense mechanisms can help to reduce anxiety |
| Once level of anxiety has diminished, assist the patient in exploring precipitating factors for the anxiety | Identifying precipitating factors can help to prevent recurrence |
| Assist the patient in identifying signs and symptoms of increasing anxiety | Being able to identify signs and symptoms facilitates early intervention |
| Work with the patient to determine usual methods of problem solving; identify effective and ineffective methods | Identifying usual methods of coping provides information about possible maladaptive strategies and opportunities for teaching more adaptive ones |
| Teach the patient various methods for reducing anxiety, such as controlled breathing, relaxation, and physical activity Assist the patient in practicing appropriate strategies; provide positive reinforcement | Using various methods for reducing anxiety provides the patient with options to manage anxiety effectively Employing breathing and relaxation techniques interferes with sympathetic nervous stimulation associated with increasing anxiety Practicing promotes success; positive reinforcement promotes self-esteem |

*(cont.)*

**PLAN OF CARE 13-1: (*CONT.*)**
**THE PATIENT WITH AN ANXIETY DISORDER (WITH PANIC) AND OBSESSIVE-COMPULSIVE DISORDER**

**NURSING DIAGNOSIS:** Powerlessness; related to perceived inability to control compulsions; manifested by worry and sense of despair regarding ritualistic behavior.

**OUTCOME IDENTIFICATION:** Patient will demonstrate a gradual increase in ability to manage anxiety.

| INTERVENTION | RATIONALE |
| --- | --- |
| Assist the patient to view situation objectively | Viewing a situation objectively helps to promote feelings of control over the situation |
| Encourage the patient to verbalize feelings associated with the performance of ritualistic behavior; suggest that the patient keep a log or diary of the behaviors to help identify possible triggers for the behaviors | Identifying feelings and triggers associated with behaviors is necessary before behaviors can be addressed |
| Initially, allow the patient to engage in behavior | Allowing behavior initially is necessary to prevent the patient from experiencing overwhelming anxiety |
| Work with the patient to gradually develop a plan or schedule to limit participation in the behavior; help the patient to make changes in small, manageable steps; assist the patient in engaging in another activity or addressing other feelings | Limiting participation promotes adaptation and gradual increase in control over behavior; using small manageable steps fosters success and promotes feelings of control |
| Assist the patient with implementing prescribed therapies such as relaxation and guided imagery | Implementing appropriate therapies helps the patient replace maladaptive coping mechanisms with adaptive ones, thus promoting feelings of control |
| Provide positive feedback for accomplishments | Providing positive feedback fosters self-esteem and feelings of control |

*Nursing Diagnosis – Definitions and Classifications 2009 – 2011. Copyright © 2011 by NANDA International. Use by arrangement with Blackwell Publishing Limited, a company of John Wiley & Sons, Inc.*

calmly intervene and work with patients who suffer with anxiety disorders. Especially important in working with patients who are anxious is the need to monitor one's own anxiety. Failure to do so may actually increase the level of anxiety in the patient. The paitent will sense the anxiety, which will fuel his or her own anxiety.

The self-aware nurse is pivotal in coming together with a patient to assess the patient's understanding of his or her anxiety symptoms. This is an essential step for developing empathy. **Consumer Perspective 13-1** provides insight into what it is like to experience an anxiety disorder from the patient's viewpoint.

**CONSUMER PERSPECTIVE 13-1:**
**A PATIENT WITH AN ANXIETY DISORDER**

*This is what is left*
*Periphery…Outline…Profile*
*A professional, perhaps*
*She knows the words*
*They make sense sometimes*
*But then she goes home*
*…void of feeling*
*…void of sense*
*imploding with rage*
*seeping feelings*
*scared to live*
*afraid to die*
*Remaining in Hell*

This was a poem written by Marie when she was 27 years old. By that time she was addicted to alcohol and marijuana. She had entered individual psychotherapy at the age of 25 and was diagnosed with PTSD related to childhood sexual abuse and ritualistic satanic abuse. She attended a year-long group conducted by two registered nurses for "survivors of incest." Experiences learned in this group motivated her to attend Narcotics Anonymous and by the age of 29 she stopped abusing alcohol and drugs. While her symptoms were slowly improving she still experienced a tremendous amount of anxiety. She therefore started cognitive behavioral therapy with a psychologist. One of her journal entries during this time reads… *"I feel lost. I'm anxious. I'm shaking. I feel very inadequate and I'm not sure why. I know I am feeling a lot of shame and*

*I don't understand the thinking that leads to this shame. I don't believe that I have any control over my feelings. They command me and take the life out of me."*

Today Marie does quite well. She is a health care professional who works full time and is involved in a healthy, committed relationship. She continues to participate in Narcotics Anonymous, attends individual psychotherapy primarily using cognitive behavioral therapy techniques and takes an SNRI and medication to help with a sleep disturbance. Marie states, "It took many different types of therapies by different professionals to help me tackle my anxiety symptoms. I needed different interventions during different times in my life. I am very grateful for the professionals that took the time to really listen to me and stick by me when I didn't believe in myself."

## Environmental Considerations

Providing a safe, comfortable environment with minimal external stimulation is necessary to establish an atmosphere of trust. Once trust is established, the nurse must provide an assessment whereby the patient feels there is genuine interest, acceptance, and positive regard. This is accomplished primarily through therapeutic communication techniques including restating, reflecting, and clarifying. (See Chapter 3 for more information on therapeutic communication.)

*Nurses need to be self-aware of feelings related to anxiety disorders and how they display anxiety during their interactions with patients to prevent adding to the patient's already heightened state.*

## Baseline Assessment

A baseline assessment is needed for a patient who is experiencing a new onset anxiety. This baseline includes a detailed physical and psychosocial symptom profile. **Table 13-1** summarizes key physical and psychosocial manifestations.

Because many medical conditions and medications can produce symptoms that mimic anxiety disorders, an assessment of anxiety must be completed after ruling out any potential medical or medication-induced etiologies. Once this is completed, it is important to obtain a detailed history including:

- Onset or precipitating factors that led to current symptoms
- Personal history including ethnic, cultural, religious, or spiritual background
- History of intake of illicit drugs, alcohol, nicotine, caffeine, herbal preparations, and over-the-counter drugs
- Current medication history
- Past psychiatric history, including co-morbid mood disorders and psychotic disorders
- Family psychiatric history

A detailed personal history is crucial because the context in which anxiety is experienced, its meaning, and responses to it are culturally mediated. It also provides information about the severity of the patient's anxiety level from which the nurse will determine the most appropriate intervention and promotes understanding of the patient's mental health beliefs and practices. For example, it is critical to understand whether a patient believe the anxiety symptoms are because he or she is a "bad person" or is being punished for past actions.

Assessing the patient from a cultural perspective will also allow the nurse to understand what is considered a cultural norm for them. Providing culturally congruent care will optimize chances for better outcomes. For example, during assessment the nurse discovers that the patient believes that meditation is beneficial and has some basic skills in performing it. This information would help the nurse apply the patient's beliefs and knowledge to the concepts of guided imagery and deep breathing techniques in managing the anxiety.

Evaluation of a patient's anxiety symptoms begins with an overall mental status examination. This includes assessment of mood, affect, speech, perceptual disturbances, thought process and content, sensorium, cognition, judgment, and insight. As with any psychiatric-mental health disorder, the nurse needs to evaluate for any suicidal, homicidal, aggressive, or self-harm tendencies at this time. If present, the nurse must intervene to ensure the safety of all involved. Once the assessment phase is completed, the nurse, together with the patient, identifies the priority problems and needs.

### TABLE 13-1: PHYSICAL AND PSYCHOSOCIAL MANIFESTATIONS OF ANXIETY

| PHYSICAL MANIFESTATIONS | PSYCHOSOCIAL MANIFESTATIONS |
|---|---|
| • Shakiness | • Jitteriness |
| • Sensation of lump in throat | • Fear of falling asleep due to disturbing dreams |
| • Trembling | • Irritability |
| • Choking sensation | • Unrealistic or excessive worry |
| • Muscle aches | • Tension |
| • Dry mouth | • Sense of impending doom |
| • Sweating | • Ritualistic behaviors |
| • Numbness and tingling of body parts | • Poor concentration |
| • Cold or clammy hands | • Avoidance |
| • Upset stomach | • Fear of being away from home |
| • Dizziness | • Isolation |
| • Nausea | • Irrational fear of strangers |
| • Vomiting | • Impatience |
| • Diarrhea | • Exaggerated startle reactions |
| • Vertigo | |
| • Fatigue | |
| • Racing or pounding heart | |
| • Decreased sexual desire | |
| • Hyperventilation | |
| • Sleep disturbances | |

Two anxiety disorders, OCD and PTSD, require additional assessment information. If the patient has OCD, assessment may reveal the presence of obsessive thoughts, words, or mental images that persistently invade his or her mind. Common obsessions include thoughts of contamination (with insects, dirt, or stool), thoughts of violence (such as staging, shooting, or beating), repetitive doubts or worries about a tragic event such as death, and repeating or counting images, words, or objects in their environment. The patient understands that these obsessions are a product of his or her own mind but feels powerless over them. The assessment may also reveal the presence of compulsions, which are irrational and recurring impulses to repeat a specific behavior. Common compulsions include repetitive touching, counting, doing and undoing (opening and closing a door for example), washing, and checking. These activities decrease the patient's anxiety level. It is important for the nurse to determine the time spent on obsessions or compulsions, the interference it causes in their daily life, the patient's level of resistance, the patient's feelings of control or lack of control over the obsessions and/or compulsions, and the distress it causes.

For the patient with PTSD, assessment may include the patient describing intense fear that cannot be "shut off." Patients often describe feelings of hopelessness, an exaggerated startle response, feeling emotionally numb and detached from the world, and nightmares of the traumatic event or intrusive thoughts and images of the event during the day. This memory can be triggered by a sound, smell, action, or image and the patient may not know what the trigger is. Reliving the event as if it is actually happening is called a flashback. A thorough history will provide information of the traumatic event such as a history of combat action, childhood abuse, criminal assault, victims of a natural disaster, or a serious accident. The difference between whether a patient is experiencing posttraumatic stress versus acute traumatic stress is that in acute traumatic stress disorder the symptoms must peak and be alleviated within one month. If the symptoms persist then the patient has posttraumatic stress disorder.

> *Patients experiencing anxiety demonstrate physical, psychological, and social symptoms. The nurse needs to be vigilant in assessment because many medical conditions and medications can present with similar symptoms.*

## Planning Appropriate Interventions: Meeting the Patient's Focused Needs

A patient seeking assistance on the basis of a need is often the first step in a dynamic learning experience from which a constructive next step in personal growth can occur (Peplau, 1991). Meeting patient-focused needs during the planning stage of the nursing process can only happen if the nurse has accurately completed an assessment of the patient and his or her perception of anxiety.

The nurse must also determine, based in part on the patient's ego strength, what treatment goals and plans would be most appropriate for the patient, thereby providing for the best outcomes. For example, planning to use desensitization for a patient who is still experiencing an acute stress reaction arising from a specific phobia could further increase anxiety to the point where the patient shuts down. Focusing on the patient's strengths identified in the assessment stage is key when planning interventions. Doing so will also allow for an increased sense of collaboration on the part of the patient.

Due to the varying assessment findings noted in and wide range of problems faced by patients with anxiety disorders, numerous nursing diagnoses would apply. Examples of possible nursing diagnoses would include:
- Anxiety related to diagnosis of terminal illness
- Ineffective coping related to difficulty concentrating, compulsive hand washing
- Risk for self-directed violence related to feelings of hopelessness
- Risk for other-directed violence related to feelings of anger
- Posttrauma syndrome related to childhood sexual abuse
- Powerlessness related to chronic illness
- Insomnia related to environmental changes
- Risk for impaired skin integrity related to compulsive hand washing
- Impaired social interaction related to ritualistic behaviors

These nursing diagnoses also will vary based on the acuity of the patient's illness, developmental stage, comorbidities, current treatment regimen, and sources of support. Based on the identified nursing diagnoses, the nurse and patient collaboratively would determine the outcomes to be achieved. For example, outcomes for the nursing diagnosis of risk of ineffective coping related to compulsive hand washing may include the following:
- The patient will express feelings of anxiety as they occur
- The patient will reduce the amount of time spent each day on ritualistic compulsions
- The patient will demonstrate techniques for interrupting ritualistic compulsions

## Implementing Effective Interventions: Timing and Pacing

Once patient-centered goals and interventions are planned, the implementation stage of the nursing process begins. For patients who suffer with anxiety disorders, the timing and pacing of interventions are critical. The key at this point is to determine how to intervene if the patient is experiencing severe, panic-level, or moderate anxiety responses.

During any phase of anxiety, nursing interventions must be protective and supportive. However, for those experiencing panic and severe levels of anxiety, patient safety is paramount. Medication administration is often an emergent intervention required. Thus, timing and pacing are critical when administering medications in this situation. Prior to medication administration, the nurse needs to understand what the patient is experiencing. For example, a patient experiencing flashbacks or intrusive imagery may have an altered perceptual state and not recognize the nurse as helpful. Patients at this level are often unable to process information clearly or use coping strategies. Thus, the nurse needs to approach the patient slowly and calmly. Additionally, the nurse needs to quickly establish a therapeutic alliance and make a human connection with the patient. Doing so will clarify that the nurse is there to support the patient and not to harm him or her. Once medication is administered, the nurse then focuses on observing for side effects, assessing vital signs, and initiating appropriate psychoeducation about the medications and management of the disorder.

In addition to administering medications to patients experiencing severe levels of anxiety, the nurse would work to decrease environmental stimuli such as by dimming the lights and reducing noise levels. The nurse also intervenes to address the patient's physical signs and symptoms of anxiety such as trembling, muscle aches, sweating, rapid breathing, increased heart rate, difficulty sleeping, and dizziness. Helpful measures include using clear, simple instructions; demonstrating slow, deep, diaphragmatic breathing techniques; guiding the patient through visualization and imagery exercises; and helping the patient through progressive muscle relaxation techniques. **Therapeutic Interaction 13-1** provides an example of an interaction between a nurse and a patient with OCD who is experiencing increased anxiety as she attempts to control her compulsive hand washing. Other appropriate interventions include identifying and modifying anxiety-provoking situations when possible and provide accepting, reassuring actions rather than those that are probing or challenging. Limiting the patient's interactions with other patients helps minimize the contagious aspects of anxiety. This action is particularly helpful on inpatient units.

When the patient's level of anxiety is reduced to a moderate or mild level, the nurse may implement insight-oriented or educative nursing interventions, which involve the patient in the problem-solving process (Stuart, 2005). These interventions may include assisting the patient to identify and describe his or her underlying feelings, encouraging physical activity to discharge energy, identifying ways to restructure thoughts and modify behaviors, using available resources, and testing new coping strategies. Throughout these interventions, the nurse maintains his or her presence with the patient to demonstrate trust and support and instill a sense of hopefulness that anxiety can be alleviated. **Patient and Family Education 13-1** highlights some helpful tips for a patient with an anxiety disorder.

Additional interventions will vary widely depending upon specific underlying anxiety responses and disorders. For example, evidenced-based treatment for patients suffering with PTSD includes interventions based on eye movement desensitization and reprocessing (EMDR) or cognitive behavioral therapies (Hamblen, Schnurr, Rosenberg, & Eftekhari, 2009). This differs from interventions for patients suffering with specific phobias who often benefit from systematic desensitization as first-line treatment. Regardless of the treatments used, nurses need to ensure that the treatments are provided at the time when they will be most effective.

> *Nurses need to time and pace interventions appropriately based on the level of the patient's anxiety to ensure that the most appropriate interventions are being used at the appropriate time.*

## Evaluating: Objective Critique of Interventions and Self-Reflection

Evaluation occurs as a continuous, cyclical, and ongoing process throughout the nursing process. Evaluation within the context of the nursing process is dynamic, involving change in the patient's mental health status over time. This requires the nurse to gather new data, re-evaluate nursing interventions, and modify the plan of care.

During the evaluation phase, the nurse reviews all activities during the previous phases and determines whether outcomes identified with and for the patient have

### THERAPEUTIC INTERACTION 13-1: INTERVENTIONS FOR OCD

Ms. Cox is admitted to an inpatient psychiatric unit for obsessive thoughts that her hands are dirty and compulsive hand washing. The compulsive hand washing has resulted in skin breakdown and impaired social and professional functioning.

| | |
|---|---|
| The nurse enters the patient's room and finds Ms. Cox sitting on her hands on her bed, rocking back and forth. The nurse gains permission to come in and sit down across from the patient. The nurse maintains a calm, pleasant demeanor and speaks in a slow, simple manner. | Showing respect strengthens the bond between the nurse and the patient and is a predictor of a successful intervention. Moving slowly and staying calm minimizes the potential for an increase in anxiety. |
| **Nurse:** "Ms. Cox, you appear anxious. I would like to show you a way to help you relax." <br><br> **Ms. Cox:** "Please, I need some help here. I'm trying not to obsess about my hands but I can't stop." (breathing rapidly) | Provides reassurance that you are there to empower the patient to learn a way to decrease her anxiety level. |
| **Nurse:** "Breathe through your nose with me." (Nurse takes three deep breaths through her nose; patient does the same) <br><br> **Nurse:** "Great job. Now let's do some more breathwork." <br><br> **Ms. Cox:** "Okay." | When anxiety levels are elevated, focus and concentration are limited. Shadowing is a simple way to demonstrate technique. Praise reinforces the behavior. |
| **Nurse:** "Breathe through your nose with me. Make your stomach move while breathing and not your chest." Nurse places her hands on her stomach and inhales for 3 seconds then exhales for 3 seconds and repeats the cycle several times until she observes a decrease in physical symptoms of anxiety (rapid breathing and rocking). Ms. Cox places her hands on her stomach and breathes with the nurse. | Slow, diaphragmatic breathing can relieve feelings of anxiety and decrease the heart rate. Placing her hands on her stomach takes the focus from sitting on them and diverts her attention to her breathing. |
| **Nurse:** "Now you continue breathing this way, inhaling for three seconds and exhaling for three seconds and repeating the cycle." | Nurse empowers Ms. Cox to do this technique independent of her. By focusing her attention on breathing and counting she is not obsessing about washing her hands. |

been met. Once again, self-reflection is an invaluable tool at this point. This can be done by asking: Have I provided the best nursing practice for my patient? Is my patient better after the planned care?

During this phase of the nurse-patient relationship, the nurse and the patient should reflect on progress made toward reaching the patient goals. Point out positives to the patient and include a plan for aftercare as

**PATIENT AND FAMILY EDUCATION 13-1:
COPING STRATEGIES FOR DEALING WITH ANXIETY**

- Decrease overwhelming stimuli in the environment by decreasing the noise level and dimming the lights

- Create a relaxing environment with music, candles, or other aromatherapy (incense, diffusers, etc.)

- Practice diaphragmatic breathing

- Go outside and breathe fresh air

- Do stretching exercises

- Exercise by talking a walk, walking your dog, walking around the yard, or going to a hiking trail

- Distract yourself by focusing on a hobby

- Call a friend or family member

- Practice guided imagery

- Practice progressive muscle relaxation

- Take a warm bath

- Watch or listen to comedy

appropriate. This phase is also part of the termination of the patient-patient relationship. Many times a patient will have a setback due to feelings of loss of this relationship. The nurse's role is to help the patient explore these feelings and ease this transition while maintaining boundaries (Peplau, 1991).

Evaluation provides a feedback mechanism for judging the quality of care given. Evaluation of the progress indicates which problems have been solved and which needs have been met, which needs require reassessment, replanning, implementation, and re-evaluation.

**SUMMARY POINTS**

- Anxiety disorders include panic disorder, obsessive-compulsive disorder (OCD), posttraumatic stress disorder (PTSD), generalized anxiety disorder (GAD), acute stress disorder, and phobias. Anxiety disorders were not officially recognized as a psychiatric illness until 1980. They are the most common and most costly psychiatric illness in the United States.

- The exact cause of anxiety disorders is not known. Psychodynamic, behavioral, and learning theories are prominent. Additionally, biological influences, including brain structures, neurotransmitters, and genetics also are proposed as contributing to these disorders.

- Pharmacological therapy for anxiety disorders includes SSRIs and SNRIs as first line treatment for many of the disorders. Benzodiazepines also are used. Other

agents used include buspirone; atypical antipsychotic agents such as venlafaxine; alpha 2 delta ligands such as gabapentin or pregabalin; tricyclic antidepressants; monoamine oxidase inhibitors (MAOIs); beta blocker propranolol; and anticonvulsants such as lamotrigine or topiramate.

- Individual psychotherapy involves a combination of supportive and insight-oriented therapy which is helpful for patients with PTSD. Eye movement desensitization and reprocessing (EMDR) is a new type of psychotherapy gaining popularity for treating PTSD. Cognitive behavioral therapy is considered the first line treatment strategy for patients with depression and anxiety disorders. Flooding or implosion therapy is a type of exposure therapy in which the patient is exposed to the anxiety-provoking stimuli all at once. It is potentially

(cont.)

## SUMMARY POINTS (*CONT.*)

dangerous and should only be used after careful consultation with a qualified practitioner.

- Caffeine is associated with an increased risk of anxiety because it increases serum epinephrine, norepinephrine, and cortisol levels. A deficiency of the amino acid tryptophan is associated with anxiety due to reductions in brain serotonin levels.

- Nurses working with patients experiencing anxiety disorders face unique challenges because symptoms may be vague or possibly not visible. Emotional problems can also be

exhibited as different symptoms arising from numerous causes. Additionally, many patients may be unable to describe their problems.

- Meeting patient-focused needs can only occur when the nurse has accurately assessed the patient and his or her perception of anxiety.

- For patients suffering from anxiety disorder, the timing and pacing of interventions is critical. The nurse needs to determine how best to intervene based on the patient's level of anxiety.

## NCLEX-PREP*

1. A patient with PTSD is exhibiting hypervigilence. Which statement would the nurse interpret as indicating this?

   a. "I'm having trouble sleeping at night."
   b. "I've been really irritable and angry."
   c. "I always have to watch my back."
   d. "I just can't seem to relax."

2. A group of nursing students is reviewing information about anxiety disorders. The students demonstrate a need for additional study when they identify which of the following as a compulsion?

   a. Hearing voices that tell a person he is the king
   b. Repeatedly washing hands
   c. Touching the door knob three times before leaving
   d. Walking in a specific pattern when entering a room

3. A patient comes to the clinic for a routine check-up and is to have laboratory testing completed. During the assessment, the

patient reveals that he is afraid of needles and begins to hyperventilate. The patient also becomes diaphoretic and complains of a lump in his throat. The nurse would suspect which of the following?

   a. Generalized anxiety disorder
   b. Posttraumatic stress disorder
   c. Acute stress disorder
   d. Specific phobia

4. A patient with panic disorder is prescribed venlafaxine. The nurse identifies this agent as which of the following?

   a. Selective serotonin reuptake inhibitor (SSRI)
   b. Serotonin/norepinephrine reuptake inhibitor (SNRI)
   c. Benzodiazepine
   d. Atypical antipsychotic

5. A nursing instructor is preparing a class on anxiety disorders and the biological influences associated with this group of illnesses. Which of the following would the instructor include as a primary

(*cont.*)

**NCLEX-PREP\*** (*CONT.*)

neurotransmitter involved in the anxiety response?

   a. Gamma-aminobutyric acid (GABA)
   b. Serotonin
   c. Dopamine
   d. Norepinephrine

6. A patient with an anxiety disorder is asked to imagine specific aspects of the feared

situation while engaged in relaxation. The nurse identifies this as which of the following?

   a. Flooding
   b. Systematic desensitization
   c. In vivo exposure
   d. Implosion therapy

\*Answers to these questions appear on page 639.

## REFERENCES

American Psychiatric Association. (2000). *Diagnostic and statistical manual of mental disorders* (4th ed., text rev.). Washington, DC: Author.

American Psychiatric Association. (2006). *American psychiatric association practice guidelines for the treatment of psychiatric disorders compendium 2006.* Washington, DC: Author.

Anderson, A. (2007). Anxiety-panic history: Anxiety, disorders and treatments throughout the ages. Retrieved July 10, 2009 from http://anxiety-panic.com/history/h-main.htm

Andreatini, R., Sartori, V., Seabra, M., & Leite, J. (2002). Effect of kava and valerian on human physiological and psychological responses to mental stress assessed under laboratory conditions. *Phytotherapy Research, 16*(7), 650–654.

Bandelow, B., Seidler-Brandler, U., Becker, A., Wedekind, D., & Rüther, E. (2007). Meta-analysis of randomized controlled comparisons of psychopharmacological and psychological treatments for anxiety disorders. *World Journal of Biological Psychiatry, 8,* 175–187.

Bell, S.J., Forse, R.A. (1999). Nutritional management of hypoglycemia. *Diabetes Education, 25*(1): 41–47.

Belmaker, R.H., Levine, J.A., & Kofman, O. (1998, May-June). *Inositol—a novel augmentation for mood disorders.* Paper presented at the 151st Annual Meeting of the American Psychiatric Association, Toronto.

Berger, W., Mendlowicz, M.V., Marques-Portella, C., Kinrys, G., Fontenelle, L.F., Marmar, C.R., & Figueira, I. (2009). Pharmacologic alternatives to antidepressants in posttraumatic stress disorder: a systematic review. *Prog Neuropsychopharmacol Biol Psychiatry, 33(2),* 169–180.

Black, D.W., Carney, C.P., Peloso, P.M., Woolson, R.F., Schwartz, D.A., Voelker, M.D., Barrett, D. H., & Doebbeling, B. N. (2004). Gulf War veterans with anxiety: prevalence, comorbidity, and risk factors. *Epidemiology,156(2),* 135–142.

Bolton, J., Cox, B., Clara, I., & Sareen, J. (2006). Use of alcohol and drugs to self-medicate anxiety disorders in a nationally representative sample. *The Journal of Nervous and Mental Disease, 194(11),* 818–825.

Brinker, F. (1998). *Herb contraindications and drug interactions* (2nd ed.). Sandy, OR: Eclectic Medical Publications.

Bruce, M.S., & Lader, M. (1989) Caffeine abstention in the management of anxiety disorders. *Psychological Medicine, 19,* 211–214.

Carr, A., & McNulty, M. (2006). *Handbook of adult clinical Psychology: An evidence-based practice approach.* London: Routledge.

Cropley, M., Cave, Z., Ellis, J., & Middleton, R. (2002). Effect of vale-potriates (valerian extract) in generalized anxiety disorder: A randomized placebo-controlled pilot study. *Phytotherapy Research, 16*(1), 23–27.

Dell'Osso, B., Nestadt, G., Allen, A., & Hollander, E. (2006) Serotonin-norepinephrine reuptake inhibitors in the treatment of obsessive-compulsive disorder: A critical review. *Journal of Clinical Psychiatry, 67,* 600–610.

Department of Veterans Affairs and the Department of Defense. (2010). *Clinical practice guideline for the management of post-traumatic stress.* Retrieved March 29, 2011from http://www.healthquality.va.gov/PTSD-FULL-2010c.pdf

Dohrenwend, B.P., Turner, J.B., Turse, N.A., Adams, B.G., Koen, K.C., & Marshall, R. (2006). The psychological risk of Vietnam for U.S. veterans: A revisit with new data and methods. *Science, 313*(5789), 979–982.

Fineberg, N.A., & Gale, T.M. (2005). Evidence-based pharmacotherapy of obsessive-compulsive disorder. *International Journal of Neuropsychopharmacology, 8*(1), 107–129.

Freud, F. (1938). *The basic writings of Sigmund Freud.* New York: Random House.

Gabriel, R.A. (1987). *No more heroes; madness and psychiatry in war.* New York: Macmillan.

Gustafsson, C., & Fagerberg, I. (2004). Reflection, the way to professional development? *Journal of Clinical Nursing, 13*(3), 271–280.

Hamblen, J.L., Schnurr, P.P., Rosenberg, M.A., & Eftekhari, A. (2009). A guide to the literature on psychotherapy for PTSD. *Psychiatric Annals, 39*(6), 348–354.

Hardesty, D.E., & Sackeim, H.A. (2007). Deep brain stimulation in movement and psychiatric disorders, *Biological Psychiatry, 61,* 831–835.

Harris, D.L. (2009). Music therapy. In Keegan, L. & Dossey, B.M. (Eds.), *Holistic nursing: A handbook for practice* (5th Ed.). Sudbury, MA: Jones and Bartlett.

Helwick, C. (2011). Unique study identifies gene associated with anxiety phenotype: Anxiety Disorder of America 31st Annual Conference. Abstract 4. Presented March 25, 2011. Retrieved April 23, 2011 from http://www.medscape.com/viewarticle/739831

Henig, R.M. (2009). Understanding the anxious mind. *The New York Times Magazine.* Retrieved October 25, 2009 from http://nytimes.com/2009/10/4/magazine/04anxiety-t.html

Herman, J. (1997). *Trauma and recovery: The aftermath of violence—from domestic abuse to political terror.* New York: Basic Books.

Kerr, T., Walsh, J., & Marshall, A. (2001). Emotional change processes in music-assisted reframing. *Journal of Music Therapy, 38,* 193–211.

Kessler, R.C., Berglund, P.A., Demler, O., Jin, R., & Walters, E. E. (2005). Lifetime prevalence and age-of-onset distributions of DSM-IV disorders in the National Comorbidity Survey Replication (NCS-R). *Archives of General Psychiatry, 62*(6), 593–602.

Kessler, R.C., Chiu, W.T., Demler, O., & Walters, E.E. (2005). Prevalence, severity, and comorbidity of twelve-month *DSM-IV* disorders in the National Comorbidity Survey Replication (NCS-R). *Archives of General Psychiatry, 62*(6), 617–627.

Keuneman, R.J., Pokos V., Weerasundera, R., & Castle, D.J. (2005). Antipsychotic treatment in obsessive-compulsive disorder: a literature review. *Australian and New Zealand Journal of Psychiatry, 39,* 336–343.

Klaassen, T., Klumperbeek J., & Deutz, N.E. (1998). Effects of tryptophan depletion on anxiety and on panic provoked by carbon dioxide challenge. *Psychiatry Resident, 77,* 167–174.

Kohnen, R., & Oswald, W.D. (1988). The effects of valerian, propranolol, and their combination on activation, performance, and mood of healthy volunteers under social stress conditions. *Pharmacopsychiatry, 21*(6), 447–448.

Kuokkanen, L., & Leino-Kilpi, H. (2000). Power and empowerment in nursing: Three theoretical approaches. *Journal of Advanced Nursing, 31,* 235–341.

Lafleur, D.L., Pittenger, C., Kelmendi, B., Gardner, T., Wasylink, S., Malison, R.T., Sanacora, G., Krystal, J.H., & Coric, V. (2006). N-acetylcysteine augmentation in serotonin reuptake inhibitor refractory obsessive-compulsive disorder. *Psychopharmacology, 184(2),* 254–256.

Leichsenring, F., Salzer, S., Jaeger, U., Kächele, H., Kreische, R., & Leweke, F. (2009). Short-term psychodynamic psychotherapy and cognitive behavioral therapy in generalized anxiety disorder: A randomized, controlled trial. *American Journal of Psychiatry, 166*(8), 875–881.

Mallet, L., Polosan, M., Jaafari, N., Baup, N., Welter, M.L., Fontaine, D., … Pelissolo, A. (2008). Subthalamic nucleus stimulation in severe obsessive-compulsive disorder. *New England Journal of Medicine, 359:* 2121–2134.

Merikangas, K.R., Ames, M., Cui, L., Stang, P.E., Bedirhan, T., Ustun, M., Von Korff, R., & Kessler, C.R. (2007). The impact of comorbidity of mental and physical conditions on role disability in the US adult household population. *Archives of General Psychiatry, 64*(10), 1180–1188.

Miller, R. (2003). Nurses at community hospital welcome guided imagery tool. *Dimensions in Critical Care Nursing, 22*(5), 225–226.

Milliken, C.S., Auchterlonie, M.S., & Hoge C.W. (2007). Longitudinal assessment of mental health problems among active and reserve component soldiers returning from the Iraq War. *Journal of the American Medical Association, 298,* 2141–2148.

NANDA International. (2009). *Nursing diagnoses: Definitions & classification 2009–2011.* Philadelphia: Author.

Paluska, S.A., & Schwenk, T.L. (2000). Physical activity and mental health. *Sports Medicine, 29,* 167–180.

Pavlov, I.P. (1927). *Conditioned reflexes.* London: Oxford University Press.

Peplau, H. E. (1991). *Interpersonal relations in nursing: A conceptual frame of reference for psychodynamic nursing.* New York: Springer Publishing Company.

Pepping, J. (1999). Kava: piper methysticum. *American Journal of Health System Pharmacy, 15;* 56(10), 957–958, 960.

Pittler, M.H., & Ernst, E. (2000). Efficacy of kava extract for treating anxiety: systematic review and meta-analysis. *Journal of Clinical Psychopharmacology, 20*(1), 84–89.

Plushner, S.L. (2000). Valerian: Valerian officinalis. *American Journal of Health Systems Pharmacy, 57*(328), 333–335.

Porter, R. (1997). *Medicine, a history of healing; Ancient traditions to modern practices.* New York: The Ivy Press.

Robins, L.N., & Regier, D.A., (Eds). (1991). *Psychiatric disorders in America: The epidemiologic catchment area study.* New York: Free Press.

Sadock, B.J., & Sadock, B.A. (2007). *Synopsis of psychiatry: Behavioral sciences/clinical psychiatry* (10th ed.). Philedelphia: Lippincott Williams & Wilkins.

Shah, L.P., Nayak, P.R., & Sethi, A. (1993). A comparative study of Geriforte in anxiety neurosis and mixed anxiety-depressive disorders. *Probe, 32,* 195–201.

Shah, D.B., Pesiridou, A., Baltuch, G.H., Malone, D.A., & O'Reardon, J.P. (2008). Functional neurosurgery in the treatment of severe obsessive compulsive disorder and major depression: Overview of disease circuits and therapeutic targeting for the clinician. *Psychiatry, 5*(9), 24–33.

Singh, Y.N., & Blumenthal, M. (1997). Kava: an overview. *Herbalgram, 39,* 33–56.

Smoller, J. W., & Farone, S. V. (2008). Genetics of anxiety disorders: Complexities and opportunities. *American Journal of Medical Genetics Part C (Seminars in Medical Genetics), 148C,* 85–88.

Stahl, S.M. (2008). *Stahl's essential psychopharmacology: Neuroscientific basis and practical applications* (3rd ed.). Cambridge: Cambridge University Press.

Stevinson, C. (1999). Exercise may help treat panic disorder. *Focus on Alternative and Complementary Therapies, 4*(2), 84–85.

Stone, M.H. (1997). *Healing the mind; A history of psychiatry from antiquity to the present.* New York: W. W. Norton.

Stough, C., Lloyd, J., Clarke, J., Downey, L., Hutchison, C., Rodgers, T., & Nathan, P. (2001). The chronic effects of an extract of *Bacopa monniera* (Brahmi) on cognitive function in healthy human subjects. *Psychopharmacology, 156,* 481–484.

Stress Management Health Center. (2007). Biofeedback topic overview. Retrieved November 2, 2009 from http://www.webmd.com/balance/stress-management/tc/biofeedback-topic-overview

Stuart, G.W. (2005). *Handbook of psychiatric nursing* (6th ed.). St. Louis: Elsevier Mosby.

Taylor, C.B., & Arnow, B. (1988). *The nature and treatment if anxiety disorder.* New York: Free Press.

Tollenaar, M.S., Elzinga, B.M., Spinhoven, P., & Everaerd, W. (2009). Psychophysiological responding in healthy young men after cortisol and propranolol administration. *Psychopharmacology, 203*(4), 793–804.

Uhde, T.W., Boulenger, J.P., Jimerson, D.C., & Post, R.M. (1984). Caffeine relationship to human anxiety, plasma MHPG and cortisol. *Psychopharmacol Bulletin, 20,* 426–430.

Volz, H. P., & Kieser, M. (1997). Kava-Kava Extract WS 1490 versus placebo in anxiety disorders—a randomized placebo-controlled 25-week outpatient trial, *Pharmacopsychiatry, 30,* 1–5.

Watson, J.B., & Morgan, J.J.B (1917). Emotional reactions and psychological experimentation. *American Journal of Psychology, 28,* 163–174.

Yates, W. (2009). Anxiety disorders. Retrieved November 2, 2009 from http://www.emedicine.medscape.com/article286227/overview

Young, R. (2007). New virtual PTSD treatment. Today in the Military. Retrieved on December 1, 2009 from http://www.military.com/features/0,15240,129993,00.html

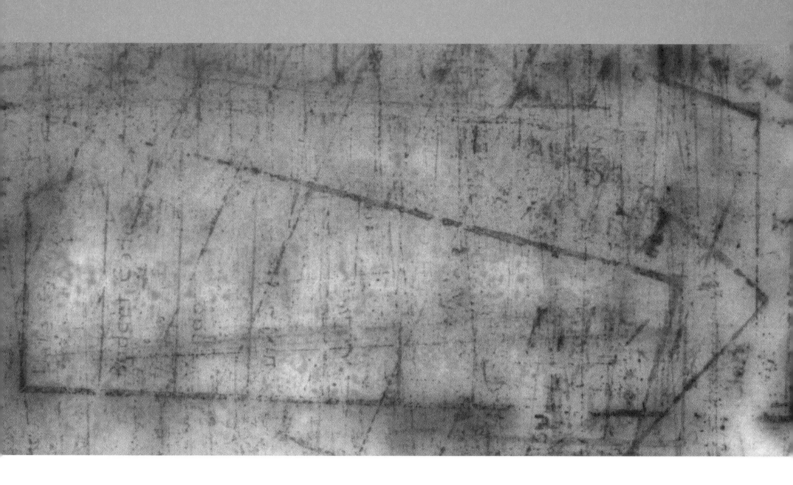

## CHAPTER CONTENTS

## EXPECTED LEARNING OUTCOMES

**After completing this chapter, the student will be
able to:**

1. Define personality.
2. Describe personality traits.
3. Identify the major personality disorders, including
   common components.
4. Describe the historical and epidemiologic
   perspectives related to personality disorders.
5. Distinguish among the characteristic behaviors
   for Clusters A, B, and C based on criteria from the
   *Diagnostic and Statistical Manual of Mental Disorders,
   4th edition, Text Revision (DSM-IV-TR).*

# CHAPTER 14
# PERSONALITY DISORDERS

Audrey Marie Beauvais

6. Discuss the behaviors of individuals with different types of personality disorders.
7. Explain current psychosocial and biologic theories related to the etiology of personality disorders.
8. Apply the nursing process from an interpersonal perspective to the care of patients with personality disorders.

## KEY TERMS

Cognitive restructuring techniques
Confrontation
Dialectical behavior therapy (DBT)
Limit setting
Magical thinking
Personality
Personality disorders
Personality traits
Splitting
Time out

PERSONALITY, essentially, refers to who a person is and how that person behaves. It influences an individual's thoughts, feelings, attitudes, values, motivations, and behaviors. Personality affects how a person deals with stressors and how he or she forms and maintains relationships (American Psychiatric Association [APA], 2000).

Everyone has a unique collection of personality characteristics or traits. **PERSONALITY TRAITS** can be defined as a distinct set of qualities demonstrated over an extended period of time that characterize an individual. The specific traits and the degree to which these traits are exhibited vary from person to person. Genetic as well as environmental factors affect personality development. People tend to react to situations in an individual but consistent way.

Personality traits are different from **PERSONALITY DISORDERS**. A personality disorder refers to a long-term maladaptive way of thinking and behaving that is ingrained and inflexible. Personality traits can be considered personality disorders when the following criteria are met: The traits are maladaptive, rigid, and enduring, and produce impairment in functioning or individual distress. Individuals with a personality disorder tend to be unbending and respond in a maladaptive way to problems. This can lead to difficulty in their relationships with others. People with personality disorders have trouble with the changes and demands of life. Most individuals with personality disorders are distressed with their life and relationships, but are generally unaware that their thoughts and behaviors are inappropriate. In addition, individuals with personality disorders tend to blame others for their circumstances. Moreover, an individual with a personality disorder demonstrates a dysfunctional pattern of coping that is not consistent with the person's culture, ethnicity, and social background (APA, 2000). Personality disorders are classified into Clusters A, B, or C based on the predominant symptoms.

- *Cluster A personality disorders*: paranoid, schizoid, and schizotypal personality disorders.
- *Cluster B personality disorders*: antisocial, borderline, histrionic, and narcissistic personality disorders.
- *Cluster C personality disorders*: avoidant, dependent, and obsessive-compulsive personality disorders.

This chapter addresses the historical perspectives and epidemiology of personality disorders as defined in the *Diagnostic and Statistical Manual, 4th edition, Text Revision* (*DSM-IV-TR*, 2000). Current psychosocial and biological etiological influences of personality disorders are addressed along with current treatment modalities. Application of the nursing process from an interpersonal perspective is presented, including a nursing plan of care for a patient with a personality disorder.

> *Personality disorders are not synonymous with personality traits. A personality disorder occurs when personality traits become maladaptive, rigid, and persistent such that the person experiences distress or impaired functioning.*

## HISTORICAL PERSPECTIVES

In the 4th century B.C., Hippocrates, known as the Father of Medicine, observed and classified four fundamental personality styles that he believed resulted from surpluses in the four bodily humors: the irritable and hostile choleric (yellow bile); the sad melancholic (black bile); optimistic and extroverted sanguine (blood); and the apathetic phlegmatic (phlegm). However, it was not until the early 19th century that formal efforts were made by American and European psychiatrists to describe abnormal personality traits. Further strides were made in 1952 with the first publication of the *Diagnostic and Statistic Manual of Mental Disorders* (*DSM-I*). This publication included seven different categories of personality disorders. In 1980, personality disorders were eventually given their own axis, Axis II, in the multi-axial evaluation system in the *DSM-III*. The *DSM-III* provided diagnostic criteria for 11 distinct personality disorders. The number of categories of personality disorders was decreased to 10 in 1994 with the publication of the fourth edition of the *DSM*. Passive-aggressive personality disorder was removed from the list and is currently being reviewed and investigated for inclusion as an official category. The list identified in 1994 did not change with the publication of *DSM-IV-TR* in 2000 (Andreasen & Black, 2005).

> *Currently there are 10 specific personality disorders, all of which are classified as a separate axis in the DSM-IV-TR.*

## EPIDEMIOLOGY

Personality disorders usually begin in early adolescence or early adulthood. Although it is unusual, children and adolescents may be diagnosed with personality disorders. However, psychiatrists will rarely give a diagnosis of personality disorder to children based on the fact that children's personalities are still developing and may change considerably by the time they achieve adulthood (Freeman & Reinecke, 2007). The intensity of personality symptoms tends to decrease with age and may in fact go into remission as a person matures (Tredget, 2001).

Although some personality disorders have been described as "common," it was not until recently that the prevalence of personality disorders in the general population of the United States became known. Approximately 9.1% of adults in the United States have a personality disorder as outlined by the *DSM-IV-TR* (Lenzenweger, et al., 2007). Estimated prevalence for Cluster A disorders is approximately 5.7%; for Cluster B, 1.5%; and for Cluster C, 6.0%. Many people with personality disorders also had co-occurring major mental disorders (Lenzenweger et al., 2007). Findings are similar in other countries. For example, the prevalence of personality disorders in adults in Australia is noted to be between 6.5% (Lewin, Slade, Andrews, Carr, & Hornabrook, 2005) and 18.6% (Moran, Coffey, Mann, Carlin, & Patton, 2006). Personality disorders in Australia were also associated with younger age, decreased functioning, and a sevenfold increase in the co-occurrence of major mental disorders. The prevalence of personality disorders in adults in South Africa is noted to be 7%. Over one-third of those individuals also had a substance abuse, anxiety, mood, or impulse disorder (Suliman, Stein, Williams, & Seedat, 2008).

An association between personality disorders and co-occurring major mental disorders has been identified by research (Lenzenweger et al., 2007; Lewin, Slade, Andrews, Carr, & Hornabrook, 2005). Personality disorders also have been linked to alcoholism. Research has shown that individuals diagnosed with alcoholism were almost two times more likely to have a personality disorder than individuals who were not alcoholic. Overall, approximately 44% of individuals diagnosed with alcoholism also met the diagnostic criteria for a personality disorder (Echeburua, De Medina, & Aizpiri, 2007).

According to the *DSM-IV-TR* (2000), antisocial personality disorder is diagnosed more frequently in men while borderline, histrionic, and dependent personality disorders are diagnosed more frequently in women. Several previous studies found that males had higher rates of personality disorder than females in the general population (Jackson & Burgess, 2000; Samuels, Nestad, Romanoski, Folstein, & McHugh, 1994). However, more recent studies suggest that personality disorders may actually be more equally distributed between the genders with the exception of antisocial, paranoid, and borderline personality disorders, which are more frequent in men (Kantojarvi et al., 2004; Torgersen, Kringlen, & Cramer, 2001).

Literature suggests that personality disorders, in particular antisocial and borderline disorders, are strongly related to violence and violent acts (Fountoulakis, Leucht, & Kaprinis, 2008). For example, individuals with antisocial personality disorders have a prevalence rate of about 2–3% in the general community in comparison to rates as high as 60% among male prisoners (Moran, 1999). Patients with borderline personality disorder comprise 10% of psychiatric outpatients and 20% of psychiatric inpatients (APA, 2000).

> *Personality disorders often occur along with another major mental disorder. They are also associated with alcoholism. Violence or violent acts are linked to the development of antisocial and borderline personality disorders.*

## DIAGNOSTIC CRITERIA

Although characteristics of personality disorders may describe traits that anyone may exhibit in varying amounts, a genuine personality disorder must meet specific criteria. The general criteria for the diagnosis of a personality disorder are presented in **Box 14-1**.

The *DSM-IV-TR* (2000) describes three different clusters of personality disorders based on characteristic features. Cluster A personality disorders include individuals who appear odd or eccentric. Cluster B personality disorders include individuals who appear dramatic, emotional, or erratic. Cluster C personality disorders include individuals who appear anxious or fearful (APA, 2000). **Box 14-2** summarizes the *DSM-IV-TR* diagnostic criteria for each personality disorder.

### Paranoid Personality Disorder

The characteristic behaviors and symptoms of a paranoid personality disorder include a persistent mistrust and suspiciousness of others. Individuals tend to believe that others are out to harm, take advantage of, or betray

---

**BOX 14-1: GENERAL DIAGNOSTIC CRITERIA FOR A PERSONALITY DISORDER**

To be diagnosed with a personality disorder, a patient must meet the following criteria:

- Demonstration of a enduring pattern that deviates markedly from that of what is expected by the individual's culture; manifested in at least two of the following areas:
  - Cognition
  - Affectivity
  - Interpersonal functioning
  - Impulse control
- Inflexible and pervasive pattern across a broad range of personal and social situations
- Clinically significant distress or impairment in social, occupational, or other areas of functioning
- Pattern that is stable and of long duration, being traced back to adolescence or early adulthood
- Enduring pattern not better accounted for as manifestation or result of another mental disorder
- Enduring pattern not the result of a substance or general medical condition

*From the Diagnostic and Statistical Manual of Mental Disorders, Fourth Edition, Text Revision. Copyright © 2000, American Psychiatric Association.*

---

**BOX 14-2: DIAGNOSTIC CRITERIA FOR PERSONALITY DISORDERS**

CLUSTER A DISORDERS

*Paranoid Personality Disorder*

- Pervasive mistrust and suspiciousness of others; motives interpreted as malevolent, as indicated by four or more of the following:
  - Suspicions that others are exploiting, harming, or deceiving person
  - Preoccupation with unjustified doubts of others' loyalty or trustworthiness
  - Reluctance to confide in others due to unwarranted fear that information will be used against person
  - Reading of hidden demeaning or threatening meanings into remarks or events
  - Grudges
  - Perception of attack on character or reputation; quick to anger or counterattack
  - Recurrent suspicions about fidelity of sexual partner
- Not occurring during other mental disorders and not due to effects of a general medical condition

*Schizoid Personality Disorder*

- Pervasive pattern of detachment from social relationships and restricted emotional expression as indicated by four or more of the following:
  - Lack of desire or enjoyment of close relationships
  - Solitary activities as consistent choice
  - Little or no interest in sexual experiences with another
  - Little if any pleasure in activities
  - Indifference to praise or criticism
  - Emotional coldness, detachment, or flattened affect
- Not occurring during other mental disorders and not due to effects of a general medical condition

*(cont.)*

## BOX 14-2: DIAGNOSTIC CRITERIA FOR PERSONALITY DISORDERS (*CONT.*)

### *Schizotypal Personality Disorder*

- Pervasive pattern of social and interpersonal deficits; acute discomfort with close relationships accompanied by cognitive or perceptual distortions and eccentricities, as indicated by five or more of the following:
  - Ideas of reference
  - Odd beliefs or magical thinking
  - Unusual perceptual experiences
  - Odd thinking or speech
  - Suspiciousness or paranoia
  - Inappropriate or constricted affect
  - Odd, eccentric, or peculiar behavior or appearance
  - Lack of close friends or confidants
  - Excessive social anxiety
- Not occurring during other mental disorders and not due to effects of a general medical condition

### CLUSTER B DISORDERS

### *Antisocial Personality Disorder*

- Pervasive disregard for and violation of the rights of others as indicated by three or more of the following:
  - Unlawful behaviors
  - Deceitfulness through lying, use of aliases, or conning others for personal pleasure
  - Impulsivity
  - Irritability and aggressiveness
  - Reckless disregard for safety (self and others)
  - Consistent irresponsibility
  - Lack of remorse
- Age of at least 18 years
- Evidence of conduct disorder with onset before age 15 years
- Not exclusive occurrence during schizophrenic or manic episode

### *Borderline Personality Disorder*

- Unstable interpersonal relationships, self-image and affect with marked impulsivity as indicated by five or more of the following:
  - Frantic efforts to avoid real or imagined abandonment
  - Alternating extremes of idealization and devaluation in unstable and intense interpersonal relationships
  - Identity disturbance
  - Impulsivity leading to potential self-damage
  - Recurrent suicidal behavior/thoughts/threats or self-mutilation
  - Affective instability
  - Chronic feelings of emptiness
  - Inappropriate, intense anger; difficulty controlling anger
  - Transient stress-related paranoid ideation

*(cont.)*

**BOX 14-2: DIAGNOSTIC CRITERIA FOR PERSONALITY DISORDERS (*CONT.*)**

*Histrionic Personality Disorder*

- Excessive emotionality and attention seeking, as indicated by five or more of the following:
  - Discomfort in situations where person is not the center of attention
  - Inappropriate sexually seductive or provocative behavior when interacting with others
  - Rapidly shifting and shallow emotional expression
  - Use of physical appearance for attention seeking
  - Excessively impressionistic style of speech that lacks detail
  - Self-dramatization
  - Easily suggestible
  - View of relationships as more intimate than actually are

*Narcissistic Personality Disorder*

- Grandiose fantasy or behavior with need for admiration and lack of empathy, as indicated by five or more of the following:
  - Grandiose sense of self-importance
  - Preoccupation with fantasies of unlimited success
  - Belief that person is special and unique
  - Need for excessive admiration
  - Sense of entitlement
  - Interpersonally exploitative
  - Devoid of empathy
  - Envious of others or belief that others are envious of person
  - Arrogant, haughty behaviors or attitudes

## CLUSTER C DISORDERS

*Avoidant Personality Disorder*

- Social inhibition, feelings of inadequacy, and hypersensitivity to negative evaluation as indicated by four or more of the following:
  - Avoidance of occupational activities involving significant interpersonal contact
  - Unwillingness to get involved with others unless certainty of being liked
  - Restraint within intimate relationships due to fear of shame or ridicule
  - Preoccupation with being criticized or rejected in social situations
  - Inhibition in new interpersonal situations due to feelings of inadequacy
  - View of self as socially inept, unappealing, or inferior
  - Reluctance to take personal risks or engage in new activities

*Dependent Personality Disorder*

- Need to be taken care of leading to submission and clinging behavior and fears of separation, as indicated by five or more of the following:
  - Difficulty in making everyday decisions
  - Need for others to assume responsibility for person's life in most major areas
  - Difficulty in expressing disagreement
  - Difficulty in initiating projects or doing things on own
  - Excessive attempts to get nurturance and support from others
  - Feelings of discomfort or helplessness when alone
  - Urgent seeking out of another care and supportive relationship when one ends
  - Unrealistic preoccupation with fears of being left to provide self-care

(cont.)

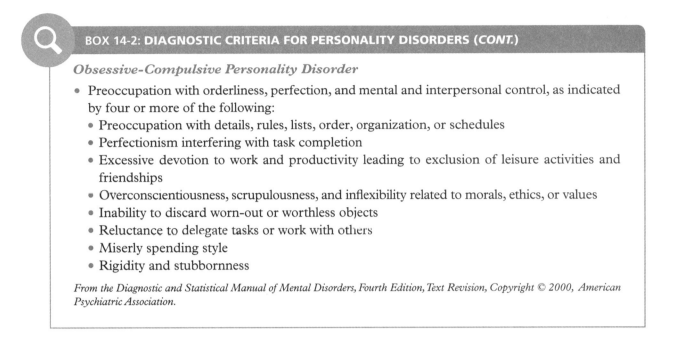

them. They feel this way despite having no evidence to support their claims. They are worried with unsubstantiated doubts about the sincerity of their colleagues and friends. They fear that the information they share will be used against them. They misinterpret benign comments as being mean or hostile and are fast to respond with anger (APA, 2000).

## Schizoid Personality Disorder

Characteristic behaviors and symptoms of a schizoid personality disorder include a persistent pattern of aloofness from relationships and decreased emotional expression. Individuals desire solitary activities and do not want or like close relationships including family relationships. They do not have many friends or pleasures in life. They appear to lack any desire for sexual experiences and appear emotionally distant and detached. They are apathetic when they receive praise or criticism from others (APA, 2000).

## Schizotypal Personality Disorder

Characteristic behaviors and symptoms of a schizotypal personality disorder include a persistent pattern involving difficulty with relationships as evidenced by severe uneasiness with and decreased ability for intimate relationships. This results in a lack of close friends. Their behavior is strange, eccentric, or peculiar. These individuals

misinterpret events as having special meaning for them. They tend to be superstitious and have odd beliefs or MAGICAL THINKING (belief that thoughts are all-powerful). They have unusual perceptions, bizarre thinking and speech, suspicious or paranoid ideation, and inappropriate or limited affect. They tend to have social anxiety and paranoid worries that persist despite familiarity (APA, 2000). When individuals with schizotypal personality disorder experience extreme stress, they may decompensate, become psychotic, and require hospitalization.

## Antisocial Personality Disorder

Characteristic behaviors and symptoms of an antisocial personality disorder include a persistent pattern of not conforming to social norms. Individuals have a disregard for and violate the rights of others. They are dishonest as evidenced by frequent lying and deceiving others for personal gain or pleasure. They are impulsive, irritable, aggressive, reckless, irresponsible, and lack remorse (APA, 2000).

Individuals with childhood or adolescent deviant behavior or conduct disorders often go on to develop a permanent antisocial psychopathology. A large percentage of individuals diagnosed with antisocial personality disorder have recognizable behaviors prior to adulthood. These behaviors include difficulty with authority figures, legal troubles, cruelty to animals, fire setting, and disregard for authority. Unfortunately, individuals diagnosed with antisocial personality disorder do not remiss as readily as some of the other personality disorders. These individuals frequently end up in prison, which only reinforces the behavior. In fact, the majority of male prisoners are diagnosed with antisocial personality disorder (Moran, 1999).

## Borderline Personality Disorder

Characteristic behaviors and symptoms of a borderline personality disorder include a persistent pattern of volatile interactions with others. Individuals are extremely impulsive and make frenzied attempts to prevent genuine or imagined abandonment. They have intense, unstable relationships that swing between extremes of admiration and deprecation. They engage in frequent repeated self-mutilating behavior or suicidal behavior or threats. In addition, they can express feelings of emptiness, intense anger, and brief, stress-related paranoid thoughts or dissociative symptoms (APA, 2000). **SPLITTING** is a common clinical manifestation in which individuals tend to view reality in polarized categories. They alternately idealize and devalue others rather than see people as a mixture of good and bad traits. In a matter of minutes, the person can go from loving an individual to hating them (APA, 2000; Bland, Tudor, & McNeil Whitehouse, 2007; Gallop & O'Brien, 2003).

There are substantial areas of clinical similarities between bipolar disorder and borderline personality disorder. This leads to the potential for misdiagnosis. It is particularly difficult to differentiate bipolar disorder and borderline personality disorder in the young adult population (Smith, Muir, & Blackwood, 2005).

## Histrionic Personality Disorder

Characteristic behaviors and symptoms of a histrionic personality disorder include a persistent pattern of extreme attention-seeking behavior. Individuals are uneasy in situations unless they are the center of attention. They are often provocative and use their physical appearance to draw attention to themselves. They are very dramatic and theatrical. They are impressionable and easily swayed by others. They tend to think relationships are closer than they really are (APA, 2000).

## Narcissistic Personality Disorder

Characteristic behaviors and symptoms of a narcissistic personality disorder include a persistent pattern of pretentiousness and need for approval and high regard. Individuals have a sense of entitlement and take advantage of other people for their own personal gain. They have no empathy and believe that people are jealous of them. They have an exaggerated sense of self worth. They are fixated on fantasies of extreme accomplishment, authority, intelligence, attractiveness, or perfect romantic involvement (APA, 2000).

When narcissistic individuals feel degraded by another person, they experience what is termed a "narcissistic injury." In response to that injury, they will fly into a "narcissist rage" in which they may scream, distort the facts, and make groundless accusations to decrease the self-worth of others and thus make themselves feel more powerful (Kieffer, 2003). The rage impairs their judgment and thinking.

## Avoidant Personality Disorder

Characteristic behaviors and symptoms of an avoidant personality disorder include a persistent pattern of shyness, feelings of incompetence, and extreme sensitivity to criticism. Individuals will avoid situations that involve interaction with other people due to fear of negative evaluation and rejection. They are different than individuals diagnosed with schizoid and schizotypal personality disorders in that the latter would desire to form relationships. They tend not to get involved with others except if they are certain they will be accepted. These individuals have difficulty forming intimate relationships. They don't like to talk about themselves and withhold their thoughts and feelings for fear of being ridiculed. They think of themselves as unattractive, inferior, and useless in comparison to others. They don't like to take risks or join in new activities for fear of embarrassment. They tend to be preoccupied with thoughts of being disparaged and unwanted (APA, 2000).

## Dependent Personality Disorder

Characteristic behaviors and symptoms of a dependent personality disorder include a persistent and extreme desire to be taken care of. Individuals tend to exhibit subservient and clinging behavior and to have fears of abandonment. They have difficulty making decisions and require lots of encouragement and guidance from others. They want others to assume responsibility for their lives. They do not like to disagree with others for fear of not being liked. They lack the self-confidence needed to start projects or do things on their own. They fear that they will not be able to care for themselves, which leads to feelings of uneasiness and helplessness. They are extremely worried about having to take care of themselves. Should their relationship end, they will immediately look for another relationship that will offer reassurance and support (APA, 2000).

## Obsessive-Compulsive Personality Disorder

Characteristic behaviors and symptoms of an obsessive-compulsive personality disorder include a persistent pattern of concern and worry over the orderliness, perfectionism, control, and details of an activity so much so that the aim of the task is lost. The need for perfectionism prevents the completion of the tasks at hand. Individuals tend to forego leisure activities and relationships because they are extremely focused on work and productivity. They tend to be painstakingly meticulous, conscientious, and rigid regarding issues of principles and values. These individuals do not like to throw away meaningless, valueless objects. They tend to save money for misfortunes that might happen later in their lives. Individuals are stubborn and rigid and do not like to delegate tasks to others unless they can guarantee that they will do it to their liking (APA, 2000). Individuals with obsessive-compulsive personality disorders usually require treatment due to complaints of anxiety and may be diagnosed with a concurrent anxiety disorder.

## Personality Disorders Not Otherwise Specified

The *DSM-IV-TR* has developed this category for those individuals who do not meet the criteria for any of the specific personality disorders already noted. The individual may not meet all the criteria for a personality disorder but have some features of more than one specific personality disorder and have significant impairment in functioning or individual distress (APA, 2000).

*Cluster A personality disorders include paranoid, schizoid, and schizotypal personality disorders characterized by odd or eccentric behavior. Cluster B personality disorders include antisocial, borderline, histrionic, and narcissistic personality disorders characterized by dramatic, emotional, or erratic behavior. Cluster C personality disorders include avoidant, dependent, and obsessive-compulsive personality disorders characterized by anxious or fearful behavior.*

## ETIOLOGY

There is no one commonly accepted understanding about the etiology of personality disorders. Most likely, it is a multifaceted process involving both genetic and environmental factors. Psychodynamic and neurobiological influences are presented here.

*Psychodynamic theories related to the etiology of personality disorders focus on an individual becoming fixated in a specific phase of psychosexual development, and thus are unable to advance to the next phase.*

## Psychodynamic Theories

According to psychodynamic theory, a lack of psychosexual development and inability to attain object constancy can lead to a personality disorder. Historically, it was thought that personality disorders arise when an individual does not successfully advance through phases of psychosexual development. For example, fixation in the oral phase was believed to cause a demanding and dependent personality such as a dependent personality disorder. Fixation in the anal phase fixation was believed to cause an obsessive, rigid, aloof personality such as an obsessive-compulsive personality disorder. Fixation in the phallic phase was thought to result in a histrionic personality in that the individual was shallow and unable to engage in meaningful relationships. However, little research supports the belief that personality disorders are correlated to fixations in any of the psychosexual development phases (Andreasen & Black, 2005).

Evidence does support that childhood abuse and trauma is a factor in development of all personality disorders but particularly in antisocial and borderline personality disorders. Children with a history of a chaotic home life including severe discipline, alcoholic caretakers, neglect, domestic abuse, separation, and/or divorce tend to be at greater risk for developing a personality disorder (Andreasen & Black, 2005; Bland, Tudor, & McNeil Whitehouse, 2007; O'Brien, 1998). Sexual abuse in childhood is also believed to be a risk factor for borderline personality disorder, as often this abuse leads one to feel emotionally abandoned (Bland, Tudor, & McNeil Whitehouse, 2007; O'Brien, 1998).

## Biological Theories

Biological theories to explain the etiology of personality disorders typically focus on genetics and neurobiology. Research involving neurobiological influences address brain structures and the neurotransmitter, serotonin.

### Genetics

In the past, personality disorders were thought to be due primarily to environmental issues including such factors as dysfunctional family life, erratic discipline by authority figures, antisocial behavior of the parents, and lack of parental involvement. However, researchers have made some strides in identifying genetic factors that may influence personality disorder (Huff, 2004). Studies involving families, twins, and adoption support the premise of involvement of a genetic factor in the development of schizotypal, antisocial, borderline, and obsessive-compulsive personality disorders (Andreasen & Black, 2005; Bland, Tudor, & McNeil Whitehouse, 2007; Huff, 2004; Moran, 1999).

### Neurobiological Influences

Little is understood about the neurobiology that contributes to personality disorders (Meyer-Lindenberg, 2009). However, efforts are being made in this regard (King-Casas, Sharp, Lomax-Bream, Lohrenz, Fonagy, & Montague, 2008; Meyer-Lindenberg, Minzenberg, New, Tang, & Siever, 2008). Brain imaging studies have recently linked a pattern of altered functioning of the frontolimbic system to functional impairment in individuals diagnosed with a borderline personality disorder (Minzenberg, New, Tang, & Siever, 2008). It appears that the portion of the brain's limbic system that controls certain components of emotions is smaller in individuals diagnosed with borderline personality disorder (Meyer-Lindenberg, 2009). The belief is that this smaller size may result in decreased control over actions and negative emotions, which, in turn, can lead to impulsivity and overly pessimistic reactions to situations (Meyer-Lindenberg, 2009). Additionally, a recent study by Brooks King-Casas and colleagues (2008) discovered neural and behavioral information that suggests that the standard rules used in perceiving social gestures are pathologically troubled or absent in individuals diagnosed with borderline personality disorder. Certain neural networks do not signal the individual to attend to behavioral cues that would lead to cooperative and collaborative social interactions. Thus, the individuals rely on their own communication rather than communication in a trusting relationship with another.

Additional strides have been made to understand the neurobiology of personality disorders (Andreasen & Black, 2005). For example, decreased levels of a metabolite of serotonin are associated with the reckless and aggressive symptoms of the Cluster B personality disorders. Some theorists believe that individuals with antisocial personality disorder are under-aroused and, hence, seek out high-risk situations to increase their arousal to a more favorable level (Andreasen & Black, 2005).

> *Genetics, a smaller-sized limbic system, and decreased levels of a metabolite of serotonin are being linked to the development of personality disorders.*

## TREATMENT OPTIONS

Until fairly recently, many in the psychology field did not feel that treatment would help individuals with personality disorders. Just as the personality traits take years to develop, so too can maladaptive personality traits and personality disorders take years to treat. There is no short-term treatment that can cure personality disorders. Likewise, no single intervention is likely to meet the various needs of individuals with personality disorders (Tredget, 2001). Many different treatment options are available such as individual, group, or family psychotherapy, cognitive behavioral therapy, dialectical behavioral therapy, and psychopharmacology (Woods & Richards, 2003). Treatment is typically long term and aimed at alleviating symptoms of self-destructive ways.

## Psychotherapy

Individual psychotherapy with a trained psychiatric-mental health professional such as an advanced practice psychiatric-mental health nurse is intended to help individuals see the unconscious conflicts that are leading to their symptoms (Bland, Tudor, & McNeil Whitehouse, 2007; Lord, 2007). It is aimed at helping the individual become more flexible, thereby decreasing the behaviors interfering with everyday life. Group therapy also may be used. It uses group dynamics and peer communication to foster an improved understanding and increased social skills. Family therapy is intended to assist families to function in a more affirming and helpful manner. This is accomplished by looking at patterns of verbal and non-verbal interactions and offering support and education. (See Chapter 9 for a more in-depth discussion of group and family therapy.)

## Cognitive Behavioral Therapy

Cognitive behavioral therapy (CBT) is designed to improve an individual's mood and behavior by focusing on distorted patterns of thinking. The goal is to assist patients in altering their usual thoughts that automatically arise and play a role in their dysfunctional thinking. This therapy helps the individual understand that thoughts produce feelings and moods that can affect behavior. CBT helps the individual recognize the underlying thoughts that have resulted in some disruptive behavior. The emphasis is in changing the patient's current thinking without attempting to determine how the patient developed his or her thinking patterns. The patient learns to substitute this thinking with thoughts that will lead to more appropriate behaviors and emotions (Lam & Gale, 2000).

## Dialectical Behavior Therapy

DIALECTICAL BEHAVIOR THERAPY (DBT) is a cognitive behavioral therapy aimed at treating individuals who have been diagnosed with borderline personality disorder or individuals who deliberately partake in self-destructive behavior or have suicidal thoughts. DBT helps individuals take responsibility for their own behavior and problems. It teaches an individual how to cope with conflict, negative feelings, and impulsivity, thereby enhancing the patient's capabilities and improving his or her motivation, which leads to a decrease in dysfunctional behavior. DBT also teaches patients how to control their emotions (Bland, Tudor, & McNeil Whitehouse, 2007; Swenson, Sanderson, Dulit, & Linehan, 2001).

> *Cognitive behavioral therapy (CBT) helps patients with personality disorders focus on their distorted patterns of thinking. Dialectical behavior therapy (DBT) focuses on helping individuals cope with conflict, negative feelings, and impulsivity.*

> *Psychopharmacology as a treatment strategy for personality disorders treats the symptoms of the disorder but not the maladaptive personality traits.*

## Psychopharmacology

Psychopharmacology is also used to treat specific symptoms of personality disorders. The American Psychiatric Association's practice guidelines for the treatment of borderline personality disorders (2005) recommend the use of psychotherapy in conjunction with symptom-targeted psychopharmacology. Psychopharmacology treats the symptoms such as anxiety and altered perceptions, not the personality traits themselves. A partial list of common medications that may be used is found in **Drug Summary 14-1**. Although additional research is necessary to help identify effective pharmacological strategies for treating personality disorders, the following classifications of medication are often used (Triebwasser & Siever, 2007):

- *Antidepressants*: treat the signs and symptoms of depression such as decreased self-esteem, suicidal thoughts, and impulsive behavior. Examples include: sertraline (Zoloft), paroxetine (Paxil), fluoxetine (Prozac), escitalopram (Lexapro), and mirtazapine (Remeron). See Chapter 12 for more information about these agents.
- *Anticonvulsants*: help balance intensity of feelings and help control impulsive and aggressive behavior. Examples include: valproic acid (Depakote), lamotrigine (Lamictal), and carbamazepine (Tegretol). See Chapter 12 for more information about these agents.
- *Antipsychotics*: treat paranoia, unstable mood, and/or unorganized thoughts. Examples include: resperidone (Risperdal), olanzapine (Zyprexa), and quetiapine (Seroquel). See Chapter 11 for more information about these agents.
- *Mood stabilizers*: treat aggression, impulsive behavior, hostility, and mood volatility. An example is lithium. (See Chapter 12 for more information about this agent.)

Benzodiazepines are not the medication of choice to treat symptoms of a personality disorder. Benzodiazepine use should be minimized due to a high potential for abuse and dependency in this population.

## DRUG SUMMARY 14-1:
## PARTIAL SELECTION OF MEDICATIONS USED TO TREAT PERSONALITY DISORDERS

| DRUG | IMPLICATIONS FOR NURSING CARE |
|---|---|
| **SELECTIVE SEROTONIN REUPTAKE INHIBITORS (SSRIs)** | |
| fluoxetine (Prozac)<br><br>paroxetine (Paxil)<br><br>sertraline (Zoloft)<br><br>fluvoxamine maleate (Luvox)<br><br>citalopram (Celexa)<br><br>escitalopram (Lexapro) | • Advise the patient to take the drug in the morning; if sedation occurs, encourage the patient to take the drug at bedtime<br>• Monitor the patient for signs of serotonin syndrome such as fever, sweating, agitation, tachycardia, hypotension, and hyperreflexia<br>• Inform the patient about possible sexual dysfunction with the drug; if this occurs and causes the patient distress, advocate for a change in the drug<br>• Discuss with patient the time to achieve effectiveness and that it may take from 2–4 weeks before symptoms resolve<br>• Emphasize the need for adherence to therapy and to not stop taking the drug abruptly to prevent withdrawal symptoms<br>• Assess the patient for evidence of suicidal thoughts, especially as depression lessens |
| **SEROTONIN/NOREPINEPHRINE REUPTAKE INHIBITORS (SNRIs)** | |
| desvenlafaxine (Pristiq)<br>duloxetine (Cymbalta)<br>venlafaxine (Effexor and Effexor XR) | • Advise the patient taking desvenlafaxine or duloxetine to have his blood pressure monitored because the drug may increase blood pressure<br>• Instruct patient taking venlafaxine to take the drug with food and a full glass of water; if the patient has difficulty swallowing capsules, suggest the patient open the capsule and sprinkle contents on an spoonful of applesauce and take immediately; reinforce the need to follow the capsule with a full glass of water<br>• Encourage the patient to check with his prescriber before taking any other prescription or over-the-counter drugs<br>• Warn patient of possible sedation and dizziness and the need to avoid hazardous activities until the drug's effects are known<br>• Emphasize the need for adherence to therapy and to not stop taking the drug abruptly to prevent withdrawal symptoms<br>• Assess the patient for evidence of suicidal thoughts, especially as depression lessens |
| **MOOD STABILIZERS** | |
| carbamazepine (Tegretol)<br>divalproex sodium (Depakote)<br>oxcarbazepine (Trileptal)<br>lamotrigine (Lamictal)<br>tiagabine HCL (Gabitril) | • Collaborate with the patient to develop a schedule for blood level testing to promote adherence<br>• Institute safety measures to reduce the risk of falling secondary to drowsiness or dizziness<br>• Emphasize the need for adherence to therapy and to not stop taking the drug abruptly to prevent withdrawal symptoms<br>• Assess the patient for evidence of suicidal thoughts, especially as depression lessens |

*(cont.)*

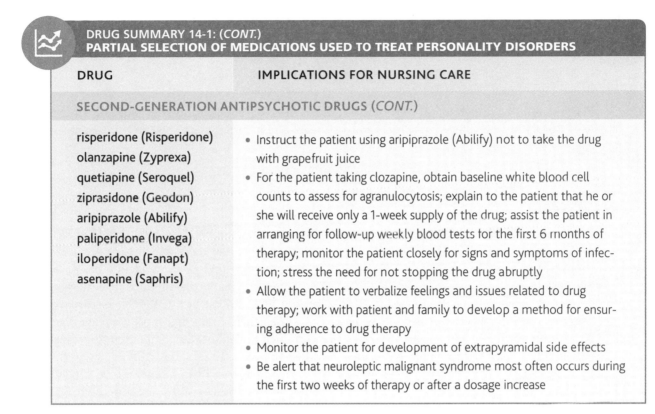

**DRUG SUMMARY 14-1:** (*CONT.*)
**PARTIAL SELECTION OF MEDICATIONS USED TO TREAT PERSONALITY DISORDERS**

| DRUG | IMPLICATIONS FOR NURSING CARE |
|---|---|
| **SECOND-GENERATION ANTIPSYCHOTIC DRUGS** (*CONT.*) | |
| risperidone (Risperidone) olanzapine (Zyprexa) quetiapine (Seroquel) ziprasidone (Geodon) aripiprazole (Abilify) paliperidone (Invega) iloperidone (Fanapt) asenapine (Saphris) | • Instruct the patient using aripiprazole (Abilify) not to take the drug with grapefruit juice<br>• For the patient taking clozapine, obtain baseline white blood cell counts to assess for agranulocytosis; explain to the patient that he or she will receive only a 1-week supply of the drug; assist the patient in arranging for follow-up weekly blood tests for the first 6 months of therapy; monitor the patient closely for signs and symptoms of infection; stress the need for not stopping the drug abruptly<br>• Allow the patient to verbalize feelings and issues related to drug therapy; work with patient and family to develop a method for ensuring adherence to drug therapy<br>• Monitor the patient for development of extrapyramidal side effects<br>• Be alert that neuroleptic malignant syndrome most often occurs during the first two weeks of therapy or after a dosage increase |

## APPLYING THE NURSING PROCESS FROM AN INTERPERSONAL PERSPECTIVE

Nurses can expect to provide care for individuals with personality disorders in all specialty areas and practice settings. In general, nurses working on inpatient psychiatric units will often encounter patients with antisocial, borderline, and schizotypal type personality disorders as a diagnosis. **Evidence-Based Practice 14-1** summarizes a study about inpatient admissions for patients with borderline personality disorder.

Recognizing the differences between normal difficulties and personality disorders can be crucial to the nurse's decision-making process in navigating the interpersonal process. Because of the difficulties these individuals have in establishing and maintaining healthy relationships, developing therapeutic interpersonal relationships with them can be challenging. Nurses will find their relationship skills challenged, boundaries tested, and patience tried. **Plan of Care 14-1** provides an example of a patient with personality disorder.

### Strategies for Optimal Assessment: Therapeutic Use of Self

When beginning a therapeutic relationship with any patient, the development of the nurse's self-awareness is essential (Duff, 2003; Kwiatek, McKenize, & Loads, 2005). This knowledge of one's own values and attitudes is especially important when working with individuals with personality disorders. The psychiatric-mental health nurse will be challenged because these patients have trouble building and sustaining healthy relationships (Duff, 2003). The nurse may feel that he or she lacks the skills to interact effectively with the patient, leading to feelings of inadequacy and failure. The nurse's self-awareness and self-reflection of knowledge, values, and attitudes can significantly impact his or her behaviors and actions. Applying the therapeutic use of self allows the psychiatric-mental health nurse to evaluate and reflect on the consequences of his or her values, attitudes, and practice in working with patients. Such awareness will help the nurse develop insight into his or her own behavior (Kwiatek, McKenize, & Loads, 2005; Duff, 2003).

### Self-Awareness

The nurse and patient meet as strangers and begin a relationship that involves getting to know one another to promote the development of trust (McNaughton, 2005; Peplau, 1991). After the nurse introduces him- or herself and describes the unit and services, the nurse assesses the patient to gain an appreciation of the situation (Feely, 1997; McNaughton, 2005; Peplau, 1991).

**EVIDENCE-BASED PRACTICE 14-1:**
**INPATIENT ADMISSION FOR PATIENTS WITH BORDERLINE PERSONALITY DISORDERS**

### STUDY

Peritogiannis, V., Stefanuou, E., Damigo, D., & Mavreas, V. (2008). Admission rates of patients with borderline personality disorder in a psychiatric unit in a general hospital. *International Journal of Psychiatry in Clinical Practice, 12*(1), 78-80.

### SUMMARY

Patients diagnosed with borderline personality disorder are frequently hospitalized. However, admission to inpatient psychiatric facilities is controversial because these patients are often disruptive to the inpatient milieu and the value of inpatient admission in this population has never been established. This study looked at the admission rates of patients diagnosed with borderline personality disorders in the inpatient psychiatric unit of a general hospital. The researchers conducted a retrospective review of medical records, which revealed that those patients diagnosed with borderline personality disorders were admitted to the hospital more often than those patients diagnosed with a major psychiatric disorder on Axis I. In fact, the difference was statistically significant. However, the length of stay for those diagnosed with borderline personality disorder and those diagnosed with a major psychiatric disorder were similar. The primary reason for admission for patients diagnosed with borderline personality disorder was suicide attempts or threats and lack of outpatient facilities.

### APPLICATION TO PRACTICE

The significance of this study for psychiatric-mental health nursing practice lies in the potential to advocate on patients' behalf for needed outpatient facilities and reorganization of mental health services. The information obtained from this study is useful in planning of appropriate services to benefit this population and to decrease the financial burden caused by inpatient psychiatric admissions.

### QUESTIONS TO PONDER

1. *How would you go about advocating for these services? Where would you start?*
2. *What obstacles might you encounter?*

Patients with personality disorders can be challenging because they can exhibit intense feelings and may evoke strong emotions in the nurse. **Consumer Perspective 14-1** provides a personal perspective of what it is like to have a borderline personality disorder. Maintain self-awareness and be alert to personal signals of frustration that the patient's behaviors can elicit. Be cognizant of personal feelings and do not allow them to interfere with the care of the patient (Feely, 1997; Peplau, 1991). Nurses need to acknowledge and accept their own emotional responses. Avoid internalizing these feelings or taking them personally.

### Environmental Management

Making the environment conducive to assessment is important to ensure that rapport and trust develop and that the information collected is comprehensive and accurate. When meeting with the patient, allow for adequate interpersonal space during the assessment process. Patients with personality disorders often experience difficulties with boundaries. Therefore, it is essential for the nurse to establish boundaries at the outset. Arrange to interview the patient in a comfortable, quiet, and safe environment that has minimal interruptions. Doing so prevents adding to the patient's already odd, dramatic, or fearful behavior. Make certain that you do not sit too close to the patient as the patient may also have some concerns about personal space. In this regard, it is often useful to ask the patient about the desired distance in order to build trust in the relationship. Also, approach the person in a calm and reassuring manner and remain nonjudgmental and nonconfrontational. If the patient's behavior starts to escalate, then offer him or her a break.

Mental health assessments often include questions that may be uncomfortable for persons with personality disorders, so priority setting is important. Brief, focused assessments may be necessary. In addition, be consistent and follow through on comments, suggestions, or promises. Doing so will help to foster a sense of trust. Also, be alert for signs of agitation or fear that can impact the patient's safety.

## Health History and Examination

The priority during the first encounter with the patient is assessment for suicidal or homicidal ideation, evidence of self-mutilation and physical injuries, as well as any

---

### PLAN OF CARE 14-1:
### THE PATIENT WITH A CLUSTER B PERSONALITY DISORDER—ANTISOCIAL OR BORDERLINE PERSONALITY DISORDER

**NURSING DIAGNOSIS:** Risk for other-directed violence; related to pervasive disregard for rights of others; manifested by unpredictable, erratic, and impulsive behavior. Risk for self-mutilation; related to impulsivity and past self-injurious behavior to reduce anxiety. Risk for suicide; related to impulsivity and feelings of low self-worth.

**OUTCOME IDENTIFICATION:** Patient will verbalize feelings related to harming self or others. Patient will refrain from engaging in activities that harm self or others.

| INTERVENTION | RATIONALE |
|---|---|
| Assess the patient's behavior for indicators suggesting potential harm to self or others; ask the patient directly about suicidal thoughts or plan; determine if the patient has access to or possesses necessary means to carry through with plan | Identifying indicators of potential harm allows for early detection and prompt intervention. Asking directly about suicidal thoughts or plan identifies real or potential risk; determining access or ability to carry through with plan identifies potential for completion of act and allows for appropriate intervention to interfere with plan |
| Observe the patient unobtrusively for wounds suggesting self-mutilation | Observing the patient unobtrusively prevents feelings of suspiciousness and "being watched" while providing information about extent of patient's behaviors |
| Develop rapport with the patient; approach the patient in a calm, nonthreatening manner, demonstrating a caring and accepting attitude | Using a calm, nonthreatening, caring, accepting attitude promotes trust and development of the therapeutic relationship |

*(cont.)*

**PLAN OF CARE 14-1: (*CONT.*)**
**THE PATIENT WITH A CLUSTER B PERSONALITY DISORDER—ANTISOCIAL OR**
**BORDERLINE PERSONALITY DISORDER**

| INTERVENTION | RATIONALE |
| --- | --- |
| Minimize the patient's exposure to stimuli; keep environment calm, quiet with little distraction; remove all hazardous items from the patient's environment; ensure the environment is safe and the patient is free of hazards | Limiting stimuli helps to prevent overwhelming the patient and avoids the patient interpreting stimuli as a threat that could lead to increased anxiety and agitation; removal of items reduces the risk of use if behavior escalates; ensuring a safe environment lessens the risk for injury and harm |
| Work with the patient to determine how the patient is feeling and what may trigger feelings of anger, aggression; assist the patient in identifying the source of anger, encouraging the patient to describe and clarify feelings and experiences | Identifying feelings and triggers allows for early intervention; identifying the source of anger and encouraging description helps increase the patient's awareness of problems |
| Contract with the patient for no self-harm | Using a no-harm contract emphasizes expectations, fosters participation in care and feelings of control over situation |
| Assist the patient in cognitive restructuring techniques | Using these techniques helps the patient recognize how his or her thoughts and feelings are contributing to the behavior |
| Reinforce use of prescribed therapies such as dialectical behavior therapy and individual psychotherapy; administer pharmacologic agents as ordered, such as antidepressants for suicidal ideation, anticonvulsants for impulsivity, and mood stabilizers for aggression, impulsivity, and/or mood volatility | Reinforcing appropriate therapy such as dialectical behavior therapy helps to promote responsibility for own behavior; using prescribed pharmacologic agents help to minimize or relieve underlying symptoms |
| Institute appropriate limits, ensuring that the patient clearly understands them; reinforce limits consistently; avoid power struggles | Setting limits and consistently enforcing them minimizes manipulation and assists patient in learning adaptive behavior |
| Provide appropriate and constructive outlets for the patient to express feelings such as anger and aggression; assist the patient in developing ways to express feelings nonviolently and problem solve | Using alternative means of expressing feelings promotes adaptive coping and learning |

(*cont.*)

**PLAN OF CARE 14-1: (*CONT.*)**
**THE PATIENT WITH A CLUSTER B PERSONALITY DISORDER—ANTISOCIAL OR BORDERLINE PERSONALITY DISORDER**

| INTERVENTION | RATIONALE |
|---|---|
| If self-mutilation or self-harm occurs, provide care to the patient and the wounds as necessary; avoid positively reinforcing maladaptive behavior | Caring for the wounds is a nursing responsibility; avoiding positive reinforcement of maladaptive behavior may help to lessen its use |
| If behavior escalation occurs toward others, place the patient in the least restrictive environment; enlist the use of time-out or confrontation as appropriate; remove others away from the area of escalation | Using the least restrictive environment is necessary to protect the patient's rights; using time out helps prevent patient from acting impulsively and allows patient to regain emotional control; using confrontation assists in reducing manipulation and helping patient gain some insight into behavior; moving others away protects their safety |

**NURSING DIAGNOSIS:** Impaired social interaction; related to unstable sense of self in relations to others; manifested by lack of trust, splitting, unstable relationships, reckless or irresponsible behavior.

**OUTCOME IDENTIFICATION:** Patient will begin to identify actions that interfere with relationships. Patient will demonstrate beginning social skills for developing a relationship.

| INTERVENTION | RATIONALE |
|---|---|
| Assist the patient in verbalizing feelings related to social situations, relationships, and interactions; help the patient understand how these feelings are connected to relationship difficulties | Verbalizing feelings promotes insight into the underlying issues |
| Help the patient identify appropriate actions and consequences related to relationships | Identifying actions and consequences is an initial step in having the patient begin to assume responsibility for his or her actions |
| Establish firm limits for relationships | Setting limits is important to facilitate control over behavior |
| Encourage the patient to communicate verbally; provide assistance with communication skills | Encouraging communication is important to promote the development of a relationship |
| Work with the patient to understand the acceptable limits involved with relationships | Understanding the limits involved with relationships is necessary for the patient to engage in a successful interaction |

*(cont.)*

### PLAN OF CARE 14-1: (*CONT.*)
### THE PATIENT WITH A CLUSTER B PERSONALITY DISORDER—ANTISOCIAL OR BORDERLINE PERSONALITY DISORDER

| INTERVENTION | RATIONALE |
| --- | --- |
| Assist the patient in using social skills training; break skills down into small discrete steps; encourage the use of role playing, social modeling, and social reinforcement | Using social skills training gradually introduces the patient to appropriate methods for developing social relationships for eventual mastery of critical social skills |
| Encourage practice of skills, emphasizing patience; provide feedback about performance | Practicing promotes the likelihood of success with a skill that takes time to develop; providing feedback promotes learning and fosters positive feelings about success |
| Assist the patient to demonstrate respect and honesty when interacting with others | Demonstrating respect and honesty with others facilitates the development of a relationship |

**NURSING DIAGNOSIS:** Chronic low self-esteem; related to identity disturbance and fears of abandonment; manifested by inability to maintain sustainable relationships.

**OUTCOME IDENTIFICATION:** Patient will identify positive aspects about self. Patient will begin to demonstrate appropriate independent decision making.

| INTERVENTION | RATIONALE |
| --- | --- |
| Assist the patient in exploring feelings, the connection of these feelings to behavior, and the effects of behavior on self-esteem | Exploring feelings associated with behaviors and effects provides insight into the disorder |
| Explore past achievements, strengths, and successes with the patient; positively reinforce actions and achievements | Exploring past achievements and reinforcing them fosters feelings of self-worth and self-esteem |
| Work with the patient to develop appropriate strategies that build on patient's strengths and assist with decision making; gradually encourage independent decision making | Building on the patient's strengths improves confidence and promotes self-esteem |
| Assist the patient with communication and social skills to promote relationships | Promoting relationships through communication and social skills enhances feelings of worth and self-esteem |

**CONSUMER PERSPECTIVE 14-1:
PERCEIVED SLIGHTS MAKE ME ANGRY**

Part of being borderline for me is going bonkers over slights or perceived slights from others. That happened last night and suddenly the whole world is against me and EVERYTHING looks bad. When I feel that way there is no relief to be found until the "storm" blows over. I was/am still a bit completely unhinged; my sense of self is torn apart, my beliefs, my interests, and EVERYTHING gets sucked in when I go down. Luckily I have managed to hide it pretty good from others and even myself at times. Someone once mentioned needing "reality checks" from others, and sometimes I feel like I can trust other people's realities and other times I don't; just depends on where I am at ... and that changes a lot.

*www.bpdcentral.com/support/stories.shtml*

history of suicidal or aggressive actions. Also assess the patient's general appearance and motor behavior closely for clues that would suggest the patient's thinking patterns. Questions and observations related to these issues are the most critical to ensure the patient's safety.

As appropriate, a detailed assessment is initiated. Areas to assess include: mood and affect; thought process and content; sensorium and intellectual processes; judgment and insight; self-concept, roles, and relationships. Also, assess the patient's physiologic status and ability to provide self-care which may be affected by the patient's personality disorder. Consider the patient's ethnic, cultural, and social background and family situation when completing the assessment. Review the patient's medical history including any use of prescribed, over-the-counter, or illicit medications. Note any financial or legal problems, whether current or in the past, which may have resulted from the patient's personality disorder.

> *Establishing a therapeutic relationship with a patient diagnosed with a personality disorder can be difficult because the patient can exhibit intense feelings that evoke strong emotions in the nurse. Nurses need to be self-aware and cognizant of these responses to prevent them from interfering with the therapeutic relationship and the therapeutic use of self.*

During the interview, ask the patient about any history of current or past physical, sexual, or emotional abuse which may be associated certain personality disorders such as antisocial personality disorder. And finally, ascertain if the patient has experienced a recent loss or a psychosocial stressor which could have exacerbated the symptoms of the personality disorder.

## Diagnosing and Planning Appropriate Interventions: Meeting the Patient's Focused Needs

The patient should be encouraged to participate in not only assessing his or her problems and needs but also be encouraged to engage as an active partner in planning his or her care (Peplau, 1991). The patient will need to begin to recognize and understand his or her current difficulties and the extent of need for help (Peplau, 1991). However, a patient with a personality disorder may not recognize that he or she has an issue. The nurse can help raise the patient's awareness that his or her behaviors related to the personality disorder are problematic.

As the patient begins to identify his or her problems, the nurse can offer appropriate suggestions for interventions to assist the patient in meeting those needs (McNaughton, 2005; Peplau, 1991). Nurses and patients need to collaborate in determining treatment goals and planning appropriate treatment interventions. All treatment team members must be aware of the plan and adhere to it (Bland, Tudor, & McNeil Whitehouse, 2007). Integrating the interpersonal process within the nurse-patient relationship helps the patient make the most of a difficult situation. Subsequently, the patient can learn different patterns of behavior that will decrease the symptoms of his or her personality disorder (Feely, 1997; Peplau, 1991).

Assessment findings and identified needs are highly variable for patients with personality disorders. When developing the plan of care for a patient, numerous nursing diagnoses would apply. Examples of possible nursing diagnoses would include:

- Risk for self-directed or other-directed violence related to impulsivity as evidenced by acting out behaviors
- Risk for self-mutilation related to unpredictable and erractic behavior as evidenced by impulsivity
- Impaired social interaction related to lack of trust as evidenced by disregard of others' feelings
- Chronic low self-esteem related to identity disturbance as evidenced by fear of abandonment
- Social isolation related to lack of trust as evidenced by superficial interactions with others

These nursing diagnoses also will vary based on the acuity of the patient's illness, developmental stage, co-morbidities, current treatment regimen, and sources of support. For example, the acutely ill person with a borderline personality disorder may have a risk for self-mutilation or self-directed violence. During periods of remission, nursing diagnoses such as impaired social interaction or chronic low self-esteem may be the priority areas to be addressed.

Based on the identified nursing diagnoses, the nurse and patient collaboratively would determine the outcomes to be achieved. For example, within the therapeutic relationship, the nurse will be able to help the patient develop a structure for daily activities and to review the expectations with the patient. If the patient does not show up for some of the scheduled activities or arrives late, this would provide an opportunity for the nurse and patient to review expectations. The patient would be helped to learn how his or her behavior affects others who are expecting their participation in the group.

> *A common priority nursing diagnosis for a patient with a personality disorder is risk for self-directed or other-directed violence.*

## Implementing Effective Interventions: Timing and Pacing

Once the nurse and patient have established treatment goals and plans for interventions, implementation of the plan occurs. The first and foremost concern is the promotion of patient safety (Bland, Tudor, & McNeil Whitehouse, 2007; Livesley, 2005; Lord, 2007). Interventions focus on ways to change the lifelong disruptive behavior associated with personality disorders to maintain a safe environment. The nurse needs to monitor the patient for suicidal ideation, a suicidal plan, lethality of plan, and intent (Livesley, 2005).

Frequently, patients with personality disorders, most particularly with borderline personality disorders, will be at high risk for suicide. One commonly used strategy to prevent suicide is the no-suicide or no-harm contract. The no-suicide contract is an agreement typically written between the patient and mental health care team in which the patient vows not to harm him- or herself. Despite common use of this intervention, there is little research to support its effectiveness (Range et al., 2002). Furthermore, some scholars have raised ethical and conceptual concerns with the use of no-harm contracts. For example, there is the potential for coercion from the mental health care team in order to protect themselves legally. In addition, ethically speaking, a no-harm contract limits a patient's choice when they are already struggling for control (McMyler & Prymachuck, 2008). Whether or not the nurse and mental health treatment team use no-harm contracts, the nurse must continuously monitor the patient's suicidal risk.

In addition, the nurse needs to create and promote a therapeutic relationship (Langley & Klopper, 2005). Patients who have been diagnosed with a personality disorder frequently display dysfunctional relationships. Therefore, the nurse must establish boundaries in the relationship, teach effective communication skills, help patients to cope, help patients to control their emotions, and assist patients in learning how to reshape their thinking patterns (Duff, 2003; Langley & Klopper, O'Brien, 1998; Lord, 2007; Woods & Richards, 2003). In general, patients with personality disorders who are on inpatient units or in partial treatment programs should be encouraged to attend the scheduled activities. Additionally, these patients should be encouraged to keep a journal. By doing so, the patient will be able to look back and potentially develop a better understanding about how feelings affect relationships and behavior. Thus, the formation of a therapeutic relationship can help promote responsible behavior.

### Interventions for Cluster A Personality Disorders
The specific interventions often vary depending on the type of personality disorder diagnosed. For example, patients diagnosed with paranoid personality disorder will benefit from nursing interventions such as frequent short interactions, a serious and straightforward approach, and education about validating thoughts prior to taking action. Patients diagnosed with schizoid personality disorder will benefit from nursing interventions aimed at helping the patient to improve his or her functioning and to locate resources in the community such as a

case manager (Hayward, 2007). Patients diagnosed with schizotypal personality disorder will benefit from nursing interventions directed at improving self-care skills, improving community functioning, and improving social skills (Hayward, 2007).

### Interventions for Cluster B Personality Disorders

Patients diagnosed with Cluster B personality disorders will benefit from different nursing interventions. For example, those individuals diagnosed with antisocial personality disorder will benefit from learning problem-solving techniques and management of anger and frustration because they tend to react impulsively when confronted with problems. **How Would You Respond?** 14-1 provides a practical example of how to deal with a patient with antisocial personality disorder.

Problem-solving techniques will help the patient learn to identify the problem, explore alternative solutions and

---

### HOW WOULD YOU RESPOND? 14-1: PATIENT WITH AN ANTISOCIAL PERSONALITY DISORDER

Dave was a 36-year-old male who was referred to an inpatient unit by the court system. He had recently served time in prison. Dave did not feel he needed treatment. When asked about his conviction, he stated that he scammed elderly individuals out of their life savings. When confronted on this behavior, he laughs out loud and says they should have known better. He is initially charming to the other individuals; however, he remains superficial and lacks genuine warmth. Dave proudly shares that as a child he frequently broke his parents' rules, started drinking alcohol at a young age, was cruel to animals, beat up other children, and was in trouble at school when he chose to attend. He has not maintained a career as he gets bored. On the unit, Dave begins to display aggressive behavior that leads to conflict with his peers. How would you respond?

#### CRITICAL THINKING QUESTIONS

1. *How does Dave reflect the diagnostic criteria for a patient with an antisocial personality disorder?*

2. *When assessing Dave, what underlying theme would be predominant?*

3. *What interventions would be appropriate for Dave to address his aggressiveness?*

---

### APPLYING THE CONCEPTS

Dave has a history of unlawful behaviors and incarceration along with a history of childhood problems involving breaking rules, cruelty to animals and other children, and trouble at school. He demonstrates a reckless disregard for himself and others and a lack of remorse, especially in relation to his scamming elderly individuals out of their life savings. In addition, he exhibits consistent irresponsible behavior in not being able to maintain a career and irritability and aggressiveness that has led to conflict with others. An underlying theme related to Dave's behavior is his impulsivity. Interventions appropriate for Dave would include limit setting, confrontation, and time out. Time out would prevent Dave from acting impulsively and having emotional outbursts. It also gives him an opportunity to reflect on his behavior and develop some more constructive alternative ways of behaving. The nurse also would need to set clear and consistent boundaries for Dave and assist him in learning problem-solving techniques. Safety measures would be a priority to prevent self-injury that might occur due to his aggressiveness and impulsivity.

related consequences, choose and implement alternatives, and evaluate the results (McMurran, Fyffe, McCarthy, Duggan, & Latham, 2001). To help patients control their emotions, the nurse can utilize a TIME OUT. Time out refers to a situation in which the nurse allows the patient to get away from the area and go to a safe, non-stimulating place to regain emotional control. This technique helps prevent the patient from acting impulsively and having emotional outbursts. It also gives the patient an opportunity to reflect on his or her behavior and develop some more constructive, alternative ways of behaving (Jones & Downing, 1991).

Other nursing interventions such as LIMIT SETTING and CONFRONTATION (technique used to help the patient take note of a behavior and examine it) will be necessary as these patients tend to try to manipulate and deceive others. Limit setting identifies for the patient what he or she can or cannot do. Several steps are involved in limit setting. First, the nurse explains which behavior is inappropriate and provides a rationale. Next, the nurse tells the patient what behavior is expected. Finally, the nurse informs the patient about the consequences for going beyond the established limit. When setting limits, use clear and concise statements phrased in a calm and non-threatening manner. Also never set a limit that cannot be enforced.

When using confrontation, the patient may respond in an angry and defensive manner. Therefore, it is important that the nurse not become defensive. Rather, the nurse needs to focus the patient on the behavior itself and not on the patient's attempts to justify his or her actions (Saper & Lake, 2002). **Therapeutic Interaction 14-1** highlights an interaction with a patient experiencing a paranoid personality disorder.

Throughout limit setting and confrontation, the nurse needs to observe the patient's behavior to enforce boundaries for inappropriate behaviors. This is very important in this population because clear boundaries often need to be established for unsafe or hostile behavior. Unfortunately, despite these efforts, the prognosis for individuals with antisocial personality disorders is poor because they often lack insight and experience a failure to conform to societal norms. Subsequently, they often become incarcerated due to criminal activity.

Like those individuals diagnosed with antisocial personality disorders, those diagnosed with borderline personality disorder will benefit from a therapeutic relationship and the establishment of boundaries and limits. However, developing a therapeutic relationship with these individuals can be challenging because persons with borderline personality disorders test the boundaries

and engage in manipulation. Thus, the nurse needs to demonstrate a firm yet supportive approach, set limits, and be consistent. Safety also is a priority. Individuals diagnosed with borderline personality disorder have difficulty coping and controlling emotions. The nurse needs to perform an ongoing thorough self-harm risk assessment and, if necessary, institute suicide precautions and administer prescribed medications. Additionally, the nurse can help the patient recognize how his or her thoughts and feelings are contributing to the behavior and then assist the patient in reshaping this thinking to result in more appropriate behaviors and emotions. This strategy is referred to as COGNITIVE RESTRUCTURING TECHNIQUES. Other useful nursing interventions involve structuring the patient's time; for example, making certain that the patient has a schedule of activity and is aware of the expectations to conform to the schedule, and teaching social and communication skills (Bland, Tudor, & McNeil Whitehouse, 2007).

Offering an empathetic response is an example of a nursing intervention used with patients diagnosed with narcissistic personality disorders. This helps to address the patient's underlying feeling of weakness and lack of self confidence (Czuchta Romano, 2004). For those patients diagnosed with histrionic disorder, a matter-of-fact approach that avoids overreaction to the patient's exaggerations is helpful (Dorgan, 2000). For patients diagnosed with narcissistic and/or histrionic personality disorders, the nurse attempts to gain the patient's cooperation with the treatment plan, providing patients with factual feedback about their behavior. Social skills training is also effective.

> *Establishment of boundaries, time out, and limit setting are effective interventions for patients diagnosed with antisocial or borderline personality disorders.*

## Interventions for Cluster C Personality Disorders

Patients diagnosed with avoidant and dependent personality disorders may benefit from nursing interventions aimed at helping the patient examine positive self-aspects and practice self-affirmations. These, in turn, may promote increased self-esteem. Nurses can provide direct feedback about social interactions and behaviors and encourage autonomy and self-reliance. Likewise, the nurse

> ### THERAPEUTIC INTERACTION 14-1:
> ### A PATIENT WITH PARANOID PERSONALITY DISORDER NEEDING CONFRONTATION
>
> Mr. C. has been transferred to the psychiatric inpatient unit from the emergency department. He presented at the emergency department with signs of severe alcohol intoxication after being involved in an auto accident and receiving minor injuries (lacerations on face). He indicated that someone had tampered with his car, causing the accident. He also voiced concern that they would follow him into this unit and would threaten his life.

| | |
|---|---|
| **Nurse:** "Mr. C, I am the nurse who will be with you today until 7 o'clock this evening. Can you tell me why you are here?" | Introduces self and begins development of interpersonal relationship. Clearly communicates role and time frame |
| **Mr. C.:** "There are people out to get me. They caused my auto accident and they will follow me here." | Communicates paranoia |
| **Nurse:** "This is a hospital and no one here will harm you. We are here to help you." | Building on the relationship, reinforces the safe environment and the therapeutic nature of the unit |
| **Mr. C:** "The only help I need is for someone to get rid of the people who are following me." | Continues to deny need for help and continues to express paranoia |
| **Nurse:** "Mr. C., can you tell me what happened last evening that led to your coming to the emergency department?" | Continues to develop therapeutic relationship and focuses on helping the patient develop beginning insight into his behavior |
| **Mr. C.:** "Someone rigged my car so that I would have an accident." | Denial of own role in behavior |
| **Nurse:** "I am very interested in helping you but first you must tell me everything that happened last evening to lead you to the emergency department. I understand that you were intoxicated and that this was related to the accident." | Directly confronts patient so as to focus the conversation on his behavior and help him develop beginning insight |

can encourage the patient to identify his or her feelings and to express them directly. Moreover, nurses can help patients learn assertiveness, problem solving, social skills, and decision making skills, as well as cognitive restructuring techniques (Stravynski, Belisle, Marcouileer, Lavallee, & Elie, 1994).

Nursing interventions for patients diagnosed with obsessive-compulsive personality disorder focus on helping the patient make timely decisions and complete work tasks. Negotiation with others is encouraged. Cognitive restructuring techniques are another useful intervention with these patients (Pretzer & Hampt, 1994). Individuals with obsessive-compulsive personality disorder desire routine and are respectful to authority figures. These characteristics, in addition to patients' compliance with rules and devotion to their professional careers, will often lead to their success. In addition, careers that call for perfectionism, a need to continually verify small details for errors, and entail micromanagement are a great fit for an individual with obsessive-compulsive personality disorder. The nurse can emphasize this aspect when working with the patient.

## Evaluating: Objective Critique of Interventions and Self-Reflection

The psychiatric-mental health nurse evaluates his or her efforts via objective critique of interventions and self reflection to ensure accountable, respectful, and nonjudgmental nursing practice. The nurse evaluates how much progress has been made toward achieving expected outcomes. During this phase, the nurse compares the patient's current level of functioning with the identified goals and outcomes. For any goals not met, the nurse needs to self-reflect on anything he or she may have done differently while providing nursing care. For example, evaluate how the patient presented upon admission and where they are at this point. Were the goals and interventions developed based on what the nurse wanted to happen, or what the patient and nurse wanted to happen? Did the nurse's buttons get pushed? Was the treatment plan reactive or proactive? During this phase of the nurse-patient relationship, both the nurse and the patient reflect on progress made toward reaching the patient goals. Point out positives to the patient and include a plan for aftercare as appropriate.

A rapid change in behavior is highly unlikely in patients diagnosed with personality disorders. It took years to develop these behaviors and patterns of thinking. Subsequently, it will take years to change. As a result, it may be difficult to determine the result of interventions because long-term treatment often is required (Shattell, 2005).

## SUMMARY POINTS

- Personality disorders are maladaptive, rigid, and enduring personality characteristics that produce impairment in functioning or individual distress.

- Personality disorders are categorized into three clusters based on the predominant symptoms. These include: Cluster A disorders, involving odd or eccentric behavior (paranoid, schizoid, and schizotypal personality disorders); Cluster B disorders, involving dramatic, emotional, or erratic behavior (antisocial, borderline, histrionic, and narcissistic personality disorders); and Cluster C disorders, involving anxious or fearful behaviors (avoidant, dependent, and obsessive-compulsive personality disorders). They occupy a separate axis in the *DSM-IV-TR*.

- Personality disorders usually begin in early adolescence or early adulthood and affect approximately 9% of the population in the United States. They are associated with other major mental disorders and alcoholism; antisocial and borderline personality disorders are strongly related to violence and violent acts.

- It is unlikely that there is a single cause for personality disorders, but rather multiple components such as psychodynamic, environmental, genetic, and neurobiological factors may converge to produce the illness.

- Many different treatment options are available and may include: psychotherapy (individual, group, and family therapy), cognitive behavioral therapy, dialectical behavioral therapy, and psychopharmacology, which is used to treat the symptoms of the disorder but has no effect on the maladaptive, rigid personality traits.

- Patients with personality disorders can be challenging because these patients can arouse intense emotions in the nurse. As a result, developing a therapeutic

*(cont.)*

## SUMMARY POINTS (*CONT.*)

relationship may be difficult. Therefore, nurses working with patients diagnosed with personality disorders need to maintain self-awareness and be alert to personal signals of frustration that a patient's behaviors can elicit and avoid internalizing feelings or taking them personally.

• Nursing interventions appropriate for patients with Cluster A personality disorders include frequent short interactions, a straightforward approach, and education about validating thoughts prior to acting on them. Emphasis is on improving the patient's functional level, locating community resources, and improving self-care and social skills.

• Nursing interventions appropriate for patients with Cluster B personality disorders include teaching problem-solving techniques, using time out, limit setting, and confrontation. An ongoing assessment of the patient's risk for self-harm is essential because the patient has difficulty coping and controlling emotions.

• Nursing interventions appropriate for patients with Cluster C personality disorders include measures to promote a positive self-aspect, encourage autonomy and self-reliance, and promote assertiveness, problem solving, social skills, and decision making.

## NCLEX-PREP*

1. A group of nursing students is reviewing class information about the different types of personality disorders. The students demonstrate understanding of this information when they identify which of the following as a Cluster A personality disorder? Select all that apply.

   a. Borderline personality disorder
   b. Paranoid personality disorder
   c. Avoidant personality disorder
   d. Schizoid personality disorder
   e. Narcissistic personality disorder
   f. Antisocial personality disorder

2. A patient is being admitted to the inpatient unit with a diagnosis of borderline personality disorder. When preparing to assess this patient, which of the following would the nurse need to keep in mind?

   a. The patient is likely to demonstrate behaviors to get attention.

   b. The patient's behavior typically reflects a need to prevent abandonment.
   c. The patient most likely has a history of involvement with law enforcement.
   d. The patient will exhibit an extreme suspiciousness about others.

3. While working with a patient diagnosed with an antisocial personality disorder, the nurse notes that the patient is beginning to exhibit signs that he is losing emotional control. The nurse assists the patient in moving to a safe, quiet area to regain his control. The nurse is using which of the following?

   a. Time out
   b. Limit setting
   c. Confrontation
   d. Cognitive restructuring

(*cont.*)

## NCLEX-PREP* (CONT.)

4. A patient with antisocial personality disorder is observed taking an other patient's belongings. Which initial nursing intervention would be most appropriate?
   a. Tell the patient's primary nurse what happened
   b. Obtain an order for an antipsychotic medication
   c. Confront the patient about his behavior
   d. Encourage the patient to discuss his angry feelings

5. The nurse is developing a plan of care for a patient diagnosed with a schizotypal personality disorder. Which of the following would be most appropriate to include in the plan?

   a. Setting specific boundaries for behavior
   b. Teaching problem-solving techniques
   c. Fostering decision-making skills
   d. Implementing social skills training

6. Which of the following would the nurse expect to assess in a patient who is diagnosed with an obsessive-compulsive personality disorder?
   a. Preoccupation with details
   b. Suspiciousness of others
   c. Exaggerated sense of self-importance
   d. Unwillingness to get involved with others

*Answers to these questions appear on page 639.

## REFERENCES

American Psychiatric Association. (1987). *Diagnostic and statistical manual of mental disorders* (3rd ed.). Washington, DC: Author.

American Psychiatric Association. (2000). *Diagnostic and statistical manual of mental disorders* (4th ed., text rev.). Washington, DC: Author.

American Psychiatric Association (2005). Guideline Watch: Practice Guideline for the Treatment of Patients with Borderline Personality Disorder. Available at: http://www.psychiatryonline.com/content.aspx?aid=148718. Accessed 2-24-2011

Andreasen, N.C., & Black, D.W. (2005). *Introductory textbook of psychiatry (4th ed)*. Washington, DC: American Psychiatric Publishing, Inc.

Bland, A.R., Tudor, G., & McNeil Whitehouse, D. (2007). Nursing care of inpatients with borderline personality disorder. *Perspectives in Psychiatric Care, 43*(4), 204–212.

Czuchta Romano, D.M. (2004). A self-psychology approach to narcissistic personality disorder: A nursing reflection. *Perspectives in Psychiatric Care, 40*(1), 20–28.

Dorgan, W.J. (2000). The histrionic personality on the job. *Modern Machine Shop, 73*(5), 132.

Duff, A. (2003). Managing personality disorders: Making positive connections. *Nursing Management, 10*(6), 27–30.

Echeburua, E., De Medina, R.B. , & Aizpiri, J. (2007). Comorbidity of alcohol dependence and personality disorders: A comparative study. *Alcohol and Alcoholism, 42*(6), 618–622.

Feely, M. (1997). Using Peplau's theory in nurse-patient relations. *International Nursing Review, 44*(4), 115–120.

Fountoulakis, K.N., Leucht, S.K., & Kaprinis, G.S. (2008). Personality disorders and violence. *Current Opinions in Psychiatry, 21*(1), 84–92.

Freeman, A.M., & Reinecke, M.A. (2007). *Personality disorders in childhood and adolescence.* Hoboken, NJ: John Wiley & Sons.

Gallop, R., & O'Brien, L. (2003). Re-establishing psychodynamic theory as foundational knowledge for psychiatric/mental health nursing. *Issues in Mental Health Nursing, 24*, 213–227.

Hayward, B.A. (2007). Cluster A personality disorders: Considering the "odd-eccentric" in psychiatric nursing. *International Journal of Mental Health Nursing, 16*, 15–21.

Huff, C. (2004). Where personality goes awry: A multifaceted research approach is providing more clues to the origins of personality disorders. *Monitor on Psychology, 35*(3), 42.

Jackson, H.J., & Burgess, P.M. (2000). Personality disorders in the community: A report from the Australian national survey of mental health and wellbeing. *Social Psychiatry and Psychiatric Epidemiology, 35*, 531–538.

Jones, R.N., & Downing, R.H. (1991). Assessment of the use of time-out in an inpatient child psychiatry treatment unit. *Behavioral Residential Treatment, 6*(3), 219–230.

Kantojarvi, L., Veijola, J., Laksy, K., Jokelainen, J., Herva, A., Karvonen, J.T., Kokkonen, P., Jarvelin, M.R., & Joukamaa, M. (2004). Comparison of hospital-treated personality disorders and personality disorders in a general population sample. *Nordic Journal of Psychiatry, 58*(5), 357–362.

Kieffer, C.C. (2003). How group analysis cures: An exploration of narcissistic rage in group treatment. *Psychoanalytic Inquiry, 23*(5), 734–749.

King-Casas, B., Sharp, C., Lomax-Bream, L., Lohrenz, T., Fonagy, P., & Montague, P.R. (2008). The rupture and repair of cooperation in borderline personality disorder. *Science, 321*(5890), 806–810.

Kwiatek, E., McKenize, K., Loads, D. (2005). Self-awareness and reflection: Exploring the "therapeutic use of self." *Learning Disability Practice, 8*(3), 27–31.

Lam, D., & Gale, J. (2000). Cognitive behavior therapy: Teaching the patient the ABC model—the first step towards the process of change. *Journal of Advanced Nursing, 31*(2), 444–451.

Langley, G.C., Klopper, H. (2005). Trust as a foundation for the therapeutic intervention for patients with borderline personality disorder. *Journal of Psychiatric and Mental Health Nursing, 12*, 23–32.

Lenzenweger, M.F., Lane, M.C., Loranger, A.W., & Kessler, R.C. (2007). *DSM-IV* personality disorders in the national comorbidity survey replication. *Biological Psychiatry, 62*, 553–564.

Lewin, T.J., Slade, T., Andrews, G., Carr, V. J., & Hornabrook, C.W. (2005). Assessing personality disorders in a national mental health survey. *Social Psychiatry and Psychiatric Epidemiology, 40*, 87–98.

Livesley, W.J. (2005). Principles and strategies for treating personality disorders. *Canadian Journal of Psychiatry, 50*(8), 442–450.

Lord, S.A. (2007). Systemic work with patients with a diagnosis of borderline personality disorder. *Journal of Family Therapy, 29*, 203–221.

McMurran, M., Fyffe, S., McCarthy, L., Duggan, C., & Latham, A. (2001). "Stop & think": social problem-solving therapy with personality disordered offenders. *Criminal Behavior and Mental Health, 11*, 273–285.

McMyler, C., & Pryjmachuk, S. (2008). Do "no-suicide" contracts work? *Journal of Psychiatric and Mental Health Nursing, 15*(6), 512–522.

McNaughton, D.B. (2005). A naturalistic test of Peplau's theory in home nursing. *Public Health Nursing, 22*(5), 429–438.

Meyer-Lindenberg, A. (2009). Perturbed personalities. *Scientific American Mind*, 40–43.

Minzenberg, M.J., Fan, J., New, A.S., Tang, C.Y., & Siever, L. J. (2008). Frontolimbic structural changes in borderline personality disorder. *Journal of Psychiatric Research, 42*(9), 727–733.

Moran, P. (1999). The epidemiology of antisocial personality disorder. *Social Psychiatry and Psychiatric Epidemiology, 34*(5), 231–242.

Moran, P., Coffey, C., Mann, A., Carlin, J.B., & Patton, G.C. (2006). Dimensional characteristics of DSM-IV personality disorders in a large epidemiological sample. *Acta Psychiatrica Scandinavica, 113*, 233–236.

O'Brien, L. (1998). Inpatient nursing care of patients with borderline personality disorder: A review of the literature. *Australian and New Zealand Journal of Mental Health Nursing, 7*, 172–183.

Peplau, H.E. (1991). *Interpersonal relations in nursing: A conceptual frame of reference for psychodynamic nursing.* New York: Springer Publishing Company.

Peritogiannis, V., Stefanuou, E., Damigo, D., & Mavreas, V. (2008). Admission rates of patients with borderline personality disorder in a psychiatric unit in a general hospital. *International Journal of Psychiatry in Clinical Practice, 12*(1), 78–80.

Pretzer, J., & Hampt, S. (1994). Cognitive behavioral treatment of obsessive compulsive personality disorder. *Clinical Psychology and Psychotherapy, 1*(5), 298–307.

Range, L.M., Campbell, C., Kovac, S.H., Marion-Jones, M., Aldridge, H., Kogos, S., & Crump, Y. (2002). No-suicide contracts: An overview and recommendations. *Death Studies, 26*(1): 51–74.

Samuels, J.F., Nestad, G., Romanoski, A.J., Folstein, M.F., & McHugh, P.R. (1994). DSM-III personality in the community. *American Journal Psychiatry, 151*, 1055–1062.

Saper, J.R., & Lake, A.E. (2002). Borderline personality disorder and the chronic headache patient: review and management recommendations. *Headaches, 42*, 663–674.

Shattell, M. (2005). Nurse bait: Strategies hospitalized patients use to entice nurses within the context of the interpersonal relationship. *Issues in Mental Health Nursing, 26*, 205–223.

Smith, D.J., Muir, W. J., & Blackwood, D.R. (2005). Borderline personality disorder characteristics in young adults with recurrent mood disorders: A comparison of bipolar and unipolar. *Journal of Affective Disorders, 87*(1), 17–23.

Stravynski, A., Belisle, M., Marcouiller, M., Lavallee, Y.J., & Elie, R. (1994). The treatment of avoidant personality disorder by social skills training in the clinic or in real-life settings. *Canadian Journal of Psychiatry, 39*(8), 377–383.

Suliman, S., Stein, D.J., Williams, D.R., & Seedat, S. (2008). *DSM-IV* personality disorders and their Axis I correlates in the South African population. *Psychopathology, 41*(6), 356–364.

Swenson, C.R., Sanderson, C., Dulit, R.A., & Linehan, M. (2001). The application of dialectical behavior therapy for patients with borderline personality disorder on inpatient units. *Psychiatric Quarterly, 72*(4), 307.

Torgersen, S., Kringlen, E., & Cramer, V. (2001). The prevalence of personality disorders in a community sample. *Archives of General Psychiatry, 58*(6), 590–596.

Tredget, J.E. (2001). The aetiology, presentation, and treatment of personality disorders. *Journal of Psychiatric and Mental Health Nursing, 8*(4), 347–356.

Triebwasser, J., & Siever, L.J. (2007). Pharmacotherapy of personality disorders. *Journal of Mental Health, 16*(1), 5–50.

Woods, P., & Richards, D. (2003). Integrative literature review and meta-analyses effectiveness of nursing interventions in people with personality disorders. *Journal of Advanced Nursing, 44*(2), 154–172.

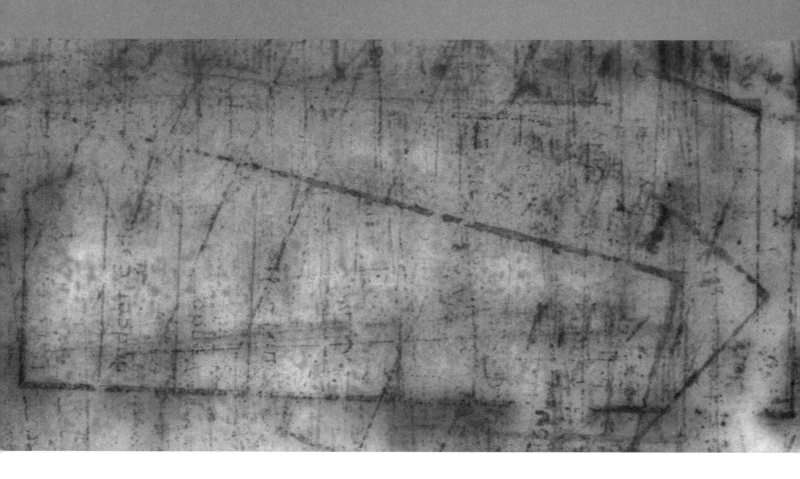

## CHAPTER CONTENTS

## EXPECTED LEARNING OUTCOMES

**After completing this chapter, the student will be able to:**

1. Define addiction.
2. Describe the historical perspective and epidemiology of addictive disorders.
3. Distinguish among the characteristic behaviors for disorders involving addiction based on criteria from the *Diagnostic and Statistical Manual of Mental Disorders, 4th edition, Text Revision* (*DSM-IV-TR*).
4. Discuss current theories of addiction and other problems related to substance use.

# CHAPTER 15
# ADDICTIVE DISORDERS

Carolyn A. Baird

5. Explain the various treatment options available for addiction disorders, including evidence-based strategies.

6. Apply the nursing process from an interpersonal perspective to the care of patients with anxiety disorder.

**A**DDICTION refers to a "chronic, relapsing brain disease that is characterized by compulsive drug seeking and use, despite harmful consequences" (National Institute of Drug Abuse [NIDA], 2010). Initially, a person voluntarily makes the choice to use a drug. However, over time, the person's ability to voluntarily choose not to use the drug becomes impaired. As a result, the person's self-control is compromised, leading to compulsive behavior to seek out and use the drug. The explanation is that addiction affects the brain circuitry, causing changes in specific areas such as those involved in reward and motivation, learning and memory, and inhibitory control over behavior (NIDA, 2009).

Addiction involves a spectrum of disorders of substance use including substance abuse and substance dependence, and substance-induced disorders including intoxication and withdrawal. Substance abuse and addiction in populations present many challenges for society in general as well as health care providers.

This chapter addresses the historical perspectives and epidemiology of addictive disorders followed by a detailed description of these disorders as defined in the *Diagnostic and Statistical Manual, 4th edition, Text Revision* ([*DSM-IV-TR*], 2000). Specific scientific theories focusing on addiction are described along with common treatment options. Application of the nursing process from an interpersonal perspective is presented, including a plan of care for a patient with an addictive disorder.

> *Compulsive drug seeking and use that leads to harmful consequences is termed addiction*

## HISTORICAL PERSPECTIVES

Any substance has the potential to become a drug of abuse, not just alcohol or illegal drugs. The U.S. Drug Enforcement Administration (DEA) statistics state that over 7 million Americans are abusing prescription drugs (Palladini, 2011). Over the past centuries, society has viewed the use of alcohol, tobacco, and other drugs in varying ways. Initially, substances were viewed from a cultural perspective and were accepted. Additionally, when individuals overindulged and their intoxicated behavior became a problem, alcohol and drug use was dealt with as a criminal offense. Thus, the theory of addiction was based on a more social model. Gradually, the view changed as

the addictive nature of substances was identified. This led to addiction being viewed through a medical or disease model. For example, notable instances of general use of a now known addictive substance are opium in paregoric and cannabis in many patent medications.

The American Medical Association (AMA) first took the position in 1958 that alcoholism was a disease. Identifying similarities in the action of various substances to produce the same dysfunction in the neurotransmitters of the brain led to a broader understanding of addiction. The introduction of the first Controlled Substances Act in 1970 came as a result of the acknowledgment of addiction as a disease of the neurotransmitters of the brain. Since that time, researchers have identified the specific neurotransmitters, areas of the brain, and response pathways that are implicated in addiction. It has been observed that abusive relationships with objects and behaviors may affect the same areas of the brain. The resulting disorder is now considered a process addiction.

Over time, a number of substance and process addictions have been noted. Each generation appears to have its own primary addictions. Consider these examples. Individuals born prior to 1943, termed the Traditional or Silent Generation, were more likely to experience alcoholism and prescription drug abuse and less likely to use illicit substances. This changed with the Baby Boomer generation, those born between 1944 and 1964. They experienced the social issues involving the Vietnam War, antiwar demonstrations, Flower Children, and Woodstock. As a result, illicit substances were brought into the forefront in the form of cannabis and lysergic acid diethylamide (LSD). Individuals of Generation X, those born from 1964 to 1978, appear to have started with cannabis, used LSD and mescaline, graduated to cocaine and methamphetamine, and then expanded into heroin (Furek, 2008). Generation Y or Millennial, those born from 1979 to 2000 and known for their preoccupation with the technology, has been noted for its use of club drugs.

> *Addiction is a disease affecting the brain and its chemistry. Both substances and behavioral or process addictions activate the same neurotransmitters and use the same reward pathways.*

## EPIDEMIOLOGY

The Substance Abuse and Mental Health Services Administration (SAMHSA) funds an annual National Survey on Drug Use and Health (NSDUH). The 2010 report reveals that the number of Americans 12 years or older who engaged in the use of an illicit drug was estimated at 21.8 million or approximately 8.7% of the population in 2009. This rate was an increase of 0.7% from 2008. Additionally, an estimated 22.5 million persons aged 12 years and older were classified as having substance dependence or substance abuse in the past year according to diagnostic criteria. Of these, approximately 3.2 million persons abused or were dependent on alcohol and illicit drugs, 3.9 million persons were dependent on or abused illicit drugs alone, and 15.4 million were dependent on or abused alcohol alone (SAMSHA, 2010). Treatment also was addressed in this report. According to SAMSHA (2010), 23.5 million persons or 9.3% (aged 12 years and older) needed treatment for an illicit drug or alcohol use problem. Out of this group, only 2.6 million received treatment at a specialty facility, with the remaining 20.9 million with a problem not receiving treatment.

Many reasons exist for this large discrepancy in the numbers receiving treatment. One reason may be that the secrecy and confusion surrounding this disease make it difficult to diagnose. There are no formal standardized definitions, terminology, and/or criteria. The terms substance use, abuse, and dependence are often used interchangeably even though they are separate terms referring to discrete patterns of behavior. The terminology used by the American Psychiatric Association (APA) in the *DSM-IV-TR* refers to substance-induced, substance-related, and substance-use disorders (SUDs). Substance abuse and dependency are the two categories under SUDs. Both relate to a maladaptive pattern of substance use. **ABUSE** is the initial stage where the individual may have recurrent substance use that leads to failure to meet obligations, puts the individual in hazardous situations, causes legal problems, or results in social, interpersonal, or professional problems. **DEPENDENCY** is the final stage and refers to a maladaptive pattern of behavior characterized by progression, tolerance, withdrawal, preoccupation with the behavior regardless of any consequences, and has the potential to be fatal (Doweiko, 2006).

## DIAGNOSTIC CRITERIA

Addiction is a disease that can occur at any time across the life span, manifesting as chronic with remissions and exacerbations, or as an isolated episode (Antai-Otong, 2006).

Many presenting core symptoms are the same across addictions while others are descriptive of the particular type of addiction. The quest for knowledge about addiction has led to the understanding that individuals may be addicted to a substance, prescribed or illicit, liquid, vapor or solid, or, they may be addicted to a particular course of action, thoughts, feelings, or behaviors known as a process addiction. Between 50% and 75% of individuals diagnosed with substance dependence have a co-occurring mental health disorder.

The *DSM-IV-TR* (2000) lists specific criteria as possible signs of a drug or alcohol addiction. Although the criteria are usually considered to refer to a physiological addiction, the criteria can be adapted to apply in the case of a psychological or behavioral addiction, better known as process addictions. To be diagnostic, any combination of four or more of these criteria must be present:

* Preoccupation with the use of the chemical between the times of use.
* Using more of the chemical than had been anticipated.
* The development of tolerance to the chemical in question.
* A characteristic withdrawal syndrome when the person stops using the chemical.
* Use of the chemical to avoid or control withdrawal symptoms.
* Repeated efforts to cut back or stop the drug use.
* Intoxication at inappropriate times (such as at work) or when withdrawal interferes with daily functioning (hangover makes the person too sick to go to work).
* A reduction in social, occupational, or recreational activities in favor of further substance use.
* Continuation of chemical use in spite of having suffered social, emotional, or physical problems related to drug use.

The *DSM-IV-TR* classifies addictive disorders into two major categories: substance-use disorders and substance-induced disorders. Use disorders broadly include **SUBSTANCE ABUSE** (recurrent substance use that leads to failure to meet obligations, puts the individual in hazardous situations, causes legal problems or results in social, interpersonal, or professional problems) and **SUBSTANCE DEPENDENCE** (maladaptive pattern of behavior characterized by progression, tolerance, withdrawal, preoccupation with the behavior regardless of any consequences, and with the potential to be fatal). Substance-induced disorders broadly include substance **INTOXICATION** (reversible substance-specific syndrome with central nervous system response and related behavioral and psychological changes after exposure or ingestion of a substance) and substance **WITHDRAWAL** (substance-specific syndrome with significant physical and psychological distress, and impairment in areas of functioning that occur after reducing or stopping heavy and prolonged use of the substance). **Box 15-1**

**Q BOX 15-1: DIAGNOSTIC CRITERIA**

SUBSTANCE USE DISORDERS

*Substance Abuse*

A. Maladaptive pattern of substance use with clinically significant impairment or distress as manifested by one or more of the following:

- Recurrent use leading to failure to fulfill major role obligations at work, school, or home
- Recurrent use in situations typically considered physically hazardous
- Recurrent substance-related legal problems
- Continued use despite persistent or recurrent social or interpersonal problems due to or increased by the substance's effects

B. Symptoms never meeting criteria for substance dependence

*Substance Dependence*

A. Maladaptive pattern of substance use with clinically significant impairment or distress as manifested by three or more of the following at any time within the same 12-month period:

- **TOLERANCE**: need for markedly increased amounts of substance to achieve effect or markedly diminished effect with continued use of same amount
- Withdrawal: characteristic withdrawal syndrome for the substance or use of same or closely related substance to relieve or avoid withdrawal symptoms
- Substance being taken in larger amounts or over a longer period than intended
- Persistent desire or unsuccessful efforts to cut down or control use
- Great deal of time spent in activities needed to obtain the substance
- Giving up of or reducing important social, occupational, or recreational activities because of use
- Continued use despite knowledge of persistent or recurrent physical or psychological problem likely due to or exacerbated by substance

SUBSTANCE-INDUCED DISORDERS

*Substance Intoxication*

A. Development of a reversible substance-specific syndrome due to recent ingestion or exposure to a substance

B. Clinically significant maladaptive behavior or psychological change due to effect of substance on central nervous system developing during or shortly after use

C. Symptoms not due to a general medical condition and not better accounted for by another mental disorder

*Substance Withdrawal*

A. Development of a substance-specific syndrome due to cessation of or reduction in heavy, prolonged substance use

B. Significant distress or impairment in social, occupational, or other important area of functioning due to syndrome

C. Symptoms not due to a general medical condition or not better accounted for by another mental disorder

*From the Diagnostic and Statistical Manual of Mental Disorders, Fourth Edition, Text Revision, Copyright © 2000. American Psychiatric Association.*

highlights the diagnostic criteria for these disorders. In addition, the *DSM-IV-TR* identifies specific criteria for 11 classes of substances associated with use and induced disorders. These classes include:

- Alcohol
- Amphetamines and similar acting drugs (amphetamine, dextroamphetamine, methamphetamine ["speed"])
- Caffeine
- Cannabis (marijuana, bhang, hashish)
- Cocaine
- Hallucinogens (lysergic acid diethylamide [LSD], morning glory seeds, phenylalkylamines [mescaline, "STP"], MDMA [ecstasy])
- Inhalants (hydrocarbons such as those found in gasoline, paint thinners, glue, and spray paints)
- Nicotine
- Opioids (morphine, heroin, codeine, hydromorphone, methadone, oxycodone, meperidine, and fentanyl)
- Phencyclidine (PCP) and similar acting drugs (such as ketamine)
- Sedatives, hypnotics, or anxiolytics (benzodiazepines, barbiturates)

> *The DSM-IV-TR classifies substance disorders as substance use and substance-induced disorders. Substance use disorders are further classified as substance abuse and substance dependence. Substance-induced disorders are further classified as substance intoxication and substance withdrawal.*

## ETIOLOGY

Many models have been used to explain the theoretical basis of addiction. Research has focused on a wide range of areas including the spiritual, systems, moral, characterological, behavioral, educational, temperance, dispositional, and medical or disease models (Doweiko, 2006; Konrad, 2005). Many of these models are based on the individual lacking knowledge or control of behavior. These are all part of what may be considered the social model and their focus is on blaming the individual for choosing bad behavior or for lacking sufficient character or a strong moral compass. For example, the spiritual model is the basis for

Alcoholics Anonymous (AA) and other 12-step programs. Following the program necessitates the individual declaring powerlessness and finding a higher power. All of the models based on individual choice support the idea that all the individual with an addiction has to do is stop using the substance or engaging in the activity. Medication is not usually a part of the treatment protocol.

While the medical or disease model is the most widely accepted within the substance abuse field, many laypeople and professionals continue to question the presence of biological markers (Doweiko, 2006). Doweiko defines the disease model of addiction as a primary medical disorder with the potential to affect an individual's social, psychological, spiritual, and economic life. Yet he also admits that "a universally accepted comprehensive theory of addiction has yet to be developed" (Doweiko, 2006, p. 20). To really understand addiction, it is important to acknowledge the role of the central nervous system, neurotransmitters, and the brain's reward pathways.

In pursuit of a comprehensive theory based on the medical or disease model, research has been conducted in a variety of areas (Shaffer et al., 2004; Koob, 2006). Evidence is emerging that suggests that addiction must be viewed or conceptualized in a much broader fashion to capture the nature, origin, and processes that comprise addiction (Shaffer et al., 2004). In reviewing the evidence, Shaffer and colleagues (2004) identified a number of interacting biopsychosocial antecedents. This study is highlighted in **Evidence-Based Practice 15-1**. Shared neurobiological antecedents include the central nervous system circuitry, neurotransmitters, and reward pathways along with the genetic vulnerability factors. Social and psychological risk factors make up the shared psychological antecedents. The last set of antecedents are shared experiences with shared manifestations and sequelae, parallel natural histories, object nonspecificity, concurrent manifestations, and treatment nonspecificity (Shaffer et al., 2004). For example, not everyone who uses a substance or engages in a behavior develops the disease, but everyone who develops an addiction displays the same symptomatology, has the same genetic vulnerability, and shares a similar life history regardless of the substance or behavior. Thus, these shared antecedents support the idea that there are common risk factors for addiction that reflect a shared origin or etiology. For these reasons, addiction can be identified as a syndrome disorder.

Viewing the disease of addiction as a syndrome may be helpful in understanding the process that the individual undergoes in relationship to a substance or a behavior. It may also explain why only some of the individuals displaying this relationship become dependent while others do

## EVIDENCE-BASED PRACTICE 15-1: MODEL OF ADDICTION

### STUDY

Shaffer, H. J., LaPlante, D. A., LaBrie, R. A., Kidman, R. C., Donato, A. N., & Stanton, M. V. (2004). Toward a syndrome model of addiction: Multiple expressions, common etiology. *Harvard Review Psychiatry, 12*, 367-374. Retrieved September 19, 2009 from http://www.expressionsofaddiction.com/docs/shafferetalsyndrome.pdf

### SUMMARY

The authors challenge the current view of the disease of addiction. Instead of relying on just the physiological action of the substances as the causal factor, they state there is strong evidence of both neurobiological and psychosocial antecedents. This suggests a syndrome model of addiction that simultaneously covers multiple expressions and common etiology. Proposals for the understanding of addiction as a syndrome have their basis in the co-occurrence of various chemical and behavioral expressions of addiction stemming from an underlying commonality of genetic and psychosocial susceptibility.

### APPLICATION TO PRACTICE

At the present time, more emphasis is put on self-report as the key to diagnosis. Using a syndrome approach to the treatment of addiction engages the clinician in an ongoing evaluation of the relationships among the various antecedents, manifestations, and consequences and the course of the illness. Rethinking the philosophy of addiction will lead to more objective diagnostic criteria, strengthen treatment approaches, and improve treatment outcomes.

### QUESTIONS TO PONDER

1. *How does viewing addiction as a syndrome challenge your current understanding of the disease?*
2. *What implications can you see for changing treatment approaches?*

not. The ability to assess the shared manifestations allows for adjusting the diagnosis and treatment to fit the course of the illness, the potential for relapse, and any addiction hopping (Shaffer et al., 2004). This is important for all health care professionals, especially psychiatric-mental health nurses. Psychiatric-mental health nurses must gain an understanding of addiction as a disease process with clearly defined characteristics and manifestations due to the increased presence of co-morbid psychopathology in the abusing and dependent population. This psychopathology takes the form of generalized anxiety, major depression, and posttraumatic stress disorder (Shaffer et al., 2004).

There is a great deal of research being conducted in an attempt to understand the genetic and neurobiological components of addiction. It is known that some individuals appear to be more genetically vulnerable and researchers have been attempting to identify the specific genes that may predispose individuals to become addicted to specific substances. It should be acknowledged that all individuals who use an addictive substance have the potential to become addicted. Genetic vulnerability may decide what substances or processes an individual is most at risk for or the extent of the cognitive damage that may occur as a result of the alteration in neurotransmitter function. The only protection from becoming addicted is to never use the substance. This is true even for individuals with genetic vulnerability. Having a positive life history, good coping and stress management skills, and a supportive environment are also protective factors.

In the late 1940s and early 1950s, Jellinek (2007) conducted some of the earliest research on substance use disorders using a population of male alcoholics. These results were then used to develop a male model of care that was used through much of the 20th century. This gender bias was not considered a problem because substance abusing men were offered treatment, while substance abusing women were often hidden, protected, or abandoned (Doweiko, 2006). It is still difficult to compare gender rates because most statistics do not identify a male to female ratio. Statistics do reveal that 4.4 million women abuse or are dependent on alcohol, one of every three individuals dependent on alcohol is female, and that two million women abuse or are dependent on illicit drugs. This is important because of the biological differences between males and females. They experience substance abuse, addiction, and co-morbid conditions differently and enter treatment through different pathways and for different reasons. Men frequently are referred to treatment by employers or the law. They also have lower incidences of depression and their substance diagnosis is primary. On the other hand, women seek treatment on their own, frequently from a mental health provider, due to a preexisting depression, anxiety, or posttraumatic stress disorder (Doweiko, 2006).

## Factors Related to Addiction and Substance Abuse

As stated previously, there is currently no one theory that explains the cause of addiction or substance use and abuse. However, several factors have been identified that increase a person's vulnerability to developing a substance abuse problem. These factors do not occur in isolation, that is, no one single factor is responsible for substance abuse. Rather it is the interplay or sharing among these factors that increases a person's vulnerability.

### Psychological Factors

Substance abuse disorders often occur in individuals with other mental health disorders. Although estimates vary depending on the population being surveyed, statistics from the Substance Abuse and Mental Health Services Administration (SAMHSA) (CSAT, Tip 42, 2005) set the number of individuals who admit to any mental health or substance use disorder at 52 million (30%) and those with both substance dependence and a severe mental illness (major depression, generalized anxiety, or posttraumatic stress disorder) at 8 million (5%). Another proposed explanation for a shared vulnerability is the prevalence of comorbid psychiatric and addictive disorders. Substance use disorders often occur as a secondary illness in those with mental health disorders; and, mental health disorders are increasing in frequency with increasing rates for substance abuse. Thus, health care professions need to understand that the interaction of mental health and substance use disorders is an expectation rather than an exception (Minkoff, 2005).

### Environmental Factors

Also common to this at-risk population are a variety of sociodemographic factors. Poverty, geography, family, and peer groups have been shown to influence the onset and course of various disorders, as do subclinical risk factors, such as impulsivity, delinquency, and impaired parenting skills (Shaffer et al., 2006). Additionally, researchers are beginning to examine the prevalence of addictive and mental health disorders in certain groups of individuals to identify additional risk factors. For example, the military came under scrutiny after the Vietnam War due to the large numbers of returning veterans who were addicted and met criteria for comorbid mental health disorders such as major depression and posttraumatic stress disorder. Military service has continued to attract interest as a risk factor. A history of trauma, domestic violence, and criminal justice involvement also appear to be risk factors for developing mental health and substance use disorders.

### Shared Experiences

Not all members of at-risk populations or individuals with risk factors develop a mental health or substance use disorder. However, being under stress, experiencing traumatic events, having poor coping skills, or having a particular genetic makeup may make individuals vulnerable to the onset of the neuroadaptive response if they are also exposed to potential objects of addiction, such as chemicals or behaviors (Shaffer et al., 2004). No particular personality traits have been identified as predictive, however, once abuse and dependency are present, common traits such as dysthmia, deceit, shame, or guilt have been identified.

A natural history appears to exist within the experience of addiction that begins with risk factors and exposure, spreads an addictive pattern across chemical and behavioral expressions, and ends with an identifiable pattern of compulsion, tolerance, withdrawal, craving, and relapse. For example, the individual grows up in a home with an alcoholic, drug-addicted, or abusive parent, conferring genetic and psychological risk factors. The peer group they belong to likes to party on the weekends. They binge drink or use drugs each weekend, then start drinking or using during the week. They find it takes more for them to relax and have fun. Soon they are drinking or using during the day, or they drink or use and drive. They are on report at work or get a driving-under-the-influence (DUI) charge. They attend treatment as ordered but return to drinking or using drugs as soon as they are out of treatment.

The addiction syndrome presentation is the same regardless of the substance or behavioral process of addiction. Both processes and substances of addiction are frequently interchangeable. These shared manifestations of compulsion, tolerance, withdrawal, craving, and relapse serve as the definitive evidence for diagnosis (Shaffer et al., 2004).

## Neurobiological Influences

Substance dependence or addiction is known to be a chronically relapsing disorder presenting with compulsive use of a substance or behavior, loss of control, and withdrawal symptoms, such as dysphoria, anxiety, or irritability (Koob, 2006). Individuals experience the use of drugs with the potential for dependence in different ways; therefore, there is current neurobiological research being conducted in an attempt to understand if there are neuropharmacological and neuroadaptive mechanisms that control this (Koob, 2006). One of the neuroadaptive mechanisms that have offered the best understanding of the addictive process is the brain reward system (Shaffer et al., 2004; Koob, 2006; NIDA, 2009).

Using functional magnetic resonance imaging, researchers have been able to track the neurobiological reward activity associated with the neurotransmitter dopamine (Shaffer et al., 2004; Koob, 2006). The dopamine reward system provides positive reinforcement for all natural rewards such as food, water, sex, and nurturing. These activities are rewarded with feelings of pleasure. Research has revealed that the use of psychoactive drugs has the ability to stimulate the same neurobiological pathways. Certain behaviors are capable of stimulating the same dopamine reward pathways, resulting in addictions that are known as process or behavioral addictions (Shaffer et al., 2004). Other pathways and neurobiological mechanisms such as the learning and memory functions of the hippocampus and the role of the amygdala in emotional regulation have been implicated as playing a role in substance abuse.

Although it is not possible to use imaging techniques to follow all the changes in the brain and predict the addictive process, researchers have used their knowledge of the brain's neurobiology to develop generalized theories of the addictive process. As addiction develops, changes occur in the neural circuits associated with the amygdala and in the function of various neurotransmitters and neuromodulators that recruit the brain stress system and reinforce dependence. The resulting dysregulation in these systems is implicated in decreases in orbitofrontal/prefrontal cortex function and brain dopamine D2 receptors (Koob, 2006). These changes are thought to explain the difficulty dependent individuals have with abstinence motivation, recurrent cravings, and frequent relapse. Shaffer et al. (2004, p.369) have proposed that "the neurobiological circuitry of the central nervous system is the ultimate common pathway for addictive behaviors."

As a companion to the study of the neurobiological antecedents for addiction, researchers have also examined the possibility of genetic markers as links and predictors to specific addictive behaviors. The evidence appears to support that a familial vulnerability transmission link for dependency is present, but that this risk is general rather than specific. This has raised the potential for the existence of a genetic link to a general increased risk for addiction (Shaffer et al., 2004; Koob, 2006). What remains to be examined is the outcome of an individual having any of these associated markers. It is known that some affected individuals will never develop an addictive disorder. Other family members may display a variety of individual process or substance disorders or multiple disorders.

One suggested explanation for these differences in the expression of addiction is the impact of varying environmental, psychosocial, ethnic, and cultural factors. Although international research into alcohol use is impacted by variations in the size and strength of drinks and the methods used to measure alcohol consumption, survey data have provided insight into rates of consumption and abstinence. Once the comparability difficulties have been resolved, additional studies may provide information on alcohol-related outcomes and differences within and across countries (Bloomfield, Stockwell, Gmel, & Rehn, 2003). Researchers have found it is easier to study some of these differences within the population of the United States, as many races, cultures, and ethnic groups are represented. While race is primarily representative of physiological responses, Straussner proposed that culture and ethnicity represent "worldviews, life patterns, institutions, languages, religious ideals, artistic expressions, and relationships shared by their group's members" (National Institute on Alcohol Abuse and Alcoholism [NIAAA], 2005, p. 3). For these reasons, trends and patterns of alcohol consumption and drug use differ greatly across various groups and manifest symptomatology according to the underlying physiological status of the individual.

> *Psychological, environmental, and neurobiological influences and shared experiences play a role in whether or not a person develops an addiction.*

## TREATMENT OPTIONS

Regardless of the origin of the addiction, substance or process, the gender of the individual, or the presence of co-morbid conditions, the treatment options are much the same. Substance abuse treatment is delivered in a variety of settings and across a broad continuum of care according to the severity of the symptoms the patient is experiencing. Patient placement criteria have been developed in order to ensure that clinical needs are matched with the correct care setting. The best known is the criteria published by the American Society of Addiction Medicine (ASAM).

Treatment usually consists of a mix of therapies including self-help programs, psychopharmacology, and psychotherapy such as cognitive behavioral therapy and insight-oriented psychotherapy. For example, the compulsive nature of addictive behavior often responds better to selective serotonin reuptake inhibitors (SSRIs) than to insight-oriented therapy. In addition, specific treatment of associated physiological disorders may be required. Another part of the treatment process often involves participation in a self-help program such as 12-step groups. Many variations on the original 12-step group have come into existence as a way of addressing the various substance and process addiction behaviors.

Treatment begins with screening, followed when indicated by a complete assessment to evaluate the presenting signs and symptoms reported by an individual as a basis of formulating a diagnosis. In October of 2003, the Center for Substance Abuse Treatment (CSAT), part of SAMHSA, awarded seven national Screening, Brief Intervention, Referral and Treatment (SBIRT) grants. The intention was the development of a continuum for

the activities of screening, intervention, and referral within medical and community settings that act as entry to treatment. This work was further supported by the 2007 National Quality Forum consensus report, "National Voluntary Consensus Standards for the Treatment of Substance Use Conditions: Evidence-Based Treatment Practices." This report broadened the responsibility for screening, brief intervention, and referral for treatment to all medical and mental health settings.

Treatment options for individuals with co-morbid psychiatric and substance use disorders are many and varied. Best practice is to address both/all disorders simultaneously in an integrated treatment program rather than in parallel or sequential treatment episodes. During the assessment phase, the severity of the disorders is determined and initial placement is made based on the American Society of Addiction Medicine (ASAM) criteria or on criteria determined by the state where treatment is being delivered. Individuals at risk for withdrawal symptoms need to be admitted to an inpatient medically managed detoxification program. Intensity of treatment steps down from there to inpatient rehabilitation, halfway house, partial hospital programming (minimum of 10 hours a week), intensive outpatient (between 5 and 9 hours a week), and outpatient (at most 5 hours a week).

Within each level of care, a patient-centered treatment plan is developed. Many facilities use a multi-disciplinary plan of care, better known as a care pathway. Care pathways are one way that evidence-based best practices can be introduced and implemented in the provision of care. The format also assists in tracking and evaluating the quality of care and the accomplishment of patient goals (Rayner, 2005). The care provided is threefold with therapy, interpersonal relationships, and neurobiological approaches. A number of modalities may be used simultaneously and treatment plans are individualized based on the specific mix of modalities and approaches. Although not considered treatment, 12-step groups and activities are included.

### 12-Step Programs

Founded in 1930, Alcoholics Anonymous (AA) is the oldest and best known of the 12-step fellowships. Everyone is welcome; all that is needed is a desire to quit drinking. Using the support of other members and the 12 steps, individuals learn how to be sober one day at a time. Attendance begins during treatment and is based on complete confidentiality and anonymity. Members choose a home group and a sponsor that best fits them. Meetings are available worldwide and around the clock, including online. Sponsors serve as their guide to completing the tasks associated with the 12 steps. Although AA meetings are open to individuals who have problems with substances other than alcohol and with process addictions, programs are available for their significant others, family members, or support persons. The 12-step movement has expanded to include meetings for most substance and process addictions, as well as for individuals experiencing pain from a loved one's addiction.

Links for the most common ones, such as Alcoholics Anonymous (aa.org), Narcotics Anonymous (naranon.org), Gamblers Anonymous (gamblersanonymous.org), Overeaters Anonymous (oa.org), Rational Recovery (rational.org), and Dual Recovery Anonymous (draonline.org), as well as similar organizations can be found on the websites of most treatment facilities or through the use of a search engine. Significant others and family members can attend Al-Anon, Alateen, and Nar-Anon. Unless the information about the meeting identifies it as closed, most meetings welcome health care providers who have an interest in understanding the role of the 12-step process in recovery. In addition, many resources are available online from the Substance Abuse Mental Health Services Administration (SAMHSA) at www.samhsa.gov, Hazelden Treatment Center at www.hazelden.org, Enter Health at www.enterhealth.com, and the National Alliance on Mental Illness at www.nami.org, to list a few.

> *Alcoholics Anonymous is the oldest and most notable of the 12-step programs. Confidentiality, anonymity, and a desire to remain sober are key components of AA.*

## Psychopharmacology

Given that dependency and many psychiatric disorders result from neurobiological changes in the brain, there has been a great deal of research into psychoactive medications that would reverse or ameliorate the changes and offer some restoration of function. Medications are specific to the psychiatric disorder and the substance of abuse. They are used to manage symptoms during periods of acute withdrawal, to assist with detoxification, and to support abstinence in early recovery and during maintenance. Some medications have shown to be effective with behaviors associated with abuse and dependence while other medications are available as substitutes to reduce harm. Harm reduction is also practiced by encouraging

controlled use at a lower level. Research is ongoing into medications and genetics in an effort to offer additional resources to treat these disorders. **Drug Summary 15-1** highlights specific agents used for substance use and induced disorders.

Medications are prescribed according to the specific symptomatology and medical need. Some drugs of abuse produce severe symptoms during detoxification. For example, alcohol withdrawal may precipitate seizures and can be treated with a variety of medications from barbiturates such as phenobarbital, benzodiazapines such as diazepam (Valium) or chlordiazepoxide (Librium), or anticonvulsants such as carbamazepine (Tegretol). Heroin is another drug with severe withdrawal symptoms. Patients may need symptom-specific medications like clonidine (Catapres) to control hypertension that may develop during withdrawal. Once the patient is past the initial withdrawal of the substance, he or she may need pharmacologic support for continued abstinence. For example, acamprosate calcium (Campral), naltrexone (Revia, Vivitrol), disulfiram (Antabuse), or quietiapine (Seroquel) may be prescribed to manage alcohol cravings. Partial opioid antagonists, buprenorphine (Subutex, Suboxone) and narcotic analgesics (methadone) may be useful in maintaining abstinence from opiates.

> *Numerous medications are used to treat addiction. Some medications are used to control the symptoms that occur during detoxification and withdrawal. Other medications are used to promote continued abstinence.*

## Psychotherapy

Another treatment approach is psychotherapy. There are many therapeutic modalities, but the most common ones include cognitive behavioral therapy, motivational enhancement (interviewing) therapy, mindfulness and meditation, community reinforcement, and contingency management. Cognitive behavioral therapy addresses thinking patterns. By assisting the patient to identify potentially flawed core beliefs, dysfunctional thought processes can be identified and redirected (Angres & Bettinardi-Angres, 2008). Motivational enhancement therapy is based on the transtheoretical or stages of change model. Individuals move

**DRUG SUMMARY 15-1:**
**MEDICATIONS USED WITH SUBSTANCE DISORDERS**

| DRUG | INDICATION | USE | IMPLICATIONS FOR NURSING CARE |
|------|------------|-----|-------------------------------|
| disulfiram (Antabuse) | Alcohol dependence | Maintenance | Emphasize the need to avoid alcohol ingestion<br><br>Inform patients that ingesting alcohol while taking this medication produces a toxic reaction that causes intense nausea and vomiting, headache, sweating, flushed skin, respiratory difficulties, and confusion |
| carbemazepine (Atretol, Tegretol)) | Alcohol dependence | Withdrawal | Inform the patient that he or she may experience dizziness or drowsiness (effect is dependent on therapeutic level)<br><br>Work with the patient to ensure that the drug is taken consistently<br><br>Advise the patient about the need to be gradually tapered off the drug to prevent seizures |
| acamprosate calcium (Campra) | Alcohol dependence | Relapse-prevention agent | Inform patients that side effects, although minimal, include diarrhea, nausea, itching, and intestinal gas |
| clordiazepoxide (Librium) | Alcohol | Increase seizure threshold; reduce withdrawal agitation | Alert the patient to potential sedation. Educate about the signs and symptoms of withdrawal, including warnings of seizure activity |
| phenobarbital (Phenobarbital) | Alcohol | Withdrawal | Warn the patient of possibility of sedation; work with the patient on ways to minimize effect on activities |
| quietiapine fumarate (Seroquel) | Alcohol dependence | Detoxification with reduced craving | Alert the patient to possible drop in blood pressure when changing position from sitting to standing. Work with the patient on measures to combat dry mouth and restlessness |
| diazepam (Valium) | Alcohol | Withdrawal | Alert the patient to potential sedation. Educate about the signs and symptoms of withdrawal, including warnings of seizure activitiy |
| naltrexone (Vivitrol, Injectable; Revia; Depade, Oral) | Alcohol<br>Opiates | Withdrawal; relapse prevention | Inform the patient that nausea is the primary side effect initially; although nausea usually goes away after first month, the patient should expect headache, feeling of sedation, and pain at the injection site with each injection |

*(cont.)*

**DRUG SUMMARY 15-1: (CONT.)**
**MEDICATIONS USED WITH SUBSTANCE DISORDERS**

| DRUG | INDICATION | USE | IMPLICATIONS FOR NURSING CARE |
|---|---|---|---|
| clonidine (Catapres) | Opiate addiction Presence of hypertension | Heroin withdrawal | Inform the patient to be alert for signs and symptoms of opioid withdrawal (tachycardia, fever, runny nose, diarrhea, sweating, nausea, vomiting, irritability, stomach cramps, shivering, unusually large pupils, weakness, difficulty sleeping, gooseflesh) and report severity. Urge the patient to take each dose as given |
| levo-alpha-acetyl methadol (LAAM) | Opiate addiction | Withdrawal and maintenance | Inform the patient this is contraindicated if pregnant or expecting to get pregnant, has experienced side effects in past treatment, or has liver damage. Explain that induction takes longer than with methadone |
| methadone hydrochloride (Methadone) | Opiate addiction | Detoxification and maintenance | Educate the patient that this is an effective but controversial drug. Explain that an induction period is required Advise the patient about possible need for safety measures initially and with higher doses because sedation is possible |
| buprenorphine (Subutex, Oral; Buprenex, Injectable; Suboxane) | Opiate addiction | Detoxification and maintenance | The patient must be in withdrawal before this medication is given Assess the patient closely for changes and anticipate that levels will be adjusted over several days Explain that therapy will usually require 9-12 months of use after which tapering will occur |
| naltrexone hydrochloride (Trexan) | Heroin Opiates Pathological gambling | Detoxification and maintenance Reduce impulsive and compulsive behaviors | Alert the patient not to increase or change dose or use opiates Work with the patient on safety measures because of possible drowsiness, dizziness, or blurred vision Suggest small, frequent meals and frequent mouth care due to nausea or vomiting Evaluate the patient for possible pregnancy or breastfeeding (contraindicated) |

(cont.)

**DRUG SUMMARY 15-1: (*CONT.*)**
**MEDICATIONS USED WITH SUBSTANCE DISORDERS**

| DRUG | INDICATION | USE | IMPLICATIONS FOR NURSING CARE |
|---|---|---|---|
| varenicline (Chantix) | Nicotine addiction | Reduce craving and withdrawal | Advise the patients to stop taking medication and call health care provider immediately if agitation, hostility, depressed mood, changes in behavior or thinking, or suicidal ideation or suicidal behavior develops<br><br>Warn the patient of possible vivid, unusual, or strange dreams |
| rimonabant (Zimulti) | Nicotine<br>Obesity | Smoking cessation<br>Maintenance of body weight | Inform the patient that this drug is known to have serious side effects if taken long term. Reports have included depression, suicidal tendencies, nausea, anxiety and nervousness, frequent unpredictable mood swings, tendency to become irritated at most things, and difficulty sleeping<br><br>Urge the patient to report any changes to health care provider immediately |
| bupropion (Zyban, includes patches, gums, lozenges, nasal sprays, and inhalers) | Nicotine | Withdrawal from smoking | Inform the patients to take with food to minimize GI discomfort<br><br>Warn the patient that agitation and insomnia are possible. Monitor anxiety<br><br>Encourage the patient not to take at bedtime or double up if doses missed |

through the process of change from the use/abuse behavior to abstaining by completing phases or stages: pre-contemplation, contemplation, preparation, and action. This model is very successful in breaking denial. Mindfulness and meditation focuses on learning to be present.

The setting used may be individual, group, or family. Family therapy is a part of substance abuse treatment because addiction does not develop in isolation. The dynamics and structural elements that have contributed to the dysfunction of the family can be addressed. Therapy is usually time limited, focuses on an expectation of change, elicits new behavior, and supports the new patterns of interaction that are developing. Families may attend therapy as individual or extended family groups, couples, or multifamily groups. Multifamily groups may be convened as a part of ongoing group therapy.

Group therapy may occur as an open group or closed group process. The same techniques or approaches will be used. The groups may be process sensitive or directive in nature and group members can support or confront each other, providing the group dynamics. The shorter the length of time that the group will meet, the more structured and goal oriented it will be. Groups can be run using the same therapeutic modalities that are used for individual therapy with the addition of psychodrama (Center for Substance Abuse Treatment, TIP 34, 1999).

Once present and motivated to complete the goals of treatment, recovering individuals have a need to be reconnected to the community and the activities that will sustain their lifestyle. Community reinforcement helps to reactivate or establish supportive relationships, employment, and educational activities. Finally, contingency management introduces rewards, which will ensure that the individual continues to follow the treatment and aftercare plans and maintains long-term sobriety.

## Detoxification and Rehabilitation

DETOXIFICATION refers to the process of managing a patient during withdrawal. Detoxification is composed of three components: evaluation, stabilization, and readiness for treatment. It can occur at five levels from ambulatory without extended onsite monitoring to medically managed intensive inpatient treatment, and may or may not involve medication.

As detoxification is normally very short term, it is important to build a therapeutic relationship with the patient to prepare him or her for entrance into treatment. The highest level of intensity for treatment is inpatient rehabilitation. Once a 28-day stay, inpatient treatment is now authorized on a week-to-week basis. During the rehabilitation stay, patients receive individual, group, and family therapy. They are introduced to the 12-step program and may attend meetings during their stay. At discharge, a referral will be made for the most appropriate level of follow-up care. Research has shown a link between the length of treatment and recovery percentages. Patients may step down into a halfway house, partial hospital program (over 9 hours a week), intensive outpatient treatment (4–9 hours a week), or outpatient treatment (up to 4 hours a week).

## APPLYING THE NURSING PROCESS FROM AN INTERPERSONAL PERSPECTIVE

Recent federal reports, such as Crossing the Quality Chasm (Institute of Medicine, Committee on Quality Health Care, 2001), have highlighted problems in the quality of care arising from silos of care that exist within physical and behavioral health treatment. These factors have complicated treatment for individuals with co-occurring mental health and substance use disorders. Both are legitimate illnesses, each deserving appropriate treatment. Current federal initiatives are attempting to address these problems with new approaches to the way patient care is provided. Thus, nurses working in all specialty areas need to be aware of the potential to see only the specific mental health issue while ignoring possible dual diagnose that can complicate the treatment regime.

The guidelines developing from these federal initiatives suggest that mental health and substance use disorders need an integrated approach and support the creation of patient-centered, recovery-oriented, evidence-based treatment systems (Snow & Delaney, 2006). This has broad implications for nursing and, in particular, for the specialty of psychiatric-mental health nursing.

Patients with addiction disorders may be seen in a variety of settings such as acute care settings, day hospitalization programs, community and outpatient centers, and long-term care facilities. Some mental health settings may have nurses or other clinicians specializing in addiction to provide continuity of care. In the event that patients need to be referred to addiction-specific services, it is critical that providers communicate, collaborate, and coordinate care. Addiction is a progressive disorder that will require ongoing relationships to prevent additional physical and behavioral health consequences and the progression of this disease. In addition, many individuals may have co-morbidities such as major depression or anxiety disorders. Additionally, the effects of substance use can lead to medical conditions. As a result, patients often can be encountered in general medical facilities, emergency departments, and specialty clinics. Therefore, psychiatric-mental health nurses need a firm understanding of the nursing process that integrates the interpersonal process when caring for patients with addiction disorders. **Plan of Care 15-1** provides an example for a patient with an addictive disorder.

## Strategies for Optimal Assessment: Therapeutic Use of Self

The hallmark of Peplau's Interpersonal Theory of Nursing is the therapeutic nurse-patient relationship. Nursing and the addiction treatment field agree that clinicians establish rapport for a therapeutic relationship during their first face-to-face session (Beeber, Caruso, & Emory, 2004; Cooke & Matarassa, 2005; Perraud et al., 2006; SAMHSA TAP 21, 2005; Stockmann, 2005). Empathy, respect or positive regard, congruence, and genuineness are necessary relationship factors for the therapeutic relationship to develop. Reflective (active) listening promotes an understanding and appreciation for the patient's world (Perraud et al., 2006). **Consumer Perspective 15-1** provides an example of what it is like to have alcohol dependency and mental health problems. The psychiatric-mental nurse becomes oriented to the patient's lived experience. Many individuals suffering from the disease of addiction will have experienced multiple losses within previous relationships. It is important to take these prior experiences into consideration in establishing this therapeutic relationship. As the therapeutic relationship is established it allows for open, ongoing communication, collaboration, and patient-centered information gathering. The information collected in the initial assessment provides the basis for patient-centered goal setting to follow.

**PLAN OF CARE 15-1:**
**THE PATIENT WITH AN ADDICTIVE DISORDER**

**NURSING DIAGNOSIS:** Risk for injury related to substance abuse, intoxication, and withdrawal.

**OUTCOME IDENTIFICATION:** Patient will remain free of injury.

| INTERVENTION | RATIONALE |
|---|---|
| Assess the patient for signs and symptoms of abuse, intoxication, and withdrawal; assess vital signs, look for indicators of impending withdrawal; assess neurologic status | Assessing for signs and symptoms provides a baseline from which to develop appropriate interventions; assessing neurologic status provides evidence for changes related to intoxication and withdrawal |
| Institute safety measures, seizure precautions, and fall precautions | Instituting safety measures are important to prevent injury due to effects of the substance |
| Maintain a calm and nonstimulating environment | Maintaining a calm, nonstimulating environment minimizes exposure to stimuli that can induce anxiety |
| Administer prescribed medications | Administering medications helps to control symptoms associated with intoxication and/or withdrawal |
| Reorient the patient as necessary; provide verbal reassurance | Reorienting and verbally reassuring the patient help to minimize anxiety related to intoxication and withdrawal |
| Continue to frequently monitor the patient's physiologic and psychologic status for changes | Monitoring the patient frequently for changes provides information about effectiveness of therapy, as well as information about possible complications needing immediate attention |

**NURSING DIAGNOSIS:** Defensive coping; related to disease process of addictions; manifested by denial and inability to perceive problems related to abuse.

**OUTCOME IDENTIFICATION:** Patient will begin to demonstrate acceptance of responsibility for behavior.

| INTERVENTION | RATIONALE |
|---|---|
| Establish a therapeutic relationship with the patient; demonstrate empathy and a nonjudgmental, caring approach | Establishing a therapeutic relationship is important in helping the patient begin to acknowledge the problem |

*(cont.)*

**PLAN OF CARE 15-1: (*CONT.*)**
**THE PATIENT WITH AN ADDICTIVE DISORDER**

| INTERVENTION | RATIONALE |
| --- | --- |
| Reinforce that the substance abuse behavior is the problem, and not that the patient is a "bad person"; educate the patient about misconceptions related to abuse | Emphasizing the behavior rather than the patient as the problem promotes feelings of self-worth and helps to reduce feelings of guilt and weakness; educating the patient fosters understanding of the problem |
| Assess the patient's usual coping strategies; identify maladaptive strategies and situations or issues that may precipitate use | Assessing usual strategies provides information on how the patient responds to problems and provides a baseline from which to provide suggestions for change |
| Help the patient identify triggers associated with substance use and abuse and connect these triggers with abuse behaviors; offer suggestions for identifying precipitating triggers and for replacing maladaptive strategies with positive coping strategies | Identifying triggers and making the connection to abuse behaviors promotes acknowledgment of the problem and lessening of denial |
| If necessary, confront the patient about behavior using a nonthreatening, caring approach | Confronting the patient may be necessary to relinquish the denial; using a nonthreatening, caring approach helps maintain trust and minimizes the possibility that the patient will become defensive |
| Help the patient practice adaptive coping techniques | Practicing adaptive coping techniques enhances the chances for success |
| Refer patient to appropriate community resources for assistance, such as self-help groups | Ensuring adequate support such as self-help groups reduces the feelings of isolation associated with addiction and facilitates sharing of feelings |

**NURSING DIAGNOSIS:** Dysfunctional family processes; related to prolonged history of substance abuse; manifested by chaotic and unstable family dynamics.

**OUTCOME IDENTIFICATION:** Patient and family will demonstrate appropriate adaptive behaviors to promote family functioning.

| INTERVENTION | RATIONALE |
| --- | --- |
| Review family history, including roles and functions of members and the relationships; involve family members in treatment plan; assist family members in identifying how each has coped with the substance problem | Assessing family history and relationships provides a baseline for developing appropriate individualized interventions; involving family members in the treatment plan is important because addiction does not occur |

*(cont.)*

## PLAN OF CARE 15-1: (*CONT.*)
## THE PATIENT WITH AN ADDICTIVE DISORDER

| INTERVENTION | RATIONALE |
|---|---|
|  | in isolation; identifying coping strategies promotes understanding of the family functioning and strategies that are maladaptive and adaptive |
| Work with family members to develop appropriate methods for expressing feelings related to patient's substance abuse problem | Using appropriate methods for expressing feelings minimizes maladaptive coping |
| Reinforce techniques related to prescribed therapy, such as family therapy | Reinforcing therapy techniques promotes continuity of care and enhances chances for success |
| Teach the patient and family appropriate techniques for problem solving and conflict management | Using appropriate problem-solving and conflict management techniques fosters trust for improved relationships |
| Encourage patient and family members to participate in the family roles and functions; assist family members in assuming new or changing roles with the patient's change in behavior | Assisting family members in assuming new roles enhances the transition to a more functional family as the patient's behavior changes |
| Refer the family to community support groups as appropriate | Ensuring adequate support such as by self-help groups reduces the feelings of isolation associated with addiction, promotes adjustment to the changes in the patient's behavior, and facilitates sharing of feelings |

*Nursing Diagnosis – Definitions and Classifications 2009 – 2011. Copyright © 2011 by NANDA International. Use by arrangement with Blackwell Publishing Limited, a company of John Wiley & Sons, Inc.*

## Self-Awareness

During the assessment process, relevant data are elicited. The nurse pays special attention to the patient's verbal and nonverbal communication skills. At the same time, the nurse needs to be aware of his or her own responses to the patient and the issues they present. During these first meetings, the nurse will establish the boundaries of the relationship, help patients clarify their issues, listen to what patients are not saying, reflect back to validate any perceptions and remain open, attentive, and nonjudgmental (SAMHSA TAP 21, 2005; Perraud et al., 2006). It is important to remember that establishing the therapeutic relationship and collecting information are the primary goals. The nurse is responsible for identifying and managing any inner conflict or countertransference through the development of his or her own self-awareness. **Therapeutic Interaction 15-1** provides an example of an interpersonal interaction.

## CONSUMER PERSPECTIVE 15-1: A PATIENT WITH SUBSTANCE ABUSE

Having a dependency on alcohol on top of mental health problems is a nightmare. The situation is bad enough with just mental health problems. Add the alcohol and it becomes the worst ever. You can't solve either problem. Every time you try to stop drinking, the mental health problems become bad and you start drinking again. It is a good day just to drink a little bit. You feel so bad about yourself because you can't stop drinking or feeling depressed and anxious. If you go to AA, it seems as though no one understands. Even having a sponsor doesn't help. They act as though you need to just stop. Someone without mental [health] problems can't understand. I take all this medication and nothing seems to help. My mouth is dry all the time. I still can't sleep without bad dreams. I just keep trying to make it through the day.

> *During assessment, the nurse must be ever vigilant in monitoring him- or herself for conflicts and countertransference. The nurse also uses active listening to gain an understanding of the patient's experience.*

## Screening

Nurses, regardless of their area of practice, need to be educated about addictive disorders and the disease of addiction. Nurses also need to be able to use screening tools and assessment skills for early detection. An accurate assessment for both mental health and substance use disorders is essential for developing a thorough treatment plan and providing quality care (Baird, 2009; Baird & Fornili, 2008; Snow & Delaney, 2006).

To screen for addictive disorders, the nurse may choose to add a question or two to the assessment process or complete a full screen. A wide variety of screening tools are available, ranging from simple to complex. Many of the tools are in the public domain and include guides to help in administering and interpreting them. Usually the screening process can be completed quickly so that a decision can be made about the need for further intervention or brief counseling. **Box 15-2** provides an example of a screening tool for alcohol abuse.

Regardless of the tool used for screening, the tool needs to be reliable and validated for use with all consumers. Communication must be clear to avoid any misinterpretation. Recognition must be given that diagnosis relies on a defined set of elements or criteria (Doweiko, 2006).

Research on the existence of an addiction syndrome determined that the same types of neuroadaptation occurred whether or not a chemical or a process was being used (Shaffer et al., 2004).

One screening tool that is commonly used is the Alcohol Use Disorders Identification Test (AUDIT). This tool consists of two parts. Part I is the core of the tool and consists of 10 questions to determine diagnosis and need for treating alcohol abuse, dependence, and/or addiction. It assesses symptoms and other problems associated with use. Specific criteria for standardizing the amount of alcohol ingested by drink to denote risky or hazardous drinking amounts have been identified in conjunction with this tool. **Table 15-1** lists the amounts that would be considered problematic. Part II of the tool is the clinical assessment, consisting of a brief physical exam, questions about trauma history, and liver function testing. The AUDIT has been the basis for many evidence-based nursing research projects and much information is available to assist nurses in conducting the AUDIT and using the information that is collected.

A different assessment tool, the CAGE, is widely used to screen for alcohol abuse. It offers an opportunity for quickly screening and determining a need for a more thorough assessment. **Box 15-3** lists the four questions used to assess patient responses. This tool can be completed by the nurse during an office visit. The information collected provides prescreening data to determine the need for continued assessment, whereby responses will be further explored to establish need for treatment with an addiction professional. The CAGE-AID is an assessment tool based on the CAGE tool that has been adapted to screen for drug use.

The psychiatric-mental health nurse could use either tool in any setting because each permits the focus to be

**THERAPEUTIC INTERACTION 15-1:**
**WORKING WITH A PATIENT WITH AN ADDICTION**

Mrs. S. is a 50-year-old female who was admitted to the drug treatment clinic for opiate addiction.

| | |
|---|---|
| **Nurse:** "Mrs. S., this is Day 4 of your stay here at the clinic and I am stopping by to see why you declined to attend the Narcotics Anonymous group you were scheduled to attend this morning." | Gathers information to assess treatment compliance |
| **Mrs. S.:** "Because it's a bunch of crap! I don't need that, I feel better now. I just need to get out of here." | Exhibits possible signs of denial of disease |
| **Nurse:** "I am glad you feel better. The first 48 to 72 hours coming off of opiates can be rough." | Provides validation and education |
| **Mrs. S.:** "You make it sound as though I was addicted! I only took the Vicoden as prescribed." | Defends and rationalize her behavior |
| **Nurse:** "I understand that you believe this. Let's talk about what happened even though you thought you took it as prescribed." | Lays the groundwork for gentle confrontation |
| **Mrs. S:** "What do you mean what happened?" | Questions the reality of her circumstances |
| **Nurse:** "Well, your doctor reported needing to increase your Vicoden, you have incurred 2 separate driving-while-impaired tickets recently, you are on the verge of losing your job because you don't seem to be able to function in the role as you used to, your family reports you are moody and irritable, you report you can't sleep, and you complain of such severe anxiety that you have gone to several emergency departments seeking Xanax. These are all signs of opiate dependence and side effects of long-term opiate use." | Provides psychoeducation and methodically lays out the facts regarding the patient's circumstances in a non-threatening, matter-of-fact way |
| **Mrs. S.:** (yelling) "But I'm in pain, you moron. You obviously don't know what it's like to live with back pain!" | Vents anger and frustration while trying to validate her use of opiates |

*(cont.)*

### THERAPEUTIC INTERACTION 15-1: (*CONT.*)
### WORKING WITH A PATIENT WITH AN ADDICTION

| | |
|---|---|
| **Nurse:** "Pain can be difficult to live with, but becoming dependant on addictive substances in the long run makes the situation even worse." | Validates the experience of pain but continues to present the reality of the situation in a calm, matter-of-fact manner and not responding to the personal attacks |
| **Mrs. S.:** (begins crying) "I don't know what to do, I can't go on like this." | Begins to show signs of accepting her situation |
| **Nurse:** "I think this would be a good time to meet others in the program who are in recovery and hear their stories of how they figured out how to move on with their lives without these substances. There is another group after lunch; I would like to introduce you to them." | Recognizes this opportunity to offer treatment in a supportive way |

## BOX 15-2: AN EXAMPLE OF A SCREENING TOOL FOR ALCOHOL ABUSE

THE RAPS4 QUESTIONS

1. Have you had a feeling of guilt or remorse after drinking?
2. Has a friend or a family member ever told you about things you said or did while you were drinking that you could not remember?
3. Have you failed to do what was normally expected of you because of drinking?
4. Do you sometimes take a drink when you first get up in the morning?

A "yes" answer to at least one of the four questions suggests that your drinking is harmful to your health and well-being and may adversely affect your work and those around you.

If you answered "no" to all four questions, your drinking pattern is considered safe for most people and your results do not suggest that alcohol is harming your health.

*From Alcohol Concern. "Primary Care Alcohol Information Service – Screening tools for health care settings." Retrieved 2007.*

## TABLE 15-1: RISKY/HAZARDOUS DRINKING FROM THE AUDIT SCREENING TOOL

One drink equals 12 ounces of regular beer (150 calories) or 5 ounces of wine (100 calories) or 1.5 ounces of 80-proof distilled spirits (100 calories)

| | MEN | WOMEN | PREGNANT | ADOLESCENTS | ELDERLY |
|---|---|---|---|---|---|
| Per day/occasion | 4 drinks | 3 drinks | Any at all | Any at all | 3 drinks |
| Per week | 14 drinks | 7 drinks | Any at all | Any at all | 7 drinks |

**BOX 15-3: CAGE ASSESSMENT TOOL QUESTIONS**

1. Have you ever felt that you should cut down on your drinking/prescription drug use/illicit drug use?
2. Have people annoyed you by criticizing your drinking/prescription drug use/illicit drug use?
3. Have you ever felt bad or guilty about your drinking/prescription drug use/illicit drug use?
4. Have you ever had a drink or used your drug the first thing in the morning to steady your nerves or get rid of a hangover (eye opener)?

This tool can be downloaded from Project Cork website www.project cork.org/clinical_tools/index.html. There is no fee for use.

on the therapeutic relationship between nurse and patient. The role of screening and providing brief interventions is one that fits Peplau's theory of the interpersonal focus that occurs between the nurse and patient. Just as Peplau's theory is focused on being able to understand one's own behavior to help others identify perceived difficulties, substance abuse counseling is focused on the ability to utilize self and the force of interpersonal processes in the therapeutic relationship, and apply principles of human relations to the problems that arise at all levels of experience (*Current Nursing*, 2009; Konrad, 2005).

> *The nurse uses reliable and validated screening tools to provide for early detection of substance disorders.*

## Physical Examination

An individual whose life is being compromised because of an addiction may present in any care setting and for many different reasons. Any of the following conditions, if present, might alert the nurse to ask additional questions about the use of substances. These conditions can be assessed while discussing the individual's lifestyle during the assessment:

- Vague physical complaints and requests for medication to improve sleep, energy, anxiety, concentration, indigestion, and others
- Requests for samples of medications or to refill prescriptions earlier than the recommended schedule, with a variety of reasons why the medication is currently not at the patient's disposal
- Unexplained bruises or injuries suggesting falls or other accidents resulting from substance-induced impairment or blackouts

- Increased frequency of visits or calls to the primary care provider's office requesting treatment for self or family member that may include prescribing a medication that has the potential for abuse
- Unexplained weight loss or symptoms of malnourishment resulting from diminished need for food or the lack of money to buy food
- Decline in oral hygiene, resulting from overall neglect of this and other activities of daily living, or eating disorders that cause dental damage
- Changes in menstrual cycle associated with weight loss or gain and other eating disorders
- Skin conditions indicating poor general hygiene, malnourishment, or injection sites
- Overall changes in appearance, presentation, or laboratory values that may include unfavorable response to previously prescribed remedies
- Unexplained tremors, ataxic gait, and poor coordination

In addition, during the physical examination, the psychiatric-mental health nurse needs to be alert for signs and symptoms of physiological problems that may suggest a substance problem. Special attention should be given to:

- Changes noted from previous physical exams (if previous patient)
- Odors on the breath and clothing or intoxicated behavior such as slurred speech and staggering gait
- Poor nutritional status
- Poor personal hygiene
- Signs of physical abuse, bruises, lacerations, scratches, burns, needle marks, sores, or abscesses
- Skin rashes or discoloration, hair loss, or excessive sweating
- Head, eyes, ears, nose, and throat status (inflammation, irritation, blanching of any of the mucosa, gum disease, sinus tenderness or sinusitis, rhinitis, or perforated nasal septum)

It should also be noted that disorders of the gastro-intestinal tract or the immune, cardiovascular, and pulmonary systems may be a result of addictive behavior and disorders of the liver, hypertension and tachycardia, lymphadenopathy, and coughing with wheezing, rales, and rhonchi are frequently present. There may be neurologic impairment that presents as cognitive deficits or sensory, motor, or memory impairment. In addition, there are a number of laboratory values and biological screens that may serve as an alert to pathological processes, indicating the presence of an addictive disorder.

## Diagnosing and Planning Appropriate Interventions: Meeting the Patient's Focused Needs

The therapeutic relationship carries over into all aspects of the planning and treatment process. It is within this nurse-patient relationship that a treatment plan is developed that is "patient-centered, recovery oriented, and evidence-based" (Snow & Delaney, 2006, p.290). The essential relationship factors of empathy, positive regard, and congruence reinforce the bond and assist the nurse in the task of goal setting (Perraud et al., 2006; SAMHSA TAP 21, 2005). Using the strengths and limitations of the patient, treatment priorities are identified and negotiated. The nurse assists in translating the information into goals, making sure to engage the patient's understanding, cooperation, and motivation. The patient needs to trust the nurse so that he or she will be motivated to follow through with the changes. The stronger the initial therapeutic relationship is, the easier this transition will be.

During this phase a great deal of emphasis and reliance is put on the knowledge, skills, and attitudes of the nurse. The psychiatric-mental health nurse needs to clarify the priorities and goals for the patient and family members, collaborate with them on the development of the goals and objectives of the plan, and then assess the patient's ability and readiness for participation and change. Key to this process is the nurse's theoretical and intuitive knowledge base (Sjostedt, Dahlstrand, Severinsson, & Lutzen., 2001). As the process evolves, awareness grows. Patient and nurse are communicating on a deeper level. With this increased sense of the patient and patient vulnerabilities comes the need to make a moral commitment to provide patient-centered quality care, be flexible to the needs of the situation, and to maintain the professional role (Sjostedt et al., 2001).

Assessment findings and identified needs are highly variable for patients with addictive disorders. When developing the plan of care for a patient, numerous nursing diagnoses would apply. Some may be dependent on the type of substance used. Examples of possible nursing diagnoses would include:

- Risk for injury related to effects of substance abuse, intoxication, or withdrawal
- Defensive coping related to denial of substance abuse, inability to perceive problems related to abuse
- Impaired social interaction related to guilt, feelings of worthlessness, anxiety, unpredictable behaviors
- Dysfunctional family processes related to history of long-term substance abuse
- Ineffective role performance related to continued use of substances
- Risk for self- or other-directed violence related to impaired judgment, unpredictable behavior, episodes of acting out resulting from substance abuse
- Disturbed sensory perception related to altered neurologic function secondary to effects of substance use and abuse

These nursing diagnoses also will vary based on the acuity of the patient's illness, developmental stage, comorbidities, current treatment regimen, and sources of support. For example, the person with substance intoxication may have risk for injury or disturbed sensory perception. Once the intoxication clears, nursing diagnoses such as defensive coping and dysfunctional family processes may be the priority areas to be addressed.

Based on the identified nursing diagnoses, the nurse and patient collaboratively would determine the outcomes to be achieved. For example, an appropriate outcome for the patient experiencing defensive coping would be that the patient verbalizes acceptance of responsibility for behavior involving substance abuse.

> *Although nursing diagnoses may vary, a common nursing diagnosis for a patient with addiction is defensive coping.*

## Implementing Effective Interventions: Timing and Pacing

The careful balance of moral commitment, flexibility, and professional role influences how the plan of care is carried out. Using the strength of the initial therapeutic relationship, interpersonal interactions occur between nurse and patient that promote the patient's growth. Beeber et. al. (2004) have proposed that these therapeutic interactions use and

Q **BOX 15-4: THE FIVE As FOR BEHAVIOR CHANGE INTERVENTION**

Assess consumption with a brief screening tool and follow with clinical assessment as needed
Advise patients in reducing consumption
Agree on individual goals for reducing use or for abstinence
Assist patients to acquire motivation, self-help skills, and supports
Arrange follow up, repeat counseling, or specialty referral

*From U.S. Preventive Services Task Force http://www.uspreventiveservicestaskforce.org/3rduspstf/behavior/behsum2.htm*

exchange units of energy to stimulate the development of new patient competencies. Peplau used the term instrumental inputs without a definition for the process that she felt occurred. In contrast, Beeber et. al. applied the term to the concept. During the work of the treatment plan within the therapeutic relationship, the patient develops vulnerabilities that produce energy units. These energy units are the instrumental inputs to which Beeber et al. refer. As the patient confronts these vulnerabilities or threats with the support of the nurse, interactions, growth, and forward movement occur. An example of integrating the interpersonal approach when intervening is the use of the Five As: assess, advise, agree, assist, and arrange. **Box 15-4** highlights the Five As for behavior change. These patient-centered interactions can be applied to any substance misuse intervention as well as to any time that behavior is evaluated and change is sought.

Competencies, the ability to use skills to perform effectively, develop through repetitive purposeful activities and distinct phases within therapeutic encounters that have clear boundaries. Psychoeducation is an important aspect for developing these competencies. **Patient and Family Education 15-1** provides an example. By completing interventions that address the prioritized needs, problems, and personal challenges, the patient develops these necessary competencies. According to Beeber and associates, in Peplau's theory the nurse-patient interactions are carefully shaped verbal exchanges. Through the use of carefully sequenced activities, words, and actions, patients begin to see cause and effect.

Ongoing assessment acknowledges the work the patient is doing, applies corrective feedback, reinforces the collaboration, and keeps the plan relevant. The nurse demonstrates understanding of the patient's suffering, accepts responsibility for a therapeutic relationship, and uses a common language to work with the individual's hopes for the future (Sjostedt et al., 2001). It is important that the nurse remember at all times that the relationship is therapeutic for the patient only as long as the process is patient-centered. All interventions must be implemented based on the patient's readiness to move to the next stage. The nurse must note

**PATIENT AND FAMILY EDUCATION 15-1:
LIVING WITH AN ADDICTION**

- Take ownership of your illness (that is, accept it and become responsible for managing it)

- Remember, the early phase of recovery is critical. Go to as many AA/NA meetings as possible. Stay in close contact with your sponsor

- Find things or activities to fill the void that may be left when you stop using (hobbies, classes, recreation)

- Take care of your body: eat well, exercise, get adequate sleep, reduce caffeine, and if you smoke, plan to stop

- Make sure your health care providers know you are in recovery and that they support your commitment to abstinence from substances of abuse (opiates, benzodiazepines, etc.)

- Become aware of your triggers and recognize what used to prompt you to use

- Take one day at a time! Recovery is a life-long process and can feel overwhelming unless broken down into smaller parts

not only the accomplishment of each step of the process, but the signs that the patient is preparing for the next step.

The nurse also needs to be familiar with the medications currently used in the treatment of individuals using substances of abuse (Drug Summary 15-1). In addition, the nurse needs to continually assess for signs and symptoms of intoxication and withdrawal resulting from the use, abuse, and dependence on each type of substance of abuse. **Tables 15-2 and 15-3** highlight the signs and

## TABLE 15-2: SIGNS AND SYMPTOMS* OF ALCOHOL INTOXICATION AND WITHDRAWAL

| BLOOD ALCOHOL LEVEL | ALCOHOL INTOXICATION CLINICAL PICTURE | ALCOHOL WITHDRAWAL CLINICAL PICTURE |
|---|---|---|
| 20–100 mg percent | • Mood and behavioral changes<br>• Reduced coordination<br>• Impairment of ability to drive a car or operate machinery | *Uncomplicated or mild to moderate alcohol withdrawal*<br><br>• Restlessness<br>• Irritability<br>• Anorexia (lack of appetite)<br>• Tremor (shakiness)<br>• Insomnia<br>• Impaired cognitive functions<br>• Mild perceptual changes |
| 101–200 mg percent | • Reduced coordination of most activities<br>• Speech impairment<br>• Trouble walking<br>• General impairment of thinking and judgment | *Severe alcohol withdrawal*<br><br>• Obvious trembling of the hands and arms<br>• Sweating<br>• Elevation of pulse (above 100) and blood pressure (greater than 140/90)<br>• Nausea (sometimes with vomiting)<br>• Hypersensitivity to noises (which seem louder than usual) and light (which appears brighter than usual)<br>• Brief periods of hearing and seeing things that are not present (auditory and visual hallucinations) also may occur<br>• Fever greater than 101°F also may be seen (care should be taken to determine whether the fever is the result of infection) |
| 201–300 mg percent | • Marked impairment of thinking, memory, and coordination<br>• Marked reduction in level of alertness<br>• Memory blackouts<br>• Nausea and vomiting | *Most extreme forms of severe alcohol withdrawal*<br><br>• Seizures<br>• True delirium tremens |
| 301–400 mg percent | • Worsening of above symptoms with reduction of body temperature and blood pressure<br>• Excessive sleepiness<br>• Amnesia | *Medical complications of alcohol withdrawal*<br><br>• Infections<br>• Hypoglycemia<br>• Gastrointestinal (GI) bleeding<br>• Undetected trauma<br>• Hepatic failure<br>• Cardiomyopathy with ineffective pumping<br>• Pancreatitis<br>• Encephalopathy (generalized impaired brain functioning). |
| 401–800 mg percent | • Difficulty waking the patient (coma)<br>• Serious decreases in pulse, temperature, blood pressure, and rate of breathing<br>• Urinary and bowel incontinence<br>• Death | |

*These may vary greatly with level of tolerance (chronic users of alcohol may show less effect at any given blood alcohol level).

*From Consensus Panelist Robert Malcolm, M. (SAMHSA TIP 45, 2006).*

symptoms associated with alcohol and opioid intoxication and withdrawal. **Box 15-5** highlights the key signs and symptoms of stimulant withdrawal.

Individuals who are under the influence or suffering from withdrawal may present in a variety of settings and require or request detoxification. This process has three components that are completed in sequence: evaluation, stabilization, and entry into treatment (SAMHSA TIP 45, 2006). The primary goal is to medically stabilize the patient. Once this occurs, clinical guidelines from the American Society of Addiction Medicine (ASAM) can be used to determine the intensity of services necessary to support

## TABLE 15-3: SIGNS AND SYMPTOMS OF OPIOID INTOXICATION AND WITHDRAWAL

| OPIOID INTOXICATION | OPIOID WITHDRAWAL |
|---|---|
| **Signs** | **Signs** |
| Bradycardia (slow pulse) | Tachycardia (fast pulse) |
| Hypotension (low blood pressure) | Hypertension (high blood pressure) |
| Hypothermia (low body temperature) | Hyperthermia (high body temperature) |
| Sedation | Insomnia |
| Meiosis (pinpoint pupils) | Mydriasis (enlarged pupils) |
| Hypokinesis (slowed movement) | Hyperreflexia (abnormally heightened reflexes) |
| Slurred speech | Diaphoresis (sweating) |
| Head nodding | Piloerection (gooseflesh) |
|  | Increased respiratory rate |
| **Symptoms** | Lacrimation (tearing), yawning |
| Euphoria | Rhinorrhea (runny nose) |
| Analgesia (pain-killing effects) | Muscle spasms |
| Calmness | |
|  | **Symptoms** |
|  | Abdominal cramps, nausea, vomiting, diarrhea |
|  | Bone and muscle pain |
|  | Anxiety |

*From Consensus Panelist Charles Dackis, M. (SAMHSA TIP 45, 2006).*

### BOX 15-5: STIMULANT WITHDRAWAL SYMPTOMS

- Depresion
- Hypersomnia (or insomnia)
- Fatigue
- Anxiety
- Irritability
- Poor concentration
- Psychomotor retardation
- Increased appetite
- Paranoia
- Drug craving

*From Consensus Panelist Robert Malcolm, MD (SAMHSA TIP 45, 2006).*

the safe withdrawal from the substance. Psychiatric-mental health nurses play an essential role in this process at all levels of intensity, from the physician's office to 24-hour care in an acute inpatient setting. Psychiatric-mental health nurses also may be involved during all three components of detoxification. For example, the psychiatric-mental health nurse would be involved in obtaining a complete assessment and providing ongoing evaluation of the type and level of severity of the patient's symptoms. Thus, the nurse needs to be knowledgeable of the signs and symptoms specific to each substance to facilitate this initial intervention and ongoing evaluation. In addition, when medications are involved, the nurse will need to provide education to the patient about what to expect, monitor him or her for side effects, and continually evaluate the patient for a response. During the third stage, the nurse engaged in the therapeutic relationship encourages reluctant patients to participate in establishing their treatment program.

When assessing a patient for possible withdrawal, the nurse can use various tools that are available. Examples of these tools are identified in **Table 15-4**. Throughout the process, the therapeutic relationship is integral in facilitating the nurse's ability to assess and manage symptomatology, determine the type of support needed for continuing abstinence, and prepare the patient to enter treatment.

> *Detoxification involves evaluation, stabilization, and entry into treatment.*

This same therapeutic relationship offers the patient an opportunity to learn how to manage relationships within his or her family when the treatment plan includes education on family dynamics, participation in family groups, or family therapy sessions. Many individuals with behavioral health issues have experienced problem relationships within their families and/or with significant others. Individuals may be estranged from family or have been part of unhealthy family dynamics. Addiction has

## TABLE 15-4: TOOLS FOR ASSESSING WITHDRAWAL

| | | |
|---|---|---|
| **CIWA-Ar:** Addiction Research Foundation Clinical Institute Withdrawal Assessment for Alcohol<br>*Contact Info:* SAMHSA Tip 24 | Tool asks patient to rate the following 9 areas using a scale from 0 to 7:<br>• Nausea and vomiting<br>• Tactile disturbances<br>• Tremor<br>• Auditory disturbances<br>• Paroxysmal sweats<br>• Visual disturbances<br>• Anxiety<br>• Headache, fullness in head<br>• Agitation<br>The 10th area is Orientation and Clouding of Sensorium and is scored between 0 and 4. | Takes 2-5 minutes to administer.<br>• Three areas are scored by observation (tremor, paroxysmal sweats, and agitation).<br>• One area, anxiety, is scored combining the response and observation.<br>• The maximum possible score is 67 points, with a score of 10 or more indicating clinical concern. |
| **SOWS:** Subjective Opiate Withdrawal Scale<br>*Contact Info:* Handelsman, L., Cochrane, K.J., Aronson, M.J., Ness, R., Ruginstein, K.J., & Kanof, P.D. (1987). Two new rating scales for opiate withdrawal. *American Journal of Alcohol Abuse.* 13:293–308. | A 16-item questionnaire seeking responses to the extent the individual is currently experiencing each of the characteristics described. | Each item is scored between 0-4. The higher the score, the greater the severity of the associated withdrawal. |
| **OOWS:** Objective Opiate Withdrawal Scale<br>*Contact Info:* Handelsman, L., Cochrane, K.J., Aronson, M.J., Ness, R., Ruginstein, K.J., & Kanof, P.D. (1987). Two new rating scales for opiate withdrawal. *American Journal of Alcohol Abuse.* 13:293–308. | Thirteen manifestations of withdrawal are identified. Staff completing this assessment must be familiar with the signs and symptoms of opiate withdrawal. The clinician completes this by direct observation of the individual. | Observation takes approximately 10 minutes. The rater scores each item on a scale of 0 to 13. The more pronounced the presenting symptom, the higher the score. The higher score indicates the risk of more severe withdrawal. |

long been recognized as a family disease. An example of problems faced by a patient with alcohol dependency and multiple health problems is illustrated in **How Would You Respond?** 15-1. Assessing the individual's family and addressing family issues and including family members in the treatment plan at the appropriate time offers the chance of better outcomes and longer periods of sobriety once the individual is discharged. If needed, the process of reunification may be started, or, if necessary, entirely new relationships or support systems may be forged.

## Evaluating: Objective Critique of Interventions and Self-Reflection

Evaluation occurs as an ongoing assessment of the timelines and objectives met. It is expected that once the therapeutic relationship is established, the process of change will move forward, and the goals of the treatment plan will be met. During the evaluation process, support for the relationship will be measured. The relationship is most effective when the nurse is seen as facilitating progress by being available, consistent, and trustworthy (Stockmann, 2005). The process of change is measured by identifying improvements in the patterns of expression, perception, and behavior that were once problematic for the patient, thus meeting the goals set for the treatment plan (Beeber et al., 2004). The nurse accomplishes this by accepting an ethical commitment to examine the "desires, trusts, hope, powerlessness, and guilt and shame" that make up the patient's suffering (Sjostedt et al., 2001, p.315).

Part of this ethical commitment is the responsibility for ongoing self-reflection to increase self-awareness, manage countertransference, and ensure that the goals and outcomes sought are patient-centered rather than geared to meet the needs of the nurse or the system. Therapeutic relationships can suffer or fail due to negative or conflicting responses or reactions, unrealistic expectations, poor boundaries, lack of respect or understanding for

### HOW WOULD YOU RESPOND? 15-1:
### A PATIENT WITH ALCOHOL ABUSE

S.L. is a 60-year-old female with a long history of depression and anxiety. During one treatment episode, she was diagnosed with attention deficit disorder. She began drinking daily in the early 1990s in an effort to manage work-related stress. After ten years, she took a forced retirement and applied for social security disability. The main people in her life are her ex-husband, her adult son and his family, her siblings, and her employer, a disabled man she assists with household chores. Her ex-husband is an end-stage alcoholic. He lives with their son, who tolerates his father's drinking but pressures his mother for sobriety. Her parents are deceased, but when alive, they experienced major depression, anxiety, and obsessive compulsive disorder and a psychotic depression. An older sister died recently. She lived out of state and suffered from major depression and alcoholism. Two brothers, residing out of state, meet the criteria for substance abuse or a mild mental health disorder. Two other brothers and a sister reside in the area. Her sister and one brother have anxiety and a form of obsessive-compulsive disorder. Her youngest brother has schizophrenia and is on disability. She is the sibling that everyone looks to for guidance.

Since her retirement six years ago, S.L. has been receiving treatment for her depression and anxiety and trying to address her alcohol use. Her current diagnoses are major depression, generalized anxiety disorder, and alcohol dependency. Although the severity of her symptomatology would indicate the need for inpatient treatment at a drug and alcohol rehabilitation facility, followed by a halfway house or partial program treatment episode, her current insurance does not cover these levels of treatment. Since she has coverage only for inpatient treatment, her treatment consists of week-long inpatient stays for medical management of her withdrawal from alcohol (detox) followed by Alcoholic Anonymous's 12-step program. Her first treatment episode was in mid-2006. She has had five more episodes since then. Her pattern is to remain abstinent for a week or so postdischarge, attend 12-step groups, and then start drinking as her anxiety increases. As her drinking increases, her AA attendance decreases. Her drink of choice is vodka by the pint, but she will substitute wine to manage intake.

Shortly after her first detox experience, she started working with her current psychiatrist, an addictionologist. He has been trying to address all three disorders with interactive and complementary medications. There have been multiple medication changes. Pharmacologic management has been impacted by her resistance to taking medications, sleep disorders including restless legs and vivid dreams, and difficulties with attention and concentration. Currently, she is on quietiapine (Seroquel) to manage anxiety and assist with sleeping; venlafaxine (Effexor) to treat her depression; gabapentin (Neurontin) for restless legs and withdrawal anxiety. Acamprosate (Campral) is prescribed but not taken consistently. In addition to her psychiatrist, outpatient counseling, and AA, she has been following up with her primary care physician for her hypertension, arthritis, hypothyroidism, seizure disorder, and recent positive hepatitis C screen.

### CRITICAL THINKING QUESTIONS

1. *What factors may have played a role in this patient's development of alcohol dependency?*

2. *How does acamprosate differ from another drug, disulfiram, used to manage alcohol abstinence?*

3. *How might the nurse involve the patient's family in the treatment plan?*

### APPLYING THE CONCEPTS

Addiction is a disease with both neurobiological and psychosocial antecedents (Shaffer, LaPlante, LaBrie, Kidman, Donato, & Stanton, 2004). The patient history described in the scenario is positive for a number of neurobiological and psychosocial factors. The family dynamics have been impacted by several generations of alcoholism and mental health disorders. In families impacted by addiction, members identify with one of several roles. This patient responded to the family's dysfunctional dynamics by identifying with the role of hero child. As the role carried over into adulthood, the individual displayed characteristics of perfectionism and caretaking in all relationships.

The most basic relationships that an individual experiences are within the family unit. Because addiction is a disease that impacts family members as well as the individual with an addiction, family therapy is an important part of the treatment. All members of the family will need to learn to relate to each other differently. Focus may be on healthier coping skills, problem solving without the substances, sharing and managing feelings, and learning to be assertive about boundaries and limit setting.

Acamprosate is used as a relapse-preventing agent that has minimal side effects. The patient does not experience the toxic reaction that occurs with disulfiram if alcohol is ingested. However, the patient should continue alcohol counseling when taking either drug.

The nurse would encourage the patient and family to continue to engage in family therapy and reinforce the skills learned. Additionally, the nurse would provide patient and family education about the disorder and treatment, including any medications prescribed.

individual's communication styles, and cultures (Beeber et al., 2004; Narayanasamy, 1999; Perraud et al., 2006; Rayner, 2005; Stockmann, 2005). Preventing the therapeutic relationship from weakening and impacting the patient's successful accomplishment of goals is a crucial task of the nurse. If all the tasks are completed, the patient will develop competencies. These competencies help make it possible for alterations to occur in problematic areas. In addition, the patient will have acquired skills that could be used to manage future problems. As the last task of evaluation, the nurse will assist the patient to complete a personal appraisal using reflective thinking and a critique of the progress of treatment. At this point, if the patient is comfortable with the competencies, the therapeutic relationship is terminated and the patient is discharged. Terminating the relationship with mutual respect and consideration for boundaries is important so that the patient can retain a positive view for future treatment opportunities.

### SUMMARY POINTS

- Addiction is defined as a chronic, relapsing condition characterized by compulsive drug seeking and use, even when harmful consequences are present. It involves a spectrum of disorders including substance abuse and substance dependence, substance intoxication, and substance withdrawal

- Eleven classes of substances are identified by the *DSM-IV-TR*: alcohol, amphetamines, caffeine, cannabis, cocaine, hallucinogens, inhalants, nicotine, opioids, phencyclidine, and sedatives, hypnotics, and anxiolytics

- Current thinking views addiction as a syndrome, which helps to explain why only some individuals become dependent and others do not

- An interplay of psychological, environmental, shared experiences, and neurobiological influences is believed to increase a person's vulnerability to substance problems. No

*(cont.)*

## SUMMARY POINTS (*CONT.*)

one theory is currently available to explain the cause of addiction

- Treatment options include a mix of therapies such as self-help programs, psychopharmacology, and psychotherapy including cognitive behavioral and insight oriented therapy

- Addiction is a progressive disorder that requires ongoing relationships to prevent additional physical and behavioral health consequences and progression of the disease. Nurses establish rapport for the therapeutic relationship and demonstrate empathy, respect or positive regard, congruence, and genuineness

- Nurses need to be able to use screening tools and assessment skills for early detection of addictive disorders

- The therapeutic relationship between the nurse and patient offers the patient the opportunity to learn how to manage relationships with his or her family

- Terminating the nurse-patient relationship with mutual respect and consideration for boundaries is important so that the patient can retain a positive view for future treatment opportunities

## NCLEX-PREP*

1. A group of students are reviewing information about the classification of addictive disorders. The students demonstrate understanding of the information when they identify which of the following as a substance use disorder?
   - a. Substance dependence
   - b. Substance-induced disorder
   - c. Susbstance intoxication
   - d. Substance withdrawal

2. The psychiatric-mental health nurse is working with a patient diagnosed with alcohol abuse and is describing the 12-step program of Alcoholics Anonymous. Which of the following would the nurse include?
   - a. Participants are selected based on their ability to attend meetings.
   - b. The desire to quit drinking is the underlying concept.

   - c. Sponsors are selected by the leader of the group meeting.
   - d. Sobriety requires that the person focus on future events.

3. A patient is experiencing heroin withdrawal and develops hypertension. Which of the following would the nurse expect to administer?
   - a. Phenobarbital
   - b. Diazepam
   - c. Clonidine
   - d. Acamprosate

4. A patient with addiction is undergoing treatment that focuses on redirecting dysfunctional thought processes. The patient is involved in which of the following?
   - a. Motivational enhancement therapy
   - b. Cognitive behavioral therapy
   - c. Mindfulnesss
   - d. Community reinforcement

*(cont.)*

## NCLEX-PREP* (CONT.)

5. A patient with alcohol intoxication and a blood alcohol level of 190 mg percent is exhibiting signs of withdrawal. Which of the following would the nurse expect to assess? Select all that apply.

   a. Restlessness
   b. Visible hand trembling
   c. Hypersensitivity to light
   d. Auditory hallucinations
   e. Pulse rate less than 89 beats per minute
   f. Seizures

6. A patient is brought to the emergency department by a friend who states, "He's been in a lot of pain and has been using oxycodone quite a bit lately." Which of the following would lead the nurse to suspect that the patient is experiencing intoxication?

   a. Tachycardia
   b. Pinpoint pupils
   c. Rhinorrhea
   d. Gooseflesh

7. A psychiatric-mental health nurse identifies a nursing diagnosis of defensive coping for a patient being treated for alcohol intoxication. Which statement would support this diagnosis?

   a. "I really just drink when my life gets really stressful."
   b. "My employer said I might lose my job if things don't change."
   c. "I just can't do anything right, I'm such a failure."
   d. "My family just seems to be falling apart lately."

8. The psychiatric-mental health nurse is using the CAGE assessment tool to screen for alcohol abuse. Which question would the nurse ask first?

   a. "Have you ever had a drink first thing in the morning to steady your nerves?"
   b. "Have people annoyed you by criticizing your drinking?"
   c. "Have you ever felt you should cut down on your drinking?"
   d. "Have you ever felt bad or guilty about your drinking?"

*Answers to these questions appear on page 639.

## REFERENCES

Agency for Health Care Research and Quality [AHRQ]. (2006). *The Guide to Clinical Preventive Services.* Recommendations of the U.S. Preventive Services Task Force. Department of Health and Human Services [DHHS].

American Psychiatric Association. (2000). *Diagnostic and Statistical Manual of Mental Disorders* (4th ed., text revision). Arlington, VA: Author.

Angres, D.H., & Bettinadi-Angres, K. (2008, October). The disease of addiction: Origins, treatment and recovery. *Disease a Month, 54(10),* 696–721. Retrieved October 25, 2009 from http://www.diseaseamonth.com/article/S0011-5029(08)00092-8/abstract

Antai-Otong, D. (2006). Women and alcoholism: Gender-related medical complications: Treatment considerations. *Journal of Addictions Nursing, 17(1),* 33.

Baird, C. (2008). Treating women with children: What does the evidence say? *Journal of Addictions Nursing, 19(3),* 83–85.

Baird, C. (2009, July/August). Spotting alcohol and substance abuse: How to start a screening program for primary care patients. *American Nurse Today, 4(7),* 29–31.

Baird, C., & Fornili, K. (2008). Effective health care delivery and integrated behavioral health screening. *Journal of Addictions Nursing, 19*(3), 174-177. Retrieved September 10, 2009 from http://dx.doi.org/10.1080/10884600802306180

Baird, C., Pancari, J.V., Lutz, P. J., & Baird, T. (2009). Addiction Disorders. In J.C. Urbanic & C.J. Groh (Eds.), *Women's Mental Health: A Clinical Guide for Primary Care Providers* (pp. 125–179). Philadelphia: Lippencott, Williams & Wilkins.

Beeber, L.S., Camuso, R., & Emory, S. (2004, October). Instrumental inputs: moving the interpersonal theory of nursing into practice. *Advances In Nursing Science, 27*(4), 275–286. Retrieved August 4, 2009, from MEDLINE with Full Text database.

Bloomfield, K., Stockwell, T., Gmel, G., & Rehn, N. (2003, Dec.) International Comparisons of Alcohol Consumption. *National Institute on Alcohol Abuse and Alcoholism (NIAAA).* Retrieved November 24, 2009 from http://pubs.niaaa.nih.gov/publications/arh27-1/95-109.htm

Center for Substance Abuse Treatment. (2005). *Addiction Counseling Competencies: The Knowledge, Skills and Attitudes of Professional Practice,* Technical Assistance Publication [TAP] Series, 21. DHHS Publication No.(SMA) 05-4087. Rockville, MD: Substance Abuse and Mental Health Services Administration.

Center for Substance Abuse Treatment. (1999). *Brief Interventions and Brief Therapies for Substance Abuse Counseling.* Technical Assistance Publication [TAP] Series, 34. DHHS Publication

No.(SMA) 99–3353. Rockville, MD: Substance Abuse and Mental Health Services Administration.

Center for Substance Abuse Treatment. (2005). *Substance Abuse Treatment for Persons With Co-Occurring Disorders,* Treatment Improvement Protocol [TIP] Series, 42. DHHS Publication No.(SMA) 05–3992. Rockville, MD: Substance Abuse and Mental Health Services Administration.

Center for Substance Abuse Treatment. (2006). *Detoxification and Substance Abuse Treatment,* Treatment Improvement Protocol [TIP] Series, 45 DHHS Publication No.(SMA) 06–4131. Rockville, MD: Substance Abuse and Mental Health Services Administration.

Committee on Quality of Health Care in America, Institute of Medicine. (2001, March). *Crossing the Quality Chasm: A New Health System for the 21st Century.* Retrieved October 19, 2007 from http:// www.iom.edu/Object.File/Master/27/184/Chasm-8pager.pdf

Cooke, M., & Matarasso, B. (2005, December). Promoting reflection in mental health nursing practice: a case illustration using problem-based learning. *International Journal Of Mental Health Nursing, 14*(4), 243–248. Retrieved August 4, 2009, from MEDLINE with Full Text database.

Current Nursing. (2009). Application of Interpersonal Theory in Nursing Practice. Retrieved December, 2011, from http:// currentnursing.com/nursing_theory/interpersonal_theory.htm

Doweiko, H.E. (2006). *Concepts of chemical dependency.* Belmont, CA: Thomson Brooks/Cole.

Furek, M.W. (2008). *The Death Proclamation of Generation X: A Self-Fulfilling Prophecy of Goth, Grunge, and Heroin.* iUniverse, Inc.: NY.

Jellinek, E.M. (n.d.). *Jellinek Curve of Alcoholism.* Retrieved Friday, March 31, 2007 from http://www.in.gov/judiciary/ijlap/docs/jellinek.pdf

Konrad, S. (2005). Addictions and Disability Counseling. In *An Introduction to Counseling in Canada.* Retrieved October 10, 2009 from http:/psych. athabascau.ca/html/Resources/Psych388/CanadianSupplement/Chapter13/print.shtml

Koob, G. F. (2006). The neurobiology of addiction: a neuroadaptational view relevant for diagnosis. *Addiction, 101 (Suppl. 1),* 23–30.

Minkoff, K. (2005). Comprehensive Continuous Integrated System of Care (CCISC): Psychopharmacology Practice Guidelines for Individuals with Co-occurring Psychiatric and Substance Use Disorders (COD). Retrieved October 22, 2009 from http:// www.kenminkoff.com/articles.html

Narayanasamy, A. (1999, June 10). Transcultural mental health nursing. 2: Race, ethnicity and culture. *British Journal of Nursing (Mark Allen Publishing), 8*(11), 741–744. Retrieved August 4, 2009, from MEDLINE with full text database.

National Institute on Alcohol Abuse and Alcoholism [NIAAA]) (2005, March). Module 10H: Ethnicity, Culture and Alcoholism. Retrieved November 25, 2009 from http://pubs. niaaa.nih. gov/publications/Social/Module10HEthnicity&Culture/Module10H.html

National Institute of Drug Abuse (NIDA). (2010). Drugs, Brains, and Behavior. The Science of Addiction. Retrieved from: http:// www.nida.nih.gov/scienceofaddiction/ Accessed 2/28/2011

National Institute of Drug Abuse (NIDA). (2009). NIDA InfoFacts Treatment Approaches for Drug Addiction. Retrieved http:// drugabuse.gov/infofacts/treatmeth.html. Accessed 2/28/2011.

National Institute of Drug Abuse (NIDA), National Institutes of Health (NIH), and U.S. Department of Health and Human Services (2009). Principles of Drug Addiction and Treatment, A Research Based Guide, 2nd ed. Bethesda, MD: NIH.

National Institute of Drug Abuse (NIDA). (2009). The Neurobiology of Drug Addiction. Section II: The Reward Pathway and Addiction. Retrieved October 11, 2009 from http://www.nida. nih.gov/pubs/teaching/teaching2/Teaching3.html

National Quality Forum. (2007). National Voluntary Consensus Standards for the Treatment of Substance Use Conditions: Evidence-Based Treatment Practices. A Consensus Report. Retrieved October 18, 2009 from http://www.qualityforum. org/Search.aspx? keyword=substance+abuse+treatment+cons ensus+document

Palladini, M. (2011). *Drugs of abuse: From doctors and dealers, users and healers.* Three Suns Publishing.

Perraud, S., Delaney, K.R., Carlson-Sabelli, L., Johnson, M. E., Shepard, R., & Paun, O. (2006, November). Advanced practice psychiatric mental health nursing, finding our core: the therapeutic relationship in 21st century. *Perspectives In Psychiatric Care, 42*(4), 215–226. Retrieved August 4, 2009, from Medline with Full Text database.

Rayner, L. (2005, August). Language, therapeutic relationships and individualized care: addressing these issues in mental health care pathways. *Journal of Psychiatrics and Mental Health Nursing, 12*(4), 481–487. Retrieved August 4, 2009, from Medline with Full Text database.

Shaffer, H.J., LaPlante, D.A., LaBrie, R.A., Kidman, R.C., Donato, A.N., & Stanton, M.V. (2004). Toward a Syndrome Model of Addiction: Multiple Expressions, Common Etiology. *Harvard Review Psychiatry, 12,* 367–374. Retrieved September 19, 2009 from http://www.expressionsofaddiction.com/docs/shafferetal-syndrome.pdf

Sjostedt, E., Dahlstrand, A., Severinsson, E., & Lutzen, K. (2001, July). The first nurse-patient encounter in a psychiatric setting: discovering a moral commitment in nursing. *Nursing Ethics, 8*(4), 313–327. Retrieved August 4, 2009, from Medline with Full Text database.

Snow, D. & Delaney, K.R. (2006, December). Substance Use and Recovery: Charting a Course Toward Optimism. *Archives of Psychiatric Nursing,* 20:6, 288–290.

Stockmann, C. (2005, November). A literature review of the progress of the psychiatric nurse-patient relationship as described by Peplau. *Issues in Mental Health Nursing, 26*(9), 911–919. Retrieved August 4, 2009, doi:10.1080/01612840500248197

Substance Abuse and Mental Health Services Administration [SAMHSA] Office of Applied Studies (OAS). (2008). *Results from the 2008 National Survey on Drug Use and Health*: National Findings. U.S. Department of Health and Human Services [DHHS]. Retrieved September 20, 2009 from http://www.oas. samhsa.gov/nsduh/2k8nsduh/2k8Results.cfm

Substance Abuse and Mental Health Services Administration [SAMHSA] (2010). Results from the 2009 National Survey on Drug Use and Health, Volume I. Summary of National Findings (Office of Applied Studies, NSDUH Series II-38A, HHS Publication No. SMA 10–4586Findings). Rockville, MD. Retrieved from: http://www.oas.samhsa.gov/nsduhLatest.htm Accessed 2/28/2011.

U.S. Preventive Services Task Force. *Evidence-Based Methods for Evaluating Behavioral Counseling Interventions.* Retrieved from http://www.uspreventiveservicestaskforce.org/3rduspstf/behavior/behsum2.htm

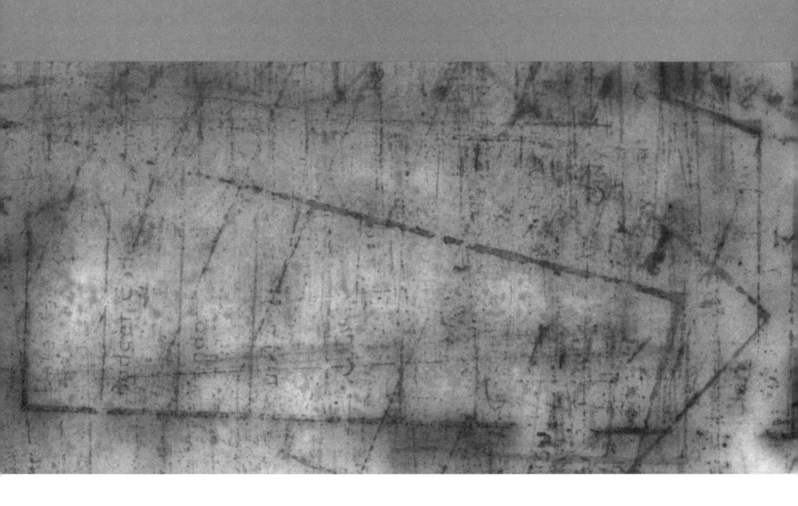

## CHAPTER CONTENTS

## EXPECTED LEARNING OUTCOMES

**After completing this chapter, the student will be able to:**

1. Define cognitive disorders.
2. Identify the major cognitive disorders.
3. Describe the historical perspectives and epidemiology of cognitive disorders.
4. Discuss current scientific theories related to the etiology and pathophysiology of cognitive disorders, specifically dementia of the Alzheimer's type.
5. Identify the diagnostic criteria for cognitive disorders.

# CHAPTER 16
# COGNITIVE DISORDERS

Mark P. Tyrrell

Geraldine McCarthy

6. Explain the pharmacological and non-pharmacological treatment options for persons with cognitive disorders.

7. Describe common assessment strategies for individuals with cognitive disorders.

8. Apply the nursing process from an interpersonal perspective to the care of patients with cognitive disorders, demonstrating an appreciation of the challenges that face family caregivers in caring for someone with dementia.

## KEY TERMS

Delirium

Dementia

Enriched model of dementia

Malignant social psychology

Neurofibrillary tangles

Positive person work

Progressively lowered stress threshold (PLST)

Reality orientation

Reminiscence therapy

Senile dementia

Validation therapy

**C**OGNITIVE DISORDERS refer to a group of disorders in which a person experiences a disruption in areas of mental function. These areas include orientation, attention, logic, awareness, memory, intellect, language, abstract thinking, and reasoning. Two major cognitive disorders identified by the American Psychiatric Association (APA) are DELIRIUM and DEMENTIA. Delirium refers to an acute disruption in consciousness and cognitive function. Dementia refers to a group of conditions that involve multiple deficits in memory and cognition. With the exception of delirium, which tends to be sudden in onset and short-lived, neurodegenerative processes characterize many cognitive disorders. Those resulting from dementia are insidious, and usually present for a number of years by the time symptoms become apparent. Moreover, symptoms may be so insidious that they are ignored or misinterpreted by the individual, or by family members or health care professionals as being insignificant or representative of normal aging. Symptoms are typically present for between one and two years before family members bring the person in for medical attention (Wilkinson et al., 2005). The average length of time from onset of symptoms until diagnosis is twenty months; however, it can be up to three years before a firm diagnosis is made (Wilkinson et al., 2005; Speechly, Bridges-Webb, & Passmore, 2008). This often results in a delay in reaching a diagnosis. Subsequently, there is a lost opportunity to initiate an early treatment plan, one that might afford sufferers additional months of cognitive competence, preserve their quality of life longer, and afford them the opportunity to put their financial and personal affairs in order before significant cognitive decline takes hold (Giaquinto & Parnetti, 2006).

This chapter focuses on dementia and delirium because these are the two most common types of cognitive disorder found in clinical practice. While both result in cognitive impairment and have profound implications for patients and their carergivers, the respective etiologies, treatments, and outcomes are distinctly different. While delirium is commonplace, particularly among the hospitalized elderly, it usually arises from an underlying medical condition. Furthermore, in a majority of cases, the cause is readily identified and treatable, thus enabling the person to return to the community. For these reasons, delirium is addressed only briefly in this chapter.

This chapter covers the historical aspects and epidemiology of cognitive disorders and includes a detailed description of the major cognitive disorders as defined in the *Diagnostic and Statistical Manual, 4th edition, Text Revision* (*DSM-IV-TR*, 2000). Relevant scientific theories related to the etiology and pathophysiology of dementia are described along with common pharmacotherapy and nonpharmacotherapy strategies used in the treatment of dementia, specifically dementia of the Alzheimer's type. Application of the nursing process from an interpersonal perspective is discussed, including a plan of care for a patient with dementia.

> *Delirium occurs suddenly and is the result of an underlying medical condition. Dementia occurs gradually and involves multiple problems of memory and cognition.*

## HISTORICAL PERSPECTIVES

Cognitive impairment has been documented as a health concern for many centuries. Indeed, there are apparent references to such conditions in the literature of ancient Greece and Rome. For example, Juvenal (AD 60–130) wrote:

> *"But worse than all bodily failing is the weakening mind which cannot remember names of slaves nor the face of a friend he dined with last evening, cannot remember the names of offspring begotten and reared...."* (Juvenal, cited in Gilliard, 1993)

Up until the 20th century, older adults with organic brain disease were generally diagnosed as having SENILE DEMENTIA. This was a term that categorized memory loss as part of normal aging. In the early part of the 20th century, neuropathologists began to recognize that a number of conditions could lead to senile dementia including Alzheimer's disease (now referred to as dementia of the Alzheimer's type [DAT]), arteriosclerotic brain disease, and neurosyphlis. In 1903, a young German physician, Alois Alzheimer, established a laboratory for brain research at the Munich Medical School. Three years later, Alzheimer presented a case study of a 55-year-old woman in which he described an unusual disease of the cerebral cortex characterized by memory loss, disorientation, and hallucinations. The woman in question died shortly afterward and Alzheimer carried out a post-mortem examination that showed various anomalies in her brain, including a thinning of the cerebral cortex, senile plaques, and neurofibrillary tangles. The disease that Alzheimer first described over a century ago bears his name to this day. In

1968, the link between the neuropathological features of DAT and the cognitive disorder of DAT were established by Blessed, Tomlinson, and Roth (1968). In the following decade, the biochemistry of DAT became more clearly understood, initially with the discovery of the cholinergic deficit, and later with the identification of beta-amyloid peptide.

Subsequent work throughout the 20th century revealed that a number of different types of dementia exist and that a myriad of other conditions could result in cognitive impairment such as that seen in senile dementia. Today, the *DSM-IV-TR* classification of cognitive disorders includes dementia, delirium, amnesic disorder, and other cognitive disorders.

## EPIDEMIOLOGY

The increase in life expectancy in industrialized countries over the past few decades has resulted in a greater incidence of cognitive disorders, particularly those resulting from neurodegenerative conditions such as dementia. One reason for the increased incidence is that dementias are age-related, hence the longer one lives, the greater the chance of being diagnosed with a dementia. Indeed, dementias account for the majority of cognitive disorders seen in mental health care, and dementia of the Alzheimer's type is by far the most common dementia in the Western world, accounting for between 55% and 65% of all cases.

Current statistics reveal that delirium is the most common cognitive disorder and is most frequently seen in the elderly, including those with dementia (Nassisi et al., 2006). It is estimated that about 50% of people with delirium have an overt psychosis (Boyle & Hands, 2009).

In both developed and developing countries, the number of people over the age of 65 is rising steeply, and as dementia is age-related this will inevitably lead to a rise in the number of people who have dementia. Indeed, recent estimates suggest that this number will double every 20 years and that by 2040, this number will amount to over 80 million people globally who have some form of dementia (Ferri et al., 2005). At age 60, the prevalence of dementia of the Alzheimer's type (DAT) is thought to be about 1%. However, this rate doubles approximately every five years, resulting in rates of 2% at age 65 and 8% at 75. By age 85, approximately one-third of individuals have the disease (Silvestrelli et al., 2006). Projections for the United States alone suggest that by 2050, the cost for treating dementia will exceed $380 billion (Katzman & Fox, 1999).

Dementia of the Alzheimer's type (DAT) accounts for between 55% and 65% of all dementias and is found in all human populations worldwide. More women than men are diagnosed with the disease probably due to the greater longevity of females. While DAT is primarily a disease of old age, occasionally people in their 40s or 50s are diagnosed with the condition.

> *Delirium is the most commonly occurring cognitive disorder. Dementia of the Alzheimer's type accounts for more than half of all dementias globally.*

Dementia of the vascular type affects men more often than women. Because the symptoms are similar to Alzheimer's, definitive diagnosis can be difficult. To complicate matters, dementia of the vascular type and DAT can coexist in the same person.

## DIAGNOSTIC CRITERIA

Cognitive disorders include delirium and dementia. Although the *DSM-IV-TR* provides diagnostic criteria for several types of dementia, four major types are presented here. These include dementia of the Alzheimer's type, dementia of the vascular type, dementia with Lewy bodies, and frontotemporal dementia. **Box 16-1** highlights the diagnostic criteria for these disorders.

While each type of dementia has its own distinctive set of clinical features, a number of common features exist. It is not unusual for some individuals to have more than one dementia at the same time; for example, someone may have both DAT and dementia of the vascular type and will present with some of the features of both conditions. In this regard, Smith and Buckwalter (2005) describe four groups of symptoms that are commonly seen in dementia. These are summarized in **Table 16-1**.

### Delirium

Delirium is a medical condition characterized by fluctuating levels of disorientation and clouded consciousness, accompanied by cognitive impairment, altered mood states, altered perception, altered self-awareness, and an inability to focus and maintain attention (APA, 2000). The person is often drowsy during the day; however, at night the person experiences sleeplessness, agitation, and restlessness. It is an acute state with a rapid onset. Some of the many causes of delirium are outlined in **Box 16-2**.

## BOX 16-1: DIAGNOSTIC CRITERIA

### DELIRIUM

A. Disturbance of consciousness with reduced ability to focus, sustain, or shift attention

B. Change in cognition such as memory deficit, disorientation or language difficulties or development of a perceptual disturbance that is not better accounted for by a pre-existing dementia

C. Disturbance develops over a short time and tends to fluctuate over the course of the day

D. Evidence of being due to a general medical condition, substance intoxication, substance withdrawal, or multiple etiologies

### DEMENTIA

*Dementia of the Alzheimer's Type*

A. The development of multiple cognitive deficits manifested by both:

- Memory impairment (impaired ability to learn new information or to recall previously learned information)
- One (or more) of the following cognitive disturbances:
  - Aphasia (language disturbance)
  - Apraxia (impaired ability to carry out motor activities despite intact motor function)
  - Agnosia (failure to recognize or identify objects despite sensory function)
  - Disturbance in executive functioning (i.e., planning, organizing, sequencing, abstracting)

B. Significant impairment in social or occupational functioning and a significant decline from a previous level of functioning resulting from cognitive deficits

C. The course characterized by gradual onset and continuing cognitive decline

D. The cognitive deficits not due to any of following:

- Other central nervous system conditions that cause progressive deficits in memory and cognition (e.g., cerebrovascular disease, Parkinson's disease, Huntington's disease, subdural hematoma, normal-pressure hydrocephalus, brain tumor)
- Systemic conditions that are known to cause dementia (e.g., hypothyroidism, vitamin B12 or folic acid deficiency, niacin deficiency, hypercalcemia, neurosyphilis, HIV infection)
- Substance-induced conditions

E. The deficits not occurring exclusively during the course of a delirium

F. The disturbance not better accounted for by another Axis I disorder (e.g., Major Depressive Disorder, Schizophrenia)

*Dementia of the Vascular Type*

A. The development of multiple cognitive deficits manifested by both:

- Memory impairment (impaired ability to learn new information or to recall previously learned information)
- One (or more) of the following cognitive disturbances:
  - Aphasia (language disturbance)
  - Apraxia (impaired ability to carry out motor activities despite intact motor function)
  - Agnosia (failure to recognize or identify objects despite sensory function)
  - Disturbance in executive functioning (i.e., planning, organizing, sequencing, abstracting)

B. Significant impairment in social or occupational functioning and a significant decline from a previous level of functioning resulting from cognitive deficits

*(cont.)*

## BOX 16-1: DIAGNOSTIC CRITERIA (*CONT.*)

C. Cerebrovascular disease as the etiology evidenced by focal neurological signs and symptoms or laboratory findings

D. Deficits not occurring exclusively during course of delirium

*Dementia With Lewy Bodies*

A. Development of multiple cognitive deficits manifested by both:

- Memory impairment
- One or more of the following: aphasia, apraxia, agnosia, or disturbance in executive functioning

B. Cognitive deficits causing significant occupational or social impairment and respresenting significant decline in functioning

C. Evidence from history, physical examination, or laboratory testing that disturbance is a direct physiological consequence of a general medication condition other than Alzheimer's disease or cerebrovascular disease

D. Deficits not occurring exclusively during the course of delirium

*Frontotemporal Dementia*

A. Dementia judged to be a direct pathophysiological result of Pick's disease

- Changes in personality early on with deterioration in social skills, emotional blunting, behavioral disinhibition, and language abnromalities
- Memory difficulties, apraxia, and other features occurring later
- Primitive reflexes possibly prominent
- Apathy or extreme agitation

*From the Diagnostic and Statistical Manual of Mental Disorders, Fourth Edition, Text Revision, Copyright © 2000, American Psychiatric Association.*

## TABLE 16-1: COMMON CLINICAL FEATURES OF DEMENTIA

| CLINICAL FEATURE | MANIFESTATIONS |
|---|---|
| Personality changes | Apathy<br>Loss of interest<br>Decreased control over one's behavior<br>Increased self-absorption<br>Apparent selfishness, with lack of ability to consider the needs of others |
| Cognitive changes | Memory loss of recent events<br>Confabulation to make up what is forgotten<br>Difficulty learning new things<br>Poor judgment<br>Deterioration of written and verbal language skills<br>Loss of the concept of time |
| Functional changes | Decreased ability to carry out skills and activities of daily living<br>Inability to put steps in correct sequence to get job done despite knowing what he or she wants to do |
| Altered stress threshold | Decreased ability to tolerate stress<br>Easy fatigue<br>Prone to anger<br>Irritation or becoming overwhelmed with situations that were not a problem previously; becoming more problematic and evident as disease progresses |

## BOX 16-2: CAUSES OF DELIRIUM

- Dehydration
- Sensory impairment
- Metabolic disorders
- Pain
- Emotional distress
- Social isolation
- Electrolyte imbalance
- Dementia
- Sleep deprivation
- Neurological conditions
- Severe medical illness
  - Diabetes mellitus
  - Myocardial infarction
  - Thyroid crisis
  - Liver or renal failure
- Anesthetic exposure
- Infections
- Hypoxia
- Fever
- Hypothermia
- Trauma
- Surgery
- Drugs and medications

## BOX 16-3: *DSM-IV-TR* CLASSIFICATION OF DEMENTIA

- Dementia of the Alzheimer's type (DAT)
- Lewy body disease (LBD)
- Vascular dementia
- Frontotemporal dementia (FTD)
- Dementia due to Parkinson's disease
- Dementia due to Huntington's disease
- Creutzfeldt-Jacob disease (CJD)
- Substance-induced persisting dementia
- Dementia due to other general medical conditions
- Dementia due to human immunodeficiency virus (HIV)
- Dementia due to multiple etiologies
- Dementia not otherwise specified

In extreme cases, delirium represents a medical emergency and carries a high morbidity and increased mortality. In some cases, it may result in a permanent cognitive impairment (Adamis et al., 2007). Therefore, a sudden onset of delirium in an otherwise healthy individual may indicate an underlying life-threatening condition.

## Dementia

Dementia is an umbrella term used to describe various conditions that cause brain cells to die, leading to a progressive deterioration in memory and the ability to carry out everyday activities such as washing, dressing, eating, and communicating. Dementia may also affect a person's mood and personality.

Many diseases can result in dementia. Twelve different types of dementia are identified by the current classification of the *DSM-IV-TR* and are listed in **Box 16-3**. However, four of these account for almost 90% of cases, with the most common being dementia of the Alzheimer's type, accounting for over half of all the cases of dementia encountered in clinical practice.

### Dementia of the Alzheimer's Type (DAT)

Dementia of the Alzheimer's type is a progressive neurological condition characterized by the build up of proteins in the brain called "plaques" and "tangles." These proteins gradually damage and eventually destroy the nerve cells. Subsequently, it becomes more and more difficult to remember and to perform higher cognitive functions such as reasoning and use of language. The loss of memory of recent events may be one of the first difficulties noticed. The person may also become disorientated, be at a loss for a word when speaking, and have increasing difficulty with simple daily tasks such as using the telephone, preparing meals, or managing money.

Although the early signs and symptoms of DAT may vary from person to person, increasing memory loss over time is often the first noticeable symptom. Other common signs include getting stuck for words or having language difficulties; forgetting things (names, dates, places, and people); loss of interest in things of interest previously; difficulty in solving problems or in performing everyday tasks; misplacing things; poor or decreased judgment; changes in mood, behavior, and overall personality; and becoming easily disorientated, even in familiar surroundings.

> *Although signs and symptoms may vary in patients with dementia of the Alzheimer's type, often progressive memory loss is noticed first.*

## Dementia With Lewy Bodies

Dementia with Lewy bodies, which accounts for approximately 20% of all causes of dementia, is characterized by progressive decline in cognitive functioning; drowsiness; lethargy; lengthy periods of time spent staring into space; disorganized speech; visual hallucinations, delusions; and motor symptoms including muscle rigidity and the loss of spontaneous movement. These latter features may result in falls. Depression is also common. This type of dementia results from the build-up of Lewy bodies (accumulated bits of alpha synuclein protein) inside the nuclei of neurons in areas of the brain that control particular aspects of memory and movement. While the reasons for this build up are unknown, what is known is that alpha-synuclein accumulation is also linked to Parkinson's disease (another movement disorder). People with dementia with Lewy bodies usually have no known family history of the disease. Average survival after the time of diagnosis is about 8 years, with progressively increasing disability (National Institute of Neurological Disorders and Stroke [NINDS], 2010a).

## Dementia of the Vascular Type

Dementia of the vascular type, also called vascular dementia, is caused by multiple mini strokes that lead to a disruption in blood flow to the brain. This disruption results in damaged brain tissue and subsequent loss of function. Some of these strokes may occur without noticeable clinical symptoms and hence are often termed "silent strokes." The onset of dementia of the vascular type is insidious. Thus, the person experiencing these mini strokes is unlikely to know that anything is wrong initially. With time, and as more areas of the brain are damaged and more small blood vessels are blocked, the symptoms become apparent. In some instances, however, the onset of symptoms may be sudden and may progress in a stepwise fashion, unlike the downward linear progression of dementia of Alzheimer's type. Common presenting symptoms include confusion, short-term memory deficits; wandering, getting lost in familiar places; rapid, shuffling gait; loss of bladder or bowel control; laughing or crying inappropriately; difficulty following instructions; and problems counting money and making monetary transactions. Unfortunately, the prognosis for those who have dementia of the vascular type is generally poor, thus emphasizing the importance of early life prevention. While some people may appear to improve for short periods, resulting in episodes of lucidity, this is often followed by further decline when the individual has another stroke, thus the stepwise nature of the disease progression (NINDS, 2010b). Typically, individuals die from one of these strokes or from associated heart disease. Thus, life expectancy with this type of dementia is typically shorter than for other forms of dementia.

## Frontotemporal Dementia

Frontotemporal dementia is characterized by changes in the frontal and temporal lobes of the brain, that control reasoning, personality, social behavior, and speech. This type of dementia was originally known as Pick's disease because of the intracytoplasmic inclusions (Pick bodies) that are found in the neurons of those with the disease. The term Pick's disease is now more commonly used in discussing the specific pathology involved in the clinical syndrome now known as frontotemporal lobar degeneration. Typically, a person with this type of dementia presents with two groups of symptoms: behavioral changes and problems with language. The behaviors involved are often anti-social in nature, including loss of social tact, inappropriate sexual behavior, lack of empathy, or lack of insight. Language problems include difficulty understanding speech or articulating what one wants to say. Frontotemporal dementia has a strong genetic component and runs in families (NINDS, 2010c). Unlike other major dementias, memory remains intact.

> *Frontotemporal dementia is manifested by changes in behavior and language.*

## ETIOLOGY

The majority of research addressing delirium and dementia focuses on the neurobiological influences for the disease. As stated earlier, delirium almost always results from a physiological disturbance that is a direct result of an underlying general medical condition. The neurobiological influences for the development of dementia of the Alzheimer's type are presented here.

### Neurobiological Influences

The progressive brain dysfunction that characterizes dementia of the Alzheimer's type occurs in a staged biological sequence beginning with neuronal injury, leading to synaptic failure, and, in time, neuronal death (Silvestrelli et al., 2006). Initially, NEUROFIBRILLARY TANGLES occur at various parts of the cerebral cortex. These tangles are thick clots of protein which reside inside damaged neurons and are made from a protein called tau ($\tau$). They spread in a sequential and generally predictable manner to other parts of the cortex.

The neurofibrils become entangled for an as yet unknown reason. In general, the denser these filaments are, the more severe the dementia is (Cummings, 2004).

The neurofibrillary tangle process typically begins in the limbic system, an area of the brain concerned with emotion and memory storage. The hippocampus, one part of the limbic system, is primarily involved in the storage of recent memories, which may explain why recent memory loss is a common feature of this type of dementia. Moreover, damage to the locus ceruleus and associated parts of the limbic system may help explain why depression is a common feature of the disease. Deterioration of long-term memory tends to be delayed probably because these memories are stored in a number of areas of the brain (Garand, Buckwalter, & Hall, 2000).

Later in the disease another major pathological feature appears. Cerebral beta-amyloid plaques (Aβ) form on the outside of dead and damaged neurons initially in poorly myelinated areas of the cortex. The plaques consist of fragments of dying cells mixed with beta-amyloid protein. It appears that Aβ plaque enters the mitochondria of affected neurons wherein it interacts with a number of enzymes resulting in cell death. Some evidence suggests that inflammation around these Aβ plaques spreads to other neurons in the vicinity, leading to their destruction (Cummings, 2004). Beta-amyloid protein is made from amyloid precursor protein (APP), which is coded on chromosome 21. Individuals with Down's syndrome have an extra copy of this chromosome, thus increasing their risk of developing dementia. Indeed, almost three quarters of people with this condition who are over age 60 have dementia.

A second protein, apolipoprotein E (Apo-E), is also implicated in the pathology of dementia of the Alzheimer's type. Apo-E plays a role in the transportation of cholesterol in the brain. Among the effects of Apo-E is the deposition of cerebral amyloid in the brain. Certain subtypes of Apo-E, specifically Apo-E3 and Apo-E4, have been found to increase the risk of dementia. However, Apo-E2 has been shown to decrease the risk.

A further feature of the etiology of dementia of the Alzheimer's type involves a deficiency of the neurotransmitter, acetylcholine (ACh), first discovered in the 1970s. ACh is manufactured in the brain from choline and acetyl coenzyme A in the presence of the enzyme choline-acetyl transferase (ChAT). Another enzyme, cholinesterase (ChE), "mops up" excess ACh at the synapse after neurotransmission has occurred. Studies have shown a deficiency in both ACh and ChAT and an excess

of ChE in people with dementia of the Alzheimer's type. This has become known as the "cholinergic hypothesis." Essentially, the cholinergic hypothesis suggests that "cognitive, functional, and behavioral dysfunction associated with DAT may be caused by an inability to transmit nerve cell impulses across cholinergic synapses (Silvestrelli et al., 2006, p. 150). ACh increases attention span and facilitates learning. Furthermore, depletion of ACh has also been shown to result in memory impairment.

While other neurotransmitters are also implicated in the etiology of Alzheimer's, the cholinergic hypothesis has been most prominent in this area of research. Other neurotransmitters have been studied. For example, serotonin (5-HT) is also decreased in patients with dementia of the Alzheimer's type, leading to anxiety, agitation, and depression. Low levels of dopamine have also been observed, which may result in problems with mobility, psychosis, and apathy (Garand, Buckwalter, & Hall, 2000). In time, the destructive processes involved in this type of dementia spread to all parts of the brain resulting in a wide variety of symptoms. In later stages of the disease, gross anatomical changes such as brain atrophy, enlarged ventricles, and widened sulky become apparent using neuroimaging techniques.

> *Pathologic changes involved with dementia of the Alzheimer's type include neurofibrillary tangles, beta-amyloid plaques, and apolipoprotein E. Acetylcholine deficiency, referred to as the cholinergic hypothesis, is also implicated in the etiology of dementia of the Alzheimer's type. Other neurotransmitters, such as a deficiency of serotonin and dopamine also may be involved.*

## TREATMENT OPTIONS

Various treatment options are available for patients with cognitive disorders, specifically dementia. These include but are not limited to: psychopharmacology, reality orientation, validation therapy, reminiscence therapy, person-centered care, the enriched model of dementia, and the progressively lowered stress threshold model. The focus of the discussion here is on dementia of the Alzheimer's type. **Table 16-2** summarizes the major treatment options for the other types of dementia.

Treatment for delirium differs somewhat from that for dementia. With delirium, the main approach to treatment is the rapid identification and elimination or management of the cause, as well as symptomatic treatment until the person's condition stabilizes. In cases where the person's behavior is very disturbed, a low-dose antipsychotic or a benzodiazepine is useful in the short-term management of psychosis associated with delirium (Boyle & Hands, 2009). In addition, management also involves a low stimulus environment, adequate hydration, normalization of the sleep-wake cycle, and the use of reality orientation.

## Psychopharmacology

Currently, there is no known cure for dementia of the Alzheimer's type or other related dementias. However, some drugs have been developed that have been shown to slow the progression of the disease.

### Cholinesterase Inhibitors

Most of the drugs that have been approved for clinical practice focus on the cholinergic hypothesis. They attempt to boost the remaining activity at cholinergic synapses. While a number of agents have the ability to do this, only cholinesterase inhibitors are currently licensed for use. These drugs delay the degradation of acetylcholine at the synapse, theoretically prolonging its effect at this site and thus augmenting neurotransmission. Three such drugs are currently in use: donepezil (Aricept), rivastigmine (Exelon), and galantamine (Reminyl). These drugs, listed in **Drug Summary 16-1**, are used mainly in patients with mild to moderate DAT. While these drugs may enhance cognitive functioning in some patients, they do not alter the overall course of the disease.

A fourth drug, memantine (Ebixa), is an N-methyl d-aspartate (NMDA) antagonist. NMDA receptor antagonists are a class of drugs that work to inhibit the action of the NMDA receptor. This drug has been developed for the treatment of people with moderate to severe dementia. It acts with a novel mechanism of action that targets glutamate, the principal excitatory neurotransmitter in the brain. Excessive activity of this neurotransmitter (excitotoxicity) has been shown to result in neuronal damage, neuronal cell death, and cognitive dysfunction. The drug

> *Cholinesterase inhibitors are used to treat dementia of the Alzheimer's type. These agents do not cure the disease; rather, they are believed to help slow the progression of cognitive decline.*

| TABLE 16-2: TREATMENT FOR DEMENTIAS OTHER THAN DEMENTIA OF THE ALZHEIMER'S TYPE | |
|---|---|
| **TYPE OF DEMENTIA** | **TREATMENT OPTIONS** |
| Dementia of Lewy bodies | Management of psychiatric, behavioral, and motor symptoms |
| | Acetylcholinesterase inhibitors (donepezil and rivastigmine) for cognitive symptoms; also helpful for psychiatric and motor symptoms |
| | Antipsychotic agents for hallucinatory symptoms are avoided due to risk of neuroleptic sensitivity worsening motor symptoms (Walling, 2004) |
| Dementia of the vascular type | Alleviation of symptoms |
| | Prevention of future mini strokes through dietary and lifestyle measures |
| | – Smoking cessation |
| | – Hypertension control |
| | – Cholesterol lowering |
| | – Diabetes management |
| | – Regular exercise |
| | Maintenance of healthy body weight (Nazarko, 2006) |
| Frontotemporal dementia | Behavior modification (some success) |
| | Antidepressant agents to manage some behavioral symptoms |

## DRUG SUMMARY 16-1:
## DRUGS USED TO TREAT DEMENTIAS

| DRUG | IMPLICATIONS FOR NURSING CARE |
|---|---|
| **CHOLINESTERASE INHIBITORS** | |
| **donepezil (Aricept)** | Explain to the patient and family that the drug does not cure the disorder but rather works to control the symptoms |
| **rivastigmine (Exelon)** | Emphasize the need to take the drug as prescribed; for example, advise the patient and family to administer donepezil at bedtime or advise the patient and family to take or give rivastigmine or galantamine in the morning and evening with food |
| **galantamine (Reminyl)** | Instruct the patient and family about dosage increases that may be necessary to promote maximum effectiveness |
| | Assist the patient and family with measures to combat nausea and vomiting |
| | Encourage the patient and family to check with the health care provider before taking any over-the-counter medications for colds or sleep that may interact with the drug |
| | Work with the patient and family on ways to promote optimal cognitive function within the limits of the patient's disease |
| | Emphasize that changes in cognition function are often subtle |
| **NMDA ANTAGONIST** | |
| **memantine (Ebixia)** | Explain to the patient and family that the drug does not cure the disorder but rather works to control the symptoms |
| | Emphasize the need to take the drug as prescribed |
| | Encourage the patient and family to check with the health care provider before taking any over-the-counter medications or herbal preparations as these may interact with the drug |
| | Work with the patient and family on ways to promote optimal cognitive function within the limits of the patient's disease |
| | Instruct the patient and family in how to use oral solution form |

acts to reduce this glutamatergic excitotoxicity. Recent research also suggests that memantine diminishes the toxic effects of Aβ and that it may also inhibit its production (Silvestrelli et al., 2006).

## Antioxidants

Free radicals are known to play a role in the aging process and, in particular, have been implicated in the etiology of some forms of dementia, including dementia of the Alzheimer's type. Antioxidants act as free radical scavengers and, among other things, appear to protect neurons from the damaging effects of Aβ. Vitamin C (ascorbic acid) and melatonin are powerful natural antioxidants.

## Hormone Replacement Therapy

The incidence of dementia of the Alzheimer's type is particularly low in postmenopausal women who take estrogen. Therefore, some authorities recommend estrogen therapy as a protective mechanism against this type of dementia.

## Non-Steroidal Anti-Inflammatory Drugs (NSAIDs)

Epidemiological evidence suggests that people who are on long-term NSAID treatment, such as ibuprofen and naproxen sodium, seem to be protected in some way from developing dementia of the Alzheimer's type. It may be that NSAIDs, particularly those that target cyclooxygenase-1, inhibit inflammation around beta-amyloid plaques, thus preventing this inflammatory process from affecting other neurons in the vicinity (Youdim & Buccafusco, 2005).

## Lipid-Lowering Agents

Cholesterol has been implicated in the etiology of both dementia of the Alzheimer's type and vascular dementia for many years now. The understanding of the role of *APO-E* further reinforces this belief. The *APO-E* gene provides instructions for making a protein called apolipoprotein E. This protein combines with fats (lipids) in the body to form molecules called lipoproteins. As a result, drugs such as statins and other cholesterol-lowering agents have become a major component of therapy as they have been shown to decrease the risk of developing dementia of the Alzheimer's type.

## Other Agents

In addition to the above, the benefits of omega-3 fish oil, lecithin for those taking niacin, selegiline, and dehydroepiandrosterone (DHEA), to name but a few, are now established and are recommended by some authorities as agents for the prevention and treatment of dementia.

Some interesting research is underway on the potential benefits of anti-amyloid pharmacotherapies, immunotherapy, substances that target mitochondrial dysfunction, and anti-apoptosis compounds.

## Herbal Remedies

For millennia, traditional herbal medicine has offered many plant-based remedies to treat age-related conditions including dementias. Some of these have been used with varying levels of success. While the pharmacology underpinning of many of these compounds has yet to be established, some compounds have been researched and their pharmacology has been validated. However, little evidence is available at the present time about their clinical application and utility. Nevertheless, a few exceptions exist, including ginkgo biloba extracts, some species of the herb sage (salvia), and the plant extracts galanthamine and huperazine A. Many of these extracts inhibit cholinesterase and are antioxidant in nature. Ginko biloba enhances cerebral circulation.

## Reality Orientation

**REALITY ORIENTATION** is a technique used to improve the quality of life of confused older adults by assisting them to gain a more accurate understanding of their surroundings. In this approach, people who are confused are regularly presented with information about time, place, and person in an effort to orientate them to the here and now. It is based on the assumption that people who are disorientated can return to the present if given sufficient information (Spector et al., 2000). The technique often entails the use of signs on bathroom and bedroom doors, for example, or the use of a reality orientation board displaying large-faced clocks and notices indicating the day, date, year, and so on. In addition, staff using this approach consistently orient the confused individual to his or her surroundings. Evidence supporting the benefits of this therapy for people with dementia is mixed, however. Some suggest that it contradicts the person's "reality" and thus increases frustration, anxiety, and anger. Consequently, it can erode the person's self-esteem and can make the individual feel as if he or she is constantly being tested (Hall & Buckwalter, 1999). One view is that reality orientation works well with people who are temporarily confused, such as those who are suffering from delirium or concussion, or who are experiencing disorientation as a result of relocation. However, it is of limited utility in dementia except perhaps in the early stages of the disease (Smith & Buckwalter, 2005).

## Validation Therapy

**VALIDATION THERAPY** is one of the most popular psycho-social interventions for people with dementia. It is based on a number of principles, including the affirmation of the person's feelings and the adoption of a nonjudgemental approach on the part of the caregiver. It was developed by Feil in the 1960s (Feil, 1967) and four stages of cognitive impairment are featured in her work: malorientation, time confusion, repetitive motion, and vegetation (Feil, 1992). Feil proposes that the disorientation observed in many people with dementia is a defense mechanism that may be a solution to past conflicts in their lives. Essentially, according to the theory, the person with dementia retreats into the past to resolve painful emotions. Therefore, validating the person's reality can assist them in resolving some of these past conflicts. Thus, the emphasis is on going with the person to his or her reality (Feil, 1993). This would mean allowing the person to express emotions such as anger or sadness and then validating that emotion.

Traditionally, many lay and professional caregivers have been taught to use principles of reality orientation. However, some such as Hall and Buckwalter (1999) argue that validation therapy principles are more useful. The person with dementia has a deteriorating short-term memory. Thus, it is difficult if not impossible for them to be in the here and now. Recent memories are not as firmly established in the brain. Once the dementia has started to progress, it becomes increasingly difficult for the person to remember what he or she have just been told or what has happened in the immediate past because the person no longer has the ability to retain this information. Long-term memories, on the other hand, appear to be stored in a number of places in the brain and are likely to survive longer after the dementia has been established. Hence, the person with dementia is often able to talk at length and in great detail about events that occurred in the distant past. If reality orientation principles are used, the person with dementia are likely to fail or be unsuccessful because the brain no longer has the capacity to allow him or her to remember enough about the present. It cannot adequately store memories of the present and recent events. This may lead to anxiety and frustration and, consequently may result in deterioration of behavior. On the other hand, because people with dementia generally have a more intact long-term memory, they can remain competent and be successful if caregivers go with them to "their reality" through the use of reminiscence therapies, for example. While the experience can be "validating," reminiscence therapy is separate from validation therapy.

> *Validation therapy focuses on the premise that past conflicts can be resolved by validating the person's reality.*

## Reminiscence Therapy

**REMINISCENCE THERAPY** involves the discussion of past activities, events, and experiences, with another person or group of people. Aids such as videos, pictures, archives, and life story books often are used (Woods et al., 2005). It can be formal or informal. Formal reminiscence is a structured activity. The caregiver schedules a reminiscence session in which the patient is prompted to recollect past events and memories. Informal reminiscence, on the other hand, is opportunistic. The caregiver engages the patient in discussion of past events or experiences, for example, after watching an old film or when the caregiver discovers the patient is perusing old family photographs (Hong et al., 2005). A systematic review of studies on reminiscence therapy (Woods et al., 2005) revealed improvements in cognition and mood four to six weeks after treatment, and lower caregiver strain when caregivers participated in a reminiscence group with their relative. Improvements in functional capacity also were noted.

> *Reminiscence therapy can be formal, using a structured activity, or informal, using a specific event to stimulate discussion of past events.*

## Person-Centered Care

The term person-centered care is used in many different contexts in health care and can mean different things to different people. Some people equate it to the individualization of care, whereas others see it as a philosophical approach with a particular value base. Still others still see it as a set of techniques to assist those who work with people with dementia (Brooker & Surr, 2005). Regardless of the definition, person-centered care is seen as an approach to delivering high-quality care. However, it can only do so if the recipient of care is placed at the heart of the care agenda

(Edvardsson, Winblad, & Sandman, 2008). The Bradford Dementia Group, established in 1992, is a multi-disciplinary, multi-professional group committed to making a difference to policy and practice in dementia care, through excellence in research, education, and training. They offer a comprehensive definition of person-centered care as it relates to caring for people with dementia. This definition emphasizes "respecting and valuing the individual as a full member of society" and recognizing that they have "all the rights of citizenship." It focuses on rooting out discriminatory practices against people with dementia and their caregivers and on individualizing a plan of care that "is in tune with people's changing needs giving increasing compensation and reassurance as cognitive disability increases." The need to try to understand the perspective of the person with dementia and the importance of providing a supportive social psychology (explained in the following) are also enshrined in the definition, as these are key to ensuring that the person can "live a life where they can experience relative well-being" (Brooker & Surr, 2005, p.13).

A number of models exist that help one understand key aspects of dementia from a psychodynamic perspective and help to ensure that the care of the person with dementia is person centered. In particular, these models help explain many of the behaviors in dementia, emphasizing that these behaviors are not just a result of the person's neurological impairment. Two such models are Kitwood's Enriched Model of Dementia and the Progressively Lowered Stress Threshold (PLST) Model.

## Kitwood's Enriched Model of Dementia

Kitwood's **ENRICHED MODEL OF DEMENTIA** acknowledges that the primary cause of problems for the person with dementia stems from the person's neurological impairment. It also argues that other factors play a role in determining how the person with dementia lives with his or her illness. These factors include the person's level of health and physical fitness, life history, personality, and social psychology. The model suggests that it is the complex interplay between these factors plus the person's degree of neurological impairment that determines how dementia affects the way the person lives.

The inspiration for the model arose from Kitwood's observation that some people with dementia who had considerable neurological impairment seemed to function better and have a better quality of life than others who had a lesser degree of neurological impairment. Kitwood hypothesized that the social and psychological environment in which the person with dementia lives could be supportive or damaging to his or her well-being. He used the term "**MALIGNANT SOCIAL PSYCHOLOGY**" to describe the damaging effects of the negative attitudes and prejudices of other people on someone's personhood. He uses an opposite term "**POSITIVE PERSON WORK**," to describe how one could uphold the personhood of an individual with dementia. These are outlined in **Table 16-3**. The goal when working with this model is to maximize interventions that incorporate aspects of positive person work and minimize those that lead to malignant social psychology.

| TABLE 16-3: FACTORS THAT SUPPORT OR DENY PERSONHOOD | |
|---|---|
| TYPES OF MALIGNANT SOCIAL PSYCHOLOGY | TYPES OF POSITIVE PERSON WORK |
| • Intimidation<br>• Withholding<br>• Outpacing<br>• Infatilization<br>• Labeling<br>• Disparagement<br>• Accusation<br>• Treachery<br>• Invalidation<br>• Disempowerment<br>• Imposition<br>• Disruption<br>• Objectification<br>• Stigmatization<br>• Ignoring<br>• Banishment<br>• Mockery | • Warmth<br>• Holding<br>• Relaxed pace<br>• Respect<br>• Acceptance<br>• Celebration<br>• Acknowledgment<br>• Genuineness<br>• Validation<br>• Empowerment<br>• Facilitation<br>• Enabling<br>• Collaboration<br>• Recognition<br>• Including<br>• Belonging<br>• Fun |

*From Brooker, D. (2007) Person centred dementia care: Making services better. London, Jessica Kingsley Publications.*

> *The Enriched Model of Dementia focuses on minimizing the damaging negative social and psychological environment (termed "malignant social psychology") and maximizing the supportive aspects (termed "positive person work").*

## The Progressively Lowered Stress Threshold (PLST) Model

The **PROGRESSIVELY LOWERED STRESS THRESHOLD (PLST)** Model proposes that a person has a stress threshold firmly established by adulthood but that can be temporarily altered during times of illness, or permanently altered during episodes of brain damage such as in dementia. Normally, adults have a relatively high threshold to stress. People with dementia, however, have a diminished ability to interact with their environment. They find things in their environment confusing because their brain is no longer able to process information accurately. Consequently, they have a heightened potential for anxiety and dysfunctional behavior. As a result, their stress threshold is lower. The model proposes that "persons with dementia need environmental conditions modified as they experience progressive cognitive decline so that cues can be more easily processed and are thus less stressful" (Smith, Gerdner, Hall, & Buckwalter, 2004, p. 1756).

The principles underpinning this model have been adapted to form the PLST intervention for lay caregivers. The main focus is on the caregiver modifying the home environment to accommodate the care recipient's diminishing stress threshold. Some of the key stressors identified by the model are fatigue; multiple competing stimuli or too many things going on at once (such as eating dinner, receiving medicines, background music playing, and visitors calling all at once); illness; side effects of medicines; and changes in caregiver, routine, or environment. The model recommends that caregivers:

- Establish simple routines and stick to them
- Assess stressors in the person's environment on an on-going basis
- Eliminate or modify environmental stressors to make the world appear less stressful

According to this model the caregiver needs to take immediate action if the patient exhibits key warning signs indicating that he or she is reaching the stress threshold. These signs include anxiety, agitation, and avoidance or escape behaviors. Actions to initiate include promoting rest, decreasing stimuli (such as noise, too many people, television, or radio), and assessing for and eliminating internal stressors such as hunger, pain, or constipation.

The PLST intervention has been shown to significantly benefit individuals with dementia and their family caregivers. Findings reveal improved patient behavior (Gerdner, Buckwalter, & Reed, 2002); reduced caregiver depression (Buckwalter et al., 1999); decreased caregiver burden, increased caregiver satisfaction (Stolley, Reed, & Buckwalter, 2002); and improved caregiver immune function (Garand et al., 2002). The PLST intervention is currently being adapted for delivery to groups of family caregivers (Tyrrell, 2011). Although yet incomplete, tentative findings indicate that family caregivers are satisfied with the dementia-specific information they are given in the group intervention. In addition, they find the care strategies to be logical and easy to implement when caring for the family member with dementia. Meeting with other family caregivers is being shown to be both a source of support and a valuable social outlet.

> *A person with dementia experiences a diminished stress threshold. The PLST Model focuses on modifying the environment to reduce stress for the patient with dementia who is nearing his or her stress threshold.*

## APPLYING THE NURSING PROCESS FROM AN INTERPERSONAL PERSPECTIVE

Patients with cognitive disorders may be seen in a variety of settings, such as acute care settings, day hospitalization programs, community and out-patient centers, long-term care facilities, and the home. Many individuals have underlying medical co-morbidities such as diabetes or cardiovascular or respiratory disorders. As a result, patients often can be encountered in general medical facilities, emergency departments, and specialty clinics. Therefore, nurses need a firm understanding of the nursing process that integrates the interpersonal process when caring for patients with cognitive disorders. The information provided here focuses on the patient with dementia. **Plan of Care 16-1** provides an example for a patient with a cognitive disorder.

### PLAN OF CARE 16-1:
### THE PATIENT WITH A COGNITIVE DISORDER

**NURSING DIAGNOSIS:** Chronic confusion; related to neurological changes; manifested by memory impairment, disorganized thinking, and impaired judgment

**OUTCOME IDENTIFICATION:** Patient will demonstrate adequate level of orientation and mental function within the limits of the disorder

| INTERVENTION | RATIONALE |
|---|---|
| Assess patient's neurological status | Assessing neurological status provides information about the degree and extent of the patient's level of confusion |
| Approach the patient calmly and from the front; address the patient by name; speak directly to the patient using a normal tone of voice | Approaching the patient calmly, from the front, and speaking directly to the patient help the patient to focus on the nurse and what is being said. Calling the patient by name helps to reorient the patient |
| Orient the patient to person, place, and time; reinforce and repeat information as necessary | Orienting the patient and reinforcing the information helps to refocus and reorient the patient |
| Use environmental cues as appropriate; provide cues to current events, seasons, locations, and names; consider using symbols instead of written signs for key locations such as the bathroom | Using cues—whether words or symbols—helps stimulate the patient's memory and assists in reorienting the patient |
| Provide a low-stimulus environment; eliminate competing stimuli; keep decorative changes in the home to a minimum | Controlling environmental stimuli promotes feelings of security and prevents overwhelming the patient, which could lead to increased anxiety and agitation |
| Provide ample time for responding to questions; do not pressure the patient to respond or assume that no response indicates lack of understanding | Allowing for ample time in responding is necessary because of the patient's diminished cognitive ability; pressuring can lead to frustration and possible agitation |
| Use simple, straightforward language when communicating with the patient; break tasks and activities down into simple steps | Using simple language and simple steps prevents overwhelming the patient, thus minimizing frustration and stress |
| Administer prescribed medications for symptomatic control | Administering medication such as that for Alzheimer's disease can slow the progression of the disease; other medications may be needed to address agitation or inability to sleep |

*(cont.)*

**PLAN OF CARE 16-1: (*CONT.*)**
**THE PATIENT WITH A COGNITIVE DISORDER**

**NURSING DIAGNOSIS:** Risk for injury; related to cognitive impairment, impaired judgment, and wandering behavior

**OUTCOME IDENTIFICATION:** Patient will remain free of harm

| INTERVENTION | RATIONALE |
|---|---|
| Institute safety measures and fall precautions | Instituting safety measures reduces the risk of injury and falls |
| Arrange the environment so that it is free of obstacles and allows for ease of access and ambulation | Ensuring the environment is free of obstacles reduces the risk for injury from falls |
| Work with patient and family to address potential hazards in the home, such as removing loose rugs, putting locks on windows and/or doors, adjusting the thermostat on the water heater, putting safety guards on electrical outlets, and removing knobs from stove and oven | Identifying potential hazards allows for action to reduce possible effects |
| Teach family members about ways to help reorient the patient; suggest the use of environmental cues | Teaching the family about ways to help the patient fosters participation in care |
| Encourage family to maintain consistency in caregivers and routines as much as possible | Maintaining consistency helps promote feelings of comfort and familiarity and decrease stimulation |
| Suggest the use of protective or adaptive devices if the patient wanders; suggest providing boundaries such as tape on the floor in front of an exit or disguising exit with drapes or wall hangings | Using protective or adaptive devices can alert the family to the patient's movement; using boundaries acts as cues to stall the patient's movement |
| Ensure that emergency telephone numbers are readily available | Ensuring ready access to phone numbers is crucial if an emergency arises |

*(cont.)*

**PLAN OF CARE 16-1:** (*CONT.*)
**THE PATIENT WITH A COGNITIVE DISORDER**

**NURSING DIAGNOSIS:** Risk for caregiver role strain; related to progression of the disease and increased care needs/demands of client

**OUTCOME IDENTIFICATION:** Caregiver will verbalize a need for help in providing care to patient to maintain own health and well-being

| INTERVENTION | RATIONALE |
|---|---|
| Assess the level of care required and the caregiver's knowledge and ability to provide care | Assessing the level of care needed and the caregiver's ability to provide that level of care provides a baseline for individualizing interventions |
| Assist the caregiver in identifying areas of needed help or support | Identifying areas of need ensures provision of appropriate services |
| Encourage the caregiver to ask for help; investigate sources for help as appropriate, such as other family members, friends, neighbors, church or organization members; provide emotional support | Determining potential sources for support enhances the chances that the caregiver will use them |
| Teach the caregiver how to manage stress and maintain physical and mental well-being; encourage the caregiver to take breaks periodically to address personal care needs | Managing stress and taking periodic breaks help to reduce anxiety and stress associated with caregiving |
| Provide positive feedback and emotional support for caregiving activities | Providing support and positive feedback promotes feelings of accomplishment and positive self-esteem even if setbacks occur |
| Refer the patient and caregiver for community support services as appropriate; arrange for respite care as indicated | Arranging for additional support and/or respite care provides time for the caregiver to recover without feeling guilty and minimizes the risk for social isolation from full-time caregiving activities |

*From Nursing Diagnosis – Definitions and Classifications 2009 – 2011. Copyright © 2011 by NANDA International. Use by arrangement with Blackwell Publishing Limited, a company of John Wiley & Sons, Inc.*

## Strategies for Optimal Assessment: Therapeutic Use of Self

Therapeutic use of self is recognized as an important therapeutic tool and a core skill of the psychiatric-mental health nurse. According to Mosey (1986), this entails "the use of oneself in such a way that one becomes an effective tool in the evaluation and intervention process" (p. 199). It involves a planned interaction with another person to alleviate fear or anxiety, provide reassurance, obtain necessary information, provide information, give advice, and assist the other individual to gain more appreciation, more expression, and more functional use of his or her latent inner resources.

At the onset of the relationship, the nurse and patient meet for the first time. Due to the cognitive difficulties involved with dementia, in most cases the nurse will also be developing the relationship with the patient's family members or caregivers. Regardless of who is involved, all are strangers to each other. The nurse can also be viewed as an authority figure for the patient. The nurse is responsible for beginning to establish trust and rapport with the patient and family. This can be done by showing concern, empathy, and honesty. Pay attention to verbal and nonverbal cues and use therapeutic verbal techniques. Be alert to the possible issues and problems associated with patients experiencing a cognitive disorder and the impact on their families. **Consumer Perspective 16-1** provides insight from the wife of a patient with dementia of the Alzheimer's type.

### Self-Awareness

To develop an effective therapeutic relationship, the nurse also must be self-aware of attitudes, beliefs, prejudices, or philosophical stances that could interfere in the relationship with a patient (Edwards & Bess, 1998). Working with a patient with dementia can be frustrating due to the demand for time. During a busy shift, having someone follow you around asking the same questions over and over can be taxing. The nurse needs to monitor his or her own frustration level and ask for assistance when needed. The nurse also needs to monitor his or her own feelings of transference if someone in his or her own family is also suffering from dementia.

### Environmental Management

Providing a safe, comfortable environment with minimal external stimulation is necessary to establish an atmosphere of trust. Minimizing stimulation and external stressors also are key to preventing the patient from becoming overwhelmed.

---

**CONSUMER PERSPECTIVE 16-1:
A WIFE'S VIEW**

Hello, my name is Ethel. My husband David and I have been married for 55 years now and we have two grown-up children, both of whom live a considerable distance from our home. I would say that overall, our marriage was a very happy one and David was always caring and kind—I suppose you could say a perfect husband! Sadly, that has all changed in the past three years. David was diagnosed with probable dementia of the Alzheimer's type six months ago but I now realize that many of the signs were there for at least a year before that. I thought he was just becoming a little forgetful and that that was normal for an 88-year-old. What really upset me, however, was that he has become very selfish and seems to be unaware of my needs and feelings. He was never like that, always caring and kind. Lately he has started to wander about the house at night. When I ask him what he is doing, he says that his father is calling to take him to the cinema and he must not be late. His father has been dead for over 30 years! I have tried telling David that and tried to get him to come back to bed, however this just makes him angry. I'm a little scared now that he might hurt me—he pushed me last week when I confronted him. He was never like that. I'm really upset and find I am getting tearful when I think about what's happening to us. Our family doctor gave us a referral to our local branch of the Alzheimer's Society. I didn't want to trouble them by telephoning—they are busy people; I'm sure others are more needy. Maybe I'll give them a call though. I do feel I need help. I'm at my wit's end trying to cope at the moment.

Once trust is established, the nurse must provide an assessment whereby the patient feels there is genuine interest, acceptance, and positive regard. This is accomplished primarily through therapeutic communication techniques including restating, reflecting, and clarifying. (See Chapter 3 for more information on therapeutic communication.)

## Data Collection

In the assessment phase, data are collected and documented using observation and interview on all aspects of the patient's illness. Occasionally, assessment scales are used to evaluate the patient's status. Typically in dementia, assessment tools or scales are used to assess a patient's cognitive and functional capacity as well as any behavioral features that are present. The Mini Mental State Exam (MMSE) (Folstein, Folstein, & McHugh, 1975) is a commonly used assessment tool to determine a patient's cognitive status. The Katz Index (Katz et al., 1963) and the Revised Memory and Behavior Problems Checklist (RMBPC) (Teri et al., 1992) are useful in assessing functional capacity and behaviors, respectively.

Data collection must also include the family and other caregivers. Due to the nature of cognitive impairments and the specific perceptual and communication limitations associated with dementia, the patient is often unable to provide sufficient data. Consequently, the nurse and other team members must rely on data from key informants such as family members and other caregivers. Information also is obtained from friends, health records, and other health care professionals. In such situations, the nurse must be mindful of the need to corroborate information from several sources because secondary sources such as these are not always accurate. Nevertheless, despite these limitations, it is imperative that the nurse makes every effort to genuinely involve the patient in the assessment process. Patients in the early stages of dementia often retain enough ability to contribute to this assessment process in a meaningful way.

Important information to gather during the assessment includes information related to:
- General appearance and behavior
- Mood and affect
- Thought processes and thought content (abstract thinking, perception, organization, delusions, hallucinations)
- Intellectual processes (memory [recent and long-term], attention span)
- Reasoning, judgment, and insight (decision-making ability)
- Self-concept
- Participation in usual roles
- Self-care capabilities

> *Assessment of a patient with dementia requires patient, family, and caregiver involvement to ensure that enough information is collected to develop a complete picture of the patient's status.*

## Diagnosing and Planning Appropriate Interventions: Meeting the Patient's Focused Needs

Once a full assessment is completed, the nurse, patient, and family proceed to develop a plan of care with mutual goals and expectations for outcomes. The nurse collaborates with the patient and family to identify their needs and specific problems and then begins a plan for care (Peplau, 1991). Focusing on the patient's strengths identified in the assessment stage is key when planning interventions. Doing so will also allow for an increased sense of collaboration on the part of the patient and family. Patient care needs are addressed in order of priority, and goals that are realistic and achievable are established. The nurse ensures that appropriate evidence-based interventions feature in the plan. Therefore, it is imperative that the nurse remains up to date with literature relevant to his/her field of practice. **Evidence-Based Practice 16-1** summarizes a study about methods to decrease wandering in patients with dementia of the Alzheimer type.

Due to the wide range of assessment findings and multiple problems faced by patients with cognitive disorders, numerous nursing diagnoses would apply. Examples of possible nursing diagnoses include:
- Acute confusion related to altered cognitive function
- Chronic confusion related to the disease process
- Disturbed sleep pattern related to wandering and altered sleep/wake cycle
- Risk for injury related to cognitive impairment and wandering behavior
- Impaired memory related to cognitive impairment
- Caregiver role strain related to demands of caring for parent with dementia
- Risk for caregiver role strain related to new diagnosis of parent with dementia
- Compromised family coping related to grieving loss of parent functioning

**EVIDENCE-BASED PRACTICE 16-1:**
**FAMILIAR ENVIRONMENT AND WANDERING**

### STUDY

Hong, G.S., & Song, J. (2009). Relationship between familiar environment and wandering behavior among Korean elders with dementia. *Journal of Clinical Nursing, 18* (9), 1365–1373.

### SUMMARY

The researchers in this study hypothesized that establishing a familiar environment would decrease purposeless wandering in a community in which people with dementia reside. They used a descriptive cross-sectional survey design and a convenience sample of 77 non institutionalized, community-dwelling persons with dementia and their family caregivers in Seoul and Wonju, South Korea. The researchers explored the relationship between wandering behavior and familiar environment in this cohort. Data were analyzed using *t*-tests and multiple regression analysis. The results indicated that providing persons with dementia with a familiar feeling in daily clinical practice through the establishment of a familiar physical as well as psychosocial environment may assist in decreasing wandering behavior.

### APPLICATION TO PRACTICE

Behavioral and psychological symptoms of dementia (BPSD) are common in patients with dementia of the Alzheimer's type. Estimates suggest that over 90% of people exhibit these behaviors at some time during their illness (Boustani & Ham, 2007). Furthermore, BPSD are documented as perhaps the greatest source of stress for both formal and informal dementia caregivers (Fauth et al., 2006). Among the most troublesome of these behaviors is purposeless wandering. The research illustrates that familiarity with a physical and psychological environment can be helpful in decreasing wandering behavior. Nurses can implement this measure in any setting. In addition, nurses can educate caregivers about how to establish a familiar environment for the patient. Doing so may help to reduce wandering behavior in patients with dementia, thereby alleviating caregivers' concerns about potential harm that might result from such behavior. The ultimate result could lead to an improved quality of life of persons with dementia and their caregivers.

### QUESTIONS TO PONDER

1. *What interventions would you include when developing a plan to make a patient's physical environment familiar?*
2. *How would you attempt to familiarize a patient's psychological environment?*
3. *What other areas of research might be appropriate to pursue related to this topic?*

- Ineffective role performance related to inability to perform activities of daily living without assistance
- Self-care deficit (bathing, dressing, feeding, toileting) related to cognitive impairment

These nursing diagnoses also will vary based on the acuity of the patient's illness, developmental stage, comorbidities, current treatment regimen, and sources of support. Based on the identified nursing diagnoses, the nurse and patient collaboratively would determine the outcomes to be achieved. For example, for a patient who was diagnosed with early dementia, the outcome may be that the patient will accept diagnosis as evidenced by use of terms "Alzheimer's" and "dementia" when describing impairments.

## Implementing Effective Interventions: Timing and Pacing

The timing of nursing interventions when caring for someone with dementia is critical. People with dementia are easily fatigued and reach their stress threshold earlier in the day compared to persons who do not have dementia (Hall & Buckwalter, 1987). It is important, therefore, that regular rest periods are built in to the person's daily routine (every 90 minutes), and that high stimulus activities are alternated with low-stimulus activities (Smith & Buckwalter, 2005). Therefore, nursing interventions must be spaced appropriately throughout the day.

The activities should occur in a low-stimulus environment with few other stimuli present so that the person can focus on what is being asked and not be distracted. In addition, Smith and Buckwalter (2005) recommend that caregivers observe the patient to determine the best time of the day for that individual. These times can then be used for interventions and aspects of care that are most problematic, such as showering or bathing, foot care, hair care, or shaving. They also recommend that the person with dementia is well rested prior to these interventions and that some pleasant activity follows afterward.

When planning activities, it is also important that only one care activity or intervention occurs at a time. Otherwise there may be too many stimuli impinging on the person with dementia with resultant negative consequences for behavior (Smith & Buckwalter, 2005). For example, it is unwise to have visitors calling during meal times, or to attempt to administer medications at the same time while the television is on in the room. It is far better to separate these activities to decrease the amount of environmental stimuli, and hence stressors, that are impinging upon the person at any given time.

The nurse also must be cognizant of the pacing of activities and interventions. Indeed, outpacing, or providing information and presenting choices at a rate too fast for the person to understand, has been identified by Kitwood as a significant contributor to malignant social psychology, as outlined earlier (Brooker & Surr, 2005). People with dementia have a decreased ability to process information and hence need more time to respond to questions or instructions. Due to their diminished cognitive capacity, it is harder for their brains to make sense of what is being asked of them and then to select an appropriate response. It is important therefore that nurses give the person adequate time to respond and do not assume that any delays in responding means that the person did not understand the instruction (Smith & Buckwalter, 2005). The nurse must avoid pressuring the patient into responding, getting angry or frustrated at a lack of response, or not waiting for a response. Reactions such as these are not only disrespectful, they may also lead to frustration and/or anger in the person with dementia who may well be trying very hard to find the correct response to what has been asked. It is also important that the nurse speaks slowly, using simple sentences which are unambiguous. **Therapeutic Interaction 16-1** highlights an interaction with a patient experiencing dementia.

As nursing care is implemented, careful documentation is maintained so that the team can establish that the interventions decided upon are being delivered, and that this is done in the manner that was intended. Clear documentation is also necessary for consistency of care delivery. If the plan is clearly written, each nurse on the team should be able to deliver care, again, in the manner that was intended by the designer of the plan. Moreover, documentation is also a necessary legal requirement.

### Safety Issues

People with dementia lose many abilities over time, among which is their ability to judge what is safe and what is dangerous. Thus, as brain functioning deteriorates, the patient's ability to maintain personal safety diminishes (National Institutes of Health [NIH] and National Institute on Aging [NIA], 2010). They may no longer be able to perceive danger. In addition, they may begin to wander, a common feature of dementia. Thus, if doors are easily opened, the person may wander off and get lost or may get into dangerous situations. Also, with dementia, the person's ability to perceive the world accurately is diminishing. Therefore, patients may misinterpret their surroundings and become fearful of what is happening

### THERAPEUTIC INTERACTION 16-1:
### COMMUNICATING WITH A PATIENT WITH DEMENTIA

George is 88 years old and has had dementia of the Alzheimer's type for over 6 years. Until recently he had been living at home with his wife Alice; however, Alice is no longer able to care for her husband because of her failing health. Eight months ago, George was admitted to St. Raphael's nursing home for long-term care. His short-term memory is particularly poor at present, as is his ability to use and understand language. Samantha, a nurse, has been caring for George over the past 6 months, taking him for a walk on the grounds as part of his daily therapeutic program. Samantha has also noticed recently that he is easily startled when approached by other residents or staff.

| | |
|---|---|
| Samantha approaches George slowly from the front and stops about 10 feet away. She ensures that George can see her and is making facial contact. | Approaching slowly from the front and allowing adequate personal space is likely to be perceived by George as less threatening. Approaching him hastily from the side is likely to have the opposite effect. Because George's short-term memory is very poor, he easily forgets people he has met before. Addressing him by name tells him that this is someone who knows him and hence decreases any perceived threat. |
| **Samantha:** "Hello George, this is Samantha." (adopts an open posture and smiles widely when speaking; also wearing own coat, hat, and scarf) | Introducing oneself by name also conveys respect for George and may help orient him. It is also important to ensure that you have the person's attention before beginning the interaction. In this instance, Samantha did not speak until she was sure that George could see her and that he was looking at her face, indicating that she had his attention. An open posture minimizes threat and risk of the patient becoming startled; adopting a broad smile sends the signal that this is someone friendly and hence, non threatening. |
| **Samantha:** "We are going for a walk." (speaks in a slow manner) | People with DAT find it increasingly difficult to process information, hence the use of simple instructions is more likely to succeed. Avoid pronouns such as "there," "that," "them," "him," "her," and "it." Also avoid sentences that have a number of components or meanings. Speaking slowly increases the chances of being understood. |

(cont.)

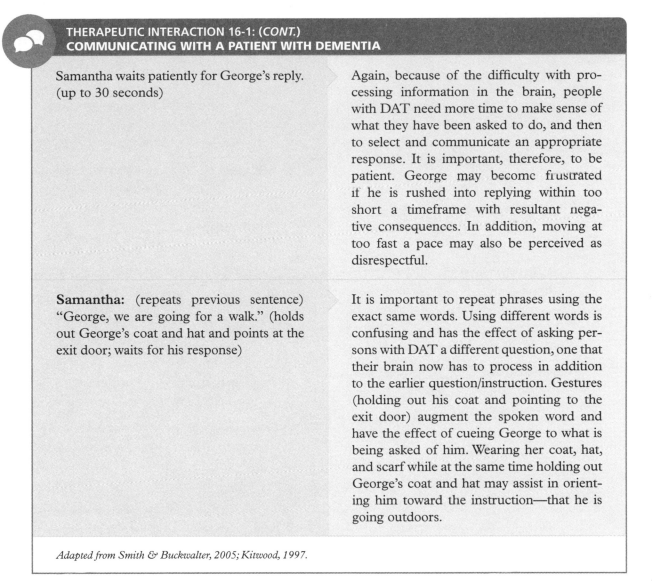

**THERAPEUTIC INTERACTION 16-1: (*CONT.*)
COMMUNICATING WITH A PATIENT WITH DEMENTIA**

| | |
|---|---|
| Samantha waits patiently for George's reply. (up to 30 seconds) | Again, because of the difficulty with processing information in the brain, people with DAT need more time to make sense of what they have been asked to do, and then to select and communicate an appropriate response. It is important, therefore, to be patient. George may become frustrated if he is rushed into replying within too short a timeframe with resultant negative consequences. In addition, moving at too fast a pace may also be perceived as disrespectful. |
| **Samantha:** (repeats previous sentence) "George, we are going for a walk." (holds out George's coat and hat and points at the exit door; waits for his response) | It is important to repeat phrases using the exact same words. Using different words is confusing and has the effect of asking persons with DAT a different question, one that their brain now has to process in addition to the earlier question/instruction. Gestures (holding out his coat and pointing to the exit door) augment the spoken word and have the effect of cueing George to what is being asked of him. Wearing her coat, hat, and scarf while at the same time holding out George's coat and hat may assist in orienting him toward the instruction—that he is going outdoors. |

*Adapted from Smith & Buckwalter, 2005; Kitwood, 1997.*

around them. Environmental safety, both physical and psychological, is a priority. For patients cared for in their homes, caregivers and family members need teaching about how to keep the patient safe and make him or her feel safe. **Patient and Family Education 16-1** highlights some important safety measures to stress with the patient and family.

## Environmental Management

In addition to the safety considerations, nursing staff and informal caregivers must also consider other aspects of the environment that need to be managed to achieve an optimal milieu for the person with dementia. A central tenet of Hall and Buckwalter's (1987) Progressively Lowered Stress Threshold (PLST) Model is that caregivers should modify the environment to make it less stressful for the person with dementia. Key points to address include:

- Provide a low-stimulus environment by eliminating multiple competing stimuli such as radio, television, too many people, and too many things going on at once. Also eliminate over-stimulation (crowds, noisy children), under-stimulation (isolation, boredom, rooms with few decorations and monochromatic colors), and misleading stimuli (television, reflections in mirrors or windows). Remove or cover mirrors if the person becomes agitated or frightened by them.
- Keep decorative changes in the home to a minimum; for example, new furniture, changing drapes, new wallpaper, or paint. Also, use minimal decorations at holiday times such as a Christmas tree or menorah.

**PATIENT AND FAMILY EDUCATION 16-1:**
**MAINTAINING PHYSICAL AND PSYCHOLOGICAL SAFETY**

### Maintaining physical safety

- Be sure to supervise the person when in the bath to prevent drowning or slips and falls; when shaving to prevent cuts; and when eating and drinking to prevent choking.

- Keep stairs and doors secure. Consider installing a stair gate or door alarms or locks. You may also have to place locks on windows, especially upstairs.

- As the dementia progresses, watch for new safety hazards and keep them under control; for example, the individual may no longer be safe with teapots, stoves, heating appliances, or hot water (faucets, kettles, hot water bottles).

- Keep medicines and household cleaning products in a locked cupboard to avoid poisoning.

- Keep sharp knives or other potentially dangerous objects or materials under lock and key.

- Clean up any spills immediately to avoid slips and falls.

- If the person has used a walking stick or some other object in a threatening way, carefully supervise his or her use of these items.

- Keep car keys in a safe place when the person can no longer safely drive (in case he or she forgets and attempts to drive).

- Keep gas or electric stoves safe; have a control switch installed in a place where the person is unlikely to reach and turn the stove off with this switch each time.

- Keep a careful eye on the person when cooking so that he or she doesn't spill hotfood on him- or herself.

- Consider installing heat sensors beside the stove.

- Keep matches and cigarette lighters in a safe place and be sure you have smoke alarms installed and that they are checked regularly.

- Be sure to lock garden sheds and to keep gardening equipment such as lawnmowers, garden shears, spades, and garden chemicals locked in the shed.

- Establish a predictable daily routine. This eliminates uncertainty and anxiety for the person with dementia.

### Maintaining psychological safety of the person with dementia

- Use non threatening body postures and movements, and use eye contact when you are speaking to the person. Slow movements, use of smiles, open palms, and a relaxed body posture are perceived as less threatening than quick hurried movements, a grimacing or scowling face, tense posture, and clenched fists.

- Avoid standing too close or standing over the person when they are sitting down. Rather, sit in front of them allowing enough space. Lean forward a little toward the person and use a gentle touch.

- Use a calm, friendly tone of voice, and gentle touch (an arm on the shoulder or holding the hand, for example); these are more likely to

make the person with dementia feel safe and less threatened.

- Explain what you are going to do before you move closer to the person. Always address the person by name and tell him or her who you are if he or she is inclined to forget you.

- If the person becomes agitated or upset when you are trying to get him or her to do something, it is probably best to stop and leave the person alone to settle down. It is far better to avoid conflict. Come back in a short while with something the person likes, such as a snack or drink, and do not try to re-engage the person in the activity that caused the previous upset unless the patient is clearly more relaxed.

- Avoid changes in caregiver and daily routines, especially when the person becomes more disabled. Consistency in caregivers, care routines, and the physical surroundings are a source of comfort to the person with dementia and gives a sense of security.
- Provide cues to current events, seasons, location, and names of people present to assist orientation.
- Consider using symbols instead of written signs to key locations such as bathroom, kitchen, or the person's bedroom.
- If wandering is a risk, provide boundaries such as red tape on the floor in front of exit doors or disguise with drapes, wall hangings, or wallpaper.
- If the person with dementia has to be transferred to a long-term care setting, ensure that personal belongings (and, if possible, items of furniture) accompany him or her in order to have some familiar objects in the new surroundings.
- Also consider the person's physical sensations (cold, pain, hunger, thirst), thoughts and beliefs (delusions, visual misinterpretations, and hallucinations), psychological and emotional needs (boredom, loneliness, or fear).

## Medication Management

Dementia has long been identified as a significant factor in poor medication management among older adults and hence is an issue that needs careful coordination and management (Kralik et al., 2008). In the interests of person-centered care and patient autonomy, however, every effort should be made to allow persons with dementia to manage their own affairs, including their medications, for as long as possible. As the disease progresses, the degree of supervision required to ensure the person can continue to do this safely will increase. A number of assessment tools exist that can assist in determining the person's competence. One such example is the Medication Administration Test (MAT), an instrument which was developed by Schmidt and Lieto (2005).

Inevitably, however, patient self-medication may no longer be possible. For those patients living in their homes, informal caregivers often assume this responsibility (Cotrell, Wild, & Bader, 2006). The extent to which these caregivers are successful and comfortable in this regard depends on a number of factors. These include their past experience of medication management, their degree of self-confidence, their level of literacy, the quality of their relationship with the patient, and the presence of negative emotional states, and cognitive impairment, and physical disability in the caregiver (Lau et al., 2010).

Therefore, a key role of the nurse in coordinating medication management of community-dwelling older adults with dementia is to assess the person's ability to self-medicate, and assess the informal caregivers' suitability to take over this role when the patient can no longer manage. In addition, the nurse plays a pivotal role in educating caregivers about the principles of medication management, key aspects of which are identified in **Patient and Family Education 16-2**.

## Caregiver Stress

In addition to the nurse serving as a therapeutic instrument, family caregivers also represent a significant therapeutic force in the care of someone with dementia. Most people with dementia live in the community and are cared for primarily by family members in the home setting. Family caregiving can be stressful, however, and can have significant negative consequences for the caregiver's physical and mental health, especially if they are inadequately supported. It is imperative that family caregivers are adequately prepared for and supported in their caregiving role. **How Would You Respond? 16-1** provides a practical example of the impact of a patient experiencing dementia on a family member.

The caregiver in the home is typically a spouse or other family member (Brodaty, Green, & Koschera, 2003). As the patient's disease progresses, many patients develop challenging behaviors such as sleep disturbances, problems with elimination, anxiety and aggression, falls, wandering, and inability to recognize familiar faces. As a result, caregiving becomes very difficult, so much so that the caregivers may jeopardize their ability or inclination to continue with their caregiving role (Acton & Kang, 2001).

> *Providing care for a family member with dementia can be highly stressful and overwhelming. Family caregivers need to receive adequate preparation and support when caring for the individual.*

Research has consistently shown that informal caregiving for a relative or friend with dementia of the Alzheimer's type can have significant negative consequences on that person's physical, psycho-emotional, social, and, indeed, spiritual well-being (Schulz, Martire,

## PATIENT AND FAMILY EDUCATION 16-2: MEDICATION MANAGEMENT

- Always store the medications in a safe place; be aware of any special requirements such as refrigeration or the need to protect the medication from light.

- Allow the person with dementia to self-medicate for as long as is safe; if there is a question, have your home care nurse evaluate the patient's ability to do this on a regular basis.

- Follow the prescribed medication plan. Do not make any changes to the person's medication regimen without talking with the patient's primary health care provider.

- Know the names of the medications, when to administer them, and the intended and unwanted effects for each medicine. Be knowledgeable about which side effects to report immediately.

- Know what to do if a dose is missed or an adverse reaction occurs.

- Check to make sure that the patient can swallow; ensure that this is assessed regularly as the disease progresses.

- Ensure that the person has swallowed each medicine; visually inspect the mouth if necessary.

- Do not to crush or break medicines or open capsules unless specifically instructed to do so. In cases where the patient is having difficulty swallowing the medicines that are prescribed, consult with the home care nurse, primary health care provider, or pharmacist so that an alternative form of the medicine can be used if available.

- Inform your home care nurse, health care provider, and/or pharmacist if any over-the-counter (OTC) medicines or herbal remedies are being taken.

- Know what to do if the person refuses to take the medication.

- Report any concerns you might have about the amount of medicines the patient is prescribed, especially if you feel this is having a damaging effect.

- Adopt as simple a dosing schedule as possible; using medicine cups, charts, or checklists as necessary to keep track.

- Where possible, use one pharmacy for all prescriptions.

---

& Klinger, 2005; Acton & Kang, 2001). To complicate matters further, research has also shown that informal caregivers in this context often feel unsupported and taken for granted (Schulz, Martire, & Klinger, 2005). Thus, interventions to reduce these difficulties associated with caregiving have been the focus of numerous studies over the past two decades (Gallagher-Thompson & Coon, 2007). **Patient and Family Education 16-3** provides some helpful tips for caregivers to maintain their health.

## Evaluating: Objective Critique of Interventions and Self-Reflection

In the evaluation phase, the nurse makes a judgment as to whether or not the plan of care is effective. The nurse evaluates how much progress has been made toward achieving expected outcomes. For any goals not met, the nurse needs to self-reflect on anything he or she may have done differently while providing nursing care. In addition, plan modification and further assessment

### HOW WOULD YOU RESPOND? 16-1:
### A PATIENT EXPERIENCING DEMENTIA

Catherine is an 84-year-old retired school teacher who lives at home with her husband George. George has contacted the family physician as he is worried about his wife's recent behavior. He reports that she has been becoming forgetful for the past 2 years and initially thought this was just a normal part of aging. Recently, on two occasions George was awakened in the middle of the night by the sound of the kitchen smoke alarm. He also noticed that Catherine was not in bed. On investigation he found an empty saucepan on the stove and the kitchen filling with smoke. After switching off the stove and opening the windows, George searched for his wife, finding her fully dressed wandering about the garden. When he asked Catherine to come back to bed, she insisted that it was daytime and that she had to get ready for work. She also indicated that she did not know who he was and why he was in her home. George tried to further persuade Catherine, but she became very agitated, angry, and began using abusive language toward him, suggesting that he was not her husband and that if he didn't leave her house, she would telephone the police. This upset George greatly, as in 52 years of marriage, he had never witnessed any such behavior from his wife. How would you respond?

### CRITICAL THINKING QUESTIONS

1. *Based on the situation, how does Catherine meet the diagnostic criteria for dementia of the Alzheimer's type?*

2. *What nursing diagnosis would be a priority for Catherine at this time? For her husband?*

3. *What suggestions would be appropriate to include in Catherine's plan of care to lower her stress threshold?*

### APPLYING THE CONCEPTS

Catherine is exhibiting several cognitive deficits. First, George has noticed a gradual onset of increasing forgetfulness. In addition, she is experiencing agnosia (not recognizing her husband) and disturbances in executive functioning (episodes of leaving an empty saucepan on the stove, insisting that it was daytime, and needing to get ready for work). Her behavior represents a significant change from her previous level of functioning as evidenced by her husband's upset.

The priority nursing diagnosis for Catherine would be risk for injury related to her wandering behavior, leaving the empty saucepan on the stove, and her agitation. The priority nursing diagnosis for George would most likely be deficient knowledge related to his upset about his wife's behavior and lack of understanding about what is happening to her and why.

To assist in lowering Catherine's stress threshold, suggestions would focus on modifying Catherine's environment. These might include establishing simple routines for her and having George adhere to them and continually evaluating her environment, making the necessary changes to reduce stress. George also would need instruction about monitoring Catherine for signs, such as increasing anxiety, agitation, and avoidance or escape behavior, that indicate she is reaching her stress threshold. George could then be taught how to take action to reduce the stress such as by promoting rest, decreasing external stimuli, and assessing for and eliminating internal stressors such as hunger or pain.

## PATIENT AND FAMILY EDUCATION 16-3: PREVENTING CAREGIVER STRESS

Caring for someone with dementia can become a round-the-clock job and it is very easy for the family caregiver to neglect his or her own health. It is also a stressful undertaking. It is important, therefore, that the caregiver give consideration to his or her own health, as failing health may mean that the caregiver will no longer be able to care for the loved one at home. Consider the following tips:

- Be sure to eat a balanced nutritious diet. This can be a challenge if the person you are caring for no longer conforms to a three-meals-a-day routine. Use periods when the person is resting or napping during the day, or if they go out to a day care facility to have a meal yourself. Your family physician or home care nurse can give you information about a balanced nutritious diet.

- Get enough sleep. Again, this can be a challenge, especially if the person with dementia wanders at night. Take advantage of any daytime naps and try to get some rest yourself at these times. Arrange for respite care periodically; try to arrange for someone else to take over caring one night per week or more often so that you can get a good night's sleep. Sleeping aids can help, but these should not be considered as a long-term solution. Discuss this with your primary care provider.

- See your own primary care provider on a regular basis to keep a check on your own health. Be sure to keep all hospital, doctor, and dental appointments. Arrange in advance for a family member or friend to care for the person with dementia so that you can maintain these appointments. Where possible, try to schedule appointments on the same day.

- Take any medicines that you have been prescribed, and if you are feeling unwell, see your health care provider promptly. Do not delay because this could jeopardize your ability to continue as a family caregiver and could delay your recovery.

- Being a family caregiver can be physically demanding. Take special care with your back if you have to help the person get in or out of bed. Ask for advice from a health care professional on how to move someone without injuring them or you.

- Engage in regular exercise. Perhaps take the person for a walk each day; this provides both you and your loved one with some healthy exercise together. This time could also be used to reminisce (to talk about old times) and to explore nature (plants, flowers, trees). If you have a secure garden, you could use gardening as a means of exercise that both of you could engage in together.

- Maintain at least one hobby and schedule time each day or week (whichever is appropriate) so that you can engage in your hobby. If necessary, get family or friends to help with care for a few hours so that you can keep up your hobby.

- Similarly, keep contact with family and friends. If you were accustomed to socializing outside of the home with family or friends, try to maintain this. Again, schedule time each week for this and get someone else to help with care for a few hours so that you can socialize.

- Plan for respite care. Discuss this with your home care nurse. You may be able to arrange some time each year so that you can go on a short holiday, or it may be possible to arrange weekend or overnight respite so that you can take a short break.

*(cont.)*

**PATIENT AND FAMILY EDUCATION 16-3: (*CONT.*)**
**PREVENTING CAREGIVER STRESS**

- Try to involve other family and friends in caring. This will not only lighten your workload, but will also enable them to maintain contact with the person with dementia and to develop some of the necessary skills to care for a person with dementia. That way, you can be confident that they know what to do when they take over caring while you are having a short break. Always accept help from family or friends when offered.

- If you say you can manage, they may not think to offer help again.

- If you find that you are becoming very stressed or depressed, talk to your primary health care provider who may recommend some counseling or other therapy. It is very important that you do not try to "soldier on" and suffer in silence. Seek help as soon as possible.

needs to be done. Evaluation should be done early and in an ongoing fashion. If not, an ineffective plan of care may be allowed to run its course even though it is not delivering the goals that were anticipated. Not only is this a waste of time, it may also be harmful to the client.

Evaluate how the patient presented initially and where he or she is as termination nears. During this phase of the nurse-patient relationship, the nurse, patient, and family should reflect on progress made toward reaching the patient goals. Point out positives to the patient and family and include a plan for aftercare and referral as appropriate.

This phase is also part of the termination of the nurse-patient relationship. Many times a patient or caregiver will have a setback due to a feeling of loss of this relationship. The nurse's role is to help them explore their feelings and ease this transition while maintaining boundaries (Peplau, 1991).

**SUMMARY POINTS**

- The major cognitive disorders that are encountered in clinical practice are delirium and dementia.

- Essential features of cognitive impairment include disorientation, confusion, impaired memory, impaired function, and behavioral symptoms such as agitation and restlessness.

- Delirium is an acute-onset, short-lived medical condition caused by an underlying illness; it can be treated by identifying and treating the cause, and by providing supportive therapy until the patient's condition has stabilized

- Several different types of dementia have been identified. Dementia of the

- Alzheimer's type accounts for more than one-half of all cases of dementia.

- Features common to all types of dementia include personality changes, cognitive changes, functional changes, and altered stress threshold.

- Neurobiological influences including neurofibrillary tangles, beta-amyloid plaques, apolipoprotein E, and neurotransmitter deficiencies. Acetylcholine, has been identified as playing a role in the development of dementia of the Alzheimer's type.

- There are no cures for dementia. Cholinesterase inhibitors are available that may slow the rate of cognitive impairment and improve the patient's overall

*(cont.)*

## SUMMARY POINTS (*CONT.*)

functioning. Other therapies available include reality orientation, environmental stress management, validation and reminiscence therapies, and maintenance of the patient's personhood.

- Assessment of the patient with dementia requires evaluation of the patient's cognitive and functional capacity along with any behavioral features. Family and other

caregivers are included in the assessment to ensure that sufficient data are collected.

- Care of the patient with dementia focuses on maintaining safety, providing a supportive environment that decreases stress and confusion, and assisting family and caregivers to understand patient behaviors and to participate in care.

## NCLEX-PREP*

1. A nurse is preparing a presentation for a local senior citizen group about dementia and delirium. When describing delirium, which of the following would the nurse include?

   a. It occurs gradually over a period of time.
   b. It is usually due to an underlying medical condition.
   c. It requires medication to slow its progression.
   d. It remains fairly constant throughout the day.

2. A group of nursing students is reviewing the different types of drugs that may be used to treat dementia of the Alzheimer's type. The students demonstrate a need for additional study when they identify which of the following as an example of a cholinesterase inhibitor?

   a. Donepezil
   b. Rivastigmine
   c. Galantamine
   d. Atorvastatin

3. The nurse is providing care to a patient with frontotemporal dementia. The nurse develops a plan of care for this patient,

integrating knowledge about which of the following?

   a. The patient has a much shorter life expectancy.
   b. The patient has probably experienced multiple ministrokes.
   c. The patient's memory will remain intact.
   d. The patient is at risk for falls due to muscle rigidity.

4. A patient with dementia of the Alzheimer's type is demonstrating increasing problems with wandering. In addition, the patient's caregiver reports that the patient has wandered into the kitchen during the night and left the stove on several times over the past few weeks. Which of the following would be a priority nursing diagnosis for this patient?

   a. Chronic confusion related to effects of dementia
   b. Risk for injury related to increased wandering
   c. Deficient knowledge related to effects of illness
   d. Disturbed sleep pattern related to frequent nighttime awakenings

(*cont.*)

≡  **NCLEX-PREP\*** (*CONT.*)

5. The nurse is implementing validation therapy with a patient diagnosed with dementia of the Alzheimer's type. Which of the following would the nurse do?

   a. Confirm the patient's version of reality
   b. Place cards on the bathroom and bedroom doors
   c. Repeatedly tell the patient what day it is
   d. Have the patient discuss past events

6. A nurse is working with a patient diagnosed with dementia to foster the patient's personhood. Which of the following would be appropriate to use? Select all that apply.

   a. Intimidation
   b. Labeling
   c. Acceptance
   d. Objectification
   e. Collaboration
   f. Recognition

\*Answers to these questions appear on page 639.

## REFERENCES

Acton, G.J., & Kang, J. (2001). Interventions to reduce the burden of caregiving for an adult with dementia: A meta-analysis. *Research in Nursing and Health.* 24, 349–360.

Adamis, D., Treolar, A., Martin, F.C., & MacDonald, A.J.D. (2007). A brief review of the history of delirium as a mental disorder. *History of Psychiatry. 18(4),* 459–469.

Adams, M., Gmünder, F., & Hamburger, M. (2007). Plants traditionally used in age-related brain disorders—A survey of ethnobotanical literature. *Journal of Ethnopharmacology, 113,* 363–381.

Algase, G.L., Beck, C., Kolanowski, A., Whall, A., Berent, S., Richards, K., & Beattie, E. (1996). Need-driven dementia-compromised behaviour: An alternative view of disruptive behaviour. *Journal of Alzheimer's Disease and other Dementias. 11,* 10–19.

American Psychiatric Association (APA). (2000). *Diagnostic and Statistical Manual of Mental Disorders (4th Ed) text revision.* Washington, D.C.: Author.

Arskey, H., Jackson, K., Crouchert, K., Weatherly, H., Golder, S., Hare, P., Newbronner, E., & Baldwin, S. (2004) *Review of respite services and short-term breaks for carers for people with dementia.* Report for the National Co-ordinating Centre for NHS Service Delivery and Organisation R&D (NCCSDO). York: University of York.

Blessed, G., Tomlinson, B.E., & Roth, M. (1968). The association between quantitative measures of dementia and of senile change in the cerebral grey matter of elderly subjects. *British Journal of Psychiatry, 114*(512), 797–811.

Boustani, M., & Ham, R.J. (2007). Alzheimer disease and other dementias. In: Ham, R.J., Sloane, P.D., Warshaw, G.A., Bernard, M.A., and Flatley, E. (Eds). *Primary Care Geriatrics: A Case-Based Approach. (5th Ed).* Philadelphia: Mosby.

Boyle, A., & Hands, O. (2009). Acute Psychosis. *General Practice Update, 2*(3), 42–45.

Brodaty, H., Green, A., & Koschera, A. (2003). Meta-analysis of psychosocial interventions for caregivers of people with dementia. *Journal of the American Geriatrics Society. 51,* 657–664.

Brooker, D., & Surr, C. (2005). *Dementia Care Mapping: Principles and Practice.* Bradford: University of Bradford.

Buckwalter, K.C., Gerdner, L., Kohout, F., Hall, G.R., Kelly, A., Richards, B., & Sime, M. (1999). A nursing intervention to decrease depression in family caregivers of persons with dementia. *Archives of Psychiatric Nursing. 13,* 80–88.

Chang, B. (1999). Cognitive-behavioural intervention for homebound caregivers of persons with dementia. *Nursing Research. 48*(3), 173–182.

Coon, D., Thompson, L.W., Steffen, S., Sorocco, K., & Gallagher-Thompson, D. (2003) Anger and depression management: Psycho-educational skills training interventions for women caregivers of a relative with dementia. *The Gerontologist. 43,* 678–689.

Cotrell, V., Wild, K., & Bader, T. (2006). Medication management and adherence among cognitively impaired older adults. *Journal of Gerontological Social Work. 47*(3/4), 31–46.

Covinsky, K.E., Newcomer, R., Fox, P., Wood, J., Sands, L., Dane, K., & Yaffe, K. (2003). Patient and caregiver characteristics associated with depression in caregivers of patients with dementia. *Journal of General Internal Medicine. 18*(12), 1006–1014.

Cummings, J.L. (2004). Advances in the neuropsychopharmacologic management of behavioral alterations in Alzheimer's disease. *Dementia and Geriatric Cognitive Disorders, 17*(1/2), 54.

Dröes, R.M., Meiland, F.J.M., Schmitz, M.J., & van Tilberg, W. (2006). Effect of the Meeting Centre Support Program on informal carers of people with dementia: Results from a multicentre study. *Aging and Mental Health. 10*(2), 112–124.

Edvardsson, D., Winblad, B., & Sandman, P.O. (2008). Person-centred care of people with severe Alzheimer's disease: Current status and ways forward. *Lancet Neurology, 7,* 362–367.

Edwards, J.K., & Bess, J.M. (1998). Developing effectiveness in the therapeutic use of self. *Clinical Social Work Journal, 26*(1), 89–105.

Fauth, E.B., Zarit, S.H., Femia, E.E., Hofer, S.M., & Stephens, M.A. (2006). Behavioral and psychological symptoms of dementia and caregiver's stress appraisals: Intra-individual stability and change over short-term observations. *Aging and Mental Health, 10*(6), 563–573.

Feil, N. (1993). *The validation breakthrough: Simple techniques for communicating with people with alzheimer's type dementia.* Cleveland: Health Professions Press.

Feil, N. (1992). The validation helping techniques can be used in each of the four stages that occur with late-onset demented populations. *Geriatric Nursing, 3,* 192–195.

Feil, N. (1967). Group therapy in a home for the aged. *The Gerontologist, 7,* 192–195.

Ferri, C.P., Prince, M., Brayne, C., Brodaty, H., Fratiglioni, L., Ganguli, M., Hall, K., Hasegawa, K., Hendrie, H., Huang, Y., Jorm, A., Mathers, C., Menezes, P.R., Rimmer, E., & Scazufca, M. (2005). Global prevalence of dementia: A Delphi consensus study. *Lancet, 366* (9503), 2112–2117.

Folstein, M.F., Folstein, S.E., & McHugh, P.R. (1975). "Minimental state." A practical method for grading the cognitive state of patients for the clinician. *Journal of Psychiatric Research, 12,* 189–198.

Gallagher-Thompson, D., & Coon, D.W. (2007). Evidence-based psychological treatments for distress in family caregivers of older adults. *Psychology and Ageing, 22,* (1): 37–51.

Garand, L., Buckwalter, K.C., Lubaroff, D.M., et al. (2002). A pilot study of immune and mood outcomes of a community-based intervention for dementia caregivers. The PLST Intervention. *Archives of Psychiatric Nursing,16,* 156–167.

Garand, L., Buckwalter, K.C., & Hall, G.R. (2002). The biological basis of behavioral symptoms in dementia. *Issues in Mental Health Nursing, 21,* 91–107.

Gerdner, L.A., Buckwalter, K.C., & Reed, D. (2002). Impact of a psychoeducational intervention on caregiver response to behavioral problems. *Nursing Research, 51,* 363–374.

Giaquinto, S., & Parnetti, L. (2006). Early detection of dementia in clinical practice. *Mechanisms of Ageing and Development, 127,* 123–128.

Gibson, F. (2006) *Reminiscence and recall: A practical guide to reminiscence work.* London: Age Concern.

Gilliard, J. (1993) On course for success. *Elderly Care, 5*(5): 32–34.

Hall, G., & Buckwalter, K. (1987). Progressively lowered stress threshold: A conceptual model for care of adults with Alzheimer's disease. *Archives of Psychiatric Nursing, 1,* 399–406.

Hong, G. S., & Song, J. (2009). Relationship between familiar environment and wandering behavior among Korean elders with dementia. *Journal of Clinical Nursing, 18*(9), 1365–1373.

Howes, M.J., & Houghton, P.J. (2003). Plants used in Chinese and Indian traditional medicine for improvement of memory and cognitive function. *Pharmacology, Biochemistry and Behavior, 75,* 523–527.

Huang, H., Shyu, Y.L., Chen, M., Chen, S., & Lin, L. (2003) A pilot study on a home-based caregiver training program for improving caregiver self-efficacy and decreasing the behavioral problems of elders with dementia in Taiwan. *International Journal of Geriatric Psychiatry, 18,* 337–345.

Katz, S., Ford, A.B., Moskowitz R.W., et al. (1963). The index of ADL: a standardized measure of biological and psychosocial function. *JAMA, 185*(12), 914– 919.

Katzman, R., & Fox, P.J. (1999). The worldwide impact of dementia: Projections of prevalence and costs. In: Mayeux, R., & Christen,

Y. (Eds). *Epidemiology of alzheimer's disease: From gene to prevention.* Berlin: Springer.

Kitwood, T. (1997). *Dementia Reconsidered.* Buckingham, England: Open University Press.

Kolanowski, A.M., Litaker, M.S., & Baumann, M.A. (2002). Theory-based intervention for dementia behaviour: A within-person analysis over time. *Applied Nursing Research, 15,* 87–96.

Kralik, D., Visentin, K., March, G., Anderson, B., Gilbert, A., & Boyce, M. (2008). Medication management for community-dwelling older people with dementia and chronic illness. *Australian Journal of Primary Health, 14*(1), 25–35.

Lau, D.T., Berman, R., Halpern, L., Pickard, A.S., Schrauf, R., & Witt, W. ( 2010). Exploring factors that influence informal caregiving in medication management for home hospice patients. *Journal of Palliative Medicine, 13*(9), 1085–1090.

Mittelman, M.S., Roth, D.L., Coon, D.W., & Haley, W.E. (2004). Sustained benefit of supportive intervention for depressive symptoms in caregivers of patients with Alzheimer's disease. *American Journal of Psychiatry, 161*(5), 850–856.

Mosey, A. (1986). *Psychosocial components of occupational therapy.* New York: Raven Press.

Nassisi, D., Korc, B., Hann, S., Bruns, J., & Jagoda, A. (2006). The evaluation and management of the acutely agitated elderly patient. *Mount Sinai Journal of Medicine, 73*(7), 976–984.

National Institutes of Health and National Institute on Aging. (2010). *Home safety for people with Alzheimer's disease.* NIH Publication No. 02–5179.

National Institute of Neurological Disorders and Stroke. (2010a). NINDS Dementia With Lewy Bodies Information Page. Downloaded from: http://www.ninds.nih.gov/disorders/dementiawithlewybodies/dementiawithlewybodies.htm; January 11th, 2010.

National Institute of Neurological Disorders and Stroke. (2010b). NINDS Multi-Infarct Dementia Information Page. Downloaded from: http://www.ninds.nih.gov/disorders/multi_infarct_dementia/multi_infarct_dementia.htm; January 11th, 2010.

National Institute of Neurological Disorders and Stroke. (2010c). NINDS Fronto-temporal Dementia Information Page. Downloaded from: http://www.ninds.nih.gov/disorders/picks/picks.htm; January 11th, 2010.

Nazarko, L. (2006). Recognizing the signs and symptoms of dementia. *Nursing and Residential Care, 8*(1), 32–34.

Neil, M., & Barton Wright, P. (2003). Validation therapy for dementia. Cochrane Database of Systematic Reviews. Art. No.: CD001394. DOI: 10. 1002/14651858. CD001394.

Pearson, A., Vaughan, B., & Fitzgerald, M. (2005). *Nursing Models for Practice.* Oxford, England: Butterworth-Heinemann.

Peplau, H.E. (1991). *Interpersonal relations in nursing: A conceptual frame of reference for psychodynamic nursing.* New York: Springer Publishing Company.

Pusey, H., & Richards, D. (2001). A systematic review of the effectiveness of psychosocial interventions for carers of people with dementia. *Aging and Mental Health, 5*(2), 107–119.

Schulz, R., Martire, L.M., & Klinger, J.N. (2005). Evidence-based caregiver interventions in geriatric psychiatry. *Psychiatric Clinics of North America, 28,* 1007–1038.

Silvestrelli, G., Lanari, A., Parnetti, L., Tomassoni, D., & Amenta, F. (2006). Treatment of Alzheimer's disease: From pharmacology to a better understanding of disease pathology. *Mechanisms of Ageing and Development, 127,* 148–157.

Schmidt, K., & Lieto, J. (2005). Validity of the Medication Administration Test among older adults with and without dementia. *The American Journal of Geriatric Pharmacotherapy, 3*(4), 255–261.

Smith, M., & Buckwalter, K.C. (2005). *When you forget that you forgot: Recognizing and managing alzheimer's type dementia. The geriatric mental health training series.* Hartford Centre for Geriatric Nursing Excellence, College of Nursing, University of Iowa.

Smith, M., Gerdner, L., Hall, G.R., & Buckwalter, K.C. (2004). History, development, and future of the progressively lowered stress threshold: A conceptual model for dementia care. *Journal of the American Geriatrics Society, 52*(10), 1755–1760.

Spector, A., Orrell, M., Davies, S., & Woods, B. (2002). *Reality orientation for dementia* (Cochrane Review). In: The Cochrane Library, Issue 2, Update Software, Oxford.

Speechly, C.M., Bridges-Webb, C., & Passmore, E. (2008). The pathway to dementia diagnosis. *Medical Journal of Australia, 189,* 487–489.

Stolley, J.M., Reed, D., & Buckwalter, K.C. (2002). Caregiving appraisal and interventions based on the progressively lowered stress threshold model. *American Journal of Alzheimers Disease and Other Dementias, 17,* 110–120.

Teri, L., Traux, P., Logsdon, R., Uomoto, J., Zarit, S.H., & Vitaliano, P.P. (1992). Assessment of behavioral problems in dementia: The revised memory and behavior problems checklist. *Psychology and Aging, 7*(4), 622–631.

Tyrrell, M.P. (2011) A group intervention to reduce burden and depression in informal dementia caregivers. Unpublished PhD thesis, University College Cork, Ireland.

Walsh, J.S., Welch, H.G., & Larson, E.B. (1990). Survival of outpatients with Alzheimer-type dementia. *Annals of Internal Medicine, 113,* 429–434.

Wilkinson, D., Sganga, N., Stave, C., & O'Connell, B. (2005). Implications of the Facing Dementia Survey for health care professionals across Europe. *International Journal of Clinical Practice, 59,* Suppl. 146, 27–31.

Woods, B., Spector, A.E., Jones, C.A., Orrell, M., & Davies, S.P. (2005). Reminiscence therapy for dementia. *Cochrane Database of Systematic Reviews 2005, Issue 2.*

Youdim, M.B., & Buccafusco, J.J. (2005). Multi-functional drugs for various CNS targets in the treatment of neurodegenerative disorders. *Trends in Pharmacological Science, 26,* 27–35.

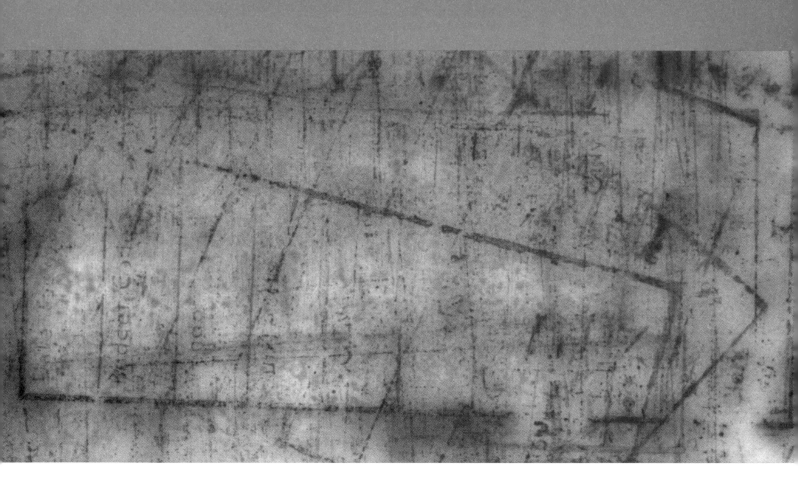

## CHAPTER CONTENTS

## EXPECTED LEARNING OUTCOMES

**After completing this chapter, the student will be
able to:**

1. Identify the disorders that can be described as
   impulse control disorders.
2. Discuss the history and epidemiology of impulse
   control disorders.
3. Distinguish among the *Diagnostic and Statistical
   Manual of Mental Disorder, 4th edition, Text Revision*
   (*DSM-IV-TR*) diagnostic criteria for impulse control
   disorders.

# CHAPTER 17
# IMPULSE CONTROL DISORDERS

Amanda Alisa Townsend

4. Describe possible theories related to the etiology of impulse control disorders.
5. Explain various treatment options for persons experiencing impulse control disorders.
6. Discuss common assessment strategies for individuals with impulse control disorders.
7. Apply the nursing process from an interpersonal perspective to the care of patients with impulse control disorders.

## KEY TERMS

Impulse control disorder (ICD)
Intermittent explosive disorder (IED)
Kleptomania
Pathological gambling (PG)
Pyromania
Trichotillomania (TTM)

A difficulty in exercising control over one's impulses occurs in a number of psychiatric-mental health disorders, including substance abuse-related conditions, conduct disorders, and psychotic disorders. However, the classification of IMPULSE CONTROL DISORDER involves those disorders whose defining feature is the inability to control or inhibit acting on impulses that might be harmful to self or others. Disorders classified by the *Diagnostic and Statistical Manual of Mental Disorders, 4th edition, Text Revision* (*DSM-IV-TR*) include: PATHOLOGICAL GAMBLING (persistent maladaptive gambling behavior), KLEPTOMANIA (recurrent failure to resist the impulse to steal), PYROMANIA (fire-setting for pleasure and gratification), INTERMITTENT EXPLOSIVE DISORDER (failure to resist aggressive impulses leading to serious property destruction or assaults) and TRICHOTILLOMANIA (recurrent pulling out of one's hair for pleasure or tension relief); (American Psychiatric Association [APA], 2000; Grant & Kim, 2003). In these disorders, there is an increasing sense of tension before acting out. However, pleasure, gratification, relief, or guilt often occurs shortly following the act.

This chapter addresses the historical perspectives and epidemiology of impulse control disorders followed by a detailed description of these disorders as defined in the *DSM-IV-TR*, 2000. Scientific theories focusing on psychodynamic and neurobiologic influences are described along with common treatment options, including pharmacotherapy and nonpharmacotherapy strategies. Application of the nursing process from an interpersonal perspective is presented, including a plan of care for a patient with an impulse control disorder.

> *Impulse control disorders are characterized by the inability to control or suppress acting on an impulse that has the potential for harm to one's self or others.*

## HISTORICAL PERSPECTIVES

Available literature in the area of impulse control disorder is sparse in comparison to other psychiatric conditions. It is generally accepted that impulse control disorder is a key feature found in many other Axis I mental disorders, such as alcohol and drug dependence and eating disorders (Fontenelle, Mendlowicz, & Versiani, 2003). When compared to other psychiatric mental health conditions, little historical information on impulse control disorders is available. Only kleptomania and trichotillomania have any specific historical prospective.

The first clinical cases of kleptomania date back two centuries, although some court cases are older. The term was modified from two Greek words meaning "to steal" and "insanity." Kleptomania was a supplementary term but was not considered a distinct diagnosis in the first edition of the *Diagnostic and Statistical Manual of Mental Disorders*. In the second edition, the term was ignored. No substantive changes were made for the diagnosis of kleptomania in the more recent *DSM* manuals (Presta, Marazziti, Dell'Osso, Pfanner, Pallanti, & Cassano, 2002).

Trichotillomania was first described by a French dermatologist over 100 years ago. In early literature, the hair was a symbolic object used to work through feelings of aggression or abandonment. This psychoanalytical approach did not prove to be helpful to patients with trichotillomania. More recent avenues of exploration in trichotillomania have noted similarities with obsessive compulsive disorder and Tourette's syndrome. Most researchers and clinicians agree the etiology of trichotillomania is multifactorial (Whitaker, Wolf, & Keuthen, 2003).

In recent psychological history, information about impulse control disorders is beginning to evolve. For example, in the 1990s some research began suggested that impulse control disorders could be viewed as part of an obsessive-compulsive spectrum. This conceptualization arose from the clinical presentation of the disorder, familial or genetic links, and the documented treatment responses. Further study and research is leading to the identification of new compulsive-impulsive disorders, such as internet usage disorder, sexual behaviors, skin picking, and excessive shopping. The impulsive features of arousal and initiation of the act or behavior, and the compulsive aspect causing the behavior to continue over time are the central focus (Dell'Osso, Altamuna, Allen, & Marazziti, 2006).

## EPIDEMIOLOGY

Reliable information related to the epidemiology of impulse control disorders is lacking. It is believed that intermittent explosive disorder is rare, but that when it occurs, it is believed to be more common in males (McClaskey, Debbenbacher, Roblett, Gollan, & Cocccano, 2008). Some nonspecific "soft" findings may present on a neurological exam like reflex asymmetries and delays in speech and coordination.

Kleptomania is rare, occurring in less than 5% of shoplifters. Most kleptomaniacs are female. Three courses of kleptomania exist in the literature. These courses are: sporadic with brief episodes and long periods of remission; episodic with prolonged periods of stealing and remission; and chronic with some fluctuation (APA, 2000). Despite convictions, the disorder continues and the items stolen are most often of little value (Grant, 2003).

Pyromania is a rare condition, occurring most often in males, with no established typical age of onset. Pyromania is found more often in those with poorly developed social skills and learning delays. Of the arson arrests in the United States, 40% are juveniles (APA, 2000).

Pathological gambling, like alcohol dependence, is more prevalent among those whose parents were pathological gamblers. However, the prevalence of this condition could be as high as 1% to 3% of the general population. One-third of pathological gamblers are female. The progression of the condition is insidious, with the urge to gamble often increasing during stressful periods of life (Grant, Kim, Calloway, Buchanan, & Potenza, 2009).

Trichotillomania is more likely to occur during reported periods of stressful life events. However, a second pattern of this disorder occurs during sedentary activity, such as while watching TV or talking on the phone. This condition, which begins in childhood, may affect 3% of the U.S. population. The condition can be self-limiting or it can progress to adulthood. Females are more often affected by this condition. The shame surrounding trichotillomania can be so great that its victims avoid basic health services for fear of discovery (Whitaker, Wolf, & Keuthen, 2003; Ferrano, Almeida, Bedin, Rosa, & Busnello, 2006).

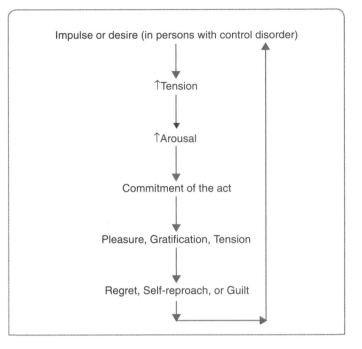

**Figure 17-1** *Cycle of impulse response.*

drive, or temptation to act in a way that is harmful to one's self or others. The individual will often report a heightened sense of stress, tension, or arousal just prior to committing the act. Following the commission of the act, the individual may report relief followed by a combination of guilt and regret (Fontenelle, Mendlowiaz, & Versiani, 2005). **Figure 17-1** depicts the cycle of the impulse response in persons with impulse control disorders. The disorders covered in this section are intermittent explosive disorder, kleptomania, pyromania, pathological gambling, and trichotillomania. **Box 17-1** highlights the major diagnostic criteria for each of these disorders as identified by the *DSM-IV-TR*.

> *Intermittent explosive disorder and pyromania are more common in males; kleptomania and trichotillomania are more common in females. Two-thirds of those with pathological gambling are male.*

> *The impulse response follows a predictable pattern: an increase in stress followed by an increase in arousal, which leads to the act and subsequent experience of pleasure, gratification, and release of tension followed by feelings of regret, self-reproach, or guilt.*

## DIAGNOSTIC CRITERIA

According to the *DSM-IV-TR*, the essential feature of impulse control disorders is a failure to resist an impulse,

## BOX 17-1: DIAGNOSTIC CRITERIA

### INTERMITTENT EXPLOSIVE DISORDER

A. Several discrete episodes of failure to resist aggressive impulses resulting in serious assaultive acts or destruction of property.

B. Degree of aggressiveness during episodes grossly out of proportion to any precipitating psychosocial stressors.

C. The aggressive episodes not better accounted for by another mental disorder and not due to the direct physiological effects of a substance or a general medical condition.

### KLEPTOMANIA

A. Recurrent failure to resist impulses to steal objects not needed for personal use or for their monetary value.

B. Increasing sense of tension immediately before committing the theft.

C. Pleasure, gratification, or relief at the time of committing the theft.

D. The stealing not done to express anger or vengeance and not in response to a delusion or a hallucination.

E. The stealing is not better accounted for by conduct disorder, a manic episode, or antisocial personality disorder.

### PYROMANIA

A. Deliberate and purposeful fire setting on more than one occasion.

B. Tension or affective arousal before the act.

C. Fascination with, interest in, curiosity about, or attraction to fire and its situational contexts (e.g., paraphernalia, uses, consequences).

D. Pleasure, gratification, or relief when setting fires, or when witnessing or participating in their aftermath.

E. Fire setting not done for monetary gain, as an expression of sociopolitical ideology, to conceal criminal activity, or express anger or vengeance, to improve one's living circumstances, in response to a delusion or hallucination, or as a result of impaired judgment.

F. Fire setting not better accounted for by conduct disorder, a manic episode, or antisocial personality disorder.

### TRICHOTILLOMANIA

A. Recurrent pulling out of one's hair resulting in noticeable hair loss.

B. An increasing sense of tension immediately before pulling out the hair or when attempting to resist the behavior.

C. Pleasure, gratification, or relief when pulling out the hair.

D. The disturbance not better accounted for by another mental disorder and not due to a general medical condition.

E. Clinically significant distress or impairment in social, occupational, or other important areas of functioning due to condition.

*(cont.)*

**BOX 17-1: DIAGNOSTIC CRITERIA (*CONT.*)**

PATHOLOGICAL GAMBLING

A. Persistent and recurrent maladaptive gambling behavior as indicated by five (or more) of the following:

- Preoccupation with gambling (e.g., preoccupied with reliving past gambling experiences, handicapping or planning the next venture, or thinking of ways to get money with which to gamble)
- Need for gambling with increasing amount of money to achieve the desired excitement
- Repeated unsuccessful efforts to control, cut back, or stop gambling
- Restlessness or irritability when attempting to cut down or stop gambling
- Gambling as a way of escaping from problems or of relieving a dysphoric mood (e.g., feelings of helplessness, guilt, anxiety, depression)
- Often return another day to get even, after losing money gambling ("chasing" one's losses)
- Concealment about extent of involvement in gambling by lying to family members, therapist, or others
- Commission of illegal acts such as forgery, fraud, theft, or embezzlement to finance gambling
- Significant relationship, job, or educational or career opportunity jeopardized or lost because of gambling
- Reliance on others to provide money to relieve a desperate financial situation caused by gambling

B. The gambling behavior not better accounted for by a manic episode.

*From the Diagnostic and Statistical Manual of Mental Disorders, Fourth Edition, Text Revision, Copyright © 2000, American Psychiatric Association.*

## ETIOLOGY

The etiology of impulse control disorders is less understood than some psychiatric-mental health disorders. Impulse control disorders and obsessive-compulsive disorders appear to be closely linked clinically (Dell'Osso, Altarmura, Allen, Marazziti, & Holland, 2006). However, no single scientific theory has been proposed to explain the cause of impulse control disorders. Many theorists suggest that the causes are multifactorial. Psychodynamic and neurobiological influences are addressed here.

### Psychodynamic Influences

The known psychodynamic influences associated with impulse control disorders vary based on the specific diagnosis. For individuals with intermittent explosive disorder, revenge for a minor injustice is often the motivation for aggression (McCloskey, Deffenbacher, Coccaro, Noblett, & Gollan, 2008). Highly aggressive individuals

with intermittent explosive disorder appear to be more treatment resistant to cognitive behavioral therapy. In children with this disorder, anger may take the form of severe temper tantrums, property destruction, and running away. Children often respond best to the use of child-centered play therapy with parental involvement (Paone & Douma, 2009).

Deviant peer groups have been linked to substance use, theft, violence, and gambling that begins in middle adolescence and continues into young adulthood. Parental supervision may have a moderating effect on the other behaviors but it does not apparently affect the youth's problem gambling. The heightened awareness of problem gambling, however, may motivate parents to seek help for their troubled youth (Wanner, Vitaro, Carbonneau, & Tremblay, 2009).

Trichotillomania generally exhibits two patterns of hair loss related to chronic hair pulling. With the binge type, the individual may extract a large amount of hair during a brief period of negative intense feelings such as anxiety or depression. The second pattern occurs when the individual is sedentary—reading, driving, watching television, or talking on the telephone. People with this second type of trichotillomania are often unaware of the behavior and pull their hair less often than those with the first type (Whitaker, Wolf, & Keuthen, 2003).

The major complication of trichotillomania is fear of discovery. This frequently leads to the avoidance of basic health care services. Research has shown this fear is so great that women will forego reporting sexual assaults due to pubic hair loss. They may also avoid dermatological follow-ups for skin cancer due to shame (Whitaker, Wolf, & Keuthen, 2003).

## Neurobiological Influences

Alterations in neurotransmitters in certain brain regions and the neural circuitry are thought to occur in impulse control disorders. Neurotransmitters in the mesocorticalimbic pathway play a critical role in reinforcement within the brain. The regions of the brain most involved are the nucleus accumbens (urges and impulses) and the amygdala (emotions). Other areas also implicated are the frontal and prefrontal cortex. These regions govern risky or compulsive behavior and control planning and judgments (Weintraub, 2008). Considerable research is still needed to determine the complex relationship between impulsivity and compulsivity (Fontenelle, Mendlowicz, & Versiani, 2005).

A decrease in serotonin has been linked to disorders characterized by poor control or impulse control issues. Thus, in more recent years, some individuals with impulse control disorders have responded to selective serotonin reuptake inhibitors (SSRIs) (Krakowski, 2003).

With intermittent explosive disorder, some features occur during or are congruent with nonspecific slowing on an EEG. Serotonin metabolism may be altered in impulsive and temper-prone individuals, but this is not a clear finding. Therefore, the diagnosis of intermittent explosive disorder is made only after other mental disorders are ruled out and the aggressive episodes, sometimes described as "spells," are determined not to be the result of mind-altering substances.

> *Alterations in neurotransmitter levels, such as serotonin, are associated with the etiology of impulse control disorders.*

## TREATMENT OPTIONS

Treatment options for impulse control disorders consist of both pharmacological and nonpharmacological therapies. However, no one therapy has been shown to be consistently effective.

## Nonpharmacological Therapies

Nonpharmacological therapies found to be helpful in the treatment of impulse control disorders include: cognitive restructuring, relaxation, anger management, family therapy, support groups, and coping skills training. The nurse can assist the patient in developing better coping skills by assisting the patient in identifying positive adaptive ways to manage stressful situations in the future and to take responsibility for wrongdoing. The use of psychosocial interventions for anger control and interpersonal aggression is well documented (McCloskey, Deffenbacher, Noblett, & Gollan, 2008). Child-centered play therapy is often used when working with children dealing with a wide range of psychiatric issues. This form of therapy has also been supported in children with intermittent explosive disorder (Paone & Douma, 2009). For the person with intermittent explosive disorder where anger management becomes a primary issue, several nonpharmological therapies may be helpful. With cognitive restructuring, patients are taught to think more useful thoughts rather than acting out in anger or impulsively. Beginning yoga may be helpful relaxation therapy. Breathing techniques can be very beneficial coping skills for those with anger impulsivity and anxiety concerns.

## Pharmacological Therapies

Currently, the primary pharmacologic treatment for impulse control disorders is with selective serotonin reuptake inhibitors (SSRIs), such as sertraline (Zoloft) and fluvoxamine (Luvox). The tricyclic antidepressant, clomipramine (Anafranil) also has been used (Lopan-Ibiz & Ruiz, 1995; see Chapter 12 for more information about antidepressants). Intermittent explosive disorder has been treated with phenytoin (Dilantin), mood stabilizers such as lithium, depakote, tegretol, SSRIs, beta-blockers such as propranolol, alpha-2-agonists such as clonidine, and atypical anti-psychotic medications, such as risperidone. Trichotillomania has responded best to SSRIs. Pathological gambling responds well to SSRIs, mood stabilizers such as lithium, and opioid antagonists such as naltrexone. See **Drug Summary 17-1** for a partial listing of medications that may be used to treat impulse control

**DRUG SUMMARY 17-1:**
**PARTIAL SELECTION OF MEDICATIONS USED TO TREAT IMPULSE CONTROL DISORDER**

| DRUG | IMPLICATIONS FOR NURSING CARE |
|---|---|
| **SELECTIVE SEROTONIN REUPTAKE INHIBITORS (SSRIs)** | |
| fluoxetine (Prozac) <br><br> paroxetine (Paxil) <br><br> sertraline (Zoloft) <br><br> fluvoxamine maleate (Luvox) <br><br> citalopram (Celexa) <br><br> escitalopram (Lexapro) | • Advise the patient to take the drug in the morning; if sedation occurs, encourage the patient to take the drug at bedtime <br> • Monitor the patient for signs of serotonin syndrome such as fever, sweating, agitation, tachycardia, hypotension, and hyperreflexia <br> • Inform the patient about possible sexual dysfunction with the drug; if this occurs and causes the patient distress, advocate for a change in the drug <br> • Discuss with patient the time to achieve effectiveness and that it may take from 2–4 weeks before symptoms resolve <br> • Emphasize the need for adherence to therapy and to not stop taking the drug abruptly to prevent withdrawal symptoms <br> • Assess the patient for evidence of suicidal thoughts, especially as depression lessens |
| **SEROTONIN/NOREPINEPHRINE REUPTAKE INHIBITORS (SNRIs)** | |
| desvenlafaxine (Pristiq) <br><br> duloxetine (Cymbalta) <br><br> venlafaxine (Effexor and Effexor XR) | • Advise the patient taking desvenlafaxine or duloxetine to have his blood pressure monitored because the drug may increase blood pressure <br> • Instruct patient taking venlafaxine to take the drug with food and a full glass of water; if the patient has difficulty swallowing capsules, suggest the patient open the capsule and sprinkle contents on an spoonful of applesauce and take immediately; reinforce the need to follow the capsule with a full glass of water <br> • Encourage the patient to check with his prescriber before taking any other prescription or over-the-counter drugs <br> • Warn patient of possible sedation and dizziness and the need to avoid hazardous activities until the drug's effects are known <br> • Emphasize the need for adherence to therapy and to not stop taking the drug abruptly to prevent withdrawal symptoms <br> • Assess the patient for evidence of suicidal thoughts, especially as depression lessens |
| **MOOD STABILIZERS** | |
| lithium carbonate (Lithobid, Lithotabs, Lithonate) <br><br> carbamazepine (Tegretol) | • Work with the patient to develop a schedule for laboratory testing of drug levels to promote compliance; remind patient that the level must be obtained 12 hours after the last dose has been taken |

*(cont.)*

**DRUG SUMMARY 17-1: (*CONT.*)**
**PARTIAL SELECTION OF MEDICATIONS USED TO TREAT IMPULSE CONTROL DISORDER**

| DRUG | IMPLICATIONS FOR NURSING CARE |
|---|---|
| **MOOD STABILIZERS** | |
| divalproex sodium (Depakote)<br>oxcarbazepine (Trileptal)<br>lamotrigine (Lamictal)<br>tiagabine HCL (Gabitril) | • Discuss with the patient the signs and symptoms of lithium toxicity:<br>-Levels 1.5 to 2.0 mEq/L: blurred vision, ataxia, tinnitus, persistent nausea and vomiting, severe diarrhea<br>-Levels 2.0 to 3.5 mEq/L: excessive dilute urine output, increasing tremors, muscle irritability, psychomotor retardation, mental confusion<br>-Levels over 3.5 mEq/L: impaired level of consciousness, nystagmus, seizures, coma, oliguria or anuria, arrhythmias, cardiovascular collapse<br>• Collaborate with patient how to ensure adequate sodium intake; reinforce the need for 6 to 8 large glasses of fluid each day; urge the patient to avoid caffeine beverages which increase urine output<br>• Advise patient to increase fluid intake if sweating, fever, or dieresis occurs<br>• Suggest the patient take the drug with food if gastrointestinal upset occurs<br>• Collaborate with the patient to develop a schedule for blood level testing to promote adherence<br>• Institute safety measures to reduce the risk of falling secondary to drowsiness or dizziness<br>• Emphasize the need for adherence to therapy and to not stop taking the drug abruptly to prevent withdrawal symptoms<br>• Assess the patient for evidence of suicidal thoughts, especially as depression lessens |
| **SECOND-GENERATION ANTIPSYCHOTIC DRUGS** | |
| risperidone (Risperidone)<br>olanzapine (Zyprexa)<br>quetiapine (Seroquel)<br>ziprasidone (Geodon)<br>aripiprazole (Abilify)<br>paliperidone (Invega)<br>iloperidone (Fanapt)<br>asenapine (Saphris) | • Instruct the patient using aripiprazole (Abilify) not to take the drug with grapefruit juice<br>• For the patient taking clozapine, obtain baseline white blood cell counts to assess for agranulocytosis; explain to the patient that he or she will receive only a 1-week supply of the drug; assist the patient in arranging for follow-up weekly blood tests for the first 6 months of therapy; monitor the patient closely for signs and symptoms of infection; stress the need for not stopping the drug abruptly<br>• Allow patient to verbalize feelings and issues related to drug therapy; work with patient and family to develop a method for ensuring adherence to drug therapy<br>• Monitor the patient for development of extrapyramidal side effects<br>• Be alert that neuroleptic malignant syndrome most often occurs during the first two weeks of therapy or after a dosage increase |

disorders. There is a lack of research on effective medication interventions for pyromania (Dell'Osso et al., 2006).

> *SSRIs are commonly used to treat impulse control disorders*

## APPLYING THE NURSING PROCESS FROM AN INTERPERSONAL PERSPECTIVE

Patients with impulse control disorders may be seen in a variety of settings, but most commonly in community and outpatient centers. If the patient has a comorbid condition or experiences injury as a result of the impulsive act, patients may be encountered in general medical facilities, emergency departments, and specialty clinics. Therefore, nurses need a firm understanding of the nursing process that integrates the interpersonal process when caring for patients with impulse control disorders. **Plan of Care 17-1** provides an example for a patient with an impulse control disorder.

### Strategies for Optimal Assessment: Therapeutic Use of Self

The therapeutic use of self as described by Joyce Travelbee is "the ability to use one's personality consciously and in full awareness in an attempt to establish relatedness and to structure nursing intervention" (Travelbee, 1971, p. 18). In this type of relationship, the nurse needs insight into his or her own behaviors and needs to possess the ability to understand the behaviors of others to ensure effective outcomes. In addition, the nurse employs the therapeutic use of self to collect data for documentation.

### Self-Awareness

Before beginning the assessment, the nurse uses this time to explore his or her own self-perceptions and fears about a patient. For example, the nurse may have gathered information from the patient's medical record that the person has a diagnosis of pathological gambling. Perhaps someone close to the nurse has struggled with gambling issues. The nurse needs to examine his or her ability to engage in a therapeutic relationship with this patient. Reflecting on one's own attitudes, values, and prejudices are a critical component of being able to calmly intervene and work with patients who suffer with impulse control disorders. Doing so will help to decrease the chance of countertransference or the emotional involvement that can interfere with the therapeutic process.

The self-aware nurse is pivotal in coming together with a patient to assess the patient's understanding of his or her condition. This is an essential step for developing empathy. **Consumer Perspective 17-1** provides insight into what it is like to experience an impulse control disorder from the patient's viewpoint.

### Data Collection

During assessment, the nurse obtains information from a patient in a goal-directed manner through observation, interview, and evaluation (**Evidence-Based Practice 17-1**). Information also is often obtained from other sources such as family members, health records, health care staff, or others on the treatment team. Throughout assessment, the nurse establishes trust and builds rapport while providing the necessary support and structure. The nurse and patient work together to set realistic goals for the relationship. In this phase, the psychiatric-mental health nurse needs to explore and investigate any patient-specific behaviors. Specifically, does anything precipitate the impulsive act or are there any antecedents or triggering phenomena that have been identified? What was the patient thinking about prior to committing the impulsive act? These specific questions may help the nurse devise an intervention plan for the client (Beck, 2009).

The nurse must treat the patient as an equal to foster the patient's regaining of control over his or her health. The nurse must trust the patient's ability to make good health decisions. This health-promoting trust encourages the patient's growth and development (Svedberg, Jormfetct, & Adividsson, 2003).

### Diagnosing and Planning Appropriate Interventions: Meeting the Patient's Focused Needs

Meeting the patient's focused needs during the planning stage of the nursing process can only happen if the nurse has accurately completed an assessment of the patient and his or her perception of the condition. Focusing on patient's strengths that were identified in the assessment stage is key when planning interventions. Doing so will also allow for an increased sense of collaboration on the part of the patient. Priorities are identified, treatment goals are established, specific actions are selected, and a plan of care is customized that is tailored to meet the individual patient's needs.

Due to varying assessment findings and the wide range of problems faced by patients with impulse control disorders, numerous nursing diagnoses would apply. Examples of possible nursing diagnoses would include:

- Risk for other-directed violence related to rage reaction/ antisocial characteristics.

**PLAN OF CARE 17-1:**
**THE PATIENT WITH AN IMPULSE CONTROL DISORDER**

**NURSING DIAGNOSIS:** Risk for other-directed violence; related to lack of impulse control, rage reaction with violent outbursts, and agitation.

**OUTCOME IDENTIFICATION:** Patient will demonstrate control of behavior to remain safe, without harm to self or others.

| INTERVENTION | RATIONALE |
|---|---|
| Approach the patient calmly; appear in control of own behavior, using a calm tone of voice and nonjudgmental attitude | Approaching the patient calmly and non-judgmentally helps to build trust and foster the nurse–patient relationship |
| Assess the patient for indicators suggesting potential for harm to self or others, such as irritability, intimidation, restlessness, shouting or loud voice, or overt threats; ensure the safety of the patient and others; be alert for these possible triggers | Identifying indicators of potential harm allows for early intervention |
| Minimize the patient's exposure to stimuli; keep environment calm, quiet with little distraction; remove all hazardous items from the patient's environment | Limiting stimuli helps to prevent overwhelming the patient, which could lead to increased anxiety and agitation; removal of items reduces the risk of use if behavior escalates |
| Set firm, reasonable expectations for patient's behavior; ensure that the patient understands the limits and the consequences associated with violating limits; Teach the patient about limits and boundaries and consistently reinforce them | Using limit setting establishes the boundaries for behavior and helps to minimize manipulation by the patient |
| Assist the patient in identifying signs and symptoms of increasing anxiety and in using measures to reduce anxiety and agitation when they occur; suggest the use of physical activity, talking about feelings, or asking for medication | Being able to identify signs and symptoms promotes early intervention; using measures such as physical activity or talking provides an outlet for reducing anxiety without harming self or others |
| Work with the patient on impulse control including explaining the benefits of control; assist the patient to employ strategies such as behavior modification to control impulses; redirect the patient to more appropriate or productive activities | Working toward impulse control provides the patient with insight about behavior and positive ways to deal with feelings rather than using violence or aggression; using behavior modification reinforces a positive method of handling feelings |
| Assist the patient in role-playing and practicing techniques; provide positive reinforcement | Using role play and practice help reinforce use of appropriate behaviors; positive reinforcement fosters self-esteem and enhances the possibility of successful use in the future |

*(cont.)*

**PLAN OF CARE 17-1:** (*CONT.*)
**THE PATIENT WITH AN IMPULSE CONTROL DISORDER**

| INTERVENTION | RATIONALE |
|---|---|
| Administer prescribed medication therapy such as selective serotonin reuptake inhibitors (SSRIs) | Using prescribed pharmacological therapies may help to control behaviors associated with the disorder |
| Ensure the development of a plan should behavior escalation occur; ensure a unified approach to the patient; contract with the patient for no self-harm | Having a plan is necessary to reduce the safety risk for all involved; employing a unified approach demonstrates control over the situation<br><br>Using a no-harm contract emphasizes expectations, fosters participation in care and feelings of control over the situation, and promotes safety |
| If behavior escalation occurs, place the patient in the least restrictive environment; move others from the area of escalation | Using the least restrictive environment is necessary to protect the patient's rights; moving others away protects their safety |

**NURSING DIAGNOSIS:** Ineffective coping related to conflict and stress; manifested by violent behavior, anger and aggression, rage reaction.

**OUTCOME IDENTIFICATION:** Patient will begin to demonstrate use of positive coping strategies to deal with underlying feelings and emotions.

| INTERVENTION | RATIONALE |
|---|---|
| Assess the patient's level of anger, aggression, and impulsivity; stay with the patient and provide for safety and security | Determining the level of the patient's anger and aggression provides a baseline from which to intervene |
| Maintain a calm, reassuring approach; keep verbal exchanges short and direct | Maintaining a calm, reassuring approach prevents adding to the patient's anger and aggression<br><br>Keeping exchanges short and direct reduces the risk of overwhelming an already overwhelmed patient |
| Once the level of aggression or anger has diminished, assist the patient in exploring feelings and precipitating factors; if necessary, encourage the patient to keep a journal or diary related to feelings associated with anger and aggression | Identifying feelings and precipitating factors can help to prevent recurrence; using a journal or diary promotes insight into possible triggers related to behavior; objectively viewing the situation can help the patient identify faulty thinking patterns |

(*cont.*)

**PLAN OF CARE 17-1: (CONT.)**
**THE PATIENT WITH AN IMPULSE CONTROL DISORDER**

| INTERVENTION | RATIONALE |
|---|---|
| Encourage the patient to discuss feelings and assist the patient in viewing situations related to feelings objectively | |
| Assist the patient in identifying signs and symptoms of increasing anger and agitation | Being able to identify signs and symptoms facilitates early intervention |
| Work with the patient to determine usual methods of problem solving; identify effective and ineffective methods; suggest appropriate methods and encourage the patient's participation in problem solving | Identifying usual methods of coping provides information about possible maladaptive strategies and opportunities for teaching more adaptive ones; encouraging patient participation promotes feelings of control over the situation, self-esteem, and self-worth |
| Reinforce use of appropriate prescribed therapies such as cognitive restructuring, relaxation techniques, and controlled breathing | Using various methods for reducing anger and aggression provides the patient with options to manage these feelings effectively |
| Assist the patient in practicing appropriate strategies; provide positive reinforcement | Practicing promotes success; positive reinforcement promotes self-esteem |

*Nursing Diagnosis – Definitions and Classifications 2009–2011. Copyright © 2011 by NANDA International. Use by arrangement with Blackwell Publishing Limited, a company of John Wiley & Sons, Inc.*

- Risk for self-directed violence related to rage reaction.
- Anxiety related to threat to or change in environmental pattern.
- Anxiety related to threat to or change in interaction pattern.
- Ineffective coping related to inadequate coping method.
- Ineffective coping related to situational crisis.
- Powerlessness related to interpersonal interactions.
- Impaired social interaction related to altered thought processes.
- Ineffective role performance related to rage reaction.

These nursing diagnoses also will vary based on the acuity of the patient's illness, developmental stage, co-morbidities, current treatment regimen, and sources of support. Based on the identified nursing diagnoses, the nurse and patient collaboratively would determine the outcomes to be achieved. For example, for the nursing diagnosis of risk for other-directed violence related to rage, an appropriate outcome would be that the patient will identify antecedents to anger and explosive behavior

in an attempt to stop escalation by a planned walking away and cooling down period.

## Implementing Effective Interventions: Timing and Pacing

In the implementation phase of the nursing process the nursing care plan is carried out. The nurse provides both nonpharmacological and pharmacological therapy and monitoring where appropriate. The care plan must ensure good documentation for legal and therapeutic reasons. The nurse is in an ongoing state of assessment to determine if the intervention is helpful or not. This phase is composed of both dependent nursing actions (giving medications) and independent/interdependent nursing actions. In this phase the patient will actively seek knowledge from the nurse and the treatment team to address the mutually identified issues. This active involvement in the therapeutic relationship shows a readiness for assistance (Beck, 2009).

### CONSUMER PERSPECTIVE 17-1:
### A PATIENT WITH KLEPTOMANIA

"Hi. My name is Jill and I take things from stores. Usually, the stuff is just junk but I see it and I've got to have it. I could buy it if I wanted to. I am 17 years old and I guess the psych diagnosis on my chart is kleptomania. I steal little things like lip gloss and earrings.

I have gotten busted before for shoplifting. It is so embarrassing but I can't stop on my own. I get so excited; it's intense, and it's kinda like getting off. I wish I could stop but sometimes I just can't help myself."

### EVIDENCE-BASED PRACTICE 17-1:
### PLAY THERAPY AND INTERMITTENT EXPLOSIVE DISORDER

#### STUDY

Paone, T.R., & Douma, K.B. (2009). Child-centered play therapy with a seven-year-old boy diagnosed with Intermittent Explosive Disorder. *International Journal of Play Therapy. 18*(1). 31-44.

#### SUMMARY

This is a case study report of the use of child-centered play therapy (CCPT) with a child with intermittent explosive disorder. Parent consultation and involvement were included throughout the therapy. Sixteen CCPT sessions were conducted; highlights of each of the sessions are described. The child did not talk to the therapist often during the therapy, but communicated most often through the type of toys he chose in the session. At the conclusion of the therapy, the child was exhibiting age-appropriate behaviors both in school and at home.

#### APPLICATION TO PRACTICE

Various forms of play therapy can be used with children and adults. For example, role playing is a form of play therapy. Patients also can be observed in recreational activities on the unit, to both assess their behaviors and learn about impulse control based on their behaviors and interactions with others in the recreational activity. Also, as part of the assessment process, patients can be asked to describe their play activities.

#### QUESTIONS TO PONDER

1. *How can nurses use modified forms of play therapy, e.g., role playing, to assess a patient's behavior?*
2. *Do you think the play therapy would have been as successful without the parents' involvement?*

> *A common priority nursing diagnosis for a patient with an impulse control disorder is risk for other-directed violence.*

In developing interventions, the nurse should consider the need for setting limits with the patient, as these individuals often test the boundaries and push the limits of rules and regulations. An important therapeutic technique is that of psychoeducation in which the focus is on teaching the patient the boundaries and the consequences of not controlling impulses (**Therapeutic Interaction 17-1**). Role play

> ### THERAPEUTIC INTERACTION 17-1:
> ### A PATIENT WITH PATHOLOGICAL GAMBLING
>
> R.B. presents for in-patient treatment after his gambling has gotten out of hand. He has depleted all of his family's savings, retirement funds, and has written a number of bad checks. The creditors are calling, he is depressed, and his wife is threatening to leave him. He has passive suicidal ideations.

| | |
|---|---|
| **R.B.:** "I have really messed up this time. I have lost everything." | Desperation stage of gambling cycle, may contemplate suicide. |
| **Nurse:** "Do you currently want to hurt yourself or others?" | Clarifying/asking directly about self-harm, a top priority for any patient who has threat-to-harm thoughts to assess/monitor safety risks. |
| **R.B.:** "No, I'm not going to kill myself, or off anybody else." | With any patient that has threat-to-harm thoughts, the nurse must attempt to get the patient to contract for safety. |
| **Nurse:** "If you feel unsafe or like you are going to harm yourself or someone else, can you let me, one of the nurses, or a psych care staff know if you feel unsafe?" | The nurse suggests a no-harm contract. |
| **R.B.:** "Ok, I will. But I wish I could stop gambling, but I can't. I drive by the casino, and before I know it, I'm in there. No one understands me." | Agrees to contract. |
| **Nurse:** "You mentioned driving by the casino. Is there another way home you could take?" | Beginning to assist the patient in cognitive restructuring. |
| **Nurse:** "You are not alone. Your treatment team will help you identify strategies to assist you to more effectively cope with your gambling addiction, like individual group therapy and gambler's anonymous (GA)." | Identifying for the patient that staff is there to help him, that he is not alone and there are strategies that have been proven helpful (support groups and therapy for addiction have been proven effective); fosters some hope without providing false reassurance. |

can also help the patient learn boundaries and consequences of the inappropriate impulsive behavior. **How Would You Respond?** 17-1 provides an example of a patient with an impulse control disorder requiring intervention.

## Evaluating: Objective Critique of Interventions and Self-Reflection

The nurse evaluates how much progress has been made toward achieving expected outcomes. For any goals not met, the nurse needs to self-reflect on anything he or she may have done differently while providing nursing care and evaluate how the patient presented initially and where he or she is at this time. During this phase of the nurse-patient relationship, the nurse and the patient should reflect on progress made toward reaching the patient's goals, with the nurse pointing out positives to the patient and including a plan for aftercare as appropriate.

Evaluation also provides a feedback mechanism for judging the quality of care given. The demand for health care services and the growing cost of these services has led to a focus on outcomes as a means for effectiveness and efficiency. Evaluation of the progress indicates which problems have been solved, which needs have been met, and which require reassessment, replanning, implementation, and re-evaluation. The ongoing process of evaluation and re-evaluation provides a realistic mechanism for judging the quality of care given (Beck, 2009).

---

**HOW WOULD YOU RESPOND? 17-1:**
**A PATIENT WITH AN INTERMITTENT EXPLOSIVE DISORDER**

Tonya is 16-year-old female who lives with her grandmother because her mother has a drug problem. Usually Tonya and her grandmother get along well, but both agree Tonya's temper is a problem. Recently, her grandmother reported that Tonya snapped after being asked to sweep the porch before Tonya's girlfriend came over to watch movies. The grandmother reports that "Tonya flipped out and took the broom handle and was knocking all the stuff off the front porch, broke it and hit me upside the head with the broom handle." The police were called and Tonya was taken to the police station. Her grandmother reports bailing Tonya out of jail the next day, but stated that Tonya must get help or she will no longer be permitted to stay with her grandmother for safety reasons. The grandmother said, "I am scared of her when she snaps." Tonya reports feeling bad afterward and crying and saying she was sorry. "I just could not stop! I just got so mad and the next thing I knew I had torn up the porch and hit my grandma. I scared myself." How would you respond?

**CRITICAL THINKING QUESTIONS**

1. *Based on the situation, how does Tonya meet the diagnostic criteria for intermittent explosive disorder?*

2. *What nursing diagnosis would be a priority for Tonya?*

3. *What suggestions might be appropriate to include in the plan of care for Tonya's explosive episodes?*

---

**APPLYING THE CONCEPTS**

Based on the situation, Tonya has a problem with her temper, suggesting that there have been other episodes of "snapping." Tonya also exhibited aggressiveness that was out of proportion to the request by her grandmother, ultimately resulting in Tonya physically assaulting her grandmother and destroying the items on the porch. Additionally, Tonya felt remorse and regretted her actions afterward.

As a result of Tonya's actions, safety, primarily for her grandmother but also for herself, is the priority. Appropriate priority nursing diagnoses would be risk for other-directed violence related to assaultive acts on her grandmother and risk for self-directed violence related to an inability to resist aggressive impulses.

Tonya might benefit from pharmacological therapy, such as SSRIs, because there is some belief that serotonin metabolism may be altered in individuals with intermittent explosive disorder. In addition, cognitive restructuring, limit setting, coping skills training, and anger management techniques would be appropriate.

## SUMMARY POINTS

- Impulse control is a common central feature in many Axis I psychiatric-mental health disorders. They include intermittent explosive disorder, kleptomania, pathological gambling, trichotillomania, and impulse control disorder not otherwise specified.

- Essential features of any impulse control disorder are (1) failure to resist the impulse to act, (2) an increasing sense of tension or arousal before committing the act, and (3) an experience of pleasure or sense of gratification or release at the time of the commission of the act.

- Impulse control disorders are treated with pharmacotherapy such as SSRIs and non-pharmacological therapies, such as cognitive restructuring, relaxation, and coping skills training.

- During assessment, the psychiatric-mental health nurse needs to explore and investigate any patient-specific behaviors, including precipitating factors, antecedents or triggers, and patient thinking prior to committing the impulsive act.

- Several interventions can be implemented by the nurse to address the symptoms and underlying causes of impulse control disorders.

## NCLEX-PREP*

1. The nurse is developing a teaching plan for a patient with an impulse control disorder. The nurse integrates knowledge of which of the following in this plan?
   a. An increase in tension leads to an increase in arousal.
   b. The act immediately leads to feelings of regret.
   c. A need for pleasure is the driving force for acting.
   d. Increased arousal leads to a rise in stress.

2. A group of nursing students are reviewing information related to impulse control disorders. The students demonstrate an understanding of the information when they identify which behavior as characteristic of trichotillomania?
   a. Fire setting
   b. Stealing
   c. Pulling out of hair
   d. Property destruction

3. A nursing instructor is preparing a class lecture about impulse control disorder. When describing kleptomania, which of the following would the instructor include?
   a. The patient needs the item for personal use.
   b. The item is too expensive for the patient to purchase.
   c. The object reflects an expression of anger.
   d. The person lacks a need for the object.

4. The nurse is assessing a patient in whom pathological gambling is suspected. Which statement(s) would the nurse interpret as reflecting the diagnostic criteria for this condition? Select all that apply.
   a. "I find myself going back to the casino the next day to get even."

(cont.)

### NCLEX-PREP* (CONT.)

b. "I started out with small amounts, but now I'm using half of my paycheck."

c. "I might bet $5 on a football pool every so often."

d. "I'm going to hit the jackpot again, like I did once before."

e. "I went to the racetrack after I told my wife I had to work late."

5. Which of the following would the nurse identify as a major issue involved with intermittent explosive disorder?

a. Fear of discovery

b. Ineffective health maintenance

c. Injury

d. Substance abuse

*Answers to these questions appear on page 639.

## REFERENCES

American Psychiatric Association (APA). (2000). *Diagnostic and Statistical Manual of Mental Disorders (4th ed) Text Revision.* Washingon, D.C.: Author.

Beck, J., (2009). The nursing process: Context of psychiatric nursing. *Mental Health Nursing.* 1–11.

Bostwick, J.M., Hecksel, K.A., Stevens, S.R., Bower, J.H., & Ahlskog, J.E. (2009). Frequency of new onset pathologic compulsive gambling or hypersexuality after drug treatment of idiopathic Parkinson's disease. *Mayo Clin Proc. 4*(84), 3110–3316.

Dell'Osso, B., Altamura, C., Allen, A., Marazziti, D., & Hollander, E., (2006). Epidemiologic and clinical updates on impulse control disorders: A critical review. *Europe Archive Psychiatry Clinical Neuroscience. 256,* 464–475.

Fontenelle, L.F., Mendlowicz, M.V., & Versiani, M. (2005). Impulse control disorders in patients with obsessive-compulsive disorders. *Psychiatry and Clinical Neurosciences. 59,* 30–37.

Grant, J.E. (2003). Family history and psychiatric comorbidity in person with kleptomania. *Comprehensive Psychiatry. 44*(6), 437–441.

Grant, J.E., & Kim, W. (2003). Comorbidity of impulse control disorder in pathological gambler. *Acta Psychiatric Scandinavia. 108,* 203–207.

Grant, J.E., Levine, L., Kim, D., & Potenza, M.N. (2005). Impulse control disorders in adult psychiatric inpatients: Brief report. *American Journal of Psychiatry 162*(11), 2184–2187.

Grant, J.E., Kim, S.W., Odlaung, B.L., Buchanan, S.N., & Potenza, M.N. (2009). Late onset pathological gambling: Clinical correlates and gender differences. *Journal of Psychiatric Research. 43,* 380–387.

Kim, Y.J., & Pork, H.A. (2005) Analysis of nursing records of candidate-surgery patients based on the nursing process and focusing on nursing outcomes. *International Journal of Medical Informatics, 75,* 952–959.

Krakowski, M. (2003). Violence and seratonen influence of impulse control, affect regulation, and social functioning. *Journal of Clinical Neurosciences, 15,* 294–305.

McCloskey, M.S., Deffenbacher, J.L., Noblett, K.L., Gollan, J.K., Coccaro, E.F. (2008). Cognitive Behavioral therapy for intermittent explosive disorder: A pilot randomized clinical trial. *Journal of Consulting and Clinical Psychology. 76*(5), 876–886.

Moro, E. (2009). Impulse control disorders and subthalmic nucleus stimulation in Parkinson's disease: Are we jumping the gun? *European Journal of Neurology. 16,* 410–441.

North American Nursing Diagnosis Association (NANDA). (2009). Nursing diagnoses: Definitions and classification 2009–2011. Philadelphia: Author.

Paone, T.R., & Douma, K.B. (2009). Child-Centered play therapy with a seven-year-old boy diagnosed with intermittent explosive disorder. *International Journal of Play Therapy. 18*(1), 31–44.

Presta, S. Marazziti, D., Dell'Osso, L., Pfarner, C., Pallanti, S., & Cassano, G.B. (2002). Kleptomania: Clinical features and comorbidity in an Italian sample. *Comprehensive Psychiatry. 43*(1), 7–12.

Svedberg, P., Jormfeldt, H., Arvidsson. B. (2003). Patients conception of how health process are promoted in mental health nursing. A qualitative study. *Journal of Psychiatric and Mental Health Nursing, 10,* 448–456.

Travelbee, J. (1971). *Interpersonal aspects of nursing.* (2nd ed.). Philadelphia: F.A. Davis.

Wanner, B., Vitaro, F., Carbonneau, R., & Tremblay, R.E. (2009). Cross-Tagged links among gambling, substance use, and delinquency from midadolescence to young adulthood: Addictive and moderation effects of common risk factors. *Psychology of Addictive Behaviors, 23*(1), 91–104.

Weintraub, D., (2008). Depamire and impulse control disorders in Parkinson's disease. *Ann Neurol. 64,* 93–100.

Whitaker, H., Wolf, K.A., & Keuthen, N. (2003). Chronic hair pulling recognizing trichotillomania. *Clinician Reviews. 13*(3), 37–44.

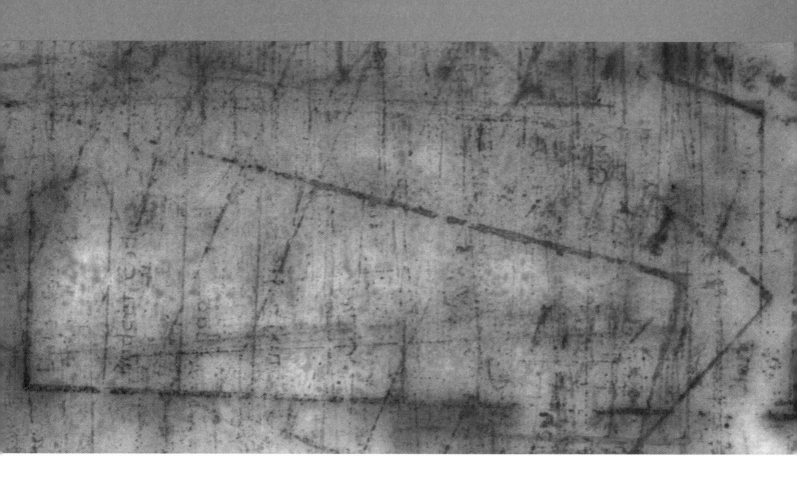

## CHAPTER CONTENTS

## EXPECTED LEARNING OUTCOMES

**After completing this chapter, the student will be
able to:**

1. Define sexuality.
2. Differentiate between a sexual dysfunction and sexual
   disorder.
3. Discuss the history and epidemiology of sexual
   disorders and dysfunctions.
4. Identify diagnoses that constitute a sexual
   disorder.Identify diagnoses that constitute a sexual
   dysfunction.
5. Describe the major diagnostic criteria for sexual
   disorders and dysfunctions.
6. Discuss possible theories related to the etiology of
   sexual disorders and dysfunction.

## CHAPTER 18

# SEXUAL DISORDERS AND DYSFUNCTIONS

Jeffrey S. Jones

7. Explain the various treatment options available for persons experiencing sexual disorders and dysfunctions.

8. Discuss the common assessment strategies for individuals with sexual disorders and dysfunctions, identifying the importance of assessing sexual functioning as part of the nursing assessment.

9. Describe the role of the nurse in promoting sexual health for patients.

10. Apply the nursing process from an interpersonal perspective to the care of patients with sexual disorders and dysfunctions, with an emphasis on boundary management when dealing with sexual health promotion of patients.

## KEY TERMS

Chemical castration

Human sexuality

Paraphilias

Sensate focus

Sexual disorders

Sexual dysfunctions

Sexual functioning

Sexual health promotion

HUMAN SEXUALITY (how people experience themselves as sexual beings) and SEXUAL FUNCTIONING (the actual act of expressing yourself sexually either for pleasure or for reproductive purposes with others) are woven into the fabric of human life throughout the life cycle. Sexuality and sexual functioning play a major role in everything from basic reproduction to childhood development, maturation, adult lifestyle, and sexual satisfaction (Fogel & Lauver, 1990). Sexual feelings, functioning, and behaviors comprise an important part of each person, no matter age or situation, and should not be neglected or ignored by health care providers. Nurses provide care for the young as well as the old and need to be comfortable in incorporating sexual health assessments and development of a treatment plan regarding SEXUAL HEALTH PROMOTION (the integration of the somatic, emotional, intellectual, and social aspects of sexual beings, in ways that are positively ensuring) for clients.

SEXUAL DYSFUNCTIONS are conditions characterized by a disturbance in the processes involved in the sexual response cycle (desire, excitement, orgasm, or resolution) or pain associated sexual intercourse (American Psychiatric Association [APA], 2000). SEXUAL DISORDERS, also called PARAPHILIAS, are characterized by recurrent, intense sexual urges, fantasies, or behaviors involving unusual objects, activities, or situations (APA, 2000).

This chapter addresses the historical perspectives and epidemiology of sexual disorders and dysfunctions, followed by a description of the major characteristics of these disorders as defined in the *Diagnostic and Statistical Manual of Mental Disorders, 4th edition, Text Revision* (*DSM-IV-TR*). Scientific theories focusing on psychodynamic and neurobiologic influences are described along with a summary of common treatment options. Application of the nursing process from an interpersonal perspective is presented, including a plan of care for a patient with a sexual dysfunction. Assessment of sexual functioning and the role of the nurse in promoting sexual health through therapeutic use of self skills such as listening and through psychoeducation are emphasized.

> *Difficulties with sexual functioning typically are classified as sexual disorders or sexual dysfunctions. Sexual disorders involve intense sexual urges, fantasies, or behaviors, whereas sexual dysfunctions involve disruptions in the sexual response cycle.*

## HISTORICAL PERSPECTIVES

The origin of modern understanding of sexual functioning from a mental health perspective can be traced to Freud (Fogel & Lauver, 1990). Freud was one of the first psychiatrists to try to understand how sexual drives and urges manifest and are expressed. In particular, his understanding of the role of the unconscious in dealing with repressed feelings continues to play a fairly prominent role in psychoanalysis. Freud's theory on psychosexual development and the oral, genital, and anal phases of development were some of the first efforts at describing the transition from infancy to childhood. More recently, scientists such as William Masters, Virginia Johnson, and Alfred Kinsey studied the human sexual response cycle, women's sexuality, and sexuality and orientation as viewed on a continuum.

> *Sexuality is viewed on a continuum from exclusively heterosexual to exclusively homosexual.*

As theories are refined and knowledge is gained from further research into human sexuality, some topics that were previously referred to as disorders are now understood to be degrees of variance on a continuum. Homosexuality is such an example. Until the 1950s in the United States, homosexuality was considered by many to be a sexual (deviant) disorder. After years of research with psychologists and psychiatrists working in the field of sex therapy, it was concluded that homosexuality is not a disorder because it does not meet the necessary criteria in terms of impairment. Additionally, the particular work of zoologist and taxonomist Alfred C. Kinsey furthered this conclusion. Kinsey, in his groundbreaking empirical studies of sexual behavior among American adults, revealed that a number of his research participants reported having engaged in homosexual behavior to the point of orgasm after age 16 (Kinsey, Pomeroy, & Martin, 1948; Kinsey, Pomeroy, Martin, & Gebhard, 1953). Furthermore, Kinsey and his colleagues reported that 10% of the males in their sample and 2% to 6% of the females (depending on marital status) had been more or less exclusively homosexual in their behaviors for at least three years between the ages of 16 and 55. This research prompted the view of sexuality as occurring on a continuum (**Figure 18-1**). In 1973, the weight of empirical data, coupled with changing social norms and the development of a politically active gay community in the United States, led the Board of Directors of the American Psychiatric Association to remove homosexuality from the *DSM*.

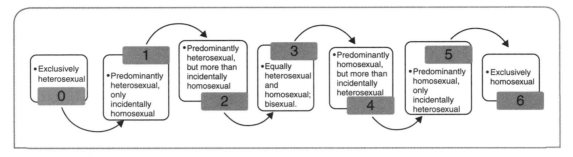

Figure 18-1 *Degrees of sexual orientation as viewed on a continuum. (Kinsey Scale. Adapted by J. Jones, 2010.)*

In discussing sexual disorders and sexual dysfunction from a historical perspective, progress on this topic has always been influenced by political, cultural, and theological aspects. The concept of monogamy or sexual fidelity within a relationship or marriage is such an example.

The Western view has been influenced heavily by the variety of religious doctrines in our culture. Most have a negative, intolerant view of affairs. In some cases, those who have or had affairs are labeled as having a compulsive sexual disorder. This view must be compared to the cultural mind-set in other countries. While not as prevalent in today's European culture, previously, certain fractions of French culture had a slotted time between the end of the workday and the beginning of evening hours that was set aside and referred to as "le temps d'affaires." During this time, a man or woman would have approximately two hours of private time between work and home in which he or she was allowed to do whatever he or she wanted to do. The partner was not to ask where the other had been. It was assumed that it was "none of their business." If the man or woman had decided to spend those hours between work and home with a lover, it was part of the accepted culture. This example is a glimpse into subtle, nuanced cultural differences on topics such as affairs that illustrate variations in perspective. However, this is not a generalization of French culture because many French couples enjoy a monogamous relationship (Ubillos, Paez, & Gonzalez, 2000).

> *Sexual problems occur in approximately 31% of men and 43% of women.*

## EPIDEMIOLOGY

Incidence and frequency of sexual disorders and dysfunctions can be difficult to obtain because this area is understudied and underreported. It is estimated that between 10% and 52% of men and 25% and 63% of women experience some sexual problems. The percentages that meet the diagnostic criteria for a sexual dysfunction are probably lower and less established (Heiman, 2002). Box 18-1 provides some statistical information about sexual disorders and dysfunctions.

## DIAGNOSTIC CRITERIA

The terms *disorder* and *dysfunction* are terms used to describe variations in sexual functioning that result in either distress when functioning sexually or inability to function sexually at all. The terms are sometimes used interchangeably in their descriptive language. In the *DSM-IV-TR*, the general category is "sexual disorders" with sexual dysfunctions, paraphilias, and gender identity disorders as the major subcategories.

In general, a sexual *disorder* will be diagnosed if the sexual behavior or pattern (such as masochism) has emerged and is causing distress for the individual interpersonally, legally, economically, or in some other way. Of course, there are cases of individuals with sexual disorders who never experience any distress; for example, an individual may have sexual masochism and have a compatible partner who may have sexual sadism.

Sexual *dysfunction* is usually diagnosed in the individual who, for either physiological or psychological reasons, cannot engage in sexual activity as desired. Dyspareunia, pain felt during intercourse, is an example. Sometimes the word "disorder" is used in the title of the diagnosis, such as male erectile disorder, but the diagnosis is actually classified as a dysfunction.

Gender identity disorders has its own subcategory in the *DSM-IV-TR* due to its unique nature. This disorder is usually characterized by the individual identifying themselves as the opposite gender. Gender identity disorder is more prevalent in childhood than in adulthood (Leiblum, 2007).

Table 18-1 summarizes the major diagnostic criteria associated with specific sexual disorders and sexual dysfunctions.

### BOX 18-1: STATISTICS ON SEXUAL DISORDERS AND DYSFUNCTIONS

- Sexual problems occur in 43% of American women.
- Sexual problems occur in 31% of American men.
- About 10% of women have never had an orgasm.
- Painful intercourse has been experienced by almost two out of three women at some time in their lives.
- It is common for breast-feeding women to have inadequate vaginal lubrication.
- About 15% of postmenopausal women experience a decrease in their sexual desire.
- The success rate for women's orgasmic dysfunction treatment by sex therapists tends to range from 65% to 85%.
- About 22% of women experience low sexual desire (compared to 5% of men).
- Some 21% of men experience premature ejaculation.
- A woman's level of androgen (a hormone that develops and maintains masculine characteristics) typically falls 50% during and after menopause (but it's unclear whether the drop translates into decreased sex drive in a large percentage of women).

*From National Library of Medicine; National Women's Health Resource Center; Journal of the American Medical Association, health. www.howstuffworks.com*

### TABLE 18-1: DIAGNOSTIC CRITERIA OF SEXUAL DISORDERS AND DYSFUNCTIONS

| SEXUAL DISORDERS (PARAPHILIAS) | KEY DIAGNOSTIC CRITERIA |
|---|---|
| Exhibitionism | Characterized by intense sexually arousing fantasies, urges, or behaviors in which the individual exposes his or her genitals to an unsuspecting stranger. |
| Fetishism | Characterized by intense sexually arousing fantasies, urges, or behaviors in which the individual uses a nonliving object (an example would be a woman's high-heeled shoe, stockings, etc.) in a sexual manner. Typically, the object is required by individual to become sexually aroused; there is an inability to be aroused without the object. |
| Frotteurism | Characterized by intense sexually arousing fantasies, urges, or behaviors in which the individual touches or rubs against a nonconsenting person in a sexual manner. Often occurring in somewhat conspicuous situations such as a crowded bus or subway. |
| Pedophilia | Characterized by intense sexually arousing fantasies, urges, or behaviors involving sexual activity with prepubescent children, typically age 13 or younger. Individual are at least 16 years old, and at least 5 years older than the child. Hebophilia, a subcategory, is sexual arousal toward children in their early teens (12 to 14 years old, specifically). |
| Sexual Masochism | Characterized by intense sexually arousing fantasies, urges, or behaviors in which the individual is humiliated, beaten, bound, or made to suffer in some way. |
| Sexual Sadism | Characterized by intense sexually arousing fantasies, urges, or behaviors in which the individual is sexually aroused by causing humiliation or physical suffering of another person. |
| Transvestic Fetishism | Heterosexual males who have sexually arousing fantasies, urges, or behaviors involved in cross-dressing (wearing female clothing). Fantasies, urges, and behaviors causing significant distress to the individual or disrupting everyday functioning. |
| Voyeurism | Characterized by intense sexually arousing fantasies, urges, or behaviors in which the individual observes an unsuspecting stranger who is naked, disrobing, or engaging in sexual activity. |

*(cont.)*

## TABLE 18-1: DIAGNOSTIC CRITERIA OF SEXUAL DISORDERS AND DYSFUNCTIONS (*CONT.*)

**SEXUAL DYSFUNCTIONS**

| | |
|---|---|
| Dyspareunia | Recurrent or persistent genital pain usually with sexual intercourse occurring in males or females. |
| Female Orgasmic Disorder | Delay of orgasm following normal excitement and sexual activity. Due to the wide variety of sexual response in women, judged by a clinician as significant, taking into account the person's age and situation. <br> Persistent or occurring frequently and causing significant distress; not a direct effect of substance abuse. |
| Female Sexual Arousal Disorder | Inability to attain or maintain, until completion of sexual activity, adequate lubrication in response to sexual excitement. <br> Significant distress; not better accounted for by another disorder, or the use of a substance. |
| Hypoactive Sexual Desire Disorder | Deficient or absent sexual fantasies and desire for sexual activity. Judgment by clinician taking into account the individual's age and life circumstances. <br> Lack of desire resulting in significant distress in the individual, and not better accounted for by another disorder. |
| Male Erectile Disorder | The recurring inability to achieve or maintain an erection until completion of sexual activity. <br> Significant distress for the individual, and not accounted for by another physical diagnosis. |
| Male Orgasmic Disorder | Delay in orgasm followed by normal excitement and activity. Due to the widely, varied sexual response in men, judgment by the clinician to be significant, taking into account the person's age and situation. <br> Persistent or occurring frequently, causing significant stress and not an effect of substance abuse. |
| Premature Ejaculation | Ejaculation with minimal sexual stimulation before or shortly after penetration and before the person wishes it. <br> Persistent or occurring frequently, causing significant distress and not the direct effect of substance abuse. |
| Sexual Aversion Disorder | Persistent or recurring aversion or avoidance of sexual activity, resulting in significant distress for the individual and not better accounted for by another disorder or physical diagnosis. When presented with a sexual opportunity, the individual possibly experiencing panic attacks or extreme anxiety. |
| Vaginismus | Recurrent or persistent involuntary spasms of the vaginal muscles that interfere with sexual intercourse. <br> Significant distress not due to a medical condition or another disorder. |

**GENDER IDENTITY DISORDERS**

| | |
|---|---|
| Gender Identity Disorder | Strong and persistent identification with the opposite gender. <br> Sense of discomfort in own gender; feelings of being born the wrong sex (Not to be confused with cross-dressing or Transvestic Fetishism, which is a distinct, separate diagnosis). |

*From the Diagnostic and Statistical Manual of Mental Disorders, Fourth Edition, Text Revision, Copyright © 2000, American Psychiatric Association.*

## ETIOLOGY

Various theories have been proposed to explain the etiology of sexual disorders and dysfunctions. These are highlighted in **Table 18-2**. Important psychodynamic and neurobehavioral influences are described here.

## Psychodynamic Influences

Professional sex therapists frequently report that the work required with patients ultimately has to do with resolution of psychodynamic conflict. Erectile dysfunction has received much attention lately with the advent

**TABLE 18-2: ETIOLOGIES ASSOCIATED WITH SEXUAL DISORDERS AND DYSFUNCTIONS**

| SEXUAL DISORDERS (PARAPHILIAS) | ETIOLOGY |
|---|---|
| Exhibitionism | Etiology relies on different theories related to exhibitionistic behavior. Many of these stem from the psychoanalytic theories. It has been suggested that childhood trauma (e.g., sexual abuse), or significant childhood experiences can manifest themselves in exhibitionistic behavior. |
| Fetishism | Many theories exist in an attempt to explain how this disorder developed. Most experts agree that there are underlying issues related to childhood, which play a major role in the etiology. Current thinking from a neurobiological perspective implicates an experience that duplicates a previous set of neurobiological scenarios that the individual is often trying to replicate (i.e., intense release of dopamine). |
| Frotteurism | There is no prominent theory as to how this disorder develops. |
| Pedophilia | A large percentage of individuals with this disorder were sexually abused as children, although the vast majority of adults who were abused do not develop pedophilic behaviors, there are also those who argue pedophilia results in feelings of inadequacy with same-age peers, and therefore transfer their sexual urges to children. New research suggests that sexual attraction to children may be an actual orientation. |
| Sexual Masochism | Theories related to sexual masochism mainly stem from the psychoanalytic perspective. They suggest that childhood trauma such as abuse or significant childhood experiences can manifest itself into masochistic behavior. |
| Sexual Sadism | Etiology is related to antisocial personality disorder. Childhood trauma such as sexual abuse is considered the primary cause. |
| Transvestic Fetishism Voyeurism | Many different theories related to this disorder. Current thinking is looking at stress reduction and anxiety management triggers. |
| **SEXUAL DYSFUNCTIONS** | |
| Dyspareunia | There is a relationship of this disorder sometimes with victims of rape or sexual abuse; can be related to vaginismus. Newest thinking relates anxiety and pain concepts to origin. |
| Female Orgasmic Disorder | Some research suggests that failure to achieve an orgasm in women is related to intimacy issues, feelings of fear or anxiety, the sense of not being safe within the intimate relationship or relationship in general. Other times medication, such as antidepressants, or medical concerns, can cause inhibited orgasm. |
| Female Sexual Arousal Disorder | Some research suggests that relationship issues or a sexual trauma in childhood may play a role in development of this disorder. Other evidence indicates hormonal imbalance (testosterone). |
| Hypoactive Sexual Desire Disorder | Life stressors or other interpersonal difficulties are suggested etiologies. There also may be medical influences, such as side effects of medication. Also, relationship issues, and sexual trauma in childhood may play a role in the development of this disorder. |
| Male Erectile Disorder | Previously referred to as impotence, medical causes of this disorder must be ruled out first. Short of any physiological cause, male erectile disorder is typically the result of performance anxiety or fears of not being able to achieve or maintain an erection. |
| Male Orgasmic Disorder | Medical causes need to be ruled out first. Male orgasmic disorder is often thought as beginning as early as adolescence, sometimes because sexual intimacy becomes related to a negative life event or aspect. |
| Premature Ejaculation | Some medical causes need to be ruled out first. Relationship stress, novelty of relationship, anxiety, issues related to control and intimacy can all play a role in the development of this disorder. |
| Sexual Aversion Disorder | Some evidence suggests that relationship issues or sexual trauma in childhood may play a role in this disorder. |
| Vaginismus | There are anxiety/relationship issues that can play a role in the development of this disorder. Sometimes victims of rape or sexual abuse or strict religious upbringing and issues of control contribute to this disorder. Prolonged dyspareunia can also lead to this. |

*(cont.)*

| TABLE 18-2: **ETIOLOGIES ASSOCIATED WITH SEXUAL DISORDERS AND DYSFUNCTIONS (*CONT.*)** | |
| --- | --- |
| GENDER IDENTITY DISORDERS | |
| Gender Identity Disorder | Theory suggests that childhood issues may play a role in this disorder, such as the parent-child relationship at an early age and the identification the child is able make with the parent of the same gender. Newer evidence suggests biological basis for the disorder. |

*From DSM Description of Sexual Dysfunctions— www.allpsych.com*

of medications aimed at resolving the problem from a physiological perspective. Often the problem is not one of physical dysfunction but of an emotional stressor such as anxiety or depression. **Evidence-Based Practice 18-1** summarizes an important study related to anxiety and sexual functioning.

Anxiety has both emotional and physical consequences that can affect erectile function. It is among the most frequently cited contributors to psychological impotence. Excessive concern about sexual performance is often referred to as performance or honeymoon anxiety and may provoke an intense fear of failure and self-doubt. It can sometimes set off a cycle of chronic impotence. In response to anxiety, the brain releases chemicals known as neurotransmitters that constrict the smooth muscles of the penis and its arteries. This constriction reduces the blood flow into and out of the penis. Even simple stress may promote the release of brain chemicals that disrupt potency in a similar way. Men in predominately Western cultures fear two things when it comes to their sexual functioning: The first one has to do with penis size; the second with ability to maintain an erection. Add to this cultural mind-set the psychodynamic influences of issues such as guilt and shame and it is not difficult to see how mounting anxiety interrupts the sexual response cycle for men.

There may be further underlying forces interfering with the sexual process for men. Some men report that they end up marrying women who have traits similar to their mother. Depending on the nature of the relationship and the strength of the attachment between the man and his mother, the relationship between the man and his wife may begin to take on characteristics of the relationship he has with his mother. He may begin to develop what is termed a "Madonna complex." According to Freudian psychology, this complex often develops when the sufferer is raised by a cold and distant mother (Freud & Gay, 1989). This man will often date women with qualities of his mother, hoping to fulfill a need for intimacy unmet in childhood. Often, the wife begins to be seen as mother to the husband—a "Madonna" figure—and thus not a possible object of sexual attraction. For this reason, in the mind

of the sufferer, love and sex cannot be mixed. The man is reluctant to have sexual relations with his wife because he thinks unconsciously that it would be incest. He will reserve sexuality for "bad" or "dirty" women, and will not develop "normal" feelings of love in these sexual relationships (Freud & Gay, 1989).

These types of psychodynamic forces influencing sexual intimacy are not exclusive to men. A disorder more frequent in woman than men is hypoactive sexual desire disorder (Leiblum, 2007). This disorder is associated with a relative deficiency or absence of sexual fantasies and/or desire to engage in sexual activity. New understanding around female sexual arousal has shed light on this phenomenon.

Previously it was thought that females followed the same arousal patterns as men, that is they felt desire, became aroused, experienced orgasm, then went through a resolution phase. It is now understood that the desire and arousal pattern for woman is much more complex and key elements such as emotional intimacy and emotional and physical satisfaction in the relationship need to exist before desire and arousal are triggered (Basson, 2001). **Figure 18-2** depicts the interplay of these elements. The belief is that females view sexual activity as an extension of these elements of the interpersonal relationship. Thus, if key relationship components of emotional intimacy, safety, or trust are absent, the female partner may find interest in sexual activity diminished.

## Neurobiological Influences

Many sexual dysfunctions, while still containing a psychological component, are biological or neurobiological in their primary cause. Many medical illnesses including cardiovascular disease and diabetes may alter the ability of the individual to function sexually. Additionally, medications that alter brain chemistry have been shown to influence sexual dysfunction. Most antidepressants that increase serotonin such as fluoxetine (Prozac), sertraline hydrochloride (Zoloft), and others potentially lower desire and inhibit or prevent orgasm. Women tend to report

## EVIDENCE-BASED PRACTICE 18-1:
## WORRY AND SEXUAL DYSFUNCTION

### STUDY

Katz, R.C., & Jardine, D. (1999). The relationship between worry, sexual aversion, and low sexual desire. *Journal of Sex & Marital Therapy,* 25(4):293–296. October–December.

### SUMMARY

In this study, the researchers attempted to assess the relationship among worry, sexual aversion, and low sexual desire. They identified the need for this research based on the understanding that the psychological trait of worry is associated with many psychiatric conditions and maladaptive ways of coping. However, its relationship to sexual dysfunctions, and desire disorders in particular, is unclear. Using a sample of 138 undergraduate college students, data were collected using the Sexual Aversion Scale, the Hurlbert Index of Low Sexual Desire, and the Penn State Worry Questionnaire. The results identified a modest but significant relationship between sexual aversion and low sexual desire. This finding correlates with the information presented in the taxonomy of the *Diagnostic and Statistical Manual of Mental Disorders, 4th Edition, Text Revision* (American Psychiatric Association, 2000), which lists sexual aversion disorder and hypoactive sexual desire disorder as separate but related conditions. The results also revealed that in contrast to the researchers' predictions, the tendency to worry was no more related to sexual aversion than it was to low sexual desire. They found that the relationship between these variables was significant, but it was also relatively weak. The researchers concluded that chronic and intense worry may predispose one to certain anxiety disorders, but it does not appear to be a risk factor for sexual desire problems in nonclinical populations.

### APPLICATION TO PRACTICE

Psychiatric-mental health nurses need to be cognizant of the influence that anxiety has on numerous areas of functioning. The results from this study help to provide some support for the role that anxiety can play in sexual disorders and dysfunctions. Thus psychiatric-mental health nurses need to integrate information from this study when obtaining a sexual history from a patient. However, nurses also need to ensure that they do not attribute anxiety as the sole reason for the patient's complaints.

### QUESTIONS TO PONDER

1. *In working with a patient who has a high level of anxiety, would it be important to assess sexual functioning to see if the anxiety is impairing this part of the patient's life?*
2. *If a patient reports during an assessment that he or she has "no desire" for sexual activity, how would you further assess this area?*

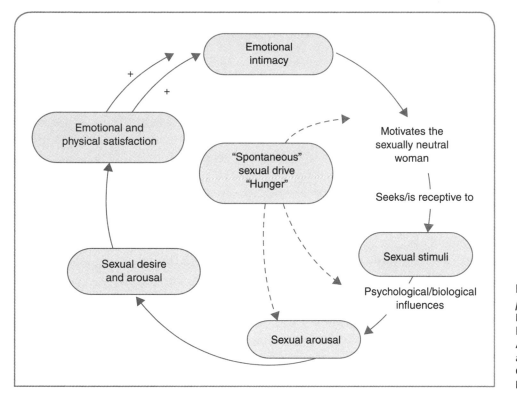

**Figure 18-2** *Desire and arousal pattern in women.*
From Basson R. (2002), Rethinking low sexual desire in women, *BJOG:* An International Journal of Obstetrics and Gynaecology, *109*, 357–63, Copyright 2002 by Blackwell Publishing Ltd.

lower desire and more orgasmic problems with this class of medication (Heiman, 2002).

The mechanism of action causing dysfunction is thought to arise from the serotonin cell bodies on the brainstem in a raphe nuclei region of the brain. Some of these project into the cortical area of the brain. Sexual dysfunctions of lower desire may result due to inhibition from selective serotonin reuptake inhibitors (SSRIs) in this region. Serotonergic projections also travel down the spine, and, when stimulated by SSRIs, inhibit aspects of sexual function such as vaginal lubrication and orgasm (Keltner, McAfee, & Taylor, 2002). The result is that intercourse may be painful and orgasm may be delayed or may not occur.

> *Emotional stressors, such as anxiety or depression, medical illnesses, and medications that alter the brain's chemistry, have been linked to development of sexual disorders and dysfunctions.*

## TREATMENT OPTIONS

Treatment options for patients with sexual disorders range from generalist interventions, such as psychoeducation and medication provided by nurses and other health care providers, to specialized intervention, such as psychotherapy from professionals credentialed as sex therapists. **Table 18-3** highlights treatment options for sexual disorders and dysfunctions.

Medications can sometimes be helpful in treating erectile dysfunction. For example, silendafil citrate (Viagra) helps treat erectile dysfunction by preventing the breakdown of a chemical called phosphodiesterase type 5 (PDE5). Normally, with arousal, nerve signals are sent from the brain to the penis, causing chemicals to be released, that relax muscles in the penis. When these muscles relax, large amounts of blood are able to enter the penis, resulting in an erection. The erection is reversed when PDE5 breaks down the other chemicals that caused the muscles to relax. When muscles in the penis constrict again, blood leaves the penis. Thus, when sildenafil prevents the breakdown of PDE5, the erection is achieved and prolonged. **Drug Summary 18-1** highlights this group of drugs.

### TABLE 18-3: TREATMENT OF SEXUAL DISORDERS AND DYSFUNCTIONS

| DIAGNOSIS | TREATMENT |
|---|---|
| Exhibitionism | Psychotherapy aimed at uncovering and working through the underlying causes of the behavior. Medications can, at times, be helpful to assist the patient in resisting urges, but are typically not utilized as the primary form of treatment. |
| Fetishism | Psychotherapy and an uncovering of or working through the underlying cause of the behavior. Anxiety may emerge as the behavior is extinguished. |
| Frotteurism | Psychotherapy aimed at uncovering and working through the underlying cause of behavior. |
| Pedophilia | Typically involves intense psychotherapy to work on deep-rooted issues concerning sexual feelings themselves and often childhood abuse. Medical treatment, such as **CHEMICAL CASTRATION** (actually a hormone medication that reduces testosterone and therefore sexual urges), has been investigated with only mixed results. New thinking is that this disorder is one of orientation. |
| Sexual Masochism | Psychotherapy aimed at uncovering and working through the underlying cause of behavior. |
| Sexual Sadism | Psychotherapy aimed in uncovering and working through the underlying cause. |
| Transvestic Fetishism | Typically involves psychotherapy or normalizing the behavior in the couple's relationship. |
| Voyeurism | Psychotherapy and sometimes a specific technique known as implosion therapy. |
| Dyspareunia | Treatment is aimed at resolving underlying anxiety and relationship issues. Also, treating the sexual pain with antidepressants often works. Specific exercises in the pelvic region aimed at strengthening muscles can often help as well. |
| Female Orgasmic Disorder | Typically involves uncovering the cause of the orgasmic dysfunction, ruling out medical contributions and then working on relationship issues, and sometimes prescribed masturbatory techniques. |
| Female Sexual Arousal Disorder | Treatment involves uncovering the conflict in the life situations. Also, hormone replacement therapy at times has been used successfully to increase sexual desire and arousal. |
| Hypoactive Sexual Desire Disorder | Ruling out medical contributions to the decreased desire and also psychotherapy that involves discovering and resolving underlying conflict. |
| Male Erectile Disorder | Erectile dysfunction medications (Viagra, etc.) are used for suspected medically based disorders. The most commonly applied treatment for non-medical-related impotence is **SENSATE FOCUS**, which involves a progression of sexual intimacy typically over the course of several weeks, eventually leading to penetration and orgasm. |
| Male Orgasmic Disorder | Once medical causes have been ruled out, working through underlying issues is very helpful. Some therapists use behavioral techniques such as sensate focus, which is a more direct approach. |
| Premature Ejaculation | Relaxation techniques, education, low dose SSRI medication, working through underlying issues. If the relationship is new, often these difficulties are self-resolving as the relationship matures. |
| Sexual Aversion Disorder | Therapy aimed at uncovering underlying conflict or life difficulties. |
| Vaginismus | Usually involves psychological counseling. Strategies involved at working through underlying issues. Other treatments such as using progressively larger dilators to help relax the muscles that prevent intercourse is sometimes helpful. Physical therapy with a therapist who can work with the patient to strengthen pelvic floor muscles is very effective. |
| Gender Identity Disorder | Psychotherapy to determine underlying cause and then, if persistent, may start the process of sexual reassignment. |

## APPLYING THE NURSING PROCESS FROM AN INTERPERSONAL PERSPECTIVE

While generalist nurses may not find themselves directly treating or caring for patients with sexual disorders, an understanding and awareness of this spectrum of disorders are helpful. More commonly, the nurse generalist will encounter patients with sexual dysfunctions, that may be uncovered through skillful questioning. Therefore, nurses need a firm understanding of the nursing process that integrates the interpersonal process when caring for patients who may be experiencing a sexual disorder or

## DRUG SUMMARY 18-1:
## AGENTS USED FOR ERECTILE DYSFUNCTION

| DRUG | IMPLICATIONS FOR NURSING CARE |
|---|---|
| sildenafil (Viagra)<br>tadalafil (Cialis)<br>vardenafil (Levitra) | • Investigate with the patient any underlying heart disease and use of nitrates as treatment; advise the patient that the drug should not be taken with nitrates because he could experience a significant drop in blood pressure.<br><br>• Work with the patient to establish ways to reduce possible anxiety associated with sexual activity.<br><br>• Encourage the patient to verbalize feelings related to sexual activity and sexual performance; reinforce use of other treatment measures as appropriate.<br><br>• If appropriate and with the patient's permission, include the patient's partner in discussion and education.<br><br>• Advise the patient to take the drug anywhere from 30 minutes to 4 hours before sexual activity; explain that the maximum benefit of the drug can be expected less than 2 hours after taking the drug.<br><br>• Encourage the patient to engage in sexual stimulation because the drug is effective only when stimulation occurs.<br><br>• Warn the patient not to use more than 25 mg of the drug within 48 hours.<br><br>• Instruct the patient to notify the prescriber or seek emergency medical attention if he experiences an erection that lasts more than 4 hours.<br><br>• Discuss potential side effects with the patient; advise the patient to notify his prescriber if he experiences any changes in vision. |

dysfunction. **Plan of Care 18-1** provides an example for a patient with a sexual dysfunction.

## Strategies for Optimal Assessment: Therapeutic Use of Self

Travelbee offered an interpersonal model to guide practice from a human-to-human perspective. The first phase of the relationship according to Travelbee is the original encounter. For many nurses, this is during the patient's admission when the nurse performs the initial assessment. The original encounter is characterized by first impressions of each other. The nurse and the patient initially perceive each other in stereotypical roles (Travelbee, 1971). The nurse needs to be able to gather data related to sexual function in a competent,

coherent, and comfortable manner. This requires that the nurse be very clear and in tune with how he or she feels about sexual functioning. The nurse must understand and acknowledge his or her own sexual feelings, biases, and beliefs. If any are negative or biased, the nurse must temporarily suspend them when working with patients.

When gathering such personal data during an assessment, the patient needs to sense unconditional acceptance by the nurse. **Therapeutic Interaction 18-1** provides an example of the therapeutic use of self when performing a sexual assessment. The moment a patient even slightly senses a prejudicial attitude, voice inflection, change of tone, or change in body posture during the interview, the chance that the person will self-disclose important information relative to this area of assessment lessens.

**PLAN OF CARE 18-1:**
**THE PATIENT WITH A SEXUAL DYSFUNCTION**

**NURSING DIAGNOSIS:** Sexual dysfunction; related to potential side effects of medication and anxiety; manifested by inability to attain or sustain an erection, concerns related to sexual performance, and decreased pleasure with sexual activity.

**OUTCOME IDENTIFICATION:** Patient will verbalize an increase in pleasure and ability to engage in sexual activity with less anxiety.

| INTERVENTION | RATIONALE |
|---|---|
| Establish rapport and provide for privacy. Demonstrate unconditional acceptance, obtain the patient's permission and begin assessment with least sensitive topics | Establishing rapport is essential for developing the nurse-patient relationship, especially in light of the sensitive nature of the topic. Obtaining the patient's permission is important for developing trust and demonstrates respect for the patient. Providing for privacy and demonstrating unconditional acceptance are important for developing trust. Beginning with the least sensitive topics first promotes the patient's comfort with the discussion |
| Review the patient's history and physical exam for possible underlying contributing factors related to the dysfunction. Assess the patient's feelings related to sexual functioning and dysfunction | Reviewing the history and physical exam provides information about possible causes, such as underlying medical conditions or use of medications that can contribute to the dysfunction; assessing the patient's feelings provides insight into the patient's view and significance of the condition |
| Provide the patient with information related to the specific disorder as appropriate. Help clarify any myths or misconceptions the patient may have | Explaining and clarifying help to provide the patient with an understanding of the condition and dispel myths or misconceptions that may be contributing to feelings |
| Explain and/or administer prescribed medications such as phosphodiesterase type 5 inhibitors (i.e., sildanifil) | Using medications may be necessary to address the underlying physiologic issue related to the dysfunction |
| Discuss methods for sexual expression other than sexual intercourse; include the patient's partner in the discussion and encourage the patient and partner to communicate openly | Discussing other methods of scxual expression can help the patient and partner attain and/or maintain intimacy. Including the partner in the discussion promotes sharing and enhances feelings of intimacy |
| Obtain referral for counseling or sex therapy if appropriate | Referring the patient and partner to a sex therapist may be necessary to promote sexual functioning |

*(cont.)*

**PLAN OF CARE 18-1: (*CONT.*)**
**THE PATIENT WITH A SEXUAL DYSFUNCTION**

**NURSING DIAGNOSIS:** Disturbed body image; related to recent mastectomy; manifested by feelings of inadequacy, shame or guilt, and sexual relationship difficulties.

**OUTCOME IDENTIFICATION:** Patient will verbalize positive statements about sexual self.

| INTERVENTION | RATIONALE |
| --- | --- |
| Assess the patient's view of self and influence of dysfunction on this view; include the patient's partner in assessment | Assessing the patient's and partner's views provide information from which to individualize interventions |
| Assist the patient in looking at him-/herself realistically; help the patient acknowledge the link between feelings, self-esteem, and sexual functioning | Assisting the patient in looking at self realistically and acknowledging the link help the patient to correct misconceptions and promote feelings of self-esteem |
| Work with the patient to refocus thinking; assist the patient in identifying strengths and resources; emphasize the patient's strengths and positive aspects of self | Assisting the patient in identifying strengths promotes feelings of self-worth and self-esteem |
| Help patient and partner discuss feelings related to body image and self-esteem and how these influence sexual activity; assist them in separating feelings from behaviors | Identifying feelings and influence on sexual activity can promote understanding of the connection and insight into behaviors |
| Work with the patient and partner on ways to alleviate feelings that can interfere with sexual activity; encourage open, honest communication | Encouraging ways to alleviate feelings related to sexual dysfunction and open honest communication can facilitate self-esteem and self-confidence |
| Assist the patient and partner in appropriate problem solving and provide positive reinforcement | Using appropriate problem solving and reinforcing it promote feelings of self-confidence and self-worth |

*From Nursing Diagnosis – Definitions and Classifications 2009–2011. Copyright © 2011 by NANDA International. Use by arrangement with Blackwell Publishing Limited, a company of John Wiley & Sons, Inc.*

*Nurses need to be aware of the messages they are sending—verbally and nonverbally—when assessing patients about their sexual functioning.*

## Sexual Health Assessment

Often, the opportunity for sexual health assessment can be performed during the initial assessment. This sometimes is awkwardly presented during the genitourinary or reproductive section of the nursing assessment. When approaching this section of the assessment, it may be

**THERAPEUTIC INTERACTION 18-1:
OBTAINING A SEXUAL ASSESSMENT**

Ms. Stevens is admitted to the unit with severe depression. The nurse is performing a nursing assessment.

| | |
|---|---|
| The nurse enters the room and introduces self while smiling; pulls the curtain closed and sits down in a chair next to the bed, facing the patient at eye level. | Provides introduction and sets the tone for the rest of the interaction; pulling the curtain closed allows for privacy; sitting at the level of the patient demonstrates a willingness to engage with the patient |
| The nurse proceeds with the assessment and is now ready to assess the patient's sexual health. | |
| **Nurse:** "Ms. Stevens, I need to learn more about your reproductive/sexual functioning now. Do you mind if I ask you questions concerning these matters?" (maintains eye contact) | Gains permission and shows respect; eye contact demonstrates interest |
| **Ms. Stevens:** "Yes that's fine." | Indicates comfortableness in proceeding |
| **Nurse:** "Are you in a sexual relationship at the present?" | Provides a beginning point without making any assumptions as to the nature of the relationship |
| **Ms. Stevens:** "Yes, I am with my husband." | Clarifies the nature of the relationship as sexual and that she is sexually active. |
| **Nurse:** "Are there any concerns related to sexual functioning?" | Focuses on concerns and provides segue into opportunities for exploration of problems and sexual health promotion. |
| **Ms. Stevens:** "Yes, he wants it more than I do." | Indicates possible area for concern. |
| **Nurse:** "Tell me more about that, for example, has it always been that way or is this a recent issue?" | Inquires about the matter to get perspective as to this being a new concern or one that was pre-existing |
| **Ms. Stevens:** "It's been more recently since I've been depressed and on medication." (starts to cry) | Provides information as to the nature of the concern and reveals the emotional impact of the problem |
| **Nurse:** "Talk about what you are feeling now." | Seeks clarification of patient's feelings |

*(cont.)*

| | |
|---|---|
| Ms. Stevens: "I worry that I'm going to lose him, he's going to have an affair or something. We used to be so close; our sex life was great when we were first married. I feel like we are drifting apart. I just have no desire at all." | Answers in a manner that reveals the enormity of the problem, indicating a broader relationship issue |
| Nurse: "Have you and you husband had a chance to seek professional help regarding these matters?" | Tries to determine if any interventions have been attempted |
| Ms. Stevens: "No, we've been too embarrassed to talk about it with anyone." | Indicates her level of discomfort around this issue |
| Nurse: "I can refer you to a local sex therapist after discharge who specializes in working with couples on such matter if you like." (smiles) | Provides opportunity for psychoeducation and sexual health promotion |
| Ms. Stevens: "Really (laughs), I didn't know there were such things out there." | Indicates curiosity and potential openness to the idea. Laughter indicates a brief shift in mood |

helpful to quickly plan ahead and consider some of the following:

- Are you alone with the patient?
- Is the spouse or significant other with the patient?
- Are there family members around?
- What is the age of the patient, spouse, or family members?
- What are the cultural beliefs?
- Have you established if there are any religious beliefs?
- What is the overall nature of the illness that has brought the patient for care?
- How has the patient answered the questions so far?
- Does the patient seem comfortable proceeding with more personal information?
- Do you need to ask others to leave the room while you finish the assessment?
- Do you need to pull the curtain or otherwise arrange for privacy?
- What is your body posture? Are you relaxed/tense? Are you making eye contact? Are your actions establishing clear and healthy boundaries?

Assuming that the nurse has gone through these questions and feels that it is appropriate to move ahead with a sexual assessment, the following statement may provide an opening:

"Mr./Mrs. Smith, I need to ask you some questions about your reproductive health. This is a chance for us to talk about any concerns you may have and a chance for me to assist you in this area. Are you ok with my discussing this with you?" Once permission is granted, proceed while conveying a comfortable, relaxed, yet interested attitude.

The ability to proceed with the discussion may signal the transition to the next phase of Travelbee's model, emerging identities. The nurse may be aware that he or she and the patient perceive each other as unique individuals. A connection has been established and the bond of a relationship is beginning to form. Now is a good time to take a quick moment to ask "What has allowed me to feel this connection?" Most important, are you ready from a boundary perspective to proceed? If so, the 10 questions included

*The nurse needs to obtain permission from the patient before proceeding with an assessment of sexual functioning.*

> ### BOX 18-2: TEN ESSENTIAL QUESTIONS FOR A NURSING SEXUAL HEALTH ASSESSMENT
>
> 1. Do you consider yourself sexually active?
> 2. If so, please discuss any concerns related to your sexual functioning; for example, pain, or any difficulty functioning as you would like.
> 3. If you are not sexually active, please share with me the reason(s) for this? (Belief system, illness, etc.)
> 4. Please discuss any illness (medical or emotional) that may be concerning you regarding your ability to function as desired sexually.
> 5. How do you maintain your sexual health, that is, breast exams, testicular exams, prostate exams, pap tests?
> 6. Please discuss any experience of sexual trauma such as rape, sexual abuse, or anything you felt was sexually abusive or exploitive.
> 7. Have there been any changes in your level of interest in sexual functioning (either increase or decrease) and if so, has this caused any difficulties?
> 8. Based on our conversation so far, what would you would like to talk about further?
> 9. Is there anything you would like more information on?
> 10. I will be developing a nursing treatment plan based on my whole assessment. Would you like me to focus one goal on an area of concern regarding sexual health promotion?
>
> *From J. Jones, 2010.*

in **Box 18-2** can help structure the experience. The flow of the questioning will depend on the facility's nursing assessment form. Box 18-2 highlights the important elements to include regardless of the structure of the form.

## Boundary Maintenance

Working with patients when the focus is on sexual issues can be uncomfortable. The subject matter combined with the expectation of practicing psychiatric-mental health nursing from a relationship-based perspective will challenge the skillful navigation of boundaries. The need to stay within the boundaries of a healthy nurse-patient relationship means that the nurse does not become overinvolved with the patient just because the treatment issue is one of a sexual nature. Conversely, the subject matter may also be awkward for the nurse. Therefore, the nurse must avoid failing to engage the patient, becoming underinvolved, or neglectful with treatment just because the treatment issue is one of a sexual nature.

## Diagnosing and Planning Appropriate Interventions: Meeting the Patient's Focused Needs

The next phase of the nursing process is planning. After concluding an interview in which assessment data were gleaned implicating a sexual dysfunction, deciding on how to incorporate this into the treatment plan must involve a sense of where the patient feels this need falls. This can be best accomplished by ensuring empathetic practice. As described by Travelbee (1971), the empathy phase is characterized by the ability to share in the other person's experience. The nurse may begin to imagine how having a sexual dysfunction has affected this patient's overall well-being. **Consumer Perspective 18-1** provides insight into what it is like to experience a sexual dysfunction.

The nurse's desire to address this issue and make it a treatment goal indicates movement into sympathy. This next phase of the therapeutic relationship, sympathy, goes beyond empathy and occurs when the nurse desires to alleviate the cause of the patient's illness or suffering. This is where the appropriate plan of care is generated. This phase requires a combination of the disciplined intellectual approach combined with the therapeutic use of self using appropriate boundaries.

For example, the nurse discovers during the course of an assessment that a patient is experiencing erectile dysfunction and this problem has never been disclosed before. Thus, the nurse, in collaboration with the patient who believes this to be a significant issue for he and his partner, includes this as part of the treatment plan. This decision is not because the nurse has determined that this is a problem. Rather, it is because the nurse has experienced sympathy and understood the importance of the

## CONSUMER PERSPECTIVE 18-1: A COUPLE EXPERIENCING VAGINISMUS

Vaginismus strikes young and old, sexually experienced and inexperienced. In our case, we were young and inexperienced. Marrying right after graduation from college, neither of us had had intercourse before and we really didn't know a lot about sex. We were basically college sweethearts that loved each other, had plans for a family, and hopes for the "American Dream." We were both brought up in caring, loving families.

We discovered vaginismus on our honeymoon—the classic primary vaginismus story about the young couple that couldn't consummate, no matter how hard they tried. Calls back home to the family physician were met with the standard advice to "Try using more foreplay or more lubricant—and just keep trying. Don't worry, you'll figure it out." We tried again and again using every method we could think of, but it was like "hitting a wall"; penetration was simply impossible. We were confused and felt utterly foolish and embarrassed.

When this happened to us, the internet was still in its infancy. Endless searches revealed little useful information. With the honeymoon over, we worked hard adjusting to our new careers in a new city. We relocated all our possessions and created a home all the while carrying on as if everything was perfect. Our family and friends had no idea what we were experiencing. We assumed somehow that we would eventually figure it out and didn't dream of suffering the embarrassment of letting anyone know about our strange honeymoon problem and ongoing failure.

As is typical for couples going through vaginismus, the passage of time began to create difficult paradoxes. How do you simply go in to a new doctor and say "By the way, we've been married for 7 months and we haven't had sex yet. Any ideas?" A person feels extreme shame and failure, to the point that it becomes very difficult to be courageous enough to seek help. In our case, we reluctantly got up our courage out of necessity and kept asking more professionals, unfortunately with little help or solutions offered.

matter to the patient because they are now in a therapeutic relationship.

Due to the wide range of assessment findings and multiple problems faced by patients with sexual disorders and dysfunctions, numerous nursing diagnoses would apply. Examples of possible nursing diagnoses would include:

- Sexual dysfunction related to painful intercourse
- Ineffective sexuality patterns related to low desire
- Situational low self-esteem related to erectile dysfunction
- Chronic low self-esteem related to changes in body following mastectomy for breast cancer

These nursing diagnoses also will vary based on the acuity of the patient's illness, developmental stage, comorbidities, current treatment regimen, and sources of support.

Based on the identified nursing diagnoses, the nurse and patient collaboratively would determine the outcomes to be achieved. For example, possible causes such as medication side effects for the erectile dysfunction will be explored and identified.

## Implementing Effective Interventions: Timing and Pacing

After the patient's needs have been identified and outcomes and goals have been set, the nurse works with the patient to implement interventions. These interventions will vary depending on the actual diagnosis. Before proceeding, the nurse needs to make sure he or she has established rapport with the patient. This last phase of Travelbee's model is characterized by nursing actions that alleviate an ill person's distress. The nurse and patient are relating as human being to human being (Travelbee, 1971). The patient exhibits both trust and confidence in the nurse. **How Would You Respond? 18-1** provides an example of a patient with a sexual dysfunction requiring intervention.

Consider the example of a patient with erectile dysfunction in which the problem is disrupting his relationship. Possibly, one of the interventions may be to rule out potential side effects of the patient's current medications. There may be a combination of medications that the patient is taking that could be contributing to this dysfunction, for example, antihypertensives or antidepressants. Several levels of intervention would be appropriate. First, the nurse would share education about potential side effects of medication to establish the patient's knowledge base and determine what would be the next course of action. The patient may have an awareness of these potential side effects, and has raised this concern with the provider on several occasions, but nothing has been changed. This may present an opportunity for the nurse, in treatment team meetings with the provider, to advocate on the patient's behalf. The timing and pacing of these interventions is a key factor. First is the manner in which the nurse approaches the patient with the suspicions about potential side effects. When does the nurse do this? Should it be done when the patient's partner is visiting? Should the nurse gather some printed information about the medication regimen and discuss it with the patient? How should the nurse begin the conversation? A possible start may go something like this:

"Hello, Mr. Smith, I am the nurse on duty today and will be meeting with you periodically throughout the shift. Do you mind if we review your treatment plan during one of those meetings to see how things are going?" Later, when the nurse senses that the timing is right, he or she might bring in the treatment plan and briefly review the problems identified. When the nurse gets to the sexual dysfunction problem, it will have been introduced within the context of his overall health and may be less threatening to discuss. The next conversation may go accordingly:

---

### HOW WOULD YOU RESPOND? 18-1: MAJOR DEPRESSION AND LOSS OF INTEREST

Mrs. Rittenour is a 47-year-old Caucasian female homemaker, mother of two teenagers, admitted to the mental health unit with a diagnosis of Major Depressive Disorder Recurrent, Most Recent Episode Severe. She had been on the antidepressant escitalopram (Lexapro) at 20 mg for over the past 3 years with good results. Recently she reported experiencing depressed mood, sleep disturbance, change of appetite, and vague suicidal ideations. Her primary mental health care provider, a psychiatric clinical nurse specialist, added aripiprazole (Abilify) 5 mg to augment the regimen. Mrs. Rittenour reported almost immediate relief of her symptoms and for approximately 1 month claimed she "felt like her old self." Unfortunately, the following month her husband announced he wanted a divorce as he had decided to pursue a relationship with someone else. Mrs. Rittenour quickly decompensated and presented to the emergency department with suicidal ideation. She was admitted for observation and possible medication reevaluation.

During the nursing assessment, Mrs. Rittenour reveals that she had lost her interest in sexual activity about three years ago and that she and her estranged husband rarely engaged in any form of intimacy. She also reported that he noted her cycles were very irregular and her moodiness seemed to correlate to her cycles. She reported increased sleep disturbance the past three years, trouble focusing and concentrating, and painful intercourse on the few occasions she did engage in sexual activity with her husband. How would you respond?

#### CRITICAL THINKING QUESTIONS

1. *During the sexual health portion of Mrs. Rittenour's history, what areas would need further exploration?*

2. *Suppose Mrs. Rittenour asks you what you would do about the marriage if you were in her shoes. How would you respond?*

3. *When working with this patient, you notice yourself becoming angry and frustrated with her at times. This seems to occur primarily when she discusses her interest in reconciling with her husband, imagining that, when you were young your father frequently left your mother and then would come back. What might you be experiencing?*

### APPLYING THE CONCEPTS

Several areas need to be addressed during the sexual health portion of the assessment. This, however, would only occur after the patient's suicidality is assessed and immediate interventions are implemented to ensure the patient's safety. Once the patient's condition stabilizes, then the nurse would continue with the assessment. Areas to address would include the patient's change of sexual function, along with her change in menstrual cycle and medications used for treating her depression. According to her statement, the patient's loss of interest occurred around the same time that she was prescribed the antidepressant.

When responding to Mrs. Rittenour about what you would do if you were her, it would be important to clarify why she is asking you. Is she doing so because she doesn't know what to do? It would be best to reflect the question back to her to encourage her to process what her options are. Another area for self reflection may be your frustration in dealing with the situation as some of the key elements mirror your own life (i.e., your father left your mother pericodically). If you do find yourself experiencing some countertransferance, it is all the more important that you not provide your opinion, but focus on the patient as you may have lost some objectivity.

"I see that one of the problems listed is sexual dysfunction related to an inability to engage in intercourse manifested by inability to achieve and/or maintain erection. One of the interventions listed is an opportunity to rule out potential side effects of medication known to cause this problem. Were you aware that some of the medication you are taking may be causing this problem?"

The nurse then assesses the patient's knowledge base, provides information as appropriate through patient education about medication and potential side effects, and together with the patient plans on the next, if any, intervention. As mentioned, this may involve the nurse advocating on the patient's behalf with the provider coordinating the medicine regimen. Again, deciding how to approach the person(s) responsible for this and in what forum will be important: approach them privately or at the nursing station? Wait until the treatment team is available or when they are making rounds, joining them in the patient's room? The nurse's assessment and judgment of when and how to do this may determine the success or failure of this intervention.

> *Psychoeducation and acting as a patient advocate are two key nursing interventions for patients with sexual dysfunction.*

## Evaluating: Objective Critique of Interventions and Self-Reflection

The nurse may have successfully provided education regarding potential medication side effects to the patient, and may have also further successfully advocated for the patient about changes in medications with the treatment team. Evaluation of successful goal attainment may not be identified immediately or ever known to the nurse because the patient may be discharged right after the interventions. The nurse would focus evaluation on the interventions, which in this case would be that the nurse provided appropriate education after identifying a problem, and successfully advocated on the patient's behalf for change in a medication regimen to try to address the identified sexual dysfunction. The resolution of the actual sexual dysfunction would have to be evaluated as "unknown or partially met."

The nurse should reflect on his or her own feelings as the scenario unfolded with regard to such intimate issues. When evaluating the treatment plan, the nurse needs to determine if the goals were reflective of the patient's needs and if healthy boundaries were maintained. The nurse also needs to determine if there were any areas at issue that became uncomfortable and, if so, how the nurse dealt with them. The nurse questions him- or herself about the possibility of self-discomfort interfering with not meeting certain goals. For any goals not met, the nurse needs to self-reflect on anything he or she may have done differently while providing nursing care.

## SUMMARY POINTS

- Sexual dysfunctions involve a disturbance in the sexual response cycle. Sexual disorders involve recurrent intense sexual urges, fantasies, or behaviors.

- Sexual dysfunctions include: dyspareunia, female orgasmic disorder, female sexual arousal disorder, hypoactive sexual disorder, male erectile disorder, male orgasmic disorder, premature ejaculation, sexual aversion disorder, and vaginismus.

- Sexual disorders include: exhibitionism, fetishism, frotterurism, pedophilia, sexual masochism, sexual sadism, transvestic fetishism, and voyeurism.

- Freud was one of the first psychiatrists to attempt to understand how sexual drives and urges are manifested and expressed.

- Political, cultural, and theological issues of the time influence the approach and discussion of sexual disorders and dysfunctions.

- Treatment options range from psychoeducation and medication administration to specialized interventions such as sex therapy.

- Assessment of a patient with a sexual disorder or dysfunction requires the nurse to understand and acknowledge his or her feelings, beliefs, and biases related to sexual functioning.

- Identifying and maintaining appropriate boundaries are priorities when caring for a patient with a sexual disorder or dysfunction.

## NCLEX-PREP*

1. When assessing a patient with dyspareunia, which of the following would the nurse expect the patient to report?
    a. Inability to attain adequate lubrication in response to sexual excitement
    b. Recurrent pain in the genital area with sexual intercourse
    c. A deficient last of desire for sexual activity
    d. An avoidance for engaging in sexual activity

2. A nurse is engaged in assessing a male patient and has determined that it is appropriate to move on to assessing the patient's sexual history. Which of the following would be most important for the nurse to do first?
    a. Make sure that the nurse and patient are alone

    b. Ask the patient about whether or not he is sexually active
    c. Question the patient about any history of sexual abuse
    d. Obtain the patient's permission to ask him questions about this area

3. A group of students are reviewing information about the various types of sexual disorders and dysfunctions. The students demonstrate understanding of this topic when they identify which of the following as examples of sexual disorders? Select all that apply.
    a. Vaginismus
    b. Exhibitionism
    c. Pedophilia
    d. Premature ejaculation
    e. Male erectile disorder

*(cont.)*

## NCLEX-PREP* (*CONT.*)

4. The nurse is reviewing the medical record of a patient, that reveals that the patient experiences intense sexual arousal when being bound and humiliated. The nurse interprets this information as characteristic of which of the following?

   a. Sexual masochism
   b. Sexual sadism
   c. Frotteurism
   d. Fetishism

5. A nurse is preparing an in-service presentation about sexual dysfunction for a group of nurses involved in a continuing education course. As part of the presentation, the nurse is planning to describe the classic male sexual response cycle. Place the phases of the cycle in the order in which the nurse would present the information.

   a. Resolution
   b. Desire
   c. Orgasm
   d. Excitement

*Answers to these questions appear on page 639.

## REFERENCES

American Psychiatric Association. (2000). *Diagnostic and statistical manual of mental disorders* (4th ed., text rev.). Washington, D.C.: Author.

Basson, R. (2001). Female sexual response: The role of drugs in the management of sexual dysfunction. *Obstetrics & Gynecology.* 98(3), 350–3.

DSM Description of Sexual Disorders/Dysfunctions–Retrieved January 7, 2012 from http://allpsych.com/disorders/paraphilias/index.html

Fogel, C.A., & Lauver, D. (1990). *Sexual health promotion.* Philadelphia: W.B. Saunders Company.

Freud, S., & Gay, P. (1989). *The Freud reader.* New York: W.W. Norton and Company.

Heiman, J.R. (2002). Sexual dysfunction: Overview of prevalence, etiological factors, and treatments. *The Journal of Sex Research.* 39(1), 73–78.

Keltner, N.L., McAfee, K.M., & Taylor, C.L. (2002). Mechanisms and treatment of SSRI-induced sexual dysfunction. *Perspectives in Psychiatric Care, 38*(3), 111–116.

Katz, R.C. and Jardine, D. (1999). The relationship between worry, sexual aversion, and low sexual desire. *Journal of Sex & Marital Therapy, 25*(4):293–296. October-December. Retrieved online 2/10/2010.

Kinsey, A.C., Pomeroy, W.R., & Martin, C.E. (1948). *Sexual Behavior in the Human Male.* Philadelphia: W.B. Saunders Company.

Kinsey, A.C., Pomeroy, W.R., Martin, C.E., & Gebhard, P.H. (1953). *Sexual Behavior in the Human Female.* Philadelphia: W.B. Saunders Company.

Leiblum, S.R. (2007). *Principals and practice of sex therapy.* (4th ed.). New York: Guilford Publications, Inc.

Travelbee, J. (1971). *Interpersonal aspects of nursing.* (2nd ed.). Philadelphia: F.A. Davis.

Ubillos, S., Paez, D., & Gonzalez, J. (2000). Culture and sexual behavior. *Psicothema.* Vol. 12, Suppl. pp. 70–82.

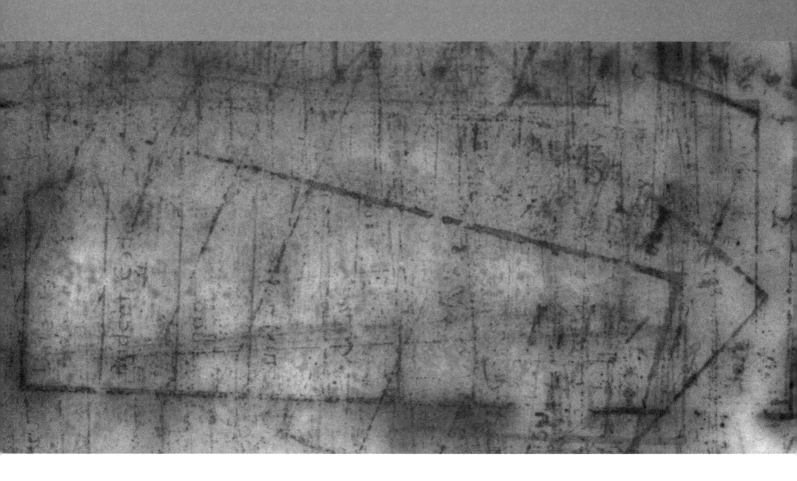

## CHAPTER CONTENTS

## EXPECTED LEARNING OUTCOMES

**After completing this chapter, the student will be able to:**

1. Define eating disorders.
2. Discuss the history and epidemiology of eating disorders.
3. Identify the different eating disorders.
4. Distinguish among the *Diagnostic and Statistical Manual of Mental Disorders, 4th edition, Text Revision* (*DSM-IV-TR*) diagnostic criteria for eating disorders.
5. Discuss possible theories related to the etiology of eating disorders, differentiating the biological, sociocultural, familial influences, psychological, and individual risk factors associated with these disorders.

# CHAPTER 19
# EATING DISORDERS

James O'Mahony

6. Explain various treatment options for persons experiencing eating disorders.
7. Apply the nursing process from an interpersonal perspective to the care of patients with eating disorders.

## KEY TERMS

Anorexia nervosa
Binge eating disorder
Bulimia nervosa
Eating disorder
Obesity
Overweight

EATING DISORDERS involve a serious disturbance in behaviors associated with eating (American Psychiatric Association [APA], 2000). They have become increasingly prevalent and of great concern to mental health professionals. Eating disorders include ANOREXIA NERVOSA (refusal or inability to maintain a minimally normal body weight), BULIMIA NERVOSA (repeated episodes of binge eating followed by compensatory behaviors), OBESITY (a body mass index greater than or equal to 30), BINGE EATING DISORDER (characterized by episodes of binge eating, i.e., eating in a discrete period of time an amount of food that is larger than most other people would eat in a similar period under comparable circumstances), and Eating Disorders Not Otherwise Specified.

To understand eating disorders, it is important to understand the concept of eating. Human eating serves many functions in addition to nutrition. Normal healthy eating is not only about what a person eats but also how and why a person eats, and the attitudes and beliefs held in relation to food and eating. How a person eats differs from individual to individual, and is dependent on many factors such as:

- Physical needs (biological)
- Cultural needs (cultural)
- Lifestyle (social)
- Emotional needs (psychological)

Healthy eating behaviors are characterized by balanced eating patterns, appropriate calorie intake, and body weight appropriate for gender, height, age, and level of activity. Nurses need to be aware of the various factors pertaining to the functions of eating and food to provide appropriate care for recovery to those who are experiencing eating disorders.

This chapter addresses the historical perspectives and epidemiology of eating disorders, followed by a detailed description of eating disorders as defined in the *Diagnostic and Statistical Manual, 4th edition, Text Revision (DSM-IV-TR;* APA, 2000). Biological, sociocultural, familial, and psychological factors that may potentially contribute to eating disorders are described along with common treatment options, including pharmacotherapy, psychoanalytical approaches, cognitive and behavioral treatments, group and family therapy, supportive therapy, and nutritional therapies. Application of the nursing process from an interpersonal perspective is presented, including a plan of care for a patient with an eating disorder.

> *Numerous factors affect an individual's eating patterns. Eating provides nutrition but also other functions.*

## HISTORICAL PERSPECTIVES

In the past 30 years, eating disorders have become more clearly defined. In Western culture, society and, in particular, the media, offer contrasting messages about food and eating (Abraham & Llewellyn-Jones, 2005). The first message is that a slim woman is a successful, attractive, healthy, happy, fit, and popular person. Most teenagers believe that being slim will help them secure a good job, find a boyfriend, be popular with their peers, be and look fit and healthy, and get on well with their family. The second message is that eating is pleasurable.

Today's society is communicating mixed messages. For example, in nearly every issue of women's magazines, there are new diets to ensure thinness followed by photographs of luscious cakes (Abraham & Llewellyn-Jones, 2005). Furthermore, the provision of food in our society is viewed as a sign of caring. The cultural imperatives place a burden on parents to provide abundant quantities of food for their children. Therefore, it is not surprising that in the face of two contradictory messages, most young women diet, with some of them developing eating disorders (Abraham & Llewellyn-Jones, 2005).

The wider societal influences of the media and popular culture have recently received much scrutiny and criticism for their negative aspects in relation to body size and its importance (Ringwood, 2010). Thinness is highly prized. People who can remain slender, lose weight, or are seen to be in control of their appetites are praised and rewarded. Celebrity culture is fixated on issues of weight and shape—the final domain where personal comments are unchallenged and not taboo. Issues such as sexual orientation, religion, race, and even age are no longer acceptable topics for derogatory remarks; however, weight and shape continue to be (Ringwood, 2010). As with families, the media itself doesn't cause eating disorders. However, it can contribute to the continuation of the myth and condition. Surrounded by hyperperfect images of celebrated thinness, individuals reinforce their strongly held belief that their weight and shape are the most important aspects of their being (Ringwood, 2010).

## EPIDEMIOLOGY

Eating disorders have long been perceived to occur primarily in women; few disorders in general medicine or psychiatry exhibit such a skew in gender distribution (Rhys Jones & Morgan, 2010). Recent research has focused on the assumption and stereotype that eating disorders in men are associated with homosexuality. Feldman and

Meyer (2007) demonstrated a much higher prevalence for eating disorders among gay and bisexual men than their heterosexual counterparts, with more than 15% of gay or bisexual men suffering from anorexia nervosa, bulimia nervosa, or eating disorder not otherwise specified. It has been suggested that gay men may be under more pressure to conform to being thin, are more dissatisfied with their bodies, and tend to diet more (Andersen, 1999). This may be related to the fact that values and norms place a heightened focus on physical appearance to which men may feel pressured to conform, ultimately influencing self-esteem and body image satisfaction (Yager, 2000). However, Morgan and Arcelus (2009) found widespread body image dissatisfaction among younger men, regardless of sexual orientation. Media and peer group influences appeared particularly relevant among gay men, but there were more similarities than differences between gay and heterosexual men, with both groups exposed to pressures to manipulate body shape and both aware of such pressures sufficient to resist them. Male beauty ideals differed from that of women in that they appeared compatible and consistent with healthy physiology, and health appeared less divorced from the aesthetic ideal for men than women.

Only a small minority of people experience an eating disorder and some people seem to be at a much greater risk of developing an eating disorder than others (Palmer, 2003).

In the late 1960s, anorexia nervosa became a much more prevalent disorder in Western societies. Young females from middle- and upper-class families were beginning to deprive themselves of food. The following decade saw the emergence of bulimia nervosa, where young women alternated self-starvation with binging usually followed by purging (Polivy & Herman, 2002). Although the number of men experiencing eating disorders is increasing, the majority of people who experience eating disorders are young women in late adolescence or early adulthood. The group at highest risk is young women between the ages of 15 and 30. Anorexia nervosa appears to strike at a younger age, with bulimia nervosa being more prevalent in the older group. Anorexia nervosa occurs in about 1% of the world population, being more prevalent among young White females under the age of 25 from middle to upper social classes in Western cultures (Abraham & Llewellyn-Jones, 2005). Men represent 10%–20% of cases of anorexia nervosa (Rhys Jones & Morgan, 2010). The age of onset for females is around 16 years of age; for males, it tends to be younger. About one-third of people experiencing anorexia nervosa become chronically ill. Anorexia has a mortality rate between 18% and 20% (Dichter, Cohen, & Connolly, 2002).

Bulimia nervosa is one of the most common eating disorders, affecting 1% to 3% of adolescents and young females. Men account for 10% to 20% of the cases (Rhys Jones & Morgan, 2010). Before being diagnosed with bulimia nervosa, nearly all sufferers, when they were between 15 and 24, had periods of severely restricting food or extreme fasting, that led to episodes of binge eating. Over time, the frequency and severity of the binge eating increased and bulimia nervosa developed (Abraham & Llewellyn-Jones, 2005). It is also believed that many people with bulimia nervosa will have met the criteria for anorexia nervosa at some time in their lives. While anorexia nervosa is more prevalent among the middle and upper socioeconomic groups, bulimia is prevalent among all groups equally (Abraham & Llewellyn-Jones, 2005). Both conditions are less common in ethnic minority groups.

The World Health Organization (WHO) defines **OVERWEIGHT** as a body mass index (BMI) $\geq$25 (kg/m²) and **OBESITY** as a body mass index (BMI) $\geq$30.0 (kg/m²) (WHO, 2000). Obesity is a global public health problem affecting both developed and developing countries (WHO, 2000). Obesity is not classified as an eating disorder in the *DSM-IV-TR* but is briefly addressed here. Approximately 1.1 billion people in the world are overweight, of which 312 million are obese (Haslam & James, 2005). In the United States, 71% of men and 65% of women are overweight or obese (Ogden et al., 2006). In the United Kingdom, 65% of men and 56% of women are overweight or obese (Zaninotto et al., 2006). Historically, Asian countries have had lower rates of obesity. However, this trend is changing. For example, in China, 29.1% of the adult population is overweight, of which 3.8% are obese (Gu et al., 2005). The Chinese now account for one-fifth of the 1.1 billion people overweight or obese in the world (Wu, 2006).

In addition, prevalence rates for conditions such as diabetes, cardiovascular disease, hypertension, and cancer are higher among those who are obese. Other adverse health conditions associated with obesity include musculoskeletal problems such as arthritis, chronic respiratory diseases, and reproductive problems such as infertility and impotence (WHO, 2003). Obesity lessens life expectancy and accounts for almost 500,000 deaths per year in the United States (Mokdad et al., 2004).

The populations affected by anorexia nervosa and bulimia nervosa are different from those affected by binge eating disorders. The prevalence rate for binge eating disorder varies between 0.7% and 6.6% for the general population (Grucza, Przybeck, & Cloninger, 2007) and 30% for persons applying for weight loss treatment (Spitzer et al., 1993). Anorexia nervosa and bulimia nervosa primarily affect women and rarely affect men. In contrast, the male to female ratio among individuals with binge eating disorder is 2:3. This disorder also occurs across ethnically diverse samples, whereas most individuals with anorexia nervosa and bulimia nervosa are Caucasians. Depression is also seen in persons with binge eating disorder, with a lifetime prevalence of about 40% (Reichborn-Kjennerud, Bulik, Sullivan, Tambs, & Harris, 2004).

> *Anorexia is more commonly found in females than in males. It occurs more frequently in adolescents and young adults, usually under the age of 25 years. Bulimia, also more common in females, occurs more frequently in individuals between the ages of 14 and 40 years.*

## DIAGNOSTIC CRITERIA

Eating disorder is characterized by severe disturbances in eating behavior (APA, 2000). The *DSM-IV-TR* categorizes eating disorders according to behavioral and cognitive characteristics. It includes anorexia nervosa, bulimia nervosa, and EDNOS. Obesity is not classified as an eating disorder in the *DSM-IV-TR*. Each disorder has a specific set of diagnostic criteria that a patient must meet for diagnosis. **Box 19-1** highlights the major diagnostic criteria as identified by the *DSM-IV-TR* (APA, 2000).

### Anorexia Nervosa

Anorexia nervosa is characterized by the maintenance of low body weight, fear of weight gain, and indifference to the seriousness of the illness (Kayne, Bulik, Plotnicov, & Thornton, 2008). It involves an intense fear of becoming obese. Therefore, the person experiencing anorexia nervosa will not eat sufficient food to maintain a normal body weight (Davidson & Neale, 1998). Anorexia can occur in two forms: the restricting type, in which the person has not participated in binge eating or purging behavior, and binge eating/purging type, in which the person has engaged in behaviors such as self-induced vomiting or misuse of laxatives, diuretics, or enemas. Although many individuals with anorexia nervosa engage in compulsive exercising, individuals with restrictive-type anorexia nervosa are distinguished by their refusal to eat (much).

> *Anorexia is characterized by a low body weight (less than 85% of minimally normal weight for age and height), intense fear of gaining weight or becoming fat, disturbed perception of the body, and amenorrhea for at least three consecutive menstrual cycles.*

### Bulimia Nervosa

Bulimia nervosa is characterized by recurrent episodes of binge eating in combination with some form of inappropriate compensatory behavior (Berkman, Lohr, & Bulik, 2007), such as frequent vomiting or diuretic and/or laxative misuse. It is important to highlight the difference between binge eating/purging type of anorexia nervosa and bulimia nervosa. Individuals with bulimia nervosa may not be able to suppress their weight below the 85% cut off and thus fail to display amenorrhea.

Bulimia is characterized by binge eating in combination with an inappropriate means to compensate for the binge eating, such as self-induced vomiting; misuse of laxatives, diuretics or enemas; fasting; or excessive exercise.

### Binge Eating Disorder

Binge eating disorder is an eating disorder that is included under the *DSM-IV-TR* category of eating disorder not otherwise specified. It is currently being reviewed for inclusion in the next edition. The proposed diagnostic criteria are provided in Box 19-1.

Binge eating disorder is associated with overweight and obesity. However, not all obese people have this disorder. Obese people with binge eating disorder display more chaotic eating habits, exhibit higher levels of eating disinhibition (i.e., eating in response to emotional states), and show substantially higher rates of psychiatric comorbidity. Individuals with binge eating disorder, like those with anorexia nervosa and bulimia nervosa, are preoccupied with shape and weight concerns, with self-worth strongly influenced. However, the characteristics of binges among individuals with binge eating disorder differ from those with bulimia nervosa. Individuals with bulimia nervosa consume more calories during a binge meal but their caloric intake is less during non-binge meals than those with binge eating disorder. Furthermore, unlike

## BOX 19-1: DIAGNOSTIC CRITERIA

### ANOREXIA NERVOSA

- Refusal to maintain at or above a minimally normal weight for age and height (e.g., weight loss leading to maintenance of body weight less than 85% of that expected; or failure to make expected weight gain during period of growth, leading to body weight less than 85% of that expected).
- Intense fear of gaining weight or becoming fat, even though underweight.
- Disturbance in the way in which one's body weight or shape is experienced, or denial of the seriousness of the current low body weight.
- In postmenarchal females, amenorrhea, the absence of at least three consecutive menstrual cycles.
- Further specified as restrictive or binge eating/purging type.

### BULIMIA NERVOSA

- Recurrent episodes of binge eating as characterized by both of the following:
  - Eating in a discrete period of time (e.g., within any 2 hour period) an amount of food that is definitely larger than most people would eat during a similar period of time under similar circumstances.
  - A sense of lack of control over eating during the episode (e.g., a feeling that one cannot stop eating or control what or how much one is eating).
- Recurrent inappropriate compensatory behavior to prevent weight gain, such as self-induced vomiting; misuse of laxatives, diuretics, enemas, or other medications; fasting; or excessive exercise.
- The binge eating and inappropriate compensatory behavior both occurring, on average, at least twice a week for 3 months.
- Self-evaluation unduly influenced by body shape and weight.
- The disturbance not occurring exclusively during episodes of anorexia nervosa.
- Further specified as purging or nonpurging type.

### BINGE EATING DISORDER*

- Recurrent episodes of binge eating, with episodes characterized by both of the following:
  - Eating, in a discrete period of time (e.g., within any 2 hour period), an amount of food definitely larger than most people would eat in a similar period of time under similar circumstances.
  - A sense of lack of control during the episodes.
- The binge eating episodes associated with at least three or more of the following:
  - Eating much more rapidly than normally
  - Eating until feeling uncomfortably full
  - Eating large amounts of food when not physically hungry
  - Eating alone because of being embarrassed by how much one is eating
  - Feeling disgusted with oneself, feeling depressed, or very guilty after eating
- Marked distress related to binge eating present.
- The binge eating occurring, on average at least 2 days a week for 6 months.
- The binge eating not associated with the regular use of inappropriate compensatory behaviors (e.g., purging, fasting, excessive exercise) and not occurring exclusively during the course of anorexia nervosa or bulimia nervosa.

*Criteria currently under investigation

*From the Diagnostic and Statistical Manual of Mental Disorders, Fourth Edition, Text Revision. Copyright © 2000, American Psychiatric Association.*

individuals with bulimia nervosa, whose binge eating takes place against a background of extreme dietary restraint, binge eating is part of a pattern of chaotic eating and general overeating for those with binge eating disorder.

## ETIOLOGY

The exact etiology of eating disorders is not fully known. Numerous research studies have attempted to address the underlying causes but without a consensus. However, various factors have been identified as contributing to the development of eating disorders.

### Biological Factors

There is evidence for the genetic transmission of eating disorders, although such evidence is not conclusive. It is argued that a hereditary predisposition to eating disorders exists in families. For example, anorexia nervosa has been found to be more common among sisters and mothers of those with the disorder than among the general population.

In addition, it has been hypothesized that a dysfunction in the hypothalamus, the "seat" of appetite, may be a factor in the development of eating disorders. Although tests of hormonal functioning and evidence of hormonal aberrations in anorexia nervosa are both prevalent, the fact that refeeding alone, leading to consistent weight gain and balanced nutrition, reverses the endocrine changes observed in anorexia nervosa. The opinion is that these aberrations are not a cause of the disorder.

### Sociocultural Factors

It is argued that an obsession with slimness, a core feature in eating disorders, is concentrated in cultures in which food is abundant. This ideal of slimness and derogation of fatness in cultures of abundance is more intense for females than males and may account for the higher incidence of eating disorders among females than males. This ideal of slimness is often portrayed in the media. However, not all individuals who are exposed to this ideal develop an eating disorder, indicating that other factors contribute to the development of eating disorders. Peer influence is also considered to be an important factor in the development of eating disorders. Adolescent girls learn certain attitudes and behaviors, such as dieting and purging, from their peers. These, in turn, may contribute to the development of an eating disorder.

### Familial Factors

Family dynamics have been implicated in the development and perpetuation of eating disorders. Studies show that individuals with eating disorders have families that tend to be enmeshed, intrusive, hostile, and negative to the individual's emotional needs or are overly concerned with parenting. Also, abnormal attachment processes and insecure attachment are recognized as common in individuals with eating disorders. Generally, individuals with eating disorders describe a critical family environment, featuring coercive parental control and a high value placed on perfectionism. The individual feels that he or she must satisfy these standards. Thus the issue of control becomes the overriding factor in the family of the individual with an eating disorder (Townsend, 2004).

Familial factors associated with eating disorders commonly involve the issue of control due to enmeshment, overly concerned parenting, abnormal attachment processes, and insecure attachments.

### Psychological and Individual Factors

Many factors specific to the individual may contribute to the development of an eating disorder. These include personality traits, self-esteem deficits, and environmental factors. Interpersonal factors that have been most frequently linked to the development of eating disorders include abuse, trauma, and teasing. Individuals experiencing eating disorders commonly report more life stresses. These stresses occur jointly with affective deficiencies such as low self-esteem, depressed mood, generalized anxiety, and irritability. This combination may be particularly significant for the development of bulimia nervosa. More recent theorists concur that an extreme need to control both eating and other aspects of behavior is a central feature of eating disorders (Palmer, 2008; Read, & Morris, 2008). Gaining a sense of control and pride in one's ability to control one's eating combats the feeling of been taken over by thoughts of food or of lacking control of one's thoughts, eating, and weight.

Other individual factors contributing to the development of eating disorders may include:

- Low self-esteem, which reflects how others react to an individual. Perceived rejection may cause lower self-esteem and maladaptive behaviors contributing to eating disorders. Dieting often results in overeating, further lowering self-esteem
- Body dissatisfaction, which occurs when negative affect and negative feelings about one's self are channeled in eating disorders, promoting further negative feelings about the body
- Cognitive factors such as cognitive aberrations, including obsessive thoughts, inaccurate judgments, and rigid thinking patterns.
- Perfectionism, which relates to the belief that one must be perfect, contributes to eating disorders by making

**DRUG SUMMARY 19-1:**
**PARTIAL SELECTION OF MEDICATIONS USED TO TREAT EATING DISORDERS**

| DRUG | IMPLICATIONS FOR NURSING CARE |
|---|---|
| **SELECTIVE SEROTONIN REUPTAKE INHIBITORS (SSRIs)** | |
| fluoxetine (Prozac)<br>paroxetine (Paxil)<br>sertraline (Zoloft)<br>fluvoxamine maleate (Luvox)<br>citalopram (Celexa)<br>escitalopram (Lexapro) | • Advise the patient to take the drug in the morning; if sedation occurs, encourage the patient to take the drug at bedtime<br>• Monitor the patient for signs of serotonin syndrome such as fever, sweating, agitation, tachycardia, hypotension, and hyperreflexia<br>• Inform the patient about possible sexual dysfunction with the drug; if this occurs and causes the patient distress, advocate for a change in the drug<br>• Discuss with patient the time to achieve effectiveness and that it may take from 2–4 weeks before symptoms resolve<br>• Emphasize the need for adherence to therapy and to not stop taking the drug abruptly to prevent withdrawal symptoms<br>• Assess the patient for evidence of suicidal thoughts, especially as depression lessens |

normal shortcomings more traumatic or by making a normal body a sign of imperfection

## TREATMENT OPTIONS

The treatment of eating disorders is complex and requires a multidisciplinary approach, drawing on a number of therapies in relation to the biological, psychological, social, and cultural needs of the individual experiencing an eating disorder. Various treatments have been employed to treat the various eating disorders, including psychopharmacological interventions with SSRIs (see **Drug Summary 19-1**), psychoanalytic approaches (self-psychology, feminist psychoanalytic approaches), cognitive and behavioral treatments, group psychotherapy, family therapies, support and educative treatment (self-help groups, support groups, and psychoeducational groups), and nutritional therapies. Table 19-1 highlights some of these modalities.

**TABLE 19-1: TREATMENT MODALITIES FOR INDIVIDUALS WITH AN EATING DISORDER**

| ANOREXIA NERVOSA | BULIMIA NERVOSA | BINGE EATING DISORDER |
|---|---|---|
| SSRIs<br>In-patient contingency management in relation to short-term weight gain (Roth & Fonagy, 2005)<br>Cognitive behavioral approaches (relapse prevention) (Roth & Fonagy, 2005)<br>Focal psychodynamic therapy (Roth & Fonagy, 2005)<br>Cognitive analytic therapy (Roth & Fonagy, 2005)<br>Nutritional counseling (dietitian) (Roth & Fonagy, 2005)<br>Motivational interviewing (Morris & Harrison, 2008)<br>Bibliotherapy (Williams & Schmidt, 2008) | Cognitive behavioral therapy (CBT) (Roth & Fonagy, 2005)<br>Dietary management/nutritional counseling (Roth & Fonagy, 2009)<br>Interpersonal therapy (Roth & Fonagy, 2005)<br>Psychoeducation with individual psychotherapy (CBT) (Roth & Fonagy, 2005)<br>Bibliotherapy (Williams & Schmidt, 2008)<br>Motivational interviewing (Morris & Harrison, 2008) | SSRIs<br>Nutritional counseling (dietitian) (Roth & Fonagy, 2005)<br>Motivational interviewing (Morris & Harrison, 2008)<br>Cognitive behavioral therapy (Roth & Fonagy, 2005)<br>Bibliotherapy (Williams & Schmidt, 2008) |

In practice, many of these therapies are used in collaboration with one another, such as cognitive behavioral therapy (CBT), family therapy, group therapy, and nutritional counseling. **Evidence-Based Practice 19-1** highlights a study demonstrating the effectiveness of family therapy. It is recommended that a combination of cognitive restructuring therapy, meal planning, the introduction of avoided foods and regular weighing is helpful in treating eating disorders (Morris & Harrison, 2008).

The National Institute of Clinical Excellence (NICE, 2004) has issued guidelines for the treatment of eating disorders based on a review of all published treatment trials and systematic reviews. It also has provided recommendations for assessing eating disorders such as anorexia nervosa, bulimia nervosa, and binge eating disorder.

A handful of studies explored the effects of CBT in treating anorexia nervosa and suggest that CBT is moderately effective in treating this disorder. However, due to the paucity of research studies, NICE cannot recommend it over other therapies. NICE recommends that treatment of anorexia nervosa requires consideration for the appropriate service setting and the psychological and physical management. Additional research is needed. In contrast, bulimia nervosa has been researched extensively and CBT, consisting of 16 to 20 sessions over 4 to 5 months, is identified as the gold standard treatment.

> *CBT is the treatment of choice for individuals with bulimia nervosa.*

## APPLYING THE NURSING PROCESS FROM AN INTERPERSONAL PERSPECTIVE

Patients with eating disorders may be seen in a variety of settings such as acute care settings, day hospitalization programs, and community and outpatient facilities. Many individuals may be encountered in general medical facilities, emergency departments, and specialty clinics because of medical problems secondary to the eating disorder. Therefore, nurses need a firm understanding of the nursing process that integrates the interpersonal process when caring for patients with eating disorders. **Plan**

of Care 19-1 provides an example of a patient with an eating disorder.

### Strategies for Optimal Assessment: Therapeutic Use of Self

When working with an individual experiencing an eating disorder, a comprehensive nursing assessment that includes biological, psychological, social, and cultural needs must be completed. Furthermore, the first few minutes of the interaction with the individual is crucial for a number of reasons. First, the nurse must use the time to begin developing the therapeutic relationship. The nurse must be cognizant of his or her own beliefs and attitudes related to eating and eating disorders. This self-awareness is critical to developing the therapeutic relationship. In addition, as the nurse is assessing the individual and the eating disorder, the individual will also be assessing the nurse. The individual will be attempting to determine whether or not the nurse is knowledgeable about eating disorders, will understand his or her experience, is willing to listen nonjudgmentally, and is trustworthy. Therefore, the nurse must have a knowledge and understanding of eating disorders and work with the individual in an open empathic manner to build a trusting therapeutic relationship.

### Assessing Physical Status

Nurses have an advantage in the treatment of eating disorders due to their knowledge and background in physical assessment. A complete assessment of vital signs, including blood pressure, pulse, respirations, and temperature, as well as the patient's weight is, carried out to determine any medical complications. In addition, the nurse assesses the patient for evidence of any serious life-threatening medical conditions that can occur as complications of the eating disorder. These complications include effects on the cardiovascular, renal, and endocrine systems as well as other body systems. These problems are highlighted in **Table 19-2**.

> *Nurses need to perform a comprehensive physical assessment of individuals with eating disorders because acute and chronic complications can occur that can affect any body system.*

## EVIDENCE-BASED PRACTICE 19-1:
## FAMILY THERAPY FOR ADOLESCENT ANOREXIA NERVOSA

### STUDY

Eisler, I., Simic, M., Russell, G.M., and Dare, C. (2007). A randomized controlled treatment trial of two forms of family therapy in adolescent anorexia nervosa: A five-year follow-up. *Journal of Child Psychology and Psychiatry,* 48 (6), 552–560.

### SUMMARY

There is growing evidence that family therapy is an effective evidence-based intervention for adolescent anorexia nervosa. The researchers aimed to ascertain the long-term impact of two forms of outpatient family intervention previously evaluated in a randomized controlled trial (RCT). This was achieved by conducting a five-year follow-up on a cohort of 40 patients who had received either conjoint family therapy (CFT) in which the whole family was seen together for treatment, or separated family therapy (SFT) in which the adolescent was seen individually, with the parents attending for separate sessions with the same psychotherapist. All patients were traced and 38 agreed to be reassessed. Overall findings revealed that there was little to distinguish between the effects of the two treatments at 5 years. More than 75% of subjects had no eating disorder symptoms. Furthermore, they identified that there were no deaths in the cohort and only 8% of those who had achieved a healthy weight by the end of treatment reported any kind of relapse. Three patients developed bulimic symptoms but only one to a degree warranting a diagnosis of bulimia nervosa. The one difference between the treatments was in patients from families with raised levels of maternal criticism. This group of patients did less well at the end of treatment if they had been offered conjoint family meetings. At follow-up, this difference was still evident, as shown in the relative lack of weight gain since the end of outpatient treatment.

### APPLICATION TO PRACTICE

In this follow-up study, the researchers demonstrated the efficacy of family therapy for adolescent anorexia nervosa, showing that those who respond well to outpatient family intervention generally stay well. In addition, their findings provide support for other studies about the long-term efficacy of family therapy in adolescents experiencing anorexia nervosa. Although the two methods of treatment (CFT and SFT) did not appear to differ in relation to the long-term outcome, the results support the conclusion that CFT is less effective in families with high levels of expressed emotion. This has practical implications, such that it may be inadvisable to use conjoint family meetings, at least early on in treatment, when raised levels of parental criticism are evident. The researchers suggest that once the family is well engaged, conjoint meetings later on in treatment may still have a useful role to play even with this group of families.

### QUESTIONS TO PONDER

1. *How important is the interpersonal therapeutic relationship between the patient and nurse?*
2. *What role does the nurse have in working with families of patients experiencing an eating disorder?*
3. *How important is it for mental health nurses to be informed on systemic (family) approaches when caring for patients experiencing an eating disorder?*

**PLAN OF CARE 19-1:**
**THE PATIENT WITH AN EATING DISORDER**

**NURSING DIAGNOSIS:** Imbalanced nutrition: Less than body requirements; related to distorted sense of self and need for control; manifested by inability/refusal to ingest food or retain food consumed, and failure to maintain weight within acceptable parameters.

Deficient fluid volume related to purging behaviors.

**OUTCOME IDENTIFICATION:** Patient will demonstrate an adequate nutritional intake to meet body requirements with gradual increase in weight to acceptable parameters for age and height.

Patient will identify the consequences of fluid loss due to self-induced vomiting and acknowledge the importance of adequate fluid intake.

| INTERVENTION | RATIONALE |
| --- | --- |
| Perform an initial assessment: obtain weight, assess usual nutritional patterns, and review results of laboratory testing such as serum electrolyte levels, serum albumin, total protein, hemoglobin and hematocrit levels | Performing an initial assessment provides a baseline from which to develop individualized interventions; evaluating laboratory test results provides objective evidence of severity of the condition |
| Work with patient to determine food preferences and collaborate with dietician related to specific nutrient and caloric requirements; encourage fluid intake; administer supplements such as electrolytes, as ordered | Identifying food preferences helps to promote compliance; working with a dietician ensures appropriate nutrient intake; encouraging fluid intake and administering supplements help restore fluid and electrolyte balance |
| If necessary, provide liquid nutrition or tube feedings if patient's status is severe | Using other methods for the ingestion of nutrients may be necessary to prevent complications secondary to refusal to eat |
| Work with the patient and dietician to establish a plan for weight gain and appropriate meal plans; employ measures for behavior modification to allow for gradual weight gain<br><br>Ensure adherence to meal plans | Working with the patient promotes participation and feelings of control over the situation, with empowerment leading to increased chances of compliance and ultimately success; employing behavior modification techniques helps to facilitate behavior change and promote compliance<br><br>Ensuring adherence to meal plans prevents manipulation or playing games with food |
| Monitor the patient for 1 hour after eating and with snacks; be firm but supportive and nonjudgmental in approach | Monitoring helps to prevent patient from engaging in not eating or purging behaviors; a firm nonjudgmental approach promotes rapport and trust |

*(cont.)*

**PLAN OF CARE 19-1:** (*CONT.*)
**THE PATIENT WITH AN EATING DISORDER**

| INTERVENTION | RATIONALE |
|---|---|
| Reinforce concepts of healthy nutrition; correct myths and misconceptions related to food intake; remind patient that physical activity is necessary for good health but that excessive exercise is unhealthy | Reinforcing healthy nutrition and physical activity helps to promote understanding and ultimately promote compliance with therapy |
| Encourage the patient to keep a journal or log of feelings, eating, and any binge/purging behaviors | Keeping a log or journal helps the patient gain insight into his or her condition and helps to identify potential triggers for behavior |
| Continually monitor vital signs, laboratory test results, intake and output, skin turgor, and trends in weight; weigh the patient at the same time and in the same clothing | Continued monitoring provides evidence of effectiveness of therapy and compliance; weighing at the same time and in the same clothing ensures accurate results |
| Provide support and positive reinforcement as the patient begins to make changes, regardless of how small the changes may be | Providing support and positive reinforcement promotes feelings of self-worth and increases the chance for compliance and a successful outcome |

**NURSING DIAGNOSIS:** Disturbed body image; related to disease process; manifested by inaccurate perception of physical appearance, preoccupation with body size, and fears of gaining weight.

**OUTCOME IDENTIFICATION:** Patient will verbalize positive statements about self.

Patient will state a realistic self-appraisal.

| INTERVENTION | RATIONALE |
|---|---|
| Assess the patient's feelings about self and appearance using a caring, nonjudgmental approach | Understanding of the patient's feelings related to self-help provides focus for individualized interventions |
| Work with the patient to help view his or her body realistically; compare actual body measurements with the patient's perception of measurement; provide objective realistic feedback | Working with the patient to view his or her body realistically, such as with actual measurements, helps to replace distorted view with realistic view |
| Help the patient identify feelings related to unrealistic high self-expectations and feelings of inadequacy. Assist the patient to identify strengths and resources; provide reinforcement of strengths | Identifying feelings related to excessive high expectations and feelings of inadequacy promotes insight into underlying feelings related to eating behaviors; reinforcing strengths promotes self-esteem and empowerment over situation and enhances motivation to change |

*(cont.)*

**PLAN OF CARE 19-1: (*CONT.*)**
**THE PATIENT WITH AN EATING DISORDER**

| INTERVENTION | RATIONALE |
|---|---|
| Reinforce prescribed therapies such as cognitive behavioral therapy; help the patient address cognitive distortions | Reinforcing prescribed therapies helps to alter the patient's current view of self to achieve a healthier, more realistic body image |
| Educate the patient about normal growth and development related to female body structure | Educating the patient helps to correct any misconceptions about the body |

**NURSING DIAGNOSIS:** Ineffective coping; related to distorted sense of cause and effect relationships; manifested by conflict avoidance and use of restricted eating to feel a sense of control in life circumstance.

**OUTCOME IDENTIFICATION:** Patient will begin to demonstrate appropriate positive coping strategies.

| INTERVENTION | RATIONALE |
|---|---|
| Use a calm, nonjudgmental approach and establish rapport with the patient | Using a nonjudgmental, calm approach with rapport promotes the development of trust and the nurse-patient relationship |
| Work with the patient to discuss feelings of anxiety, fear, powerlessness, and helplessness. Assist the patient in identifying feelings related to family role, functioning, and possible issues related to conflict, independence, and dependence | Discussing feelings associated with eating behaviors and family provides insight into behavior |
| Assist the patient in objectively appraising the situation | Identifying feelings objectively helps to restructure faulty beliefs |
| Help the patient identify the connection between feelings and eating behavior | Identifying the connection helps the patient to gain insight into behavior in the hopes of changing that behavior |
| Reinforce prescribed therapies, such as cognitive behavioral therapy, supportive therapy, and family therapy | Reinforcing therapies helps to promote success |

*From Nursing Diagnosis – Definitions and Classifications 2009–2011. Copyright © 2011 by NANDA International. Use by arrangement with Blackwell Publishing Limited, a company of John Wiley & Sons, Inc.*

## TABLE 19-2: MEDICAL COMPLICATIONS ASSOCIATED WITH EATING DISORDERS

| BODY SYSTEM | PROBLEMS |
| --- | --- |
| Gastrointestinal | Bloating secondary to delayed gastric emptying<br>Gastric dilation and perforation<br>Parotid enlargement<br>Dental erosion<br>Gastroesophageal reflux<br>Esophagitis and bleeding<br>Rupture of the esophagus<br>Unexplained diarrhea |
| Reproductive/ endocrine/ metabolic | Amenorrhea<br>Infertility<br>Irregular menses<br>Low estrogen, luteinizing hormone, and follicle stimulating hormone<br>Reduced uterine size; immature multifollicular or follicular pattern of ovarian structure<br>Hypothyroidism<br>Hypoglycemia<br>Electrolyte abnormalities |
| Musculoskeletal | Osteoporosis<br>Loss of muscle mass |
| Cardiovascular | Postural hypotension<br>Bradycardia<br>Cold intolerance; complaints of chills due to poor peripheral circulation and loss of subcutaneous fat<br>Dysrhythmias, including those related to electrolyte imbalances such as potassium<br>Heart failure |
| Hematologic | Anemia<br>Thrombocytopenia<br>Leukopenia |
| Renal | Hematuria<br>Proteinuria<br>Renal insufficiency |

Complications requiring immediate medical attention include dehydration, hypokalemia, or both, resulting in cardiac dysrhythmias; an esophageal tear resulting in hemorrhage from the mechanical trauma of vomiting; and decreased glomerular filtration rate, resulting in renal insufficiency. Serious complications of the endocrine system include abnormal thyroid function, abnormal female hormone levels, and the potential for sterility. Amenorrhea is an important indicator for anorexia nervosa.

## Assessing Psychosociocultural Status

It is also necessary to assess the psychological, social, and cultural status of the patient to aid in providing a baseline for the patient's current status in relation to his or her motivation to make psychological and behavioral changes. **Box 19-2** describes the stages associated with motivation for change.

At this time, the nurse needs to assess the behaviors that the individual engages in related to eating, such as binge eating, fasting, purging, and/or excessive exercise. The nurse also needs to obtain a history of the weight loss and/or weight gain and current eating habits. Some important questions to ask include:

- What is it about your weight that makes you unhappy?
- When did you first become concerned about your weight?
- When did you first start dieting/overeating/binge eating and what prompted you to do so?
- What has been your highest weight and how did you feel about yourself at that time?
- What has been your lowest weight and how did you feel about yourself at that time?
- What weight would you like to be?
- What is a typical day's eating to you?
- Do you avoid any foods? Do you binge eat, fast, purge, engage in excessive exercise?
- How do you feel about your body?
- What do you feel would happen if you didn't control your eating?

By asking these questions the nurse will be able to gather a comprehensive assessment of the psychological and cultural factors contributing to the patient's eating disorder. **Consumer Perspective 19-1** provides insight into what it is like to have bulimia nervosa.

## Assessing for Motivation for Change

Motivation for change or readiness for change is in many ways an interpersonal process, the product of an interaction between people, which in this situation is the patient and the nurse (Miller & Rollnick, 2002). As stated previously, the nurse determines the patient's current stage related to his or her motivation for change. Next, the nurse assesses the patient's readiness for change. One simple way to accomplish this is to use a ruler with gradations from 0 to 10, with 0 being not at all important to change and 10 being extremely important to change. This same method can be used to assess a patient's confidence in making the change, with 0 being not at all confident and 10 being extremely confident of making the change (Miller & Rollnick, 2002). The nurse, in collaboration with the patient, can assess the importance of bringing about change and also assess how confident the patient is

### BOX 19-2: MOTIVATION AND STAGES OF CHANGE

The Transtheoretical Model suggests that individuals may be thought of as occupying a number of positions with regard to the prospect of psychological or behavioral change. The person is described as being in one of 5 stages.

**STAGE 1 Precontemplation:** The person does not see a problem and does not consider attempting to change.

**STAGE 2 Contemplation:** The person can see that the issue is problematic but may also be aware of the advantages of staying as he or she is, however, he or she is thinking about the possibility of change.

**STAGE 3 Preparation:** Person is convinced of the need to change and is planning to do something.

**STAGE 4 Action:** Stage of doing something and actively changing.

**STAGE 5 Maintenance:** Change is accomplished and person makes it part of his or her life.

*Adapted from Palmer, B. (2003). Helping people with eating disorders. New York: John Wiley & Sons.*

### CONSUMER PERSPECTIVE 19-1: A PATIENT WITH BULIMIA NERVOSA

I have been living with bulimia nervosa since I was 17 years old. I am now 27 years old. I always felt that my life was disorganized and out of control. I never felt good enough and felt that everyone else had their lives in order and were happy. I believed that if I was thinner, I would have one less thing to worry about and I would be happier. I believed that thin people were happier people. The only way I had control in my disorganized life was when I purged myself after I engaged in binge eating. I felt most relaxed at this time. Before I finally admitted that I could no longer live my life like this, I wondered if I could make the change. Since I have sought help, I now understand more about myself and my relationships with food and those around me. I know that I will always struggle with food during my life but I don't want to go back to that dark place. I realize now that I need to trust and accept myself more and also I accept that bulimia is something I will struggle with at times but feel stronger now more than ever to cope with it.

in bringing about change. This measure can be repeated throughout the treatment process in order to evaluate progress and to identify any further obstacles in the patient's recovery.

> *A key component of assessment is determining how motivated the patient is to change and his or her readiness to change.*

## Diagnosing and Planning Appropriate Interventions: Meeting the Patient's Focused Needs

Meeting the patient's focused needs during the planning stage of the nursing process can only happen if the nurse has accurately completed an assessment of the patient, his or her perception of the eating disorder, and motivation for change. When planning appropriate interventions, all members of the team must be involved. The team commonly includes the nurse, dietitian, medical colleagues, psychologists, clinical nurse specialist (CNS) or nurse practitioners (NP) with a speciality in eating disorders, psychotherapists, and occupational therapists. Due to the varying assessment findings noted and wide range of problems faced by patients with eating disorders, numerous nursing diagnoses would apply. Examples of possible nursing diagnoses would include:

- Imbalanced nutrition less than body requirements related to anorexia nervosa
- Imbalanced nutrition more than body requirements related to bulimia nervosa and binge eating disorder
- Deficient fluid volume related to anorexia nervosa
- Risk for electrolyte imbalance related to anorexia nervosa
- Disturbed body image related to eating disorder
- Chronic low self-esteem related to eating disorder
- Ineffective coping related to eating disorder
- Powerlessness related to eating disorder

These nursing diagnoses also will vary based on the acuity of the patient's illness, developmental stage, any underlying co-morbidities, current treatment regimen, and sources of support. Based on the identified nursing diagnoses, the nurse and patient collaboratively would determine the outcomes to be achieved. For example, an outcome related to deficient fluid volume would be to ensure that the individual would be able to identify the consequences of fluid loss due to self-induced vomiting and acknowledge the importance of adequate fluid intake. When planning nursing interventions it is helpful to integrate the objectives of treatment, which include the following:

- To eliminate maladaptive patterns of eating such as fasting, binge eating, purging
- To establish a more normal eating pattern with regular balanced meals
- To address any physical complications of the illness, such as dental enamel erosion or fluid and electrolyte abnormalities
- To address the psychological issues that accompany the illness, including low self-esteem, body dissatisfaction, and other dysfunctional thinking patterns
- To address comorbid conditions such as mood disorders
- Finally, and over time, to prevent relapse (Mitchell, Agras, & Wonderlich, 2007)

When planning care, the nurse also needs to consider the treatment setting. Most eating disorders are treated in outpatient settings. However, if the individual's physical state deteriorates to a dangerous level, inpatient treatment is necessary. Outpatient treatment is helpful as it avoids the difficulties associated with admission. These include separation from family and friends and excessive dependency on the staff because patients typically are admitted for several months. Outpatient treatment also allows the individual to take responsibility for his or her own recovery and ensures that the individual is ready to make the change, thereby increasing the chances for recovery.

## Implementing Effective Interventions: Timing and Pacing

To be effective, interventions must be implemented at the appropriate time and in a manner that does not overwhelm the patient. **How Would You Respond 19-1** provides an example of a patient with an eating disorder who requires implementation. Effective interventions can include:

- *Enhancing the patient's motivation to change (motivational interviewing)*: Helping the patient acknowledge that he or she has a problem and then determining the stage related to change (see Box 19-2); the individual is then encouraged to consider the positive and negative aspects of changing or staying the same
- *Monitoring the physical and psychological status of the patient*: Evaluating for acute and chronic complications; monitoring weight and body mass index and keeping a weight chart; assessing for possible depression with or without suicidal ideation
- *Assisting with dietary measures*: Working with a dietitian and the individual to plan meals; assessing for any nutritional defects
- *Assisting with supportive therapy*: Supportive therapy by a counselor or a nurse trained in eating disorders; providing psychoeducation and supportive therapy in managing eating disorders
- *Reinforcing CBT*: CBT performed by advanced practice nurses to bring about change for individuals experiencing eating disorders and to help improve coping skills and self-esteem; assisting the patient in keeping a dietary diary, and learning techniques to deal with other problems such as binge eating, purging, laxative use, and excessive exercise; challenging cognitive distortions related to self-esteem and body image (summarized in **Box 19-3**)
- *Encouraging family intervention*: Exploring family issues and providing education about eating disorders; encouraging family to be supportive
- *Addressing social and occupational issues*: Identifying any social or occupational problems that may be exacerbating

## HOW WOULD YOU RESPOND? 19-1: A GIRL WITH ANOREXIA NERVOSA

Ann was the younger daughter of two girls. Her mother worked as a nurse and her father as a teacher. When she was younger, she had a happy settled life. At age 13, Ann's father was in a car accident and lost both of his legs. Following this, he suffered bouts of depression and anxiety. It was difficult for all members of the family and the strain was evident between her parents, as they often argued. Ann spent much time caring for her father and feared upsetting him because she felt that it may lead to a deterioration in his mood. She believed that if she worked hard at her studies and went to a university, she would make her father happy and proud. At age 15, Ann began dating a boy from her school. This became a source of conflict between her and her father. Finally, Ann began spending less and less time with this boy and he eventually began dating another girl. Ann was very hurt and angry with her father but she did not express this to him. Instead she focused on her school work and also decided to lose some weight. So she began dieting. At first she lost some weight and felt happy about this. Over the next year, her weight went from 127 lbs to 92 lbs. Ann then began fasting for long periods, then binge eating, and then purging. She also began exercising excessively. She thought about food a lot and studied and exercised to distract herself from food. Her weight continued to fall; she ceased menstruating, and her weight fell to 82 lbs. At this point her parents brought her to her general practitioner. How would you respond?

### CRITICAL THINKING QUESTIONS

1. *Based on the scenario, which eating disorder would you suspect and why?*

2. *What factors have played a role in contributing to Ann's eating disorder?*

### APPLYING THE CONCEPTS

Ann has lost 45 pounds and has been engaging in dieting, fasting for long periods, binge eating, and purging along with excessive exercise. Additionally, she has ceased menstruating, suggesting anorexia nervosa. Her other behaviors indicate binge eating/purging type of anorexia. Based on her initial weight of 127 pounds, considered appropriate for her height and weight, her current weight of 82 pounds is significantly lower than 85% of her 127 pounds.

Possible factors contributing to her eating disorder include her desire to be the perfect daughter for her father, her inability to verbalize her feelings to her father about losing her boyfriend, and probably issues related to self-esteem based on the boyfriend dating another girl, and the conflicts with her father.

the eating disorder; for example occupations such as modeling, dancing, acting, and athletics may make an individual prone to developing eating disorders

When working with individuals with an eating disorder it is important to include the individual's family (be sure consent is given if the patient is over the age of 18 years). Abraham and Llewellyn-Jones (2005) advocate that the family/parents "fight the illness, not the person," "don't blame yourself for causing the illness," "try to normalize family life," "educate yourself about the illness," "give unconditional love and support," and "give respect to the person with the illness." The nurse can ensure that literature pertaining to the eating disorder is given to the family and can support family members in being proactive in their loved one's recovery.

> *When implementing interventions, a strong trusting interpersonal relationship between the nurse and individual experiencing the eating disorder is necessary to ensure effective outcomes.*

# EVALUATING: OBJECTIVE CRITIQUE OF INTERVENTIONS AND SELF-REFLECTION

Evaluating the nursing care provided is of vital importance not only for the individual experiencing an eating disorder, but also for the psychiatric-mental health nurse's practice. By evaluating and reflecting on the process of care, the psychiatric-mental health nurse can identify areas of effective practice and areas that need to be improved upon, thereby developing and promoting best nursing practice.

During the evaluation phase, review all of the activities during the previous phases and determine whether outcomes identified with and for the patient have been met. Once again, self-reflection is an invaluable tool at this point. This can be done by asking: Have I provided the best nursing practice for my patient? Is my patient better after the planned care?

During this phase of the nurse-patient relationship, the nurse and the patient should reflect on progress made toward reaching the patient's goals. Point out positives to the patient and include a plan for continued care as appropriate.

This phase is also part of the termination of the nurse-patient relationship. The patient may experience a setback due to a patient feeling of loss of this relationship. The nurse's role is to help the explore his or her feelings and ease this transition while maintaining boundaries (Peplau, 1991). Additionally, reflecting on the therapeutic relationship as described by Peplau (1952) is of vital importance, as studies show that the therapeutic relationship is paramount in recovery from eating disorders.

## SUMMARY POINTS

- Eating disorders are characterized by severe disturbances in eating behavior. Eating disorders include anorexia nervosa, bulimia nervosa, and eating disorders not otherwise specified. Binge eating disorder is currently under review for inclusion in the next edition of the *DSM*.

- The majority of individuals who experience eating disorders tend to be female and most appear to be in their late adolescence or early adulthood, although the amount of men experiencing eating disorders is on the increase. The group at highest risk is young females between ages 15 and 30, with anorexia striking at a younger age and bulimia nervosa more common in the older range.

- Numerous factors have been implicated in the development of eating disorders. These include biological, sociocultural, familial, and individual risk factors.

(cont.)

### SUMMARY POINTS (*CONT.*)

- Cognitive behavioral therapy (CBT) is the standard of care for treatment of bulimia nervosa; more research is needed to determine its effectiveness as a treatment modality for anorexia nervosa.

- When working with an individual experiencing an eating disorder, a comprehensive nursing assessment that includes physical, psychological, social, and cultural needs must be completed.

- All members of the treatment team must be involved in the delivery of care to the patient with an eating disorder. The nurse works closely with the dietitian, medical colleagues, psychologists, clinical nurse specialists or nurse practitioners trained in eating disorders or psychotherapy and occupational therapists.

- The implementation of effective nursing interventions is necessary to aid recovery, such as enhancement of the motivation to change, supportive therapy, CBT techniques, family intervention, and the identification of any social or occupational issues that may be affecting recovery.

### NCLEX-PREP*

1. A patient with anorexia is admitted to the in-patient facility because of cardiovascular problems. The patient's minimal normal acceptable weight is 125 pounds. Which weight would the nurse interpret as indicative of anorexia?

   a. 118 pounds
   b. 112 pounds
   c. 107 pounds
   d. 100 pounds

2. A group of students are reviewing information about eating disorders. The students demonstrate an understanding of the topic when they identify which of the following as being associated with bulimia nervosa?

   a. Greater occurrence in males
   b. Use of severe fasting rituals
   c. More common in women in their 20s and 30s
   d. High correlation with overweight and obesity

3. A patient with anorexia nervosa disorder engages in binge eating and purging behaviors. Which of the following would the patient be least likely to use for purging?

   a. Diuretics
   b. Enemas
   c. Laxatives
   d. Antiemetics

4. A nurse is assessing a patient with an eating disorder for complications. Which of the following might the nurse assess?

   a. Hypertension
   b. Increased muscle strength
   c. Cold intolerance
   d. Tachycardia

5. While performing a routine health checkup on a teenager who is 5 feet tall and 100 lbs, a nurse begins to suspect that a patient may be experiencing an eating disorder. Which statement by the patient would lead the nurse to suspect this?

   a. "Look at me, look at how fat I am."
   b. "My last period was about 6 weeks ago."
   c. "I just lost 5 pounds so I could fit into my prom dress."
   d. "I usually like to swim about 3 times a week."

*Answers to these questions appear on page 639.

# REFERENCES

Abraham, S., & Llewellyn-Jones, D. (2005). Eating disorders: the facts. New York: Oxford University Press.

American Psychiatric Association. (1994). *Diagnostic and statistical manual of mental disorders* (4th ed). Washington, DC: Author.

American Psychiatric Association. (2000). *Diagnostic and statistical manual of mental disorders* (4th. ed), *Text Revision (DSM-IV-TR)*. Washington, DC: Author.

Andersen, A.E. (1999). Gender-related aspects of eating disorders: a guide to practice. *Journal of Gender Specific Medicine, 2* (1) 47–54.

Berkman, N.D., Lohr, K.N., & Bulik, C.M. (2007). Outcome of eating disorders: a systematic review of the literature. *International Journal of Eating Disorders, 40* (4), 293–309.

Clarkin-Watts, A. Eating disorders. In Fortinash K., Holoday-Worret (Eds), *Psychiatric mental health nursing,* St. Louis, MO: Mosby.

Davidson, G., & Neale, J. (1998). *Abnormal psychology.* New York: John Wiley and Son.

De la Rie, S., Noordenbos, G., Donker, M., and Furth, E. (2006). Evaluating the treatment of eating disorders from the patient's perspective. *International Journal of Eating Disorders, 39* (8) 667–676.

Dichter, J.R., Cohen, J., & Connolly, P.M. (2002). Bulimia nervosa: knowledge, awareness, and skill levels among advanced practice nurses. *Journal of the American Academy of Nurse Practitioners. 14* (6), 269–275.

Eisler, I., Simic, M., Russell, G.M., and Dare, C. (2007). A randomised controlled treatment trial of two forms of family therapy in adolescent anorexia nervosa: a five-year follow-up. *Journal of Child Psychology and Psychiatry 48* (6) 552–560.

Fairburn, C.G., Cooper, Z., Doll, H.A., & Welch, S.L. (1999). Risk factors for anorexia nervosa: three integrated case-control comparisons. *Archives of General Psychiatry, 56,* 468–476.

Fairburn, C., Pkil, M., & Beglin, S. (1990). Studies of the epidemiology of bulimia nervosa, *American Journal of Psychiatry, 147,* 401–408.

Feldman, M.B., & Meyer, I.H. (2007). Eating disorders in diverse lesbian gay, and bisexual populations. *International Journal of Eating Disorders 40* (3) 218–226.

Garner, D., Olmsted, M.P., & Polivy, J. (1983). Development and validation of a multidimensional eating disorders inventory for anorexia nervosa and bulimia, *International Journal of Eating Disorders, 2.*

Garner, D.M., & Bemis, K.M. (1985). In Garner, D.M. & Garfinkel, P.E. *Handbook of psychotherapy for anorexia nervosa and bulimia nervosa* (pg 107–146). New York: Guilford Press.

Gibbs, G. (1998). *Learning by day: A guide to teaching and learning,* London: Further Education Unit.

Grothaus, K.L. (1998). Eating disorders and adolescents: an overview of a maladaptive behavior. *Journal of Child and Adolescent Psychiatric Nursing, 11* (3), 146–156.

Grucza, R.A., Przybeck, T.R., & Cloninger, C.R. (2007). Prevalence and correlates of binge eating disorder in a community sample. *Comprehensive Psychiatry, 48,* 124.

Gu, D., Reynolds, K., Wu, X., Chen, J., Duan, X., Reynolds, R.F., Whelton, P.K., & He, J. & InterASIA Collaborative Group (2005). Prevalence of the metabolic syndrome and overweight among adults in China. *Lancet, 365,* 1398–1405.

Kanye, W.H., Bulik, C.M., Plotnicov, K., & Thornton, L. (2008). The genetics of anorexia nervosa collaborative study: methods and sample description. *International Journal of Eating Disorders, 41* (4), 289–300.

Lucas, A.R., Beard, C.M., O'Fallon, W.M., & Kurland, L.T. (1991). 50-year trends in the incidence of anorexia nervosa in Rochester, Minn: a population-based study. *American Journal of Psychiatry, 148,* 917.

Mitchell, J.E., Agras, S., & Wonderlich, S. (2007). Treatment of bulimia nervosa: where are we and where are we going? *International Journal of Eating Disorders, 40* (2), 95–101.

Mokdad, A.H., Marks, J.S., Stroup, D.F., & Gerberding, (2004). Actual causes of death in the United States, 2000. *Journal of American Medical Association, 291*(24):2941.

Morgan, J.F., & Arcelus, J. (2009). Body image in gay and straight men: a qualitative study. *European Eating Disorders Review. 17* (6) 435–443.

Morris, J., and Harrison, N. (2008). Psychological support within general practice cited in ABC of eating disorders. British Medical Journal Books. UK: Wiley-Blackwell.

National Institute for Clinical Excellence (NICE). (2004). *Treatment of anorexia nervosa, bulimia nervosa and related eating disorders: a clinical guideline.* London: National Institute for Clinical Excellence.

Ogden, C.L., Carroll, M.D., Curtin, L.R., McDowell, M.A., Tabal, C.J., & Flegal, K.M. (2006). Prevalence of overweight and obesity in the United States, 1999–2004. *Journal of American Medical Association, 295,* 1549–1555.

Palmer, B. (2008). Causes of eating disorders cited in ABC of eating disorders. British Medical Journal Books. UK: Wiley-Blackwell.

Palmer, B. (2003). *Helping people with eating disorders.* New York: John Wiley & Sons.

Peplau, H.E. (1991). *Interpersonal relations in nursing: A conceptual frame of reference for psychodynamic nursing.* New York, New York: Springer Publishing Company.

Peplau, H.E. (1952). *Interpersonal relations in nursing.* New York: GP Putnam.

Polivy, J., & Herman, C.P. (2002). Causes of eating disorders. *Annual Review Psychology 53,* 187–213.

Read, G., & Morris, J. (2008). Body image disturbance in eating disorders cited in ABC of eating disorders. British Medical Journal Books. UK: Wiley-Blackwell.

Reichborn-Kjennerud, T., Bulik, C.M., Sullivan, P.F., Tambs, K., & Harris, J.R. Psychiatric and medical symptoms in binge eating in the absence of compensatory behaviors. *Obes Res, 12,* 143–151.

Rhys Jones, W., and Morgan, J.F. (2010). Eating disorders in men: a review of the literature. *Journal of Public Mental Health 9* (2), 23–31.

Ringwood, S. (2010). Eating disorders: your guide to todays mental health issues. *Mental Health, 10,* 21–23.

Robinson, P.H. (2000). Review article: recognition and treatment of eating disorders in primary and secondary care. *Aliment Pharmacology Therapy,* 14.

Roth, A., and Fonagy, P. (2005). What works for whom; a critical review of psychotherapy research. New York: Guilford Press.

Spitzer, R.L., Yanovski, S.Z., Wadden, T., Wing, R., Marcus, M., Stubkard, A. et al. (1993). Binge eating disorder: a multisite field trial of the diagnostic criteria. *International Journal of Eating Disorders, 13,* 191–203.

Townsend, M.C. (2004). *Nursing diagnoses in psychiatric nursing: care plans and psychotropic medications.* Philadelphia, F.A.: Davis Company.

Wilfley, D.E., Wilson, T., & Agras, W.S. *The clinical significance of binge eating disorder,* Wiley InterScience, www.interscience.wiley.com.

Williams, C., and Schmidt, U. (2008). Advice, education and self-help cited in ABC of eating disorders. British Medical Journal Books. UK: Wiley-Blackwell.

Wu, Y. (2006). Overweight and obesity in China. *British Medical Journal, 333,* 362.

Yager, J. (2000). Weighty perspectives: contemporary challenges in obesity and eating disorders. *American Journal of Psychiatry 157* (6) 851–853.

Zaninotto, P., Wardle, H., Stamatakis, E., Mindell, J., & Head, J. (2006). Forecasting obesity to 2010. *National Centre for Social Research, Department of Health,* London, UK.

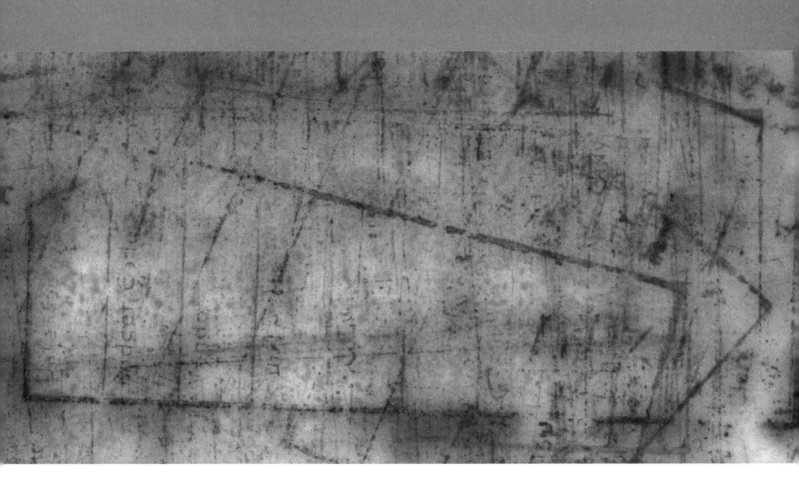

# CHAPTER CONTENTS

Suffering and the Therapeutic Use of Self

Special Issues Related to Mental Health and Physical Illness

The Nurse's Role in Breaking Bad News

End-of-Life Care

The Role of the Mental Health Liaison/Consultation Nurse

Applying the Nursing Process from an Interpersonal Perspective

Strategies for Optimal Assessment: Therapeutic Use of Self

# EXPECTED LEARNING OUTCOMES

**After completing this chapter, the student will be able to:**

1. Describe how mental and physical health are intertwined.
2. Define suffering.
3. Identify the key concepts of suffering.
4. Explain how compassion fatigue can impact the nurse.
5. Describe issues related to mental health that impact physically ill individuals, and applying mental health care concepts to other physically ill patient populations.
6. Demonstrate understanding of the nurse's role in addressing end-of-life issues.

## CHAPTER 20

# PSYCHOLOGICAL PROBLEMS OF PHYSICALLY ILL PERSONS

Patrice E. Rancour

7. Describe the role of the mental health liaison/consultation nurse.
8. Apply the nursing process from an interpersonal perspective to a physically ill patient with mental health issues.

## KEY TERMS

Assisted suicide

Bad news

Compassion fatigue

Courageous conversations

Critical incident debriefing

Delirium

Endorphins

Psychoneuroimmunology

Suffering

ental and physical health are deeply intertwined. A relationship exists between the two. Stress leads to physical changes in the body that ultimately affect the mental health of the person. In turn, the person's mental health can result in changes to that individual's physical health.

Consider this statement, "Every nurse is a mental health nurse." In every interaction that nurses have with patients who are experiencing physical illness, for example, whether in the home or inpatient or outpatient medical-surgical settings, the nurse must care for the whole person by rendering competent mental health care. Doing so can often make the difference between successful and unsuccessful outcomes for the patient and his or her family.

This chapter addresses the concept of suffering as it relates to the therapeutic use of self and its impact on the nurse. It describes the most common issues that affect the mental health of physically ill patients, end-of-life care, and the role of the mental health liaison/consultation nurse. The chapter concludes by applying the nursing process from an interpersonal perspective to promote the mental health of patients with physical illness.

## SUFFERING AND THE THERAPEUTIC USE OF SELF

**SUFFERING** is often defined as the experience of distress or pain, which can be emotional or physical. It is often synonymous with words such as agony, torment, and torture. Several theorists have addressed this concept as it relates to mental health.

### Theoretical Views of Suffering

Recall from Chapter 2 that suffering is a key concept identified by Joyce Travelbee's interpersonal theory of nursing. Travelbee built her theory on the works of existentialists including Viktor Frankl, noting that his work, *Man's Search for Meaning,* (Frankl, 1959) played a significant role in the development of her own theory. Frankl believed that in a world over which humans have little control, the way a person chooses to respond to his or her experience determines whether and how that person survives and/or thrives. These beliefs were the result of his observations while being incarcerated in a World War II concentration camp. He noticed that some of the prisoners lived while others did not, although camp conditions were the same for both groups.

Travelbee's definition addresses suffering as ranging from simple mental, physical, or spiritual discomfort to extreme anguish. She also describes phases beyond

anguish, which include the malignant phase of despairful not caring, and a terminal phase of apathetic indifference (Travelbee, 1971, p. 62). Travelbee insisted that suffering is a key element in the exploration of illness. Therefore, suffering can be addressed within the scope of the nurse-patient relationship. According to Travelbee, if the patient's meaning of suffering is found within the nurse-patient therapeutic relationship, then use of therapeutic communication is the vehicle used to relieve the suffering. (See Chapter 2 for a more in-depth discussion of Travelbee's theory and suffering.)

> *According to Travelbee, suffering must be explored as part of the nurse-patient relationship.*

Travelbee's concepts were further expanded by Shinoda Bolen, a physician who adhered to Carl Jung's beliefs. Jung felt that as a person goes through life, he or she develops abilities of inner exploration that provide meaning. He also identified archetypes or organizing principles related to the things a person does or sees. Shinoda Bolen built upon these thoughts with her contention that illness often can be experienced as an archetypal descent into the underworld. She likened common occurrences such as receiving a life-threatening diagnosis or passing the threshold of the treatment center (e.g., hospital entrance, etc.) to being ferried across the River Styx (Shinoda Bolen, 1996). Frequently, nurses are witnesses to patients experiencing such crossroads. Thus, nurses can employ the therapeutic use of self to suggest ways that the patient can reframe these periods of physical suffering into opportunities for expansion. When this happens, patients are better able to bear the burdens of such suffering because they are being assisted to find meaning in experiences that otherwise would be experienced as futile, mundane, or banal (Rancour, 2008).

Another psychotherapist, Miriam Goodman, continues Travelbee's concepts of dealing with suffering; that is, transforming suffering by attending to it and, as a result, growing in compassion with others:

> *...we carry this mistaken belief that enlightenment means we do not suffer anymore. But it is possible to suffer with calm, loving heart. These two are not mutually exclusive. Enlightenment for me is about growing in compassion, and* compassion *means "suffering with." Enlightenment has something to do*

*with not running from our own pain or the pain of others. When we don't turn away from pain, we open our hearts and are more able to connect to the best part of ourselves and others — because every human being knows pain.* (Platek, 2008, p.5)

Goodman's view suggests that nurses work on their own healing by refusing to turn away from the pain of others; that nurses recognize their call to service as the way they have decided to manifest their own purpose in the world.

Unless nurses have a relationship basis for their practice, what Travelbee calls "the therapeutic use of self," it is fairly easy to medicalize normal human experiences such as birth, illness, and death, and the subsequent pain and suffering that accompany them. When this occurs, the humanness of the experience and the potential for healing by transformation and self-actualization can be lost. Compassion as the essential human trait is replaced with pharmacology and the starkness of procedure. Vigilance toward making one's own self a therapeutic tool is often one's only defense in a world that too often depends on technology alone to save individuals from the inevitability of the human condition.

Adopting such a perspective encourages the patient and the nurse to seek meaning in traditionally painful experiences such as illness, thereby helping each bear the ordeal of the patient's suffering. Within the context of the relationship the patient is not only able to survive, but to thrive as well.

## Suffering and the Impact on Nurses

It would be an error in judgment to believe that nurses are not affected by the suffering of their patients. Providing care to people who are ill and in pain challenges nurses to be mindful of their own mental health and the mental health of their colleagues. The provision of mental health care is especially challenging because one needs to maintain watch for the unconscious tendency to allow tasks and procedures to distract and distance one's self from the suffering of those for whom one cares. The very nature of the therapeutic use of self transports the nurse directly into the very heart of suffering so that its effect upon the caregiver becomes inescapable (Pendry, 2007).

Nurses need to understand generally that **COMPASSION FATIGUE**, or the emotional and physical burnout that may interfere with caring, is an occupational hazard and does not constitute a character defect. When nurses begin to exhibit symptoms of such occupational stress or recognize it in others, a rapid response is necessary to help the nurse achieve rebalance. **CRITICAL INCIDENT DEBRIEFING**

is a formally recognized program with trained staff that allows staff to vent and process feelings in a structured way after particularly stressful patient contacts. It helps nurses acknowledge the special nature of the work in which they are engaged and to regain balance. Reaching for balance includes making sure that nurses are eating healthy foods, getting rest and exercise, and making sure that other parts of their lives are also in balance.

Within the context of the therapeutic relationship itself, experienced nurses understand the value of simultaneously moving in close and letting go. In other words, nurses understand how to stay attached to the process of providing care and to let go of the need to control the outcome. The experienced nurse would not become emotionally involved with the patient to the extent that the relationship overshadows expert clinical judgment, but would always review his/her own reactions to the interpersonal relationship with the patient and use that learning to monitor the interactions.

> *The therapeutic use of self places nurses at risk for compassion fatigue because they are directly involved in the patient's experience of suffering.*

Healing is a very complex process that occurs within the framework of the relationship and is affected by multiple variables existing outside of the nurse's control. At times, nurses may not even be aware of some of these variables, such as therapeutic interactions that have occurred with other patients or with significant others, or information that the patient has obtained via the internet. Since the relationship includes the nurse, the nurse needs to pay attention to his or her own needs for the relationship to remain therapeutic. For example, if the nurse is tired, frustrated, defensive, angry, anxious, or sad, and is not aware of these feelings, the likelihood is high that such feelings will be acted out within the context of the nurse-patient relationship rather than being worked through properly. When this happens, the nurse is unable to perceive accurately what the patient needs and how to meet those needs. As a result, the nurse is in danger of meeting his or her own needs at the expense of the patient.

Nurses need to develop self-awareness about compassion fatigue. This self-awareness helps the nurse identify the physical, emotional, and spiritual needs that he or she has and to give him- or herself permission to get these legitimate needs met. **Box 20-1** lists questions to assess compassion fatigue and ways to intervene. Doing so frees the nurse to participate in the dynamics of a therapeutic relationship more fully with the patient. When one loses the connection to the meaning of one's work, one loses the energy to accomplish it.

Therapeutic use of self and possible compassion fatigue also extend to colleagues. Compassion fatigue makes them vulnerable to burnout as well. Responding to the emotional exhaustion of co-workers in compassionate ways helps to forge strong interdisciplinary teams.

## SPECIAL ISSUES RELATED TO MENTAL HEALTH AND PHYSICAL ILLNESS

Nurses are involved routinely in procedural interventions such as collecting vital signs, administering medications, and performing treatments for individuals with physical illness. However, nurses also must continually assess the mental health of their patients. The nurse regularly assesses patient orientation, comprehension, memory, cognition, mood, and reasoning judgment. These areas are vital, for example, when determining potential cognitive dysfunction related to therapies or the capacity for informed consent. However, assessing a physically ill patient's mental health is additionally important because stress, loss, changes in body image, or pain can impact the patient's physical status as well as place the patient at risk for developing depression, anxiety, or delirium, the most common mental health comorbidities of physical illness.

## Impact of Stress

Just as patients with schizophrenia and bipolar disease present with physical illnesses, numerous patients without identifiable mental health disorders must contend with mental health distress that occurs during the course of their physical illness. This distress may be secondary to the physical illness itself. Additionally, it may be the result of the hospitalization and treatments required. As much as 75%–90% of all visits to primary care providers are due to stress-mediated causes (The American Institute of Stress, 2011).

### Adverse Childhood Events and Stress

The impact of mental health on physical health has been identified in numerous research studies. One research study, known as the Adverse Childhood Experiences (ACE) study (www.acestudy.org), has demonstrated this strong relationship. This research addresses the relationship between adverse childhood experiences and adult health (Anda et al., 2006). It has documented that unhealthy adults' lifestyle behaviors, such as tobacco use, alcoholism, poor nutritional choices, sedentary lifestyles, and stress, contribute to at least 50% of all morbidity and mortality in this country. According to the study,

---

### BOX 20-1: COMPASSION FATIGUE: ASSESSMENT AND INTERVENTION

#### ASSESSMENT

- What physical, mental, emotional, social, spiritual signs, and symptoms of compassion fatigue do I most commonly exhibit when I am distressed?
- Who/what has helped me in the past to prevent such compassion fatigue?
- Who/what has helped me in the past to heal such compassion fatigue once it presents?
- Are there any new beliefs or practices that could help me prevent or heal compassion fatigue?

#### INTERVENTIONS

- Adopt healthy lifestyle behaviors to ensure that I can successfully inoculate myself against stress in general (healthy nutrition, exercise, social support, etc.).
- Once compassion fatigue is identified, get help as soon as possible from identified resources.
- Reach out to colleagues who exhibit signs and symptoms of compassion fatigue and recognize this as a part of the mental health care rendered in the work environment.

these lifestyle behaviors actually originated as behaviors designed to protect people who as children were victims of sexual, physical, or emotional abuse.

Consider the popular truism: "While genetics loads the gun, lifestyle choices pull the trigger." Thus, for example, focusing exclusively on calorie counts with morbidly obese individuals who cannot seem to shed their weight or tobacco users who cannot seem to stop smoking lacks the more holistic approach needed for such public health problems.

Stress when not addressed in childhood results in poor stress management and lifestyle choices later in life. Such stress and unhealthy behavioral choices then contribute to the development of chronic illnesses. These chronic illnesses then increase the likelihood of increasing stress and, subsequently, psychosocial distress, setting up a recurring cycle of events. Developmentally throughout the lifespan, nurses are in excellent positions to intervene in such feedback loops and to interrupt the cascade effect such cycles can produce.

> *Adverse childhood events have been shown to lead to unhealthy lifestyle behaviors.*

## Mind-Body Interactions and Stress

Stress is well known to be directly linked to many chronic illnesses prevalent today and is often considered the primary cause of the illness (Cohen & Janicki-Deverts, 2007). Chronic stress can trigger insulin-resistance diseases such as diabetes, auto-immune diseases such as asthma, and cancers due to unremitting immunosuppression resulting from perpetually high circulating cortisol levels. Such relentlessly high cortisol levels contribute to chronic inflammation in the body. (Kiecolt-Glaser, 2002). These levels interfere with the immune system's ability to repair itself and can contribute to a cascade effect of neuroendocrine, immune, and metabolic problems resulting in the numerous chronic illnesses of today (Cohen & Janicki-Deverts, 2007).

Scientists such as C. Pert, have helped to explain the biochemical molecule responsible for translating psychoemotional phenomena into anatomical-physiological phenomena and vice-versa (Pert, 1997). These molecules, called neuropeptides, which are located throughout the entire body, are concentrated in selected areas such as the hypothalamus and the gastrointestinal tract. Information about their action forms the basis for **PSYCHONEUROIM-MUNOLOGY**, the study of the connection among the immune, nervous, and endocrine systems.

Another basis for the interrelationship of mental health with physical health issues arises from the study of complementary and alternative medicine (CAM) therapies. These therapies use physical, psychological, spiritual, and nutritional means to strengthen a person's capacity to heal. While allopathic approaches to healing tend to be disease focused, CAM approaches are more holistic in nature.

The National Institute of Health's Center for Complementary and Alternative Medicine (NCCAM) has identified five principal domains of such practices:

1. *Mind-body therapies*, such as meditation, guided imagery, visualization, and prayer
2. *Biologically based practices*, such as the use of herbal supplements, biologicals and nutriceuticals, chelation therapy, aromatherapy, and macrobiotics
3. *Manipulative and body-based practices*, such as massage, yoga, cranio-sacral therapies, reflexology, feldenkrais, and tai chi
4. *Energy biofield therapies*, such as acupuncture, reiki, and therapeutic touch
5. *Whole systems of healing*, such as traditional Chinese medicine, naturopathy, homeopathy, ayurveda, chiropracty, and native/tribal-based medicine (http://nccam.nih.gov/).

Increasingly, the population is using these modalities because of dissatisfaction with the current allopathic (medical) model. They are also being used to counter the side effects of allopathically prescribed treatments and as a way to foster balance to prevent illness initially. An integrative approach to patient care incorporates and customizes the best of CAM practices with the best of allopathic practices.

> *The mind-body interaction is demonstrated by research showing that stress can disrupt the functioning of the nervous, immune, and endocrine systems and with the study of complementary and alternative medicine therapies.*

## Nurse's Role

To address the impact of stress on patients, nurses need to assess the patient and family carefully. Questions that can help focus the assessment include the following:

• What is the patient's perception of the current stressors he or she and family are presently facing? *"Of everything happening to you right now, what seems to be the hardest?"*

- How do the patient and family typically cope with stress? *"When you have faced difficult times in the past, what has worked the best for you?"*
- What resources are the patient and family missing that could help them in the current situation? *"What is it that you think you need to help you get through the current situation?"*

Within the context of the therapeutic relationship, the nurse uses active listening skills to assist the patient and family to identify their feelings and put them into words to foster communication. A statement such as, *"You sound scared. Would you like to talk about it?"* demonstrates concern for the patient and allows the patient the opportunity to share his or her feelings if he or she wishes. Providing empathetic responses to distressed patients and families, such as, *"I understand how difficult this is; you don't have to go through this alone,"* helps to validate their emotional distress and to provide support. The nurse collaborates with the patient and family about those people or resources that can assist them to successfully navigate the current situation. For example, the nurse could ask, *"Is there someone from your faith community you would like for me to call for you?"* Again, the nurse demonstrates a concern and interest in the patient.

Nurses also may use mind-body interventions within the context of the therapeutic relationship. Since the immune system has the capacity to learn, these interventions form the basis of psychiatric-mental health nursing care designed to induce relaxation responses during which the immune system can repair itself. The subsequent release of **ENDORPHINS**, chemicals in the body that are responsible for increasing the sense of well-being, are potent mood elevators and lay the groundwork for healing responses.

Nurses incorporate many CAM therapies into their nursing care to tend to the whole person. However, the nurse needs to assess the patient's health beliefs and practices before implementing specific therapies. **Box 20-2** highlights appropriate assessment questions and provides suggestions for interventions.

---

**Q** | **BOX 20-2: COMPLEMENTARY AND ALTERNATIVE MEDICINE (CAM) THERAPIES: ASSESSMENT AND INTERVENTION**

**ASSESSMENT**

- Determine the patient's belief about what made him/her sick and what s/he believes would heal the sickness. *"Tell me about why you think you became sick and what you think will heal you."*
- Assess the patient's current use of complementary and alternative therapies. *"What healing practices, beliefs, preparations, or herbs do you currently use to help you heal?"*
- Assess the patient's willingness to explore new healing practices based on whether or not the current healing practices are helping him or her cope. *"It sounds like your pain is getting worse. Would you be willing to try something new to see if we could get a better result from the medication?"*

**INTERVENTIONS**

- Provide evidence-based information on the clinically demonstrated effectiveness of CAM therapies, how to locate credentialed practitioners, and how to assist patients become savvy health care consumers of these services. *"Looks like that massage helped you maximize the benefit from your pain medication. When it's time for you to go home, let's check with your insurance company to determine if they have any licensed massage therapists on their provider network that you can use after your discharge."*
- Integrate as many evidence-based CAM modalities into your practice by becoming credentialed in modalities that add value to the care you provide. *"While we talk about how you can cope with fatigue since your heart attack, if you like, I can give you a reiki treatment, which should boost your energy level."*
- Teach patients the value of inducing the relaxation response (meditation, prayer, reiki, etc.) as a means of assisting them to reduce circulating cortisol levels on a regular basis, thereby reducing systemic inflammation which contributes to disease. *"What do you usually do to relax?"*

The use of CAM interventions with patients presenting with physical illness can provide teachable moments whereby nurses can use their counseling skills to influence not only the patient's mental health, but physical health as well. Nurses interested in learning more about such integrative practices can search the Internet for numerous clinical, educational, and research resources that are available (e.g., www.wholehealthmd.com, www.drweil.com, www.nccam.nih.gov, www.consumerlab.com, www.naturalstandard.com). In addition, many nurses become licensed and certified in complementary and alternative therapy practices to extend the reach of their healing into areas such as the patient's bio-energy field, tapping into the mind-body connection to evoke a healing response, and making use of more psycho-spiritual approaches in their work.

## Loss and Grief

Physical illness changes people's lives often in ways that are not readily self-evident to anyone except the patient. Consider the many losses that are inherent in illness: loss of well-being, autonomy, time, body parts and functions, money, relationships, jobs, a predictable future, mobility, freedom from pain, body image, lifestyle, role changes, and time to name but a few.

The normal response to all such loss is the healing, yet painful, experience of grief. It can manifest itself in many ways, such as shock, denial, anger, anguish, and deep sadness. A grief model, developed by Bailey, a hospice nurse, illuminates the trajectory of the grief journey (Bailey, 1986). This model is highlighted in **Box 20-3**.

Nurses need to assess for signs and symptoms of the grief response in all patients facing illness. Acknowledging the validity of these feelings is important to promote working through them. Otherwise these feelings can interfere with the patient's ability to adhere to a treatment regimen. For example, a patient who is newly diagnosed with diabetes continues to deny the illness despite his or her symptoms. As a result, the patient is likely to experience morbidity from failure to come to terms with the necessary lifestyle changes required by the diagnosis. If the nurse is not attending to the patient's grief response, diabetic teaching is likely to be ineffective.

Nurses who understand the nature of such deep emotions as denial, anger, and intense sadness are better able to develop plans of care that incorporate attention to these emotions in addition to providing disease-related treatments. Assisting patients to identify what they are feeling helps to minimize the potential for acting out. In addition, the ongoing use of active listening skills such as reflection

---

> ### 🔍 BOX 20-3: BAILEY'S JOURNEY OF GRIEF MODEL
>
> - *Loss occurs*
> - *Protest*: Characterized by shock, numbness, confusion, anger, and physical symptoms
> - *Searching*: A preoccupation with what will or what has been lost, presence of vivid dreams
> - *Despair*: Anguish, depression, social withdrawal, hopelessness, slowing thinking and behavior
> - *Reorganization*: Bursts of energy, intermittent interest, indifference, fatigue, detachment, apathy, survivor guilt
> - *Reinvestment*: Integration of the old with an emerging new way of life, learning to live with the loss
>
> *From Bailey, B. (1986). Strategies for coping with loss. The Connecticut Hospice, Inc.*

---

and paraphrasing dynamically facilitates grief work. Active listening skills also provide ego strength and indicate confidence in the patient's ability to adapt (Rancour & Cluxton, 2000).

Nurses also need to consider the family, because just as patients grieve their losses, so too do their families. High rates of morbidity and mortality often occur with family caregivers as well as those who lose life partners. Providing family-focused care signifies the nurse's recognition that family members will be at varying stages of their own grief cycles in coping with and adapting to the patient's illness. In addition, the culturally competent nurse will address these responses in such a way that communicates an understanding of and empathy with families whose culture and spiritual outlooks—and therefore whose mourning and its rituals—are different from his/her own.

> *Grief and loss affect not only the patient but the family as well. Active listening skills are important to help patients and families identify their feelings and put them into words.*

## Body Image Changes and Stigma

In a culture that prizes youth and beauty, there is little room for individuals whose physical illnesses create diversions from some imagined or idealized norm. Many losses that prompt grief responses may involve changes in body appearance and functioning. Experiences such as chemotherapy-induced alopecia (hair loss), amputations, or ostomies can provoke body image disturbances with subsequent stigma. Difficulties adapting to one's changed body can create self-esteem issues, making acceptance of one's new body and its functioning challenging. For example, when does a young woman mention to her new dating partner that she has had a mastectomy? Often, patients are angry about what is happening to them, asking "Why me?" When seen as a grief response, the nurse can help the patient reframe his or her relationship with the injured or changed body part from one of anger to one of forgiveness and even compassion, that can be visualized as being sent to the injured body part (Rancour, 2006; Rancour & Brauer, 2003). **Box 20-4** highlights appropriate assessments and interventions for dealing with changes in body image and the attached stigma.

> *Changes in body image and the stigma attached to the change can elicit a grief response. Nurses need to help the patient reframe his or her relationship to the change.*

## Pain and Other Physical Symptoms

Pain, as an indicator of the presence of disease, must be addressed because it is associated with so many physical illnesses. Pain is a complex and subjective phenomenon requiring nurses to recognize that pain is whatever the patient says it is. Pain needs to be assessed frequently. Palliative care or symptom management, with special attention to pain management, is one of the most important psychosocial interventions that can be employed to assist patients with physical illness to heal. As one patient put it, "I'm in so much pain that I don't have any energy left to deal with anything else" (Fink & Gates 2001).

Pain is associated with increased mortality. The presence of pain stimulates high levels of circulating stress hormones, most importantly cortisol, which disrupt immune system function. At times of illness, such interference can result in additional cascades of stress responses leading to further debility and even death (Paice & Fine, 2001). Therefore, nurses need to assess pain thoroughly using numerical scales and/or patient descriptions of their pain and symptoms and provide appropriate pharmacological and nonpharmacological measures for pain and symptom management, including patient education about assessing, anticipating, and intervening in their own pain management.

After pain, fatigue is one of the most distressing symptoms affecting patients with physical illness. Persons who are fatigued lack energy and often do not want to do normal activities. They also pay less attention to personal appearance, have trouble thinking or concentrating, and trouble finding words to express what they want to communicate. Interventions designed to address fatigue include teaching patients the importance of energy conservation through the balance of activity with rest, nutritional support, restoration of disturbed sleep patterns, and other symptom management strategies (Dean & Anderson, 2001).

Other physical symptoms that need to be regularly assessed include headache, gastrointestinal distress (nausea and vomiting, diarrhea, constipation), anorexia and cachexia, dyspnea, hydration, skin problems, and fever. All of these symptoms affect one's physical and mental health. Energy is depleted and thus the person may not be able to engage in personal and interpersonal healing processes. Rather, the body's energy is centered on the symptoms that are causing the person distress.

> *Nurses need to assess a patient's pain and understand that pain is highly subjective.*

## Anxiety and Depression

Physical illness is acute or chronic. While acute illness is often accompanied by high levels of anxiety, and chronic illness may be attended by depression, anxiety and depression are frequently co-morbid conditions occurring during physical illnesses. The inflammatory responses of the body to persistently high levels of stress found in patients with anxiety and depression can often result in physical illness. Several studies have documented this relationship.

One study demonstrated correlation between worsening anxiety and depression and congestive heart failure in patients (Jiang, 2004). The Safety and Efficacy

> ### BOX 20-4: CHANGES IN BODY IMAGE AND STIGMA: ASSESSMENT AND INTERVENTIONS
>
> #### ASSESSMENT
>
> - Assess patient's emotional response toward the threatened or lost body part or function. *"You mention that since your stroke, the right side of your body doesn't feel like it belongs to you anymore. Can you help me better understand how you feel about it?"*
>
> - Assess for evidence of pathological grief response, which might interfere with the integration of a new body image. *"Nancy, I notice that since you were diagnosed with your epilepsy several months ago, you've shown little interest in your friends or your job. Tell me how you are feeling about all of this."*
>
> - Explore patient's concerns about how s/he will be perceived by others. *"What are you most concerned about how other people will respond to you once your Parkinson's disease becomes more evident?"*
>
> #### INTERVENTION
>
> - Acknowledge and normalize patient's concern about altered body image. *"Most people facing a colostomy express the same kinds of concerns that you do. Tell me more about what worries you the most."*
>
> - Provide patient education materials and resources that demonstrate how people cope with such an altered body image. *"I wanted to show you this video of how one of our patients won a golf championship recently while wearing a prosthetic leg."*
>
> - Re-people the patient's social world with other survivors who have gone on to live full and productive lives. *"John, would you be interested in meeting another man who had his laryngectomy five years ago and still runs his own company?"*
>
> - Use creative interventions such as guided imagery, expressive arts, or journaling to help patients work through their feelings toward their altered physical body. *"If you could write a letter to your heart right now, what would it say?"*
>
> - If the patient is angry, assist him/her to identify this and work toward generating forgiveness and compassion to the part of the self that is in pain. *"I realize you are frustrated that your arthritis flare-up is interfering with your travel plans, but I wonder if you might stop, take some deep breaths, and open your heart a little to sending your joints some warmth and tenderness since they seem to be in so much pain right now."*

of Sertraline for Depression in Patients with Congestive Heart Failure (SADHART–CHF) study showed that a nurse relationship-based intervention was superiorly more effective than the use of selective serotonin reuptake inhibitors.

*The enormous impact that the nurse facilitators had on this patient population and the reduction in the [Hamilton] scale within a two-week period of about 40%, from a very high level, was just extraordinary and points out what simply seeing these patients, the laying-on of hands, will do for these depressed heart-failure patients. It's really quite striking.* (Stiles, 2008)

Other studies have shown that patients with anxiety and depression have demonstrated increased serum cholesterol, triglycerides, and low density lipoprotein cholesterol (LDL-C) and reduced high density lipoprotein cholesterol (HDL-C) levels, increasing the patients' risk for coronary artery disease (Gabriel, 2007). **Evidence-Based Practice 20-1** highlights this research study. Another study revealed that patients with cancer who present with high anxiety and depression rates early on often suffer from extremely high rates of these disorders throughout treatment (Nordin, 2001). A third study showed that the treatment of patients with diabetes, especially related to medication and diet adherence, is

## EVIDENCE-BASED PRACTICE 20-1: TREATMENT EFFECTS

### STUDY

Gabriel, A. (2007). Changes in plasma cholesterol in mood disorder patients: Does treatment make a difference? *Journal of Affective Disorders, 99*(1), 273–278.

### SUMMARY

The research reported on preliminary findings involving the impact of treatment for acute episodes of major depression and manic or hypomanic episodes and co-morbid anxiety symptoms, on the total cholesterol blood levels of patients. Fifty-six patients completed the 4-week study. These patients were treated with antidepressants, mood stabilizers, or both. The results indicated that there was a significant increase in cholesterol levels of patients with major depression and a decrease among the patients with other diagnoses.

### APPLICATION TO PRACTICE

The researchers caution that the results require additional study before being judged as clinically significant. At the same time, it is important for psychiatric-mental health nurses to understand the interrelationships between treatments and the potential resulting negative consequences of therapeutic interventions.

### QUESTIONS TO PONDER

1. *Why would it be important to understand the interrelationship between physical and psychological symptoms in patients for whom you are providing care?*
2. *How would your knowledge of the interrelationship of mind and body influence your nursing interventions and your therapeutic relationship?*

frequently affected by high rates of anxiety and depression (Wagner & Tennon, 2007).

Assessment tools such as the Beck Depression Inventory, Hospital Anxiety and Depression Scale, Patient Health Questionnaire (PHQ-9), Symptom Checklist (SCL-90), and Hamilton Depression Rating Scale have long been used for their reliability and validity. However, asking the patient direct questions, such as "Do you feel depressed?" or "Do you feel anxious?" has also proven to be reliable. Many patients are readily able to distinguish the difference between sadness and depression, and often respond accordingly.

When assessing a patient, the nurse needs to be able to distinguish clinical depression from grief and complicated grief. Table 20-1 provides a comparison. Normal grief requires facilitation, complicated grief requires intervention, whereas depression requires active treatment. For example, it would be inappropriate to sedate a patient who is upset upon receiving bad news such as the diagnosis of cancer. Such sedation would impair the patient's ability to move ahead in his or her adaptation to an altered health status. However, if that patient experiences suicidal ideation months later, it would be critical to ensure that he or she is assessed for and receives any treatment necessary

### TABLE 20-1: COMPARISON OF NORMAL GRIEF, PATHOLOGICAL GRIEF, AND DEPRESSION

|  | NORMAL GRIEF | PATHOLOGICAL GRIEF | DEPRESSION |
|---|---|---|---|
| *Time:* | Self-limiting | No resolution | Longer than 2 months |
| *Preoccupation:* | Variable | Active | With self |
| *Emotional states:* | Variable | Hope for reunion | Consistent dysphoria |
| *Sleep/eat problems:* | Episodic | Persistent | Persistent |
| *Energy level:* | Moderate | Stressful | Extreme lethargy |
| *Extent of loss:* | Can identify | Avoids | Cannot identify |
| *Presence of crying:* | Evident | Avoidant | Absent or persistent |
| *Social response:* | Responsive | Avoidant | Socially unresponsive |
| *Dreams:* | Vivid | Rescue fantasies | No memory of dream |
| *Presence of anger:* | Open expression | Variable | No expression |
| *Recovery:* | No professional treatment | Requires professional treatment | Requires professional treatment |
| *Reality testing:* | Intact | Not intact | Latent |
| *Approach/avoidance:* | Willing to accept | Avoids acceptance | Avoidant |

to resolve any depression that could be as lethal as any malignancy.

Continued anxiety and/or depression without relief can be life-threatening. In addition, as medical treatments have become more toxic, such as radical surgeries or chemotherapies, many patients find them increasingly burdensome. Thus, **ASSISTED SUICIDE** has emerged as a potential option for patients whose physical illness has pushed them beyond their ability to cope. It is considered a direct consequence of failing to respond to the need for aggressive palliative care and management of symptoms such as pain and depression.

Assisted suicide refers to providing a person with an available means for death such as pills or weapons, with the knowledge of the person's intent to use those means to die but without acting as the direct agent for the death. This issue is highly controversial and the subject of much debate. In the United States, two states, Oregon and Washington, permit physician-assisted suicide, while 34 states have statutes that specifically classify assisted suicide as a crime. Another nine states identify it as a crime through common law statutes. The American Nurses Association, in their Position Statement (1994), states that "the nurse should not participate in assisted suicide. Such an act is in violation of the *Code for Nurses with Interpretive Statements* and the ethical traditions of the profession. Nurses are obligated to provide comprehensive and compassionate end-of-life care which includes the promotion of comfort and the relief of pain." If a patient is considering assisted suicide or verbalizes a request for it, the nurse employs the therapeutic use of self to understand the meaning of the request, demonstrating respect for and commitment to the patient. In addition, continued assessment can help to uncover factors that may be contributing to the patient's feelings, such as unrelieved pain, feelings related to loss of control, fear of isolation, or hopelessness. As factors are identified, the nurse can explore the patient's feelings and work with the patient and family in measures to address these problems. Thus, nurses need to be vigilant in assessing patients experiencing anxiety and depression regularly for suicidal ideation or thoughts of assisted suicide so that these issues can be addressed promptly.

> *Depression differs from grief and complicated grief. It requires active treatment, whereas grief requires facilitation and complicated grief requires intervention.*

Moreover, traumatizing periods of illness and treatment such as bone marrow transplant may be accompanied by another anxiety disorder, posttraumatic stress disorder (Pasacreta, 2001; Mundy, 2000). Patients may remark that their hospitalization was a "blur" or that they have nightmares of the treatment period that will not resolve on their own. Cognitive behavioral therapy in conjunction with anti-anxiety and anti-depressant medication is frequently effective. Of all the anti-depressants, the selective seratonin reuptake inhibitors seem to be tolerated best by patients with multiple physical problems. Their mild side-effect profile often makes them the drug of choice.

## Delirium

DELIRIUM is another common mental health issue associated with physical illness. It is often characterized by changes in levels of alertness, perception, awareness, sleep patterns, confusion, disorientation, memory deficits, disorganized thinking, problems with attention as well as mood lability that may be laced with agitation, anxiety, or lethargy. This rapid change in mentation and mood can be intense. To complicate matters further, the etiology of delirium can be complex and include a multitude of problems such as self-administered or prescribed medication, thyroid disorders, liver, kidney or heart failure, psychiatric conditions, sensory deprivation, infections, anemia, hypoxia, fluid and electrolyte disturbances (especially dehydration), urinary or stool retention, sleep deprivation, stress, neurological disorders, and disturbances having to do with circadian rhythms (e.g., sundowner's syndrome). Typically, eliminating or reversing the underlying cause is effective.

Nursing focuses on assessing the patient for the cause of the delirium, implementing interventions to correct the cause, and performing mental health status exams frequently for changes. In addition, nurses need to provide a calm, restful environment so that care is provided by as few people as possible to reduce confusion, provide for consistency, and communicate to the patient that he or she is safe while the diagnosis is being made and the treatment plan is implemented. Nurses should make sure that the lighting is adequate but not so bright as to startle or overwhelm the patient. It is important to ensure that the patient has any sensory aids such as eyeglasses in place. The administration of anti-anxiety or sedative agents may be indicated if environmental and interpersonal interventions are ineffective. However, these should be used selectively because they may exacerbate the delirium in some patients (Kuebler, English, & Heidrich, 2001).

## THE NURSE'S ROLE IN BREAKING BAD NEWS

An old adage has it that patients enter doctors' offices with symptoms, but leave with diseases. What happened in those doctors' offices was that people received **BAD NEWS**. Bad news is defined as any new information that the patient interprets as representing significant loss. Examples of such news might include a diagnosis of diabetes, news that the injury sustained in an automobile accident will require an amputation, an amniotic fluid test that reveals that the baby a mother is carrying has trisomy-21 (Down's syndrome), that a patient's brain tumor is not resectable, or that the pain the patient was experiencing was not heartburn after all, but a myocardial infarction. And of course, one of the most extreme kinds of bad news one receives is that one has a severe life-threatening illness or that a loved one has died of such an illness. Sometimes the way in which the news is delivered can be so problematic that the patient loses faith in the messenger, thus interfering with treatment. **Therapeutic Interaction 20-1** provides an example of applying the interpersonal process when delivering bad news.

> *Nurses can use the SPIKES protocol to deliver bad news therapeutically. The SPIKES protocol addresses setting, perception, invitation, knowledge, emotions and empathy, and summary and strategy.*

Often, bad news is delivered to patients who are in the hospital. As such, these facilities become places where nurses often find themselves on the forefront of helping to deliver or helping patients cope with such bad news. To foster a more therapeutic approach for delivering bad news, a structured format, called Buckman's SPIKES Protocol, was developed (Buckman, 1992). The SPIKES Protocol, described in **Box 20-5**, is an acronym that stands for: setting, perception, invitation, knowledge, emotions and empathy, and summary and strategy.

The nurse can use the following strategies to assist in breaking bad news:

- Provide for privacy and confidentiality. *"I have some important information for you and wondered who you want with you and who you don't."*
- Assess for what patient already understands about his or her health status alteration. *"Tell me what you already know about your illness."*
- Assess for what the patient is ready to hear. *"What is it that you would like to know about your illness and its treatment today?"*
- Provide information in small chunks. *"Now that we've talked about your illness, let's review what your treatment options are."*
- Regularly determine the patient's comprehension of information that he or she receives during the interview. *"Can you please repeat to me what you just heard me say?"*

**THERAPEUTIC INTERACTION 20-1:
DELIVERING BAD NEWS**

The nurse is meeting with Mary R., a 60-year-old, whose 25-year-old son has been brought to the emergency department following a car accident. The son, David, was dead on arrival, and Nurse Jane is the first one to meet Mary when she comes to the emergency department.

| | |
|---|---|
| **Nurse:** "Hello, Mrs. R. I know you must want to see your son, but I have to let you know that the car accident was terrible and your son did not survive." (establishes eye contact, and takes Mary's hand) "I know you must be very upset. Is there anyone else you would like to have come with you when you go to see him?" | Initiating the interaction and providing direct information, as Mary will want to know her son's status. Also, she needs to be prepared for the shock of seeing the bodily trauma that has occurred.<br><br>Eye contact and a warm response to Mary by taking her hand is a way of demonstrating concern for Mary and the shock she must be experiencing. The nurse also is trying to determine who could be helpful in supporting Mary; perhaps she will want to wait for another family member to come. |
| **Mary:** (crying) "This could not have happened to him; he was so careful whenever he drove. He was all I had in the world. He cannot be gone." | Expressing shock and disbelief |
| **Nurse:** "Please let me take you to his side. I will stay with you." (guides her down the hallway with an arm around her shoulders). | Providing support and staying with Mary so she will not be alone, especially since she has indicated that there is not anyone else that she can expect to be here |
| **Mary:** "David is all I have. He cannot be gone. He is my life." | Still in shock |
| **Nurse:** "This must be extremely difficult for you. Is there anything that you would like to know about what happened? I know that the policemen who found the car are still here and will want to talk with you." (maintaining eye contact). | Validating Mary's need for information statement; demonstrating empathy and showing concern and interest for Mary by continuing to stay with Mary in this time when she needs support |
| **Mary:** "Yes, I would like to know. I would like to talk with the police and the ambulance drivers and anyone else who was with my son." | Acknowledging her need for information |

*(cont.)*

## THERAPEUTIC INTERACTION 20-1: (*CONT.*) DELIVERING BAD NEWS

| | |
|---|---|
| **Nurse:** "Is there someone I can call for you, perhaps a friend who can come here, or someone from your church?" | Further exploration to gather information about who might be able to provide support to Mary in her time of great need. Encouraging Mary to identify someone who can be here with her |
| **Mary:** "Would you please call my friend Bess and ask her if she can come here to meet me?" | Reaching out to a friend |
| **Nurse:** "Of course I will. And please know that I will stay with you until she comes. I also will help you find out any information that you want about what happened." | Acknowledging the patient's feelings, encouraging the patient to describe feelings further |

## BOX 20-5: BUCKMAN'S SPIKES PROTOCOL

- *Setting*: Provide for privacy. Ensure that only those people the patient wants involved in the discussion are present. Sit down at eye level without using furniture as barriers. Provide eye contact and physical touch such as a hand on arm or shoulder according to the patient's comfort level. Manage interruptions.

- *Perception*: Ask the patient what he or she already knows about the condition and listen for any misunderstanding. Assess for denial and correct any information deficits to ensure that the patient understands correctly and has realistic expectations.

- *Invitation*: Ask the patient what he or she wants to know today. The patient will relay what he or she is *ready to hear* and ways to hear it, i.e., not at all today, in small chunks, or as much as the patient can tolerate.

- *Knowledge*: Alert the patient that bad news is coming. Use words that are part of the patient's own vocabulary and avoid technical jargon. Avoid making blunt statements. Assess for patient's comprehension regularly before moving on. Assess for what patient is hoping for. *Never say: "There is nothing more that we can do for you."* While the illness may be incurable, suffering can always be addressed and alleviated.

- *Emotions and Empathy*: Be alert that patients will have verbal and nonverbal emotional reactions to the news. When this happens, stop giving information and begin to identify the feeling and respond empathetically until the patient indicates he or she is ready to proceed further. Use of active listening skills such as reflection, paraphrasing, and reframing are all helpful.

- *Strategy and Summary*: Know that patients cope better, even in the face of bad news, when they have a plan based on shared decision making. Summarizing the news and developing a plan to cope with it serves as a touch-point in the ongoing relationship with the patient. This communicates to the patient that he or she will not be abandoned despite the bad news.

*From Buckman, R. (1992). How to break bad news; a practical guide for health care professionals. Baltimore, Maryland: Johns Hopkins.*

- Assess patient's affective response to the information by noting nonverbal behavior and other cues. *"I notice that you started crying when I mentioned the surgical option. How do you feel about that?"*
- Demonstrate empathy throughout the interview by employing active listening skills. *"I hear you saying that you are more afraid of pain than you are of dying. We can do a lot to help you with your pain."*
- Summarize the strategy. *"While your baby's diagnosis of cerebral palsy may feel overwhelming to you right now, we'll have the entire team meet with you and your husband next time to help you develop a comprehensive plan of care. Do you have any more questions right now?"*

## END-OF-LIFE CARE

Although not everyone will experience a heart attack, develop tuberculosis, have a baby, or fracture a pelvis, it is true that everyone will eventually die. Death is universal and, as such, deserves special mention because it remains such an emotionally laden topic for so many people, including many health care professionals. Despite wishes to the contrary, death still happens frequently in the hospital rather than in the home.

The first step in becoming proficient in providing care for those facing end-of-life and their families is to become familiar and comfortable with one's own mortality. Developing a philosophy that helps the nurse find meaning in the larger picture will ultimately inspire end-of-life care practice that is not only competent, but also compassionate, which is a prerequisite to any relationship-based intervention.

Institutions in the United States are staffed with health care providers who unfortunately fear death. In the mid-1990s, the historic SUPPORT Study (Moskowitz & Nelson, 1995; Hardwig, 1995) identified the poor state of care being delivered to the dying in this country and called for changes. Since that time, despite numerous efforts to rectify this problem, end-of-life care is still fraught with many difficulties. One area is the training and education of health care providers to deal with end-of-life care more effectively, thereby simultaneously improving cost effectiveness and delivery of quality care.

Over the course of acute and chronic illnesses, certain turning points occur in conversations held so that the patient and family are able to successfully navigate the predictable and sometimes not-so-predictable pitfalls that accompany such illness journeys. Referred to as "COURAGEOUS CONVERSATIONS," they require communication skill sets that can be learned (Rancour & Cluxton, 2000).

Such communication skills are part of the palliative care competencies that all nurses need to be able to respond to their patients' illness experiences.

Nurses are in the ideal position to engage in these "courageous conversations" with patients and their families. Doing so can help prevent merely "sad" experiences from becoming "bad" experiences. As with any other care, the nurse needs to consider the patient's and family's spiritual and cultural background, including religious rituals, special dietary regimens, prayers, and votives, that may help to enrich the meaning of this important life event. Nurses engaged in courageous conversations often address these key areas: death and dying, code status, shift from curative to palliative care goals, and hospice care.

### Conversations About Death and Dying

Patients often know they are dying before others do. Questions they might ask, such as "Am I dying?" or "When will I die?" more often reflect the need for human connection rather than a plea for an exact and precise answer. When asked such questions, the nurse should first center, that is, the nurse should take the time to concentrate their energy and attention to the present situation (often, remembering to breathe deeply can assist before proceeding). The therapeutic goal of such conversations should be to keep the line of communication open. Conversations can frequently be accomplished by asking open-ended questions designed to elucidate more information and provide support through therapeutic contact with the nurse. For example, responses to the above questions might be: *"What makes you believe you are dying?" "How long have you been thinking of this?"* or *"Tell me more about what you are thinking."*

### Conversations About Code Status

Seriously ill patients should never be allowed to reach advanced stages of illness without exploring their end-of-life care preferences. Waiting until a patient with dementia of the Alzheimer's type is too cognitively impaired to explore whether he or she will want to have a feeding tube placed for the inevitable gag reflex failure is inappropriate. It also creates needless suffering, expense, and futile treatment. A courageous conversation can be as simple as asking a patient: *"I know you understand how seriously ill you are. In the event you should stop breathing or your heart should stop beating, what would you like for us to do for you?"* This is a process of exploration. It can also include the completion of advance directives (living will and durable power of attorney for health care) to fully document the patient's preferences. A free and complete listing of the advance directives of all states can be located at http://www.caringinfo.org/stateaddownload.

## Conversations Involving a Shift From Cure-Driven Care to Palliative Care

Patients often give their caregivers cues that they are ready to stop curative-driven care if its burdens begin to outweigh its benefits. The patient might say, "I can't take much more of this," or "I'm tired of living from one emergency room visit to the next." Failing to explore these statements leaves the patient feeling isolated rather than cared for in their illness journey. Conversations that help them explore whether they are more interested in quality versus quantity of life, how their values align with proposed treatment goals, and what they hope for the future are indicated. Such courageous conversations can begin with statements such as: *"I know you understand how sick you are. We are all disappointed that your illness has not responded to the treatment as we had all hoped. Given that, what is it that you are hoping for now?"* The patient hears the truth of the real situation, and experiences a sense of comfort rather than abandonment. The health care provider is working to develop a new plan because the cure-driven plan is no longer achieving desired outcomes.

## Conversations About Hospice Care

Conversations about palliative care can become the time to introduce hospice care. Hospice care is considered the gold standard of end-of-life care, allowing patients to remain at home in their own community. Hospice care is associated with a higher quality of life. More recently, research has indicated that hospice care is also often associated with a longer life (Connor, 2007).

Hospice is an emotionally laden word. Therefore, the nurse can help the patient and family adjust to its introduction by speaking to what it can accomplish for them first before naming it. *"Would you like to discuss a home care program that can help ensure you stay in your home, receive care provided by nurses, social workers, doctors, aides, and chaplains? Would you be interested in care that is focused on you and your family in terms of keeping you as functional and symptom free as possible? Would you like more information about a program that makes all these services available to you 24/7? If so, that program is hospice. Would you like me to give you more information?"*

> *Nurses involved in end-of-life care need to be prepared to have courageous conversations about death and dying, code status, palliative care, and hospice care.*

## THE ROLE OF THE MENTAL HEALTH LIAISON/CONSULTATION NURSE

In numerous facilities nationwide, recognition that medical-surgical patients present with psychosocial distress due to their illnesses, treatments, and hospitalizations has led to the creation of the mental health liaison/consultation nurse role and similar interdisciplinary mental health teams. These teams are usually composed of a psychiatrist, psychologist, psychiatric clinical nurse specialist, and a social worker. As patient acuity and volume have increased, so too have the negative effects of high-tech treatment. This, coupled with the fragmentation of care, has made delivering care that is also therapeutic even more challenging. One response to these developments is to ensure that hospital staff has access to clinical experts who have demonstrated capability in this arena. Such clinicians deliver direct care to patients, develop programs for patient groups and sub-populations, and provide consultation and education to health care professionals delivering hospital-based care. Such nurses often function in an advance practice capacity (Harrison & Hart, 2006; Rancour & Brauer, 1993).

## APPLYING THE NURSING PROCESS FROM AN INTERPERSONAL PERSPECTIVE

The therapeutic nurse-patient relationship derived from Peplau's Interpersonal Theory of Nursing is the cornerstone of intervention. The nurse will use the interpersonal process throughout to not only develop the relationship with the patient but also to move through the stages of the nursing process. The specific interventions that are initiated will depend on the mental health disorder that the patient is experiencing along with their physical illness.

Patients experiencing mental health disorders in conjunction with physical illness can be seen in any type of setting. Therefore, nurses need a firm understanding of the nursing process that integrates the interpersonal process when caring for patients experiencing mental health issues and physical illness.

## STRATEGIES FOR OPTIMAL ASSESSMENT: THERAPEUTIC USE OF SELF

As previously stated, the first step in providing any kind of patient care is to ensure that the nurse knows him- or herself. This knowledge is necessary to perceive the patient's need accurately and provide a balanced outflow of effort on the nurse's part. Thus, the patient most likely will receive what he or she needs and the nurse will maintain a balance of personal energy needs, thereby preventing compassion fatigue.

Nurses need to be mindful of their body language, especially in terms of the effect the patient's illness has on them, because it impacts the nonverbal communication sent to the patient. Unpleasant bodily functions and appearance or anticipation of serious losses such as death, can provoke personal feelings that impact the nurse-patient relationship. Look for support from more experienced practitioners if necessary to explore these issues, keeping in mind that this exploration is a life-long learning process.

Physical illness involves many psychospiritual issues as patients come to terms with what the illness means for them on many levels. Ascertaining how their cultural and spiritual backgrounds influence their values can help in developing the nurse-patient relationship quickly when faced with these crisis situations.

Conducting assessment interviews in a busy unit is challenging due to the need to control for interruptions and to protect the patient's privacy. Nurses must clarify with the patient which individuals he or she wants present and ensure that only they are included. Doing so promotes the development of trust.

When conducting the assessment, the following questions may be helpful:
- Overall, what would you say has been the hardest part of this illness for you?
- What symptoms are you having right now that interfere with your ability to cope with your illness?
- What are you discovering about yourself through this illness experience that perhaps you might have been unaware of before?
- What special healing beliefs, rituals, or practices do you usually use that we could incorporate into your plan of care here?
- When you think about your illness, what are your primary feelings about it?
- Are you feeling anxious or depressed?

- What do you already know about your illness and what would you like to know today?
- Are you having any strong feelings about a particular part of your body or how it is functioning that makes this illness even more difficult?
- When you think of the future, what are you hoping for?
- As we develop your care plan, are there any other special issues you would like for us to address?

> *The therapeutic use of self is an important skill used throughout the nursing process when dealing with mental health issues in patients with physical illnesses.*

### Diagnosing and Planning Appropriate Interventions: Meeting the Patient's Focused Needs

Prioritizing and meeting patient needs when the presenting problems are medical usually requires that emergent physical needs be met before emotional or spiritual needs. However, at end-of-life, this may not hold true, and in fact, doing so can often interfere with a healing outcome for patient and family if futile treatment that prolongs dying is chosen over the need to assist patient and family to navigate this transition well. Participating in such care can often put nurses in ethically compromising positions and can precipitate professional burnout.

Once a full assessment is completed the nurse and the patient proceed to develop a plan of care with mutual goals and expectations for outcomes. Due to the wide range of assessment findings noted and multiple problems faced by patients with affective disorders, numerous nursing diagnoses would apply. Examples of possible nursing diagnoses would include:
- Hopelessness related to inability to live independently
- Powerlessness related to inability to control own bodily functions
- Death anxiety related to terminal illness
- Grieving related to anticipation of dying and death
- Ineffective coping related to lack of support resources
- Situational low or chronic low self-esteem related to change in physical appearance

These nursing diagnoses also will vary based on the acuity of the patient's illness, developmental stage, co-morbidities, current treatment regimen, and sources of support. For example, the acutely ill person may have more nursing diagnoses addressing physiological concerns such as imbalanced nutrition, nutrition less-than body requirements, or acute pain. As the patient's condition stabilizes, nursing diagnoses such as ineffective coping, situational low self-esteem, or grieving may be the priority areas to be addressed.

Based on the identified nursing diagnoses, the nurse and patient collaboratively would determine the outcomes to be achieved. For example, if the patient is experiencing death anxiety related to diagnosis of terminal illness, the outcome to be achieved would be a better understanding of the illness trajectory that can be expected, including the preparation for dying. The

### PLAN OF CARE 20-1:
### THE PATIENT WITH A SERIOUS MEDICAL ILLNESS

**NURSING DIAGNOSIS:** Grieving; related to recent diagnosis of terminal illness; manifested by expression of anger and depression.

**OUTCOME IDENTIFICATION:** Patient will demonstrate movement toward acceptance of illness.

| INTERVENTION | RATIONALE |
|---|---|
| Schedule private time with the patient to discuss the illness beginning with an educational approach | Sometimes patients aren't ready to discuss the emotional part of their experience. Starting off with informal information sharing can be less threatening |
| Look for opportunities to begin asking "How do you feel about all of this?" and encourage expressions of emotion to better gauge where the patient is in the grieving process | Slowly easing into the emotional realm of care and inviting patients to discuss their feelings often is more comfortable for patients with a serious medical problem |
| Look for feelings of empathy and sympathy within yourself and begin expressing them to the client during the discussion with statements such as "I am so sorry this is happening to you" | Patients are more likely to open up if they feel "connected" to their health care provider |
| Assess for the kind of support the patient would like at the present (i.e., clergy, family meeting, reading material, etc.) | Providing the appropriate level of support will help facilitate grieving |
| Provide education on the stages of grieving | Educating the patient about the phases of grieving helps them understand their experience |
| Continue to assess the patient daily through one-on-one conversation regarding where the patient thinks he or she is with the process | Continuing to be present and available to discuss this subject reassures the patient that this is an ongoing process |

*(cont.)*

**PLAN OF CARE 20-1: (*CONT.*)**
**THE PATIENT WITH A SERIOUS MEDICAL ILLNESS**

**NURSING DIAGNOSIS:** Powerlessness; related to perceived lack of control of life circumstances; manifested by indecisiveness and dependency on others in decision making.

**OUTCOME IDENTIFICATION:** Patient will begin verbalizing awareness of areas of life for which he or she is still has control.

| INTERVENTION | RATIONALE |
|---|---|
| Assist the patient in identifying the underlying reasons for feeling hopeless and powerless; encourage the patient to discuss feelings; listen actively in an accepting, nonjudgmental manner | Expressing feelings helps to identify the patient's view of the situation and to plan appropriate interventions; active listening provides opportunities for validation and clarification and helps promote trust and the nurse-patient relationship |
| Provide education to the patient regarding the medical illness and highlight areas for which he or she still is in control (type of end-of-life care want, etc.) | Identifying more realistic interpretations or ways to address the situation promote feelings of control and self-confidence; pointing out realities helps clarify the patient's perception of the situation |
| Work with the patient to identify situations that can precipitate feelings of helplessness and lack of control; assist the patient in interpreting situations objectively | Identifying precipitating situations can facilitate the patient's ability to control them; objectively interpreting situations fosters control over them |
| Assess the patient's usual methods for problem solving and decision making; help the patient identify problematic or maladaptive methods; offer suggestions for more adaptive methods; encourage the patient's participation in care and decision making, addressing one item or issue at a time | Helping the patient change maladaptive methods to adaptive ones promotes feelings of success and control; encouraging the patient's participation provides the patient with a "voice" and fosters feelings of control; focusing on one item or issue prevents overwhelming the patient and enhances the chances of success |

**NURSING DIAGNOSIS:** Disturbed body image; related to recent leg amputation; manifested by refusal to look at the stump, refusal to care for the wound, and distraught emotional expression.

**OUTCOME IDENTIFICATION:** Patient will acknowledge the loss of the leg.

| INTERVENTION | RATIONALE |
|---|---|
| Assess the patient's feelings about self and appearance using a caring, nonjudgmental approach | Understanding of the patient's feelings related to self-help provides focus for individualized interventions |

*(cont.)*

---

**PLAN OF CARE 20-1: (*CONT.*)**
**THE PATIENT WITH A SERIOUS MEDICAL ILLNESS**

| INTERVENTION | RATIONALE |
|---|---|
| Work with the patient to help view his or body realistically; engage the patient in discussion of expectations of life after amputation; provide objective realistic feedback | Working with the patient to view his or her body realistically helps to replace distorted view with realistic view |
| Work with the patient to establish where he or she is comfortable beginning to address the stump. Invite the patient to assist you with dressing changes. Provide education in a matter-of-fact manner | Discovering where the patient is able to begin allows the process of acceptance to start on the patient's terms. Inviting the patient to watch or assist you as you provide care to the stump creates collaborative experience for the patient rather than something to deal with alone. Providing matter-of-fact education encourages objective assessment of the situation for the patient |
| Provide the patient with positive reinforcement and recognition for gradual increased completion of stump care activities | Providing positive reinforcement promotes feelings of self-worth and enhances the chances for continued participation, compliance, and success |

*From Nursing Diagnosis – Definitions and Classifications 2009 – 2011. Copyright © 2011 by NANDA International. Use by arrangement with Blackwell Publishing Limited, a company of John Wiley & Sons, Inc.*

---

nurse would assist the patient to develop knowledge and understanding of the particular disease progression, and prepare him- or herself and family members for the eventual outcome (no matter the time frame) of dying and death. The patient would be encouraged to maintain hope and to engage in any therapeutic interventions that seem desirable and helpful, even if the interventions are primarily aimed at reducing the symptom burden. The ultimate desirable outcome is a peaceful death.

## Implementing Effective Interventions: Timing and Pacing

In many situations, providing psychosocial care can be accomplished as the nurse provides physical care for the patient. For example, a dressing change may prompt a conversation about how the patient is coming to terms with the loss of the leg from the amputation. Changing a syringe on a patient-controlled analgesia (PCA) pump can prompt discussions on how fatigue and pain may be contributing to a patient's anxiety or depression. Assisting a patient to ambulate down a hallway can be an opportunity to explore how his lack of progress may be signaling him to move from a curative to a more palliative care plan goal. The integration of such conversations with physical care communicates to the patient that he or she is being viewed as a whole person, and not just a person with a physical disorder or illness.

At other times, the significance of events at various turning points in the patient's illness may suggest the need for carving out time specifically dedicated to "courageous conversations." These conversations may be aimed at helping the patient to focus on making important treatment decisions or on communicating thoughts and feelings with family or other health care providers. The conversations do not need to be lengthy. As the nurse becomes more comfortable addressing these areas, the nurse will be able to focus the conversations more directly and therapeutically.

## Evaluating: Objective Critique of Interventions and Self-Reflection

Evaluation is a function that involves asking the following questions:

- Is the patient learning to adapt to any health status changes triggered by the illness experience?
- Is the patient's grief response to the sustained losses fluid or fixed?
- Is the patient able to identify his/her feelings regarding the illness experience and is he or she able to communicate them to caregivers and family/friends to receive the support needed to mobilize for recovery?
- Is the patient gaining insight into how he or she might use the illness experience to emerge at a higher level of wellness than when the patient entered it?
- Are the patient and health care team incorporating the patient's spiritual and cultural beliefs and practices into the plan of care to facilitate healing?

- Are the patient's physical and psycho-spiritual symptoms being alleviated?
- Does the patient have a realistic perception of the illness and its treatment?
- Is the patient knowledgeable about the illness and its treatment?
- Is the patient's body image adapting, such that he or she can accept an altered body image with compassion and understanding?
- Does the patient express hope for the future?

All such evaluations should also encourage self-reflection, including whether or not the nurse capitalized on his or her strengths. Look for mentorship in areas that need improvement and continue to seek to refine critical thinking skills.

---

### SUMMARY POINTS

- Mental health and physical illness are closely interrelated such that physical illness can affect a person's mental health, and changes in mental health can affect a person's physical health.

- Suffering is a key component of a person's illness and can be addressed within the scope of the therapeutic nurse-patient relationship. However, nurses can experience compassion fatigue resulting from this intense relationship. A nurse's self-awareness of personal needs and permission to meet these needs aids in preventing compassion fatigue.

- Research has demonstrated that adverse childhood events are associated with unhealthy adult lifestyle behaviors and that biochemical phenomena and disruptions in various body systems contribute to physical illness.

- Illnesses involve a loss of something to some degree; thus all patients normally experience grief in response to the loss.

- Changes in body image, pain, and other physical symptoms can impact the mental health of a person with a physical illness. Anxiety and depression are often comorbid conditions occurring during physical illness.

- The SPIKES protocol can be used to therapeutically deliver bad news.

- A familiarity and a feeling of being comfortable with one's own mortality is important when providing end-of-life care.

- The mental health liaison/consultant nurse has expertise in dealing with patients experiencing psychosocial distress due to illness, treatments, and hospitalizations.

- Self-awareness is important for the nurse when engaging in the therapeutic nurse-patient relationship with a patient who has a physical illness and is experiencing mental health issues.

## NCLEX-PREP*

1. When describing Travelbee's view of suffering to a class, which of the following would the instructor include?
   a. It is confined to situations involving physical illness.
   b. It is easily controlled through communication.
   c. It can range from simple discomfort to extreme anguish.
   d. It determines how a person will survive.

2. The following are the steps of Bailey's Journey of Grief Model. Place the steps in their proper sequence after the experience of loss.
   a. Searching
   b. Reinvestment
   c. Protest
   d. Reorganization
   e. Despair

3. The nurse is assessing a patient and determines that the patient is experiencing a normal grief response based on which of the following?
   a. Openly expresses anger
   b. Non-intact reality testing
   c. Persistent sleeping problems
   d. Consistently dysphoric

4. A nurse is planning to implement complementary and alternative medicine therapies with a patient. In which of the following would the nurse include energy biofield therapies?
   a. Meditation
   b. Visualization
   c. Aromatherapy
   d. Acupuncture

5. A group of students are reviewing information about the numerous issues that impact the mental health of physically ill patients. The students demonstrate a need for additional study when they identify which of the following?
   a. Unhealthy lifestyle practices as an adult can be traced to negative events in childhood.
   b. Grief is an abnormal response that interferes with a person's ability to heal.
   c. Neuropeptides and their actions are addressed with psychoneuroimmunology.
   d. Pain causes increased secretion of cortisol, which disrupts the immune system.

*Answers to these questions appear on page 639.

## REFERENCES

Adverse Childhood Experiences (ACE) Study. Available at: www.acestudy.org

American Institute of Stress (2011). Available at http://www.stress.org

American Nurses Association (1994). Position Statement: Assisted Suicide. Available at: http://www.nursingworld.org/MainMenuCategories/EthicsStandards/Ethics-Position-Statements/prtetsuic14456.aspx (retrieved April 8, 2011).

Anda, R.F., Feletti, V.J., Walker, J., Whitfield, C.L., Brenner, J.D., Perry, B.D., Dube, S.R., Giles, W.H. (2006). The enduring effects of abuse and related adverse experiences in childhood; a convergence of evidence from neurobiology and epidemiology. *European Archives of Psychiatry and Clinical Neurosciences, 56*(3), 174–86.

Bailey, B. (1986). *Strategies for coping with loss.* The Connecticut Hospice, Inc.

Buckman, R. (1992). *How to break bad news; a practical guide for health care professionals.* Baltimore, Maryland: Johns Hopkins.

Cohen., S, & Janicki-Deverts, D. (2007). Psychological stress and disease. *Journal of the American Medical Association, 298*(14); 1685–7.

Connor, S. (2007). Comparing hospice and nonhospice patient survival among patients who die within a three year window. *Journal of Pain and Symptom Management, 33*(3), 238–246.

Dean, G., & Anderson, P. (2001). Fatigue. In B. Ferrell & N. Coyle (Eds.) *Textbook of palliative nursing,* (pp. 91–100). New York: Oxford University Press.

Fink, R., & Gates, R. (2001). Pain assessment. In B. Ferrell and N. Coyle (Eds.) *Textbook of palliative nursing,* (pp. 53–71). New York: Oxford University Press.

Frankl, V. (1959). *Man's search for meaning.* Boston: Beacon Press.

Gabriel, A. (2007). Changes in plasma cholesterol in mood disorder patients: Does treatment make a difference? *Journal of Affective Disorders, 99*(1), 273–278.

Hardwig, J. (1995). SUPPORT and the invisible family. Special Supplement, *Hastings Center Report, 25*(6), S23-S25.

Harrison, A., & Hart, C. (2006). *Mental health care for nurses, applying mental health skills in the general hospital.* Hoboken, NJ: Blackwell Publishing.

Jiang, W. (2004). Prognostic value of anxiety and depression in patients with chronic heart failure. *Circulation, 110,* 3452–3456.

Kiecolt-Glaser, J.K. (2002). Psychoneuroimmunology and psychosomatic medicine: back to the future. *Psyhcosom. Med 64*(1), 15–28.

Kuebler, K., English, N., & Heidrich, D. (2001) Delirium, confusion, agitation and restlessness. In B. Ferrell & N. Coyle (Eds.) *Textbook of palliative nursing,* (pp. 290–308). New York: Oxford University Press.

Liebeskind, J.C. (1991). Pain can kill. *Pain, 44*(1), 3–4.

Moskowitz, E., Nelson, J.L. (1995) Dying well in the hospital: lessons of SUPPORT, Special Supplement, *Hastings Center Report, 25*(6), S3-S6.

Mundy, A. (2000). Posttraumatic stress disorder in breast cancer patients following autologous bone marrow transplantation or conventional cancer treatments. *Behaviour Research and Therapy, 38*(10), 1015–1027.

Nordin, K. (2001). Predicting anxiety and depression among cancer patients: a clinical model. *European Journal of Cancer, 37*(3), 376–384.

Paice, J., & Fine, P. (2001). Pain at the end-of-life. In B. Ferrell & N. Coyle (Eds.) *Textbook of palliative nursing* (pp. 76–90). New York: Oxford University Press.

Pert, C. (1997). Molecules of emotion, the science behind mind and body medicine. New York: Simon & Schuster.

Pasacreta, J.V., (20021). Anxiety and depression. In B. Ferrell & N. Coyle (Eds), *Textbook of Palliative Nursing* (pp. 269–289). New York: Oxford University Press.

Pendry, P. (2007). Moral distress: recognizing it to retain nurses. *Nurs Econ, 25*(4):217–221.

Platek, B. (2008). Through glass darkly, Miriam Greenspan on moving from grief to gratitude. *Sun, 385,* 4–11.

Rancour, P. (2008). *Tales from the Pager Chronicles.* Indianapolis: Sigma Theta Tau International.

Rancour, P. (2008). Integrating complementary and alternative therapies into end-of-life care. *In Touch, A Hospice and Palliative Care Resource.* Ohio Hospice and Palliative Care Organization, *12,* (4), 8–10.

Rancour, P. (2008). Using archetypes and transitions theory to help patients move from active treatment to survivorship. *Clinical Journal of Oncology Nursing, 12*(6), 935–940.

Rancour, P. (2006). Clinical treatment for body image disturbances: variations on a theme: interactive guided imagery, empty chair work, and therapeutic letter-writing. In *Body Image: New Research.* New York: Nova Science Publications.

Rancour, P., & Brauer, K. (2003). A matched set: a case study in the use of letter-writing as a means of integrating an altered body image in a patient with recurrent breast cancer. *Oncology Nursing Forum, 30*(5), 841–848.

Rancour, P., & Cluxton, D. (2000). Standing with the bereaved: a comprehensive bereavement program in a tertiary care setting. *Journal of Oncology Management, 9,* (6), 10–12.

Rancour, P. (1994). Interactive guided imagery with oncology patients: a case illustration. *Journal of Holistic Nursing, 12* (2), 148–154.

Rancour, P. (1993). The development of a comprehensive psychosocial oncology program. *The Journal of Oncology Management, 2*(5), 33–35.

Schneider, J.M. (1980). Clinically significant differences between grief, pathological grief and depression. *Patient Counseling Health Educ, 4,* 267–275.

Shinoda Bolen, J. (1996). *Close to the Bone, Life-threatening illness and the search for meaning.* New York: Simon & Schuster.

Stiles, S., (2008). SADHART-CHF: Nurse intervention impresses for depression in heart failure, SSRI doesn't, Sept 23, 2008, HFSA News, http://www.theheart.org/article/906715.do

Those tough conversations. (2000) *American Journal of Nursing,* Critical Care Supplement. 100(4), April, 24HH-24LL.

Travelbee, J. (1971). *Interpersonal aspects of nursing* (2nd edition), Philadelphia: FA Davis.

Wagner, J., & Tennen, H. (2007). Coping in diabetes: Psychological determinants of behavioral and physiological outcomes in diabetes. In Martz, E. & Livneh, H. (Eds.), *Stress Reactions to and Coping with Chronic Illness and Disability: Theoretical, Empirical, and Clinical.* New York: Springer.

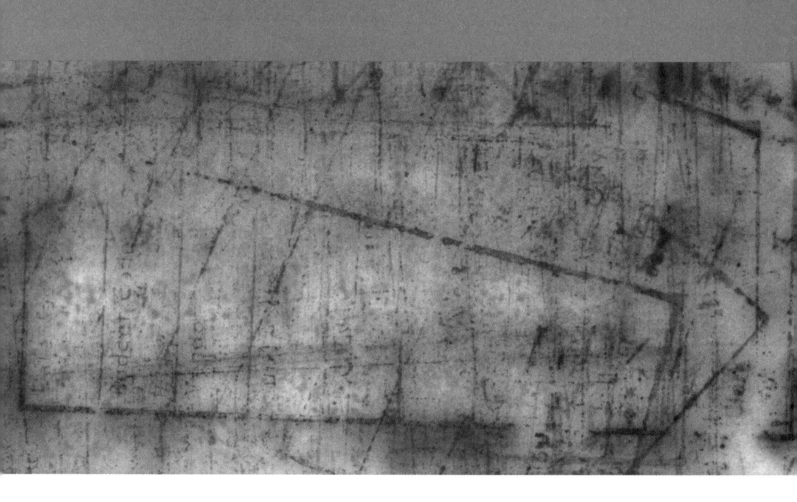

## CHAPTER CONTENTS

## EXPECTED LEARNING OUTCOMES

**After completing this chapter, the student will be able to:**

1. Discuss the major theories related to growth and development in children.

2. Identify normative versus non-normative behavioral patterns in relation to developmental milestones.

3. Describe the major mental health disorders found in children.

4. Identify the *Diagnostic and Statistical Manual of Mental Disorders, 4th edition, Text Revision* (*DSM-IV-TR*) diagnostic criteria for the major childhood mental disorders.

## CHAPTER 21
# WORKING WITH CHILDREN

Emily K. Johnson

5. Identify the primary treatment options available for mental disorders found in children.

6. Apply the nursing process from an interpersonal perspective that addresses the developmental needs of children experiencing mental health disorders.

## KEY TERMS

Autism

Circular reactions

Classical conditioning

Cognitive development

Conservation

Echolalia

Libido

Magical thinking

Object permanence

Operant conditioning

Pica

Play therapy

Reversibility

Symbolic play

Childhood behavior varies significantly with developmental stage, psychosocial environment, and genetic influence. Due to differences between childhood and adult behavior, emotional problems and mental health disorders in children can be difficult to determine. As with adults, psychiatric diagnoses in children are made by skilled professionals trained to observe particular signs and symptoms. However, in children, the signs and symptoms must be considered in the context of developmental level and physical and social environment. The signs may be significantly different from those seen in adolescents and adults. Moreover, a young child's inability to express symptoms clearly makes the determination even more challenging. For example, children with depression often display significant irritability and express nonspecific physical complaints (Fassler & Dumas, 1997). Children commonly find it more difficult to verbalize to an adult that they are feeling sad. As a result, reports from parents, other caretakers, and/or teachers are often used to supplement information gathered during a psychiatric assessment. Accurate diagnoses and effective treatment require a solid knowledge base involving childhood development, specific criteria, and assessment techniques.

This chapter addresses the unique and challenging issues involved in working with children who have a mental disorder. Major theories related to growth and development are reviewed and some of the more common mental health disorders are described. The nursing process is applied from an interpersonal perspective to provide a framework when caring for a child with a mental health disorder.

## GROWTH AND DEVELOPMENT THEORIES

In all scientific fields, theory guides clinical practice and forms the basis for reasoning behind particular treatments. Chapter 10 provides an in-depth discussion of theories in general, including those specifically related to mental

illness. This chapter describes the major theories related to an individual's development through the lifespan. These theories help to provide a foundation from which to explain the reasons why particular disorders affect particular individuals and to assist in understanding the appropriate treatment options and care.

## Piaget's Theory of Cognitive Development

Knowledge and understanding of cognitive, emotional, and psychological growth is imperative to the assessment and nursing care of children. COGNITIVE DEVELOPMENT refers to one's ability to understand the world, including interaction with stimuli and objects in the environment, social interactions related to thinking patterns, and how one receives and stores information (Bornstein & Lamb, 1999). Perhaps the most influential theory associated with cognitive development is that of Jean Piaget, a Swiss theorist who began studying childhood development in the 1920s using his own children as subjects (Sadock & Sadock, 2007). Although this method provided grounds for criticism, his observations of his children's errors in reasoning formed Piaget's theory of cognitive development.

Piaget identified four major developmental stages that children progress through when moving from infancy and continuing into early adolescence. **Table 21-1** summarizes these four stages.

The first stage is known as the sensorimotor stage and spans from birth until age two. Significant growth in this stage occurs as an infant is born with little knowledge beyond instincts and reflexes. Soon after, the newborn's cognition develops into exploration of the environment, curiosity, and mental representation (problem solving using previously experienced events and/or objects) (Bornstein & Lamb, 1999). Key features of the sensorimotor stage include CIRCULAR REACTIONS and OBJECT PERMANENCE. Circular reactions initially involve motor reflexes, such as thumb sucking and hand grasping. These then develop into object manipulation that invokes a

| TABLE 21-1: PIAGET'S THEORY OF COGNITIVE DEVELOPMENT | | |
|---|---|---|
| STAGE | AGE | KEY COMPONENTS |
| Sensorimotor | Birth–2 years | Circular reactions<br>Object permanence |
| Preoperational | 2–7 years | Symbolic play<br>Magical thinking |
| Concrete operational | 7–12 years | Reversibility<br>Conservation |
| Formal operational | 12 years–Adulthood | Abstract thinking<br>Logical thinking |

response from people or the environment (rattle shaking). By 18 months, a circular reaction no longer involves initiating behavior to elicit a response but to produce a different outcome, such as trying to place a block in a hole until it fits and falls through. Object permanence refers to the ability of the child to realize that an object is no longer visible despite the fact that it still exists (Bornstein & Lamb, 1999). For example, a child will attempt to lift a blanket they know is covering a toy instead of believing the toy has disappeared.

The second stage, preoperational stage, takes place between ages two and seven. This stage is credited for development of motor skills and language. Key developmental features of the stage include **SYMBOLIC PLAY** and **MAGICAL THINKING**. Symbolic play involves the child's ability to separate behaviors and objects from their actual use and instead use them for play (Bornstein & Lamb, 1999). For example, a child takes a wooden block and moves it through the air, stating that it is an airplane. To do this, the child must have a mental representation of an airplane and be able to replace reality (the object is a block) with the mental representation of an airplane. Magical thinking results from the child's belief that a circumstance or event may be brought on by wishing for it or thinking about it. A child exhibiting magical thinking may feel responsible for a friend falling on the playground if the child had been mad at the friend earlier that day.

The third stage is the concrete-operational stage. Adult-like characteristics begin to emerge through flexible reasoning, logical thought, and organization. The stage begins around age seven and continues until age 11 or 12 (Sadock & Sadock, 2007). Key features of this stage include **REVERSIBILITY**, in which the child realizes that certain things can turn into other things and then back again, such as water and ice, and **CONSERVATION**—the ability to recognize that despite something changing shape, it maintains the characteristics that make it what it is (clay). Both of the features of the concrete-operational stage are made possible by

*According to Piaget, a child's cognitive development occurs over four developmental stages from infancy through adolescence: sensorimotor, preoperational, concrete operational, and formal operational.*

increased ability to understand spatial operations, distance, time, velocity, and space (Bornstein & Lamb, 1999).

Finally, the formal operational stage is differentiated based on the child's ability to think abstractly. Usually occurring around age 12, this stage transitions a child into adolescence as he or she demonstrates the ability to use logic and reasoning to hypothesize, problem solve, and comprehend information (Bornstein & Lamb, 1999).

## Erikson's Theory of Emotional and Personality Development

Various theories have been used to describe the development of emotional well-being and personality, but Erik Erikson's stages of human development is commonly used. Although the stages progress throughout the lifespan, the majority of developmental "crises," as Erikson calls them, occur within the first 20 years of life (Sadock & Sadock, 2007). **Table 21-2** summarizes the major stages of Erikson's theory.

Mastery of the initial stage is dependent upon the child feeling nurtured and loved, ensuring the development of a sense of security, trust, and a basic optimism. Children who are mishandled, neglected, or abused, often become insecure in their environment and mistrustful of others. Progression of development continues into the second stage in early childhood. A well-adjusted child emerges from this stage with a sense of pride and self-control instead of shame and self-doubt (Bornstein & Lamb, 1999). The child demonstrating normal development through this stage displays willpower through tantrums and stubbornness. This is not necessarily a sign of poor development, but rather an indication of testing wills and temperament. Children experiencing poor parenting may show a lack of independence, willpower, and self-esteem.

As children move into late childhood, this newfound independence from the previous stage progresses into self-directed behavior and ability to form goals. This progression is often demonstrated through play. According to Erikson, a healthy developing child will increase imagination through fantasy play, learn to cooperate with others, and lead as well as follow (Bornstein & Lamb, 1999). Children demonstrating poor development will continue to depend on adult figures, show restrictions in play and imagination, and fail to participate fully in groups.

Children moving into school-age development begin to master more formal skills as rules are enforced, structured activity increases, and the need for

**TABLE 21-2: ERIKSON'S STAGES OF HUMAN DEVELOPMENT**

| DEVELOPMENTAL STAGE | AGE | DEVELOPMENTAL TASK | NORMAL DEVELOPMENT | DELAYED DEVELOPMENT |
|---|---|---|---|---|
| Infancy | 0–1 year | Trust vs. mistrust | Relationship formation; trust in others | Suspiciousness of others; lack of relationships |
| Early childhood | 1–3 years | Autonomy vs. shame and doubt | Self-esteem; self-control; willpower | Self-doubt; low self-esteem; lack of independence |
| Late childhood | 3–6 years | Initiative vs. guilt | Self-directed behavior; goal formation | Little sense of purpose; no goal formation |
| School age | 6–12 years | Industry vs. inferiority | Sense of competency and achievement | Difficulty working/learning; sense of inferiority |
| Adolescence | 12–20 years | Identity vs. role confusion | Beginnings of self-discovery; identity formation | Identity confusion; difficulty in group settings |
| Early adulthood | 20–35 years | Intimacy vs. isolation | Committed relationships; ability to give and receive love | Emotional isolation; egocentrism |
| Middle adulthood | 35–65 years | Generativity vs. self-absorption or stagnation | Ability to care for others; giving of time to others | Self-absorption; inability/refusal to care for others |
| Late adulthood | Older than 65 years | Integrity vs. despair | Fulfillment in life; willingness to face and accept death; balanced perspective on life events | Bitterness/dissatisfaction with life; despair over impending death |

self-discipline becomes important. A child successful in this stage gains autonomy by showing competence in self-directed activities and appreciating reward for achievements (Bornstein & Lamb, 1999). However, failure at the school-age stage will reveal difficulty learning in traditional settings and subsequently a sense of inferiority.

> *According to Erikson, the majority of an individual's emotional and personality development occurs during the first 20 years of that person's life. This development forms the foundation for continued development in adulthood.*

Over the rest of an individual's lifespan, the remainder of Erikson's stages emerge based on personality formation in the initial childhood stages. Failure to develop

mastery at any stage may result in failure at subsequent stages. The progression through stages can be compared to building a house. The foundation is essential for the structure of the house as a whole, and each floor's stability is dependent on proper construction of the floors below it. Through adulthood, an individual will discover intimacy through lasting friendships and marriage and generativity through lasting marriage, productivity, and child-rearing. The individual will also learn to maintain integrity through experiencing aging and death (Sadock & Sadock, 2007). Inability to satisfactorily complete any of the adult stages leads an individual to show signs of isolation, egocentrism, and an overall dissatisfaction with life.

## Freud's Theory of Psychological Development

Like the development of emotional well-being and personality, a variety of theories exist to outline the psychological development of children. The most notable theories include Sigmund Freud's theory of psychosexual development, and Ivan Pavlov and B.F. Skinner's behavioral theories.

> *According to Freud, if an individual does not resolve issues in an early stage, he or she becomes fixated in that stage. Fixation results in unhealthy behavior.*

Freud's psychosexual development theory is one of the best known theories in psychology. He identified five childhood stages: oral, anal, phallic, latent, and genital. Each of these stages are guided by the pleasure-seeking energy of the id. The id, commonly known as the LIBIDO, is the driving force behind specific behaviors (Bornstein & Lamb, 1999). Healthy psychosexual development occurs when each stage is successfully completed, whereas unresolved issues in a particular stage cause fixation and unhealthy behavior (Sadock & Sadock, 2007). Table 21-3

summarizes Freud's theory. Refer to Chapter 10 for additional information about Freud.

## Sullivan's Theory of Interpersonal and Personality Development

Harry Stack Sullivan, a psychoanalytically trained psychiatrist, believed that children develop a self-system through childhood and adolescence (Rioch, 1985). This system develops over a period of six stages and is based on how an individual interacts with others. Table 21-4 summarizes Sullivan's six stages.

According to Sullivan, the self-system is composed of personality traits that have been reinforced and maintained through interpersonal relationships, into adulthood, at which point they become rigid and dominant. A person has a need for satisfaction and security. If these needs are not met, anxiety develops (Sullivan, 1953). The purpose of the self system is to decrease anxiety and sustain security (Rioch, 1985). (See Chapter 2 for additional information on Sullivan.)

### TABLE 21-3: FREUD'S STAGES OF PSYCHOSEXUAL DEVELOPMENT

| STAGE | AGE | BEHAVIOR | RESULT OF FIXATION |
|-------|-----|----------|--------------------|
| Oral | 0–18 months | Rooting and sucking reflex<br>Trust, comfort | Substance abuse, eating disorders, schizophrenia |
| Anal | 18 months–3 years | Bladder and bowel control (toilet training)<br>Control, independence | Destructive personality disorders, OCD, depression |
| Phallic | 3–6 years | Discovery of opposite gender; focus on genitals<br>Identification with same-sex parent | Sexual identity disorders |
| Latent | 6 years–puberty | Sexual drives calmed; focus on peer relationships<br>Social/communication skills, self-confidence | Social phobias, anxiety |
| Genital | Puberty forward | Strong sexual interest in opposite sex<br>Balance, concern for others | Sexual perversion disorders |

### TABLE 21-4: HARRY STACK SULLIVAN'S STAGES OF INTERPERSONAL AND PERSONALITY DEVELOPMENT

| STAGE | TIME PERIOD | DEVELOPMENTAL TASK |
|-------|-------------|---------------------|
| Infancy | Birth–18 months | Oral gratification; anxiety occurs for the first time |
| Childhood | 18 months–6 years | Delayed gratification |
| Juvenile | 6–9 years | Forming of peer relationships |
| Preadolescence | 9–12 years | Same-sex relationships |
| Early adolescence | 12–14 years | Opposite-sex relationships |
| Late adolescence | 14–21 years | Self-identity development |

*From Sadock & Sadock, 2007.*

> *According to Sullivan, children develop a self-system from infancy through late adolescence based on their interactions with others.*

## Behavioral Theories of Pavlov and Skinner

Behavioral theories of child development are based only on observable behaviors influenced by interaction with the environment. Development is a reaction to rewards, reinforcement, and punishment and is described in theories of classical conditioning and operant conditioning. Pavlov made famous the theory of **CLASSICAL CONDITIONING** with his experiment on salivation in dogs. Classical conditioning refers to a learned behavioral response to a stimulus.

Pavlov's theory consists of four basic principles. The unconditioned stimulus is a naturally occurring event that illicits an unconditioned response, which is unlearned. The conditioned stimulus, although previously neutral, becomes a trigger for the conditioned response after associating with the unconditioned stimulus (Bornstein & Lamb, 1999). Simply put, Pavlov measured salivation (unconditioned response) in dogs when they were presented with food (unconditioned stimulus). He then rang a bell (unconditioned stimulus) multiple times as he presented the dogs with food; soon, the dogs would begin to salivate at the sound of the bell in expectation of receiving food (conditioned response). Pavlov's theory became the basis of behavioral psychology and is often used in child therapies for phobias, anxiety, panic disorders, and behavioral modification (Bornstein & Lamb, 1999).

> *The behavioral theories of Pavlov and Skinner form the basis for many of the therapies used for childhood disorders.*

Skinner's behavioral theory involving **OPERANT CONDITIONING** holds that learning takes place through rewards (used to increase desired behavior) and punishments (to decrease undesirable behavior). Operant conditioning is used frequently throughout the lifespan but more commonly as a parenting technique and in the classroom (Bornstein & Lamb, 1999). Examples include: time-outs for misbehavior, grounding for missing curfew, candy or praise for success in toilet training, stickers for perfect scores on spelling tests—the list could easily continue. (See Chapter 10 for a more in-depth discussion about the work of Pavlov and Skinner.)

## OVERVIEW OF DISORDERS OF CHILDHOOD

Historically, mental illness in children was rarely studied because the general population believed that psychiatric illnesses did not occur in that population. Currently diagnosis in children is more common and inclusion of childhood mental illnesses was included in the *Diagnostic and Statistical Manual of Mental Disorders, 4th edition, Text Revision (DSM-IV-TR)*. The rates of childhood psychiatric diagnoses has been on a steady rise (National Institutes of Mental Health [NIMH], 2008). Whether the increase is due to actual increases in childhood mental illness or related to increased comfort and acceptance with diagnoses from providers is unclear. Regardless, disorders of childhood are important to recognize and understand.

In the *DSM-IV-TR*, over 40 diagnoses often discovered in infancy, childhood, or adolescence are described and divided into categories. These categories include:
- Mental retardation
- Learning disorders
- Motor skills disorder
- Communication disorders
- Pervasive developmental disorders
- Attention-deficit and disruptive behavior disorders
- Feeding and eating disorders
- Tic disorders
- Elimination disorders
- Category for other disorders

A few of the more common disorders are described in this chapter.

## PERVASIVE DEVELOPMENTAL DISORDERS

The category of pervasive developmental disorders (PDD) contains five separate but similar diagnoses: autism, Rett's disorder, childhood disintegrative disorder, Asperger's disorder, and PDD not otherwise specified. Not otherwise specified (NOS) is a diagnosis classification used when significant impairment is evident, but complete criteria are not met for a specific diagnosis. The category of PDD is under debate because some practitioners feel the disorders within the category are not clearly differentiated, increasing the possibility of diagnostic errors (Gupta, 2004). The term autistic spectrum disorder has been proposed to replace PDD; it is likely that PDD criteria and terminology in the next edition of the DSM will differ from the current version. Autism and Asperger's are the most common disorders from this category. Refer to the *DSM-IV-TR* for information about the other disorders.

## Autistic Disorder

The term **AUTISM** literally means "living in self" and was first used in 1911 to describe poor social relatedness in schizophrenics. However, signs of autism are apparent in reports of children with distortions of the developmental process as early as 1867. In the early 1940s, autism was considered a subtype of childhood psychosis carrying the label "childhood schizophrenics of the pseudo-defective type" (Gupta, 2004). Over time, however, autism began to distinguish itself as a unique and independent disorder with two distinct criteria: inability to relate to people and situations, and failure to learn to speak or convey meaning to others through language.

Before the release of the third edition of the *DSM*, problems arose in the clinical setting because of similarities between autism and schizophrenia. The third edition included autistic disorder under the category of PDD, not under psychotic disorders. Although clinicians acknowledge the similarities between the diagnostic criteria, there are two significant differences:

- Schizophrenia occurs after a period of normal development, whereas autism is likely present from birth (APA, 2000).
- Positive symptoms such as hallucinations and delusions and higher intelligence levels are associated with schizophrenia but not autism (APA, 2000).

Over the past 30 years, the categories, diagnostic criteria, and subtypes of autistic disorder have undergone many changes due to increased research and diagnoses of the disorder. It is likely that features of autism will continue to change over the next 30 years. The severity of autism varies widely and exists on a spectrum from mild to severe.

Autistic disorder is the second-most common serious developmental disorder, after only mental retardation (Newschaffer et al., 2007). Prevalence studies revealed an average rate of 3.4 cases per 1000 children, with a four to five times higher rate in boys than in girls. The onset typically occurs before three years of age with a chronic course into adulthood (NIMH, 2008). Over the past 10 years, there has been an increased focus on autistic disorders in the popular media leading to research, speculations, and controversy about what causes autism. Heredity, environment, brain abnormalities, postnatal infection, and prenatal conditions may lead to an increased risk of autism.

Research demonstrates that genetic factors may play a role in the etiology of autism based on both twin and non-twin sibling studies (NIMH, 2002). However, no specific genes have been identified. Current research is exploring a number of biomarkers associated with autism, which may aid in the discovery of specific genetic markers (Newschaffer et al., 2007). Environmental influences thought to contribute to autism are assumed to be related to the interaction between the environment and genes, not environment alone. Additionally, specific risk factors have not been identified.

Abnormalities in the structure and function of the brain are generally accepted as the underlying cause of autism (NIMH, 2002). Sophisticated imaging techniques have shown that autistic children have alterations in the amygdala, which influences social interaction and processing. Defects have also been noted in the areas of the parietal lobes associated with emotion, empathy, and sight-based learning (NIMH, 2002). Researchers have yet to identify a primary deficit associated with autism.

Several early developmental problems, both prenatal and postnatal, have been linked to autistic disorders. For example, prenatal viral infections, such as rubella or cytomegalovirus, are thought to activate the maternal immune response. Antibodies from the mother passed through the placenta may react with the fetal brain and cause particular symptoms associated with autism (Dalton, Deacon, & Blamire, 2003). Additionally, gestational diabetes, teratogenic medications, pesticides, thyroid issues, folic acid deficiencies, and stress are other maternal influences that possibly contribute to autism. A large list of potential postnatal environmental causes of or associations with autism exists and includes everything from viral infections to lead exposure to excess rainfall. One issue related to the development of autism that has raised much debate is the use of vaccines. **Box 21-1** describes this issue. Over the years, most research has not been able to demonstrate a statistically significant relationship among these factors and the development of autism. However, current research into the etiology of autism is showing many possibilities and may show promising results in the near future.

> ### 🔍 BOX 21-1: DO VACCINES CAUSE AUTISM?
>
> Many studies have researched whether there is a relationship between vaccines and autism. The majority of scientific research has concluded that vaccines are not associated with autism and the risk of not immunizing children against disease supersedes the risk of potentially damaging ingredients in vaccines. In a 2007 court case, three families with autistic children sought compensation from the Vaccine Injury Compensation Program for allegedly triggering autism with an MMR vaccine containing thimerisol, a mercury-based preservative. The court ruled that the three cases presented did not prove a link between autism and particular childhood vaccines, citing insufficient evidence (Hitti, 2009).
>
> Autism Speaks, a well-known autism advocacy organization, supports continuing examination of the factors contributing to autism and encourages increased scientific research to determine the cause. Celebrity influence from Jenny McCarthy and Holly Robinson Peete, both mothers who believe vaccines were the cause of autism in their children, has made the vaccine/autism debate increasingly sensitive. Both women, along with anti-vaccine groups, trace the emergence of autism in their children to the time when thimerisol-containing vaccines were administered.
>
> Future research will likely focus on genetics and environment to determine the true etiology of autism. Until then, the debate continues in both science and the popular media.

> *Genetics, environment, structural and functional alterations of the brain, and prenatal and postnatal problems have been linked to autism.*

Children with autism will show marked impairment in social interactions and communication that is sustained throughout childhood and beyond (APA, 2000). Although the individual may speak, there will likely be an inability to initiate or carry on a conversation. It is common for the pitch, intonation, rate, and rhythm of the speech to be abnormal and inappropriate to the context of conversation. Rhyming, ECHOLALIA (repeating spoken words like an echo), peculiar languages, and referring to themselves in the third person are common (APA, 2000). A child with autism will also display repetitive and restricted behavior. They may seem to exist in their own world where repetitive routines and fantasy are apparent. Occasionally, a child with autism may exhibit a particular talent in art, music, mathematics, or another area. They are known as savants. **Box 21-2** highlights the *DSM-IV-TR* diagnostic criteria.

By definition, autism must involve delays or abnormal functioning prior to age three years. If a period of normal development occurs after age three, the child may better fit the criteria for another developmental disorder (APA, 2000). Parents can often trace abnormalities in social interaction back to birth or shortly afterward.

## Asperger's Disorder

Asperger's disorder was named after a Viennese pediatrician in 1944 when a condition similar to autism was discovered, but independently described with a lesser severity of symptoms and presence of oddity in the child's gaze (Merkel, 2006). This disorder is similar to autism but differs in several ways (see Box 21-2 for diagnostic criteria). Children with Asperger's disorder do not experience a significant delay in early cognitive and language skills. In addition, the preoccupation with objects and rituals that are common in autism are less often observed in Asperger's disorder (APA, 2000). The social isolation is much less severe in Asperger's, and individuals may display motivation for approaching others despite the eccentric, verbose, and insensitive nature of their conversation (APA, 2000). Mental retardation is far less common with Asperger's disorder, whereas it is frequent with autism. Diagnostically, it can be difficult to distinguish between Asperger's and a mild form of autism.

## BOX 21-2: DIAGNOSTIC CRITERIA OF PERVASIVE DEVELOPMENT DISORDERS

### AUTISTIC DISORDER

A. A total of six (or more) items from the following:
- Qualitative impairment in social interaction, as manifested by at least two of the following:
  - Marked impairment in the use of multiple nonverbal behaviors such as eye-to-eye gaze, facial expression, body postures, and gestures to regulate social interaction
  - Failure to develop peer relationships appropriate to developmental level
  - A lack of spontaneous seeking to share enjoyment, interests, or achievements with other people (e.g., by a lack of showing, bringing, or pointing out objects of interest)
  - Lack of social or emotional reciprocity
- Qualitative impairments in communication as manifested by at least one of the following:
  - Delay in, or total lack of, the development of spoken language (not accompanied by an attempt to compensate through alternative modes of communication such as gesture or mime)
  - In individuals with adequate speech, marked impairment in the ability to initiate or sustain a conversation with others
  - Stereotyped and repetitive use of language or idiosyncratic language
  - Lack of varied, spontaneous make-believe play or social imitative play appropriate to developmental level
- Restricted repetitive and stereotyped patterns of behavior, interests, and activities, as manifested by at least one of the following:
  - Encompassing preoccupation with one or more stereotyped and restricted patterns of interest that is abnormal either in intensity or focus
  - Apparently inflexible adherence to specific, nonfunctional routines or rituals
  - Stereotyped and repetitive motor mannerisms (e.g., hand or finger flapping or twisting, or complex whole-body movements)
  - Persistent preoccupation with parts of objects
B. Delays or abnormal functioning in at least one of the following areas, with onset prior to age 3 years:
- Social interaction
- Language as used in social communication
- Symbolic or imaginative play
C. The disturbance is not better accounted for by Rett's Disorder or Childhood Disintegrative Disorder.

### ASPERGER'S DISORDER

A. Qualitative impairment in social interaction, as manifested by at least two of the following:
- Marked impairment in use of multiple nonverbal behaviors
- Failure to develop appropriate peer relationships based on developmental level
- Lack of spontaneous seeking to share enjoyment, interests, or achievements with others
- Lack of social or emotional reciprocity
B. Restricted repetitive and stereotyped patterns of behaviors, interests, and activities, as manifested by at least one of the following:
- Encompassing preoccupation with one or more stereotyped and restricted patterns of interest abnormal in intensity or focus
- Apparently inflexible adherence to specific nonfunctional routines or rituals

*(cont.)*

> **Q** BOX 21-2: DIAGNOSTIC CRITERIA OF PERVASIVE DEVELOPMENT DISORDERS (*CONT.*)
>
> - Stereotyped and repetitive motor mannerisms
> - Persistent preoccupation with parts of objects
> C. Clinically significant impairment in social, occupational, or other important areas of functioning
> D. No clinically significant delay in language
> E. No clinically significant delay in cognitive development or development of age-appropriate self-help skills, adapative behavior, and curiosity about the environment
> F. Criteria not met for another PDD or schizophrenia
>
> *From American Psychiatric Association. (2000). Diagnostic and statistical manual of mental disorders, 4th ed., text revision. Copyright ©, American Psychiatric Association.*

*Asperger's disorder is similar to autism but the symptoms are less severe. Early cognitive and language skills are not significantly delayed and preoccupation with objects and rituals are less often noted.*

## ATTENTION-DEFICIT AND DISRUPTIVE BEHAVIOR DISORDERS

Disruptive behavior disorders involve a pattern of behavior in which an individual consistently bends or breaks rules. It is normal for children to test authority by breaking the rules and demonstrating oppositional behavior in childhood and adolescence. However, serious and routine oppositional defiance extends beyond normal. Three primary disorders are described in this section: attention deficit hyperactivity disorder (ADHD), conduct disorder (CD), and oppositional defiant disorder (ODD). All three disorders are closely linked with impulses (action without reflective thought of consequences) and the ability to manage or control those impulses (APA, 2000).

Similar to other mental illnesses, disruptive behavior disorders have been around for a long time, but were known by different names throughout history. The first documented mention of disruptive behavior disorder-like symptoms occurred in 1902 with a description of impulsiveness in children believed to have a defect of moral control (Londrie, 2006). Throughout the early 1900s, more name changes occurred and, in 1937, the hyperactivity associated with ADHD was singled out as a pharmacologically treatable symptom. Experiments began testing stimulant drug use in hyperactive children, and a short time later, methylphenidate (Ritalin) was widely accepted as the drug of choice for treatment of hyperactivity. It was not until 1980 that ADHD was documented in the *DSM-III* and accepted as a formal diagnosis (Londrie, 2006). At that time, it was known as attention deficit disorder (ADD) and classified as with or without hyperactivity.

Around 1987, researchers began noticing that the hyperactivity and impulse control associated with ADHD had a significant correlation with behavioral issues (Foley et al., 2004). As a result, conduct disorder and oppositional defiant disorder emerged with identified criteria encompassing the hostility and aggression seen with some, but not all impulsive individuals. Since that time, diagnosis of CD and ODD has been steadily increasing (APA, 2000). As with ADHD, CD and ODD have likely existed for many years without formal diagnostic criteria.

### Attention-Deficit Hyperactivity Disorder

Attention-deficit hyperactivity disorder is characterized by inattention and/or hyperactivity-impulsivity that is more frequent and severe than what would be expected for that developmental state. For example, toddlers frequently present with excessive motor activity. However, many of these children will not go on to develop ADHD. Therefore, differentiating normal overactivity from hyperactivity becomes important.

Actual prevalence of ADHD is estimated at 3–7% in school-age children. However, these rates vary significantly depending on location, nature, and method of ascertainment of the population surveyed (APA, 2000).

The actual cause of ADHD is not known. However, considerable evidence exists to suggest a strong genetic influence, especially related to symptoms of hyperactivity, impulsivity, and inattention. Siblings and children of individuals with ADHD are more likely to have the disorder (NIMH, 2000). Additionally, neurochemical studies show alterations in the neurotransmitter levels of dopamine, norepinephrine, and possibly serotonin—these alterations may be associated with disruptive symptoms. Moreover, prenatal, perinatal, and postnatal factors such as exposure to toxic substances, fetal hypoxia and/or prematurity, and central nervous system abnormalities have also been implicated as potential causes of disruptive behavior disorders (Popper, Gammon, West, & Bailey, 2003).

Formal diagnosis of ADHD usually is not made until the child starts school. At that time, maladjustment to school environment, whether hyperactive or inattentive, is better observed. Many children will display behaviors seen in ADHD. Careful diagnostic strategies must be used to distinguish those children who would benefit from pharmacological and therapeutic treatment, and those who would benefit more from increased parental guidance.

The diagnosis of ADHD has three possible subtypes: predominantly hyperactive-impulsive type (active, impulsive behavior), predominantly inattentive type (inability to pay attention), and the combined type (behavior from both types). Each subtype has specific criteria but are treated in a relatively similar way. **Box 21-3** highlights the diagnostic criteria of the *DSM-IV-TR*.

> *Inattention and/or hyperactivity-impulsivity are characteristics of ADHD, which is not diagnosed until after the child starts school.*

## Conduct Disorder

Children with CD display a repetitive and persistent pattern of behavior that violates the rights of other people, age-appropriate societal norms, or rules (APA, 2000). The prevalence of CD has been on the rise over the past few years and is estimated to occur in anywhere from 1–10% of the population (APA, 2000). CD may be diagnosed as early as preschool and is one of the most frequently diagnosed conditions in child mental health facilities. A common precursor to childhood onset of CD is a diagnosis of ODD, which is typically diagnosed first.

The underlying cause of CD is not known. However, like ADHD, similar neurologic influences are possible but environmental influence from family, school, and peers appears to be stronger based on research trends and increased prevalence in urban areas. The impact of social groups on child development is remarkable as peers play an essential role in development of interpersonal and social skills. Consistent peer rejection and poor social relationships were strongly correlated with deviance and maladaptive behavior (Ladd, 1999). Poor family dynamics and home environment also have a tremendous effect on childhood behavior. Primary factors contributing to the development of CD include: parental rejection or neglect; parental permissiveness or overly harsh punishment; foster care and early institutional living; absent father; marital conflict or divorce; and parents with antisocial personality disorder or substance abuse (Foley et al., 2004).

Temperament is another factor that may influence the development of CD. Personality characteristics that predict future mood and behavior often appear early in life, possibly even at birth. These characteristics can be referred to as the individual's temperament. Studies show that difficult temperaments in children before age three are significantly associated with development of CD (Bagley & Mallick, 2000).

To diagnose child-onset subtype of CD, the individual must exhibit one criterion before reaching age 10 (see Box 21-3). Children with CD are more commonly boys and may display physical aggression in conjunction with ADHD. The child also often has a diagnosis of ODD and will meet full CD criteria before reaching puberty. Children with child-onset subtype of CD are more likely to develop adult antisocial personality disorder (see Chapter 14 for more information on personality disorders) than those with adolescent-onset CD (see Chapter 22 for more information) (Bagley & Mallick, 2000).

Key features of children with CD include: aggression to people and animals, destruction of property, deceitfulness, theft, and serious violations of rules. The last characteristic is particular to children under the age of 13 and involves staying out late at night despite parental prohibitions and school truancy (APA, 2000).

## BOX 21-3: DIAGNOSTIC CRITERIA FOR ATTENTION-DEFICIT AND DISRUPTIVE BEHAVIOR DISORDERS

### ATTENTION-DEFICIT/HYPERACTIVITY DISORDER

A. Six (or more) of the following symptoms of inattention, persisting for at least 6 months to a degree that is maladaptive and inconsistent with developmental level:

*Inattention:*

- Often fails to give close attention to details or makes careless mistakes in schoolwork, work, or other activities
- Often has difficulty sustaining attention in tasks or play activities
- Often does not seem to listen when spoken to directly
- Often does not follow through on instructions and fails to finish schoolwork, chores, or duties in the workplace (not due to oppositional behavior or failure to understand instructions)
- Often has difficulty organizing tasks and activities
- Often avoids, dislikes, or is reluctant to engage in tasks that require sustained mental effort (such as schoolwork or homework)
- Often loses things necessary for tasks or activities (e.g., toys, school assignments, pencils, books, or tools)
- Is often easily distracted by extraneous stimuli
- Is often forgetful in daily activities
- Six (or more) of the following symptoms of hyperactivity-impulsivity, persisting for at least 6 months to a degree that is maladaptive and inconsistent with developmental level:

*Hyperactivity:*

- Often fidgets with hands or feet or squirms in seat
- Often leaves seat in classroom or in other situations in which remaining seated is expected
- Often runs about or climbs excessively in situations in which it is inappropriate (in adolescents or adults, may be limited to subjective feelings of restlessness)
- Often has difficulty playing or engaging in leisure activities quietly
- Is often "on the go" or often acts as if "driven by a motor"
- Often talks excessively

*Impulsivity:*

- Often blurts out answers before questions have been completed
- Often has difficulty awaiting turn
- Often interrupts or intrudes on others (e.g., butts into conversations or games)

B. Some hyperactive-impulsive or inattentive symptoms that caused impairment present before age 7 years

C. Some impairment from symptoms present in two or more settings (e.g., at school [or work] and at home)

D. Clear evidence of clinically significant impairment in social, academic, or occupational functioning

E. The symptoms not occurring exclusively during the course of a pervasive developmental disorder, schizophrenia, or other psychotic disorder and are not better accounted for by another mental disorder (e.g., mood disorder, anxiety disorder, dissociative disorder, or a personality disorder)

*(cont.)*

## BOX 21-3: DIAGNOSTIC CRITERIA FOR ATTENTION-DEFICIT AND DISRUPTIVE BEHAVIOR DISORDERS (*CONT.*)

### CONDUCT DISORDER

A. Repetitive and persistent pattern of behavior involving a violation of the basic rights of others or major age-appropriate societal norms or rules, as manifested by three or more of the following in the past 12 months with at least one present in the past 6 months:
- Aggression to people or animals (bullying, threatening, intimidating; initiating physical fights; using a weapon possible of causing serious physical harm; being physically cruel to people and/or animals; stealing while confronting a victim; forcing someone into sexual activity
- Destruction of property (deliberately engaging in fire setting to cause physical harm; deliberately destroying others' property)
- Deceitfulness or theft (breaking into another's house, building, or car; lying to obtain goods or favors or avoid obligation; stealing of nontrivial-valued items without confronting victim)
- Serious violations of rules (staying out at night despite parental prohibition [beginning before age 13]; running away from home overnight at least twice while living in parental or parental surrogate home; being truant from school before age 13)

B. Clinically significant impairment in social, academic, or occupational functioning.

C. Criteria not met for antisocial personality disorder if age 18 or older.

### OPPOSITIONAL DEFIANT DISORDER

A. Pattern of negativistic, hostile, and defiant behavior lasting at least 6 months, during which four (or more) of the following are present:
- Often loses temper
- Often argues with adults
- Often actively defies or refuses to comply with adults' requests or rules
- Often deliberately annoys people
- Often blames others for his or her mistakes or misbehavior
- Is often touchy or easily annoyed by others
- Is often angry and resentful
- Is often spiteful or vindictive

**Note:** Considered a criterion met only if the behavior occurs more frequently than typically observed in individuals of comparable age and developmental level.

B. The disturbance in behavior leading to clinically significant impairment in social, academic, or occupational functioning

C. The behaviors not occurring exclusively during the course of a psychotic or mood disorder

D. Criteria not met for conduct disorder, and, if the individual is age 18 years or older, criteria not met for antisocial personality disorder

*From American Psychiatric Association. (2000). Diagnostic and statistical manual of mental disorders (4th ed., text revision). Copyright ©, American Psychiatric Association.*

*Conduct disorder involves behavior that violates the rights of others or major societal norms or rules. It typically involves aggressive behavior toward individuals or animals, property destruction, deceitfulness or lying, or serious violations of rules.*

## Oppositional Defiant Disorder

Oppositional defiant disorder (ODD) is similar to CD and often precedes a CD diagnosis. The major difference between the two disorders is that ODD does not include more serious aspects of CD in which the rights of others or age-appropriate societal norms and rules are violated (APA, 2000). Individuals with ODD typically do not display aggression toward people and animals, destroy property, or show a pattern of theft or deceit—characteristics associated with CD. If a child meets the criteria for both CD and ODD, CD becomes the primary diagnosis (APA, 2000).

Rates of ODD range from 2–16% and vary greatly by population (APA, 2000). Like ADHD and CD, the cause of the disorder is not known. Like CD, environmental influence from family, school, and peers has been identified as a strong contributing factor. ODD, as with CD, has an increased prevalence in urban areas. Neurochemical influences are likely contributors but to a lesser degree.

Features of ODD vary with age and development. The most common characteristics appear to be mood lability, low frustration tolerance, swearing, and substance use (APA, 2000). Other common symptoms including running away, truancy, temper tantrums, and fighting (see Box 21-3). Appearance of these symptoms is first noted in the home environment, usually before the age of eight years. Individuals with ODD may not display oppositional behavior in a clinical setting, but behavior may be observed when they interact with a parent or other authority figure.

*Oppositional defiant disorder involves negative, hostile, or defiant behavior usually noted before the child reaches 8 years of age.*

## MOOD DISORDERS

Affective and anxiety disorders fall into the general category of mood disorders and affect children in precise ways. Common mood disorders observed in children include: depression, adjustment disorder, and post-traumatic stress disorder (PTSD).

### Depression

Depressive symptoms in children are often more subtle than adults, because children may be unable to express sadness, hopelessness, and despair in concrete terms. Instead, behaviors such as irritability, difficulty sleeping, social isolation, non-specific somatic complaints (i.e., stomachaches), bad dreams, lack of smiling or laughing, anger, and fighting, may be more significant for childhood depression (Fassler & Dumas, 1997).

The risk for depression in children increases with a family history of depression or other psychiatric disorders, and stressful life events often involving significant changes in family dynamic or lifestyle (Fassler & Dumas, 1997). In addition, childhood depression increases the risk for suicide. Although once believed that children with the inability to understand death could not attempt suicide, it is now realized that children as young as six may attempt suicide as a way to escape painful situations or gain attention, whether or not they truly understand death (Fassler & Dumas, 1997). Younger children may believe that death is temporary or reversible.

The criteria used to diagnose depression in children are the same as those used for adults. The criteria specify continuous symptoms for two weeks. However, children's symptoms often come and go over a period of time (Fassler & Dumas, 1997).

Diagnosing depression in children can be difficult. Some practitioners believe that depression can develop at any time, including in infancy and early childhood, but instead of assigning a diagnosis of depression, terms such as attachment disorder or a generalized failure to thrive may be used. Lack of motor activity, blank facial expression and/or limited eye contact, and excessive or limited crying are key symptoms of depression in infancy (Fassler & Dumas, 1997). However, due to the inability of the infant to describe symptoms, it becomes increasingly important to rule out medical conditions, abuse, or neglect before assuming infant depression. Also, side effects of various medications or an underlying somatic condition can be mistaken for depressive symptoms. The reverse is also true. Therefore, a careful, skilled assessment is important.

## Adjustment Disorder

Adjustment disorder is defined as a psychological response to a stressor resulting in significant emotional or behavioral symptoms (APA, 2000). Common stressors leading to development of adjustment disorder in children include single events such as a friend moving away or parental divorce; recurrent events such as parental substance abuse, peer rejection and bullying; or continuous events, such as living in a high crime neighborhood (Children, Psychology, and Mental Health, 2007). This disorder can occur at any age, and is diagnosed in up to 8% of children and adolescents (APA, 2000). **Box 21-4** highlights the diagnostic criteria for adjustment disorder.

## Post-Traumatic Stress Disorder

Similar to adjustment disorder, post-traumatic stress disorder (PTSD) results from the exposure to a stressor. However, PTSD differs from adjustment disorder in that PTSD is characterized by an extreme stressor with a specific constellation of symptoms, as opposed to any severe stressor and a wide range of possible symptoms associated with adjustment disorder (APA, 2000).

Stressors associated with PTSD must be extreme and traumatic, and must involve exposure to or experience of actual or threatened death or serious injury, threat to one's physical integrity, or witnessing an event that involves death or significant injury. Response to the event involves fear, helplessness, and/or horror, and can be observed as disorganized or agitated behavior in children (APA, 2000).

Events preceding the development of PTSD in children usually involve sexual or physical abuse, natural or manmade disasters, or the witnessing of harm or death to loved ones (APA, 2000). Most younger children experience symptoms similar to those in adults, with some slight differences. Although children may have specific nightmares that repeat the traumatic event, generalized nightmares of monsters or other threats are more common. Rather than verbally describing the repetition of the event, art, or play such as inappropriately touching dolls to suggest sexual abuse, or repetitively crashing play cars together following a car accident are more common. As with other childhood disorders, verbal description of symptoms is not likely, and therefore observation of changes in behavior, somatic complaints, and the waxing and waning of symptoms is common.

---

### Q BOX 21-4: DIAGNOSTIC CRITERIA FOR MOOD DISORDERS

#### ADUSTMENT DISORDER

A. Emotional or behavioral symptoms in response to an identifiable stressor within 3 months of the onset of the stressor

B. Clinically significant symptoms or behavior as evidenced by either of the following:
- Marked distress in excess of what would be expected from stressor exposure
- Significant impairment in social or occupational (academic) functioning

C. Stress-related disturbance not meeting the criteria for another disorder and not an exacerbation of pre-existing disorder.

D. Symptoms not representative of bereavement.

E. Termination of stressor or consequences leading to symptoms not persisting for more than an additional 6 months

Further classified by subtype as with:
- Depressed mood
- Anxiety
- Mixed anxiety/depression
- Conduct disturbance
- Mixed emotional/conduct disturbance
- Unspecified

> *Adjustment disorder and PTSD both result from exposure to a stressor. However, with PTSD, the stressor is extreme and traumatic.*

## FEEDING AND EATING DISORDERS

A small group of disorders in childhood are characterized by persistent feeding and eating disturbances. These are identified in the *DSM-IV-TR* and include: pica, rumination disorder, and feeding disorder of infancy or early childhood. **Box 21-5** highlights the diagnostic criteria for these three disorders. Traditional eating disorders of anorexia and bulimia are extremely rare in children until they reach puberty. (Chapter 19 provides information on these two eating disorders.)

### Pica

PICA is defined as persistent eating of one or more non-nutritive substances for a period of at least one month (APA, 2000; see Box 21-5). It is seen in all ages and cultures. Individuals affected by pica have an abnormal appetite for nonnutritive substances such as clay, soil, chalk, or soap, and may crave substances such as flour, starch, ice cubes, or salt, that most consider food but still carry little nutritional value (Ellis, 2009). The disorder most commonly affects small children, pregnant women, and those with mental retardation, obsessive-compulsive disorder, autism, and/or developmental disabilities. In some instances, the presence of pica is associated with a vitamin or mineral deficiency, where the consumed substance is thought to contain the deficient material (APA, 2000).

The exact prevalence of pica is unknown (Ellis, 2009). However, it has been reported as occurring in as many as 15 percent of those with severe mental retardation (APA, 2000). The disorder is often unrecognized until accompanied by medical sequelae, such as electrolyte disturbances or intestinal obstruction or perforation, or parasitic or bacterial infections. Frequently, intervention by mental health professionals is not involved.

The danger of pica comes with consumption of toxic substances, such as lead paint, metal, or rocks that may contain sharp edges and cause stomach or intestinal damage, and animal droppings or dirt that may contain parasites or harmful bacteria. Diagnostically, the eating of

nonnutritive substances associated with pica must be inappropriate to developmental level, meaning a toddler putting toys in their mouth and attempting to swallow them is not considered pica, even if continues for a month.

> *Pica involves the ingestion of substances such as clay, soil, chalk, soap, flour, starch, ice cubes, or salt, none of which are considered to have any nutritional value.*

### Rumination Disorder

Rumination disorder has existed in clinical documentation since the early 1600s (Olden, 2001). Although initially classified as a disorder for adults, it is now more commonly associated with infants, toddlers, and those with mental retardation or pervasive developmental disorder. Rumination disorder is described as the repeated regurgitation and rechewing of food occurring after a feeding (see Box 21-5). Infants affected by rumination disorder generally display symptoms of irritation and hunger between feedings as a result of malnutrition. Weight loss, failure to thrive, and even death can occur if untreated (APA, 2000).

The vomiting associated with rumination is typically described as unforced and effortless, and not preceded by nausea. Because the food has been recently ingested (within 30 minutes of a meal), it lacks the odor and taste of stomach acid (Chial, Camilleri, & Williams, 2003). Food that has been regurgitated is most commonly chewed and reswallowed, but can also be ejected (APA, 2000).

Generally, rumination is poorly understood. The most widely documented mechanism involves a learned, voluntary relaxation of the lower esophageal sphincter, which allows food to effortlessly pass from the stomach to the mouth. Despite the voluntary relaxation, the overall process of rumination is believed to be psychological in nature, and involuntary (Ellis, 2009). Rumination is commonly misdiagnosed as bulimia. However, the disorders differ based on cause and intention. Although symptoms may appear similar in adolescents, bulimia occurs as a result of a distorted body image, is self-inflicted, and often hidden from others. Rumination is not self-inflicted and affected individuals are generally unable to control the reflex to vomit (LaRocca & Della-Fera, 1986). The disorder is largely thought of as uncommon

> **BOX 21-5: DIAGNOSTIC CRITERIA: FEEDING AND EATING DISORDERS**
>
> ### PICA
>
> A. Persistent eating of nonnutritive substances for a period of at least 1 month
> B. The eating of nonnutritive substances inappropriate to developmental level
> C. The eating behavior not part of a culturally sanctioned practice
> D. If the eating behavior occurs exclusively during the course of another mental disorder (e.g., mental retardation, pervasive developmental disorder, schizophrenia), disorder sufficiently severe to warrant independent clinical attention
>
> ### RUMINATION DISORDER
>
> A. Repeated regurgitation and re-chewing of food for a period of at least 1 month following a period of normal functioning
> B. The behavior not due to an associated gastrointestinal or other general medical condition (e.g., esophageal reflux)
> C. The behavior not occurring exclusively during the course of anorexia nervosa or bulimia nervosa. If the symptoms occur exclusively during the course of mental retardation or a pervasive developmental disorder, it is sufficiently severe to warrant independent clinical attention
>
> ### FEEDING DISORDER OF INFANCY OR EARLY CHILDHOOD
>
> A. Feeding disturbance as manifested by persistent failure to eat adequately with significant failure to gain weight or significant loss of weight over at least 1 month
> B. The disturbance not due to an associated gastrointestinal or other general medical condition (e.g., esophageal reflux)
> C. The disturbance not better accounted for by another mental disorder (e.g., rumination disorder) or by lack of available food
> D. Onset before age 6 years
>
> *From American Psychiatric Association. (2000). Diagnostic and statistical manual of mental disorders, 4th ed., text revision. Copyright ©, American Psychiatric Association.*

and usually spontaneously remits with age and maturity. In severe cases, rumination disorder can be continuous (APA, 2000).

*The vomiting associated with rumination disorder is not self-inflicted and is not under the individual's voluntary control, making it different from the vomiting associated with bulimia nervosa.*

## Feeding Disorder of Infancy or Early Childhood

Significant weight loss or significant failure to gain weight as a result of inadequate eating can be attributed to various causes. Gastrointestinal or other medical conditions, poor living conditions with lack of available food, and malnutrition are some possibilities. The symptoms also may be associated with a psychological feeding disorder.

Approximately 1–5% of pediatric hospital admissions can be attributed to failure to thrive (lack of growth and development at a normal rate); approximately half of those admissions cannot be attributed to any general medical condition (APA, 2000). As a result, psychological issues may be involved. For example, in some cases of feeding disorders, parent-infant interaction is the primary predisposing factor. These interactions may be as innocent as inappropriately presenting food or responding inappropriately to the child's rejection of the food. The child may be unusually temperamental or have preexisting developmental impairments or psychological conditions that can explain the difficulty with feeding. With severe problems in parent-infant interaction, such as parental psychopathology, child abuse, and child neglect, the risk for long-term medical and developmental problems increases (APA, 2000). Most infants and young children diagnosed with feeding disorders experience improved growth over time, although they often remain smaller than normal through adolescence (APA, 2000).

Common symptoms associated with feeding disorders include: irritability and difficulty in consoling during feedings, apathy, withdrawal, and developmental delays (APA, 2000). Children with feeding disorders may also show symptoms of dehydration and malnutrition with associated laboratory findings and possible growth retardation (see Box 21-5 for diagnostic criteria).

## TREATMENT OPTIONS

Various treatment options may be used for childhood disorders. Options include: play therapy, behavioral therapy, cognitive behavioral therapy, family therapy, and psychopharmacology.

### Play Therapy

PLAY THERAPY is a method of psychotherapy that uses fantasy and symbolic meanings expressed during play as a medium for communicating and understanding a child's behavior. It is an effective treatment for a broad range of children's problems from the loss of a pet to PTSD. Play therapy is most commonly seen in treatment of young children with aggressive behavior, self-isolation, and children who have experienced abuse, neglect, or loss of a family member (British Association of Play Therapists, 2007).

The goal of play therapy is to focus on the child as a guide for the course of play, not on the child's presenting problem. In other words, it's not meant to cure a disorder, rather to ease the symptoms that the child finds most difficult in his or her life. Because of this method surrounding the therapy, it can be effective for essentially any child with overwhelming issues the child can't manage on his or her own (British Association of Play Therapists, 2007).

Evidence-Based Practice 21-1 highlights a study evaluating the efficacy of play therapy.

Play therapy requires extensive knowledge of normal developmental and emotional stages and knowledge of behavior and cognition in children. Typical play therapy sessions last around 45 minutes and occur one or two times per week (British Association of Play Therapists, 2007). The therapist or counselor meets with the child alone for sessions and then holds separate sessions to update and inform the parents on progress. Parent meetings are important to gain information on the child's developmental, medical, and social history and the current progress the patients are seeing at home, as well as to assist the parents with communication and parenting techniques.

A session of play therapy is child-lead, that is, the child is told that he or she may play with whatever he or she would like. Because young children don't usually communicate thoughts and feelings verbally until later in childhood, patterns and themes expressed in play will likely express relevant issues better than the child would. Over time, the clinician helps the child to create a meaning when playing, subsequently helping the child handle the difficulties. Play is not guided, and statements made by the child require the clinician to use therapeutic communication techniques such as reflection and validation (British Association of Play Therapists, 2007). Play therapy is a successful treatment option that will often reduce or eliminate presenting problems, as well as improve functioning at school, home, and in social settings.

> *Play therapy provides children with a means of communicating thoughts and feelings that they are unable to put into words.*

### Behavioral Therapy

Operant and classical conditioning techniques described earlier in this chapter provide the foundation for the techniques used in behavioral therapy. Various techniques used include exposure and response, flooding, and systematic desensitization. However, the most commonly used technique is behavior modification, which involves positive and negative reinforcement for good or bad behavior. Positive reinforcement encourages repetition of good

## EVIDENCE-BASED PRACTICE 21-1: EFFICACY OF PLAY THERAPY

### STUDY

Bratton, S.C., Ray, D., Rhine, T., & Jones, L. (2005). The efficacy of play therapy with children: A meta-analytic review. *Professional Psychology: Research and Practice, 36*(4), 376–339.

### SUMMARY

A meta-analysis was conducted to assess the overall efficacy of play therapy, based on criticism that the treatment lacked an adequate research base. A total of 93 controlled outcome studies were reviewed to look at overall efficacy of play therapy, as well as factors that influence the effectiveness. Results revealed that play therapy is a statistically viable intervention regardless of age, gender, and presenting issue, and can be effective in areas of self-concept, behavioral change, cognitive ability, social skills, and anxiety. Humanistic approaches to play therapy (development of self-concept, non-directive) yielded higher outcomes than non-humanistic approaches. Specific factors attributed to success were difficult to identify.

### APPLICATION TO PRACTICE

The meta-analytic review of play therapy outcomes is important for psychiatric-mental health nurses because it shows that play, used correctly and with appropriate patients, is an effective treatment option. It can be difficult to decide how to care for a child with issues of self-concept, social skills, anxiety, or posttraumatic stress disorder. Many therapies require insight and cognitive ability that children do not have, and providers and parents alike are reluctant to use medications on children. There are a limited number of proven approaches for treatment, and play therapy is one of them that is specific to children and their developmental needs. Play therapy is effective across modalities, settings, age and gender, clinical and nonclinical populations, and theoretical schools of thought. Implementing play therapy requires knowledge of which children may benefit and which would not, and skill at carrying out the therapy professionally and correctly.

### QUESTIONS TO PONDER

1. *How might a psychiatric-mental health nurse implement concepts of play therapy without crossing the professional lines of a trained therapist?*
2. *What types of patients may not necessarily benefit from play therapy?*

behavior and negative reinforcement discourages repetition of bad behavior. The technique of behavioral modification is often taught to parents to manage disruptive behavior disorders. Unfortunately, it may not be as useful a technique for depression or anxiety disorders.

## Cognitive Behavioral Therapy

Cognitive behavioral therapy (CBT) is one of the most popular techniques used with children It arose in the second half of the 20th century when behavioral therapy was combined with cognitive therapy (Rachman, 1997). The objective of this therapy is to identify thoughts, assumptions, and beliefs that are related to problematic emotions and further related to dysfunctional behaviors (Rachman, 1997). After the negative thoughts are identified, resulting dysfunctional emotions and behaviors can be replaced with functional ones.

The primary technique of this therapy commonly used with children is journaling of significant events or thoughts with recording of corresponding emotions and behaviors. Depending on the age of the child, art may be used in place of written words using a similar theoretical focus as play therapy. This focus is that the expression of thoughts and feelings at certain ages may be expressed more clearly through art.

## Family Therapy

Using family therapy with mentally ill children can be an extremely useful intervention because it emphasizes the importance of family relationships on a child's psychological state. Conflict within the family, inconsistencies in parenting, impact of the child's mental illness on the family dynamic, and maladaptive coping styles can be addressed during the family therapy session (Bowen, 1978). The broad range of issues addressed makes family therapy an effective treatment approach in almost every category of mental illness.

A typical family therapy course will begin with the therapist meeting with the entire family, parents, siblings, and affected child to get a feeling for how the family interacts at home. Accurate assessment of the family dynamic may require the creation of genograms to analyze roles the family members serve and any existing conflicts that exist within the family unit. Psychoeducation about the identified illness, communication techniques, relationship building, coping techniques, and psychotherapy may be components addressed over the course of family, therapy that can last anywhere from 5 to 20 sessions. The expectation is not that the individual will be cured, but rather that the family will be better able to cope effectively with the situation and solve problems that may occur as a result of poor family dynamics. (See Chapter 9 for a more in-depth discussion of family therapy.)

## Psychopharmacology

Using psychiatric medications in children remains a controversial topic. As more medications are gaining Food and Drug Administration (FDA) approval for use in children, the controversy will likely continue. Growth of psychopharmacology in children is a result of increases in scientific knowledge about behavioral and emotional disorders in children, and the presence of more rigorous scientific studies testing medication use in younger age groups (Connor & Meltzer, 2006). Despite increasing scientific knowledge and outcome studies showing positive results, the controversy continues because there are very limited data on the safety of most medications in children. In most instances, the efficacy and expected side effects with medication use is based on research and experience in adults (Connor & Meltzer, 2006). Currently there are less than 20 medications approved for use among children, with many of them approved only for use in ages 12 and up (Sipress, 2006).

The controversy is further fueled by the beliefs of some holistic parenting groups and providers. They believe that psychiatric medication use in children is never warranted because most behavioral and emotional symptoms are a result of growth and development, not symptomatic of a mental illness. Either way, treatment with psychotropic medications is monumentally more effective when combined with therapy.

Central nervous system stimulants are used to treat children with ADHD. They are the most commonly prescribed agents with certain age restrictions. Examples include methylphenidate (Ritalin, Concerta), amphetamine/dextroamphetamine (Adderall), and atomoxetine (Strattera). **Drug Summary 21-1** highlights these drugs. Additional medications that are prescribed include antidepressants, such as fluoxetine (Prozac) and sertraline (Zoloft); see Chapter 12 for more information. It cannot be stressed enough that combination treatment with medications and therapy will provide significantly better results than medication alone (NIMH, 2009).

> *Central nervous system stimulants are used as treatment for ADHD.*

## Applying the Nursing Process From an Interpersonal Perspective

Children experiencing mental health problems may be seen in a variety of settings, such as acute care settings, day hospitalization programs, community and outpatient facilities, as well as general medical facilities, emergency departments, and specialty clinics. Therefore, nurses need a firm understanding of the nursing process that integrates the interpersonal process when caring for children with mental health disorders.

In addition, nurses need a firm knowledge base about childhood development because different developmental age groups/stages represent a different stage of interpersonal relationship formation as defined by Hildegard Peplau (see Chapter 2 for more information). Peplau, drawing on the work of Sullivan (described earlier in this chapter), identified four age groups: infancy, toddlerhood, early childhood, and late childhood. Each of these groups corresponds with a stage of development, and major developmental tasks in terms of relationships

## DRUG SUMMARY 21-1: DRUGS USED TO TREAT ADHD

| DRUG | IMPLICATIONS FOR THE INTERPERSONAL PROCESS |
|------|---------------------------------------------|
| methylphenidate (Ritalin, Concerta) | • Ensure that parents/child understand how to take the drug, which comes as capsules, tablets, and transdermal patch<br><br>• If the child is using the patch form, instruct the child and parents to apply it to the child's hip and to alternate hips daily<br><br>• Advise the parents and child that the drug may be discontinued periodically after responding to the therapy to assess the child's condition and need for continued therapy<br><br>• Assist parents and child in measures to reduce the risk for insomnia; suggest that the last daily dose of tablet or capsule form be given several hours before bedtime<br><br>• Reinforce need to continue with specific interventions to address ADHD |
| atomoxetine (Strattera)<br><br>amphetamine/dextroamphetamine (Adderall) | • Assist child in understanding that the drug can cause problems with sleeping; work with the child and parents to develop an effective bedtime routine and to take the drug in a single morning dose or in divided half-doses in the morning and late afternoon or early evening<br><br>• Encourage the parents to monitor the child for changes in mood and behavior<br><br>• Urge parents to provide nutritious meals and snacks, including possible supplementation to help minimize or prevent weight loss<br><br>• Suggest small frequent meals to reduce risk of gastrointestinal upset<br><br>• Inform the parents that drug has been associated with unusual changes in behavior (increased irritability, agitation) and suicidal thinking; encourage parents to monitor the child closely for changes and to contact the prescriber immediately if any occur<br><br>• Reinforce need to continue with specific interventions to address ADHD<br><br>• Ensure that parents/child understand how to take the drug; work with them to develop a schedule that works best for the child |

*(cont.)*

**DRUG SUMMARY 21-1: (*CONT.*)**
**DRUGS USED TO TREAT ADHD**

| DRUG | IMPLICATIONS FOR THE INTERPERSONAL PROCESS |
|------|--------------------------------------------|
| atomoxetine (Strattera)<br><br>amphetamine/dextroam-phetamine (Adderall) | • Urge parents and child not to administer the drug in the evening because it may interfere with sleep<br><br>• Advise the parents and child that the drug may be discontinued periodically after responding to the therapy to assess the child's condition and need for continued therapy<br><br>• Encourage continued adherence to follow-up appointmentsto monitor the child's growth and weight<br><br>• Inform parents that drug has been associated with unusual changes in behavior (increased irritability, agitation) and suicidal thinking; encourage parents to monitor the child closely for changes and to contact the prescriber immediately if any occur<br><br>• Reinforce need to continue with specific interventions to address ADHD |

with others (Peplau, 1991). These age groups and tasks are summarized in **Table 21-5**. For example, late childhood typically involves children between the ages of six to nine, an age that frequently corresponds with diagnosis of ADHD. In this stage, the child begins to develop skills of participation by learning to compromise, compete, and cooperate (Peplau, 1991). According to Peplau, how the child will progress through illness and treatment can be correlated to the stage of personality development. Thus, the psychological tasks related to the stages of personality development can be viewed as developmental lessons required for maturity. Although this section uses ADHD as an example, the concepts can be individualized to apply to any childhood disorder.

## Strategies for Optimal Assessment: Therapeutic Use of Self

During the assessment phase, the nurse implements a therapeutic use of self (an ability to understand and interpret one's own behavior, in order to understand the dynamics of others' behavior (Truvelbee, 1971). The nurse integrates this understanding to facilitate recognizing a problem, so that an accurate assessment of the child's needs can be made. Various techniques can be used to develop a therapeutic relationship with the child and the family. **Therapeutic Interaction 21-1** provides

**TABLE 21-5: PEPLAU'S AGE GROUPS AND DEVELOPMENTAL TASKS**

| AGE GROUP | DEVELOPMENTAL TASK |
|-----------|--------------------|
| Infancy | Reliance on others |
| Toddlerhood | Delay of satisfaction |
| Early childhood | Self-identification |
| Late childhood | Skill development for participation |

an example of an interaction between the nurse and the mother of a child who has oppositional defiant disorder.

During assessment, the nurse needs to demonstrate current knowledge about causes, symptoms, and treatments to help facilitate trust. This knowledge also provides the nurse with a framework for identifying key signs and symptoms in the child. Additionally, the nurse needs to investigate which symptoms are most distressing as well as those that interfere with the child's daily functioning. For example, a child in the late childhood stage of interpersonal development begins to view him- or herself through the eyes of their peers. If the child is experiencing ADHD, behaviors such as fidgeting or squirming, difficulty playing or engaging in leisure activities, excessive talking, difficulty awaiting turn, and interrupting others may begin to negatively influence a child's relationship with siblings and peers.

**THERAPEUTIC INTERACTION 21-1:**
**WORKING WITH THE MOTHER OF A SON WHO HAS OPPOSITIONAL DEFIANT DISORDER**

J. is a 10-year-old male recently diagnosed with oppositional defiant disorder (ODD) after a few years of disruptive behavior, and most recently a fight at school resulting in suspension. His mother felt he was getting too out of control and decided to admit him to a child/adolescent psychiatry unit for stabilization and respite. Staff felt that medications were not indicated and instead implemented a behavioral plan. The RN is helping J.'s mom prepare to take him home.

| | |
|---|---|
| **RN:** "Hello, my name is M., and I am an RN on the unit. I have been caring for J. over the past few days." | Introduction and declaration of role |
| **Mom:** "Hi, I hope J. hasn't been too much of a problem. I just didn't know what to do with him anymore." | Embarrassment of child's behavior, some guilt present with justification for bringing him to the hospital—common in parents of children with behavioral disorders |
| **RN:** "It sounds like it has been a difficult time. J. has been doing well here and has not been a problem." | Validation, empathy, as well as providing some reassurance that her son is capable of good behavior. Beginning to build trust |
| **Mom:** "Oh, thank goodness, but I still don't know what I should do at home." | Relief, hope |
| **RN:** "If you would find it helpful, I can help you understand how we have been working with J. on his behavior." | Offering self, working on establishing trust, but avoiding any judgment or negative terms |
| **Mom:** "That would be wonderful, thank you for taking time to help me." | Starting to feel connection and build trust with the nurse |
| **RN:** "This is something you can do at home with J., and it has been working well here. It is called a (Behavioral Plan). It rewards J.'s good behavior and discourages negative behavior." | Putting behavioral modification strategies into simple terms, avoiding complicated explanation |
| **Mom:** "Well, I try to do that at home, but nothing seems to work." | Displaying some continued frustration and justification about parenting, feeling that she has done something wrong (this is common) |
| **RN:** "It sounds like it has been frustrating for you and that you've been doing your best. What kinds of things does J. enjoy doing at home?" | Validation, support; redirection to focus on J., looking for tools to use in behavioral plan |

*(cont.)*

**THERAPEUTIC INTERACTION 21-1:** (*CONT.*)
**WORKING WITH THE MOTHER OF A SON WHO HAS OPPOSITIONAL DEFIANT DISORDER**

| | |
|---|---|
| **Mom:** "Well, he loves his bike, and his video games…but I don't like him to play it too much. He's also on a baseball team." | Continued justification |
| **RN:** "Those are all good things we can use to develop a plan for him. With this behavioral plan, you can give him (tokens) to reward good behavior, and take the tokens back for negative behavior. You can choose together what you would like to use as your tokens." | Validation—often more necessary to continuously validate parents displaying high amounts of "guilt" with justifying action. Avoiding using the word "bad"<br><br>Education for developing behavioral plan. |
| **Mom:** "Okay, that sounds simple, but I don't really understand." | Seeking clarification. |
| **RN:** "Let's see if I can make it clearer. Some parents choose to put M&Ms in a jar each time their child demonstrate good behavior. When the M&Ms add to a certain number, he gains a reward such as more time on his bike." | Providing an example to help clarify concept in simple terms, using mother's words in example |
| **Mom:** "Oh, I see, so if he gets 20 M&Ms he gets 20 extra minutes on his bike?" | Further clarification, beginning to understand |
| **RN:** "Yes, that's a great example. For negative behaviors, M&Ms can be taken out of the jar and may indicate loss of privileges, such as the video game time." | Encouragement, validation, continued explanation |
| **Mom:** "Wow—that has really been working with him? I can certainly do it at home; it sounds so easy!" | Some surprise at effectiveness, but relief and hope about implementing |
| **RN:** "It works quite well with J., and you can definitely do it at home. You and J. can work together to develop the plan, and even pick the rewards together." | Continued encouragement, reassurance of plan working. Suggestion to spend time individually with J.—this will also help him invest in the plan |
| **Mom:** "Oh gosh, maybe I'll tell him that at 50 M&Ms, he can get a new baseball glove! He would be so happy about that." | Excitement, understanding, and building confidence |

*(cont.)*

**THERAPEUTIC INTERACTION 21-1: (*CONT.*)**
**WORKING WITH THE MOTHER OF A SON WHO HAS OPPOSITIONAL DEFIANT DISORDER**

| | |
|---|---|
| **RN:** "That sounds like a great idea! J. can go home today; you can work together developing your plan, and begin using it as soon as tonight." | Validating, solidification of confidence and mom's ability to implement |
| **Mom:** "I can't wait to take him home and work on this. Thank you." | Resolution, confidence |

Another key aspect of assessment is self-awareness on the part of the nurse. The nurse needs to be aware of how he or she may respond to a child who is hyperactive or impulsive or one who is willfully destructive or continually defiant and hostile. These behaviors can engender strong negative feelings in others, including the nurse. Therefore, the nurse needs to identify these feelings and how they might interfere with the therapeutic relationship.

## Diagnosing and Planning Appropriate Interventions: Meeting the Patient's Focused Needs

After completing the assessment, the nurse, child, and family proceed to develop a plan of care with mutual goals and expectations for outcomes. The nurse can help the patient identify his or her needs and specific problems and begin a plan for recovery (Peplau, 1991). For example, target outcomes for a child with ADHD should address multiple areas: social skills, education, self-esteem, and motivation (American Academy of Pediatrics [AAP], 2001).

Due to the wide range of assessment findings noted in and multiple problems faced by children with mental health disorders, numerous nursing diagnoses would apply. Examples of possible nursing diagnoses for the child with ADHD would include:

- Risk for injury related to impulsive behavior
- Impaired social interaction related to intrusive behavior
- Noncompliance with task expectations related to short attention span
- Chronic low self-esteem related to impaired social and familial support system

Based on the identified nursing diagnoses, the nurse, child, and parents collaboratively determine the outcomes to be achieved. For the child with ADHD, improvement in three to six behaviors is recommended initially and should include how the behavior is measured and what denotes success for the outcome. An example of an outcome for the child would be that he or she exhibits a decreased frequency of disruptive behaviors in peer groups.

> *A thorough understanding of childhood development is necessary when conducting an assessment of a child with a mental health disorder.*

## Implementing Effective Interventions: Timing and Pacing

Implementing mutually decided upon interventions again requires a therapeutic use of self. It is increasingly important during this stage that the timing and pacing of interventions meets expectations and abilities of the child, the family, and the provider. For the child with ADHD, stimulant medications or specific behavioral therapy may be instituted. Most children in the age range of 6 to 12 years respond favorably to stimulant medication use. However, it is not appropriate for every child with ADHD symptoms (AAP, 2001). The decision to use medication should be based on clinical judgment as well as the family beliefs and preferences. Behavioral modification therapy alone or in conjunction with medication is an effective treatment for ADHD.

Psychoeducation is a key intervention. The child and family need information about the disorder and how best to manage it. **Patient and Family Education 21-1** provides some helpful suggestions. The family also needs reliable information to dispel any myths or controversies associated with the child's disorder. **Box 21-6** provides information about the role of food additives in ADHD.

**PATIENT AND FAMILY EDUCATION 21-1:**
**IMPLEMENTING A BEHAVIORAL MODIFICATION PLAN USING A TOKEN REWARDS SYSTEM**

- Use positive reinforcement to encourage continued repetition of good behavior. Use negative reinforcement for discouragement of bad behavior.

- To develop the plan, decide the theme together. Use your imagination and that of your child to make it fun and he or she is more likely to invest in and follow the plan. Together, decide what you will use as "tokens." You can use M&Ms in a jar, stickers on a chart, checkmarks, points, or whatever you decide.

- Every time a positive behavior is demonstrated (completing chores, good grade on an assignment, saying a nice thing, etc.), add a token. Every time a negative behavior is demonstrated (hitting, swearing, talking back, etc.), take a token away.

- Be creative in deciding rewards. One reward may be 10 tokens equals 10 extra minutes outside playing. Make sure the rewards are realistic and reachable. The plan will not work if your child has to obtain 500 tokens for 10 extra minutes of outside time.

- Depending on age and maturity of the child, allow him or her to keep building tokens to gain bigger rewards. For example, 100 tokens equals a new baseball glove.

- The older child could use points how they want, so if they have 20 tokens, they can use 10 for some extra time outside, but save the other 10 to work toward the baseball glove. Again, make sure the reward can be produced.

- Younger kids may need smaller, more frequent rewards to stay interested. It is also a good idea to start with smaller and more frequent rewards at the beginning of any plan to build understanding and make the child want to continue following the plan.

- Set daily limits for negative reinforcement if the positive reinforcement doesn't seem to be doing enough. For example, 10 tokens removed in one day for bad behavior equals 10 less minutes of video game time.

- Be consistent! Hitting a sibling and removal of 5 tokens one day cannot turn into hitting a sibling and removal of 10 tokens the next day. The child will get confused and frustrated, and likely quit following the plan altogether. Make the expectations clear.

Throughout this phase, interventions are designed to help a child and family develop problem-solving skills to reach appropriate resolution. A child with ADHD in this stage of interpersonal/personality development must use interventions to help develop skills of competition, compromise, cooperation, consensual validation, and love of self and others.

## Evaluating: Objective Critique of Interventions and Self-Reflection

The nurse evaluates how much progress has been made toward achieving expected outcomes. For any goals not met, the nurse needs to self-reflect on anything he or she may have done differently while providing nursing care.

During this phase of the nurse-patient relationship, the nurse, child, and parents should reflect on progress made toward reaching the patient goals. Point out positives to the patient and family and include a plan for aftercare as appropriate. For example, the child with ADHD who is successful learns to participate collaboratively with others, demonstrating compromise, competition, and cooperation (Sullivan, 1953). If the initial treatment plan does not meet outcomes, the plan needs to be reevaluated to determine why, and appropriate changes must be made. Evaluation should include initial diagnosis, appropriateness of treatments, adherence to the treatment plan, and the possibility of co-existing conditions. In the case of the child with ADHD, if therapy alone was the family's choice, medication or a different form of therapy may need to be considered. If medication is not useful, trials of two to

---

**BOX 21-6: MYTH OR FACT: CAN ADHD BE CURED BY CHANGING A CHILD'S DIET?**

It has been suggested that particular food additives, namely certain food dyes and preservatives, are associated with the hyperactivity component of ADHD in children. In 2007, a study conducted in the United Kingdom found varying degrees of hyperactivity in children after they consumed a fruit drink containing a mixture of food dyes and preservatives. Because the study was unable to determine which dyes or preservatives may have been associated with the hyperactivity, and the study was not limited to children with ADHD, the U.S. Food and Drug Administration (FDA) declined to post a formal warning (Hoecker, 2008).

Most researchers speculate that ADHD is due to a combination of changes in the structure of the brain as well as particular environmental factors, largely ignoring the question of food additives. Some providers will suggest eliminating certain foods if a parent feels that they are affecting the child's behavior, while others will use diet changes as an initial intervention in ADHD children before prescribing stimulant medications. Research in this area will likely grow significantly in the near future, with results that could change current practice standards.

---

three different medications should be completed before considering a different class of medication (AAP, 2001).

Systematic follow-up and monitoring is important to assess continued progress toward target outcomes. Information continues to be gathered from parents, teachers, and the child. Additionally, ongoing and consistent communication between involved parties is incredibly important to accurately assess progress (AAP, 2001).

---

**SUMMARY POINTS**

- Theories related to growth and development include: Piaget's theory of cognitive development, Erikson's theory of emotional and personality development, Freud's theory of psychosexual development, Sullivan's theory of interpersonal and personality development, and the behavioral theories of Pavlov and Skinner.

- Autistic disorder and Asperger's disorder are the two most common pervasive developmental disorders. A child with autistic disorder exhibits significant impairment in social interactions and communication, with repetitive and restricted behavior before the age of three years. A child with Asperger's disorder does not experience the significant early delay in cognitive and language skills and preoccupation with objects or rituals.

- Attention-deficit hyperactivity disorder (ADHD) is diagnosed once a child starts school and experiences problems with adjustment to the school environment.

- A child with conduct disorder (CD) is often diagnosed with oppositional defiant disorder (ODD) first. Environmental influences from family, school, and peers seem to play a key role in the development of both disorders.

- Mood disorders in children include affective disorders of depression, and anxiety disorders of adjustment disorder and post-traumatic stress disorder (PTSD).

- Feeding and eating disorders in children include: pica, rumination disorder, and feeding disorder of infancy and early childhood. In some cases of feeding

*(cont.)*

## SUMMARY POINTS (*CONT.*)

disorders, parent-infant interaction is the primary predisposing factor.

- Play therapy is commonly used to treat a wide range of mental health problems in children. It helps to ease the symptoms that the child finds most difficult.

- Other treatment options include: behavioral therapy, cognitive

behavioral therapy, family therapy, and psychopharmacology.

- Caring for the child with a mental health problem requires a thorough understanding of growth and development, and collaboration with the child and family to establish an appropriate course of action.

## NCLEX-PREP*

1. A nurse is observing the behavior of an 18-month-old child. The child is playing with a toy that involves placing different shaped blocks into the appropriately shaped opening. The child is attempting to place a round block into the round hole. The nurse interprets this as indicating which of the following?

 a. Circular reaction
 b. Object permanence
 c. Symbolic play
 d. Magical thinking

2. The following tasks reflect the stages of growth and development as identified by Sullivan. Place them in the order in which they would occur beginning with infancy.

 a. Self-identity development
 b. Delayed gratification
 c. Same-sex relationships
 d. Oral gratification
 e. Opposite-sex relationships
 f. Peer relationships

3. The nurse is working with the parents of a child with a mental health problem in developing a system of rewards and punishments for the child's behavior. The nurse is demonstrating integration of which theorist?

 a. Freud
 b. Pavlov

 c. Skinner
 d. Erikson

4. A nurse is interviewing a child diagnosed with a conduct disorder. Which of the following would the nurse expect to assess?

 a. Repetitive, stereotypical behaviors
 b. Difficulty organizing tasks
 c. Lack of follow-through with directions
 d. Bullying behaviors

5. A child is diagnosed with ADHD. When reviewing the child's history, which of the following would the nurse expect to find?

 a. Exposure to a traumatic event
 b. Difficulty engaging in quiet leisure activities
 c. Frequent losses of temper
 d. Previous diagnosis of oppositional defiant disorder

6. A group of nursing students is reviewing information about adjustment disorders in children. The students demonstrate a need for additional study when they identify which of the following as a possible stressor?

 a. Witness to the death of a parent
 b. Moving away of a close friend
 c. Parental divorce
 d. Bullying by a classmate

*Answers to these questions appear on page 639.

# REFERENCES

American Academy of Pediatrics, (2001). Clinical practice guideline: Treatment of the school-aged child with Attention-Deficit/Hyperactivity Disorder. *Pediatrics, 108*(4), 1033–1044.

American Psychiatric Association. (2000). *Diagnostic and statistical manual of mental disorders (4th ed., text revision)*. Arlington, VA: Author.

Bagley, C., & Mallick, K. (2000). Prediction of sexual, emotional and physical maltreatment and mental health outcomes. *Child Maltreatment, 5*(3), 218–226.

Bornstein, M.H., & Lamb, M.E. (1999). *Developmental psychology (4th ed.)*. Mahwah, NJ: Lawrence Erlbaum Associates.

Bowen, M. (1978). *Family therapy in clinical practice*. New York: Jason Aronson.

British Association of Play Therapists. (2007). *A history of play therapy*. Retrieved on August 30, 2009 from: http://www.bapt.info/historyofpt.htm

Chial, H.J., Camilleri, M., & Williams, D.E. (2003). Rumination syndrome in children and adolescents: Diagnosis, treatment, and prognosis. *Pediatrics, 111*(1), 158–162.

Children, Psychology, and Mental Health. (2007). *Adjustment disorders in children and adolescents*. Retrieved on November 2, 2009 from: http://www.children-psychology-and-mental-health.com/adjustment.html

Connor, D.F., & Meltzer, B.M. (2006). *Pediatric psychopharmacology: Fast facts*. New York, NY: W.W. Norton & Company.

Dalton, P., Deacon, R., & Blamire, A. (2003). Maternal neuronal antibodies associated with autism and a language disorder. *Annals of Neurology, 53*(4), 533–537.

Ellis, C.R. (2009). Eating disorder, pica, rumination. *Pediatrics: Developmental and Behavioral on eMedicine.com*. Retrieved on November 14, 2009 from: http://emedicine.medscape.com/article/914765-overview./index.html

Fassler, D.G., & Dumas, L.S. (1997). *Help me, I'm sad*. Harmondsworth, England: Penguin Books.

Foley, D.L., Eaves, L.J., Wormley, B., Silberg, J.L., Maes, H.H., Kuhn, J., Riley, B., (2004). Childhood adversity, monoamine oxidase a genotype, and risk for conduct disorder. *Archives of General Psychiatry, 61*(7), 738–744.

Gupta, V.B. (2004). *Autistic spectrum disorders in children*. London: Informa Health Care Publishing.

Hitti, M. (2009). Vaccine court rejects autism claims. WebMD. Retrieved January 16, 2012 from http://webmd.com/binior/autism/news/20090212/naccine-court-rejects-autism-claims

Hoecker, J.L. (2008). Can special diets help children who have autism. Retrieved January 16, 2012 from http://mayoclinic.com/health/autism-treatment/AN01519

Ladd, G.W. (1999). Peer relationships and social competence during early and middle childhood. *Annual Review of Psychology, 50*, 333–359.

LaRocca, F.E., & Della-Fera, M.A. (1986). Rumination: Its significance in adults with bulimia nervosa. *Psychosomatics, 27*(3), 209–212.

Londrie, K. (2006). *History of ADHD*. Retrieved August 23, 2009 from: http://ezinearticles.com/Historyof ADHD&id=217254

Merkel, H. (2006). The trouble with Aspergers Syndrome. *Medscape Pediatrics, 8*(1). Retrieved on August 20, 2009 from: http://www.medscape.com/viewarticle/529208

National Alliance on Mental Illness. (2008). *Early onset schizophrenia*. Retrieved on August 20, 2009 from: http://www.nami.org/Template.cfm?Section=by_illness &template=/ContentManagement/ContentDisplay.cfm&ContentID=10430

National Institutes of Mental Health. (2001). *Childhood-onset schizophrenia: An update from the National Institutes of Mental Health*. Rockville, MD: U.S. Department of Health and Human Services.

National Institutes of Mental Health. (2002). *Mental health: A report of the Surgeon General—Executive summary*. Rockville, MD: U.S. Department of Health and Human Services.

National Institutes of Mental Health. (2008). *The numbers count: Mental disorders in America*. Rockville, MD: U.S. Department of Health and Human Services.

National Institutes of Mental Health. (2009). *What medications are used to treat ADHD?* Rockville, MD: U.S. Department of Health and Human Services.

Newschaffer, C.J., Croen, L.A., Daniels, J., Giarelli, E., Grether, J.K., Levy, S.E., Mandell, D.S.,…Windham, G.C. (2007). *The epidemiology of the autism spectrum disorders. Annual Review of Public Health, 28*, 235–258.

Olden, K.W. (2001). Rumination. *Current Treatment Options in Gastroenterology, 4*(4), 351–358.

Peplau, H.E. (1991). *Interpersonal relations in nursing*. New York: Springer.

Popper, C.W., Gammon, G.D., West, S.A., & Bailey, C.E. (2003). Disorders usually first diagnosed in infancy, childhood, or adolescence. In R.E. Hales & S.C. Yudofsky. *Textbook of clinical psychiatry* (4th ed.). Washington, DC: American Psychiatric Publishing.

Rachman, S. (1997). A cognitive theory of obsessions. *Behaviour Research and Therapy, 36*(4), 385–401.

Rioch, D.M. (1985). Recollections of Harry Stack Sullivan and of the development of his interpersonal psychiatry. *Psychiatry, 48*(2), 141–158.

Sadock, B., & Sadock, V. (2007). *Kaplan and Sadock's synopsis of psychiatry (10th ed.)*. New York: Lippincott Williams & Wilkins.

Sipress, R. (2006). *Psychiatric medications for children and adolescents*. Department of Human Services: Oregon. Retrieved on November 2, 2009 from: http://www.oregon.gov/DHS/ mentalhealth/child-mh-soc-in-plan-grp/subcommittees/csac/psych-med4child-adol.pdf

Sullivan, H.S. (1953). *Interpersonal theory of psychiatry*. New York: William-Frederick Press.

Travelbee, J. (1971). *Interpersonal aspects of nursing*. Philadelphia: F.A. Davis Company.

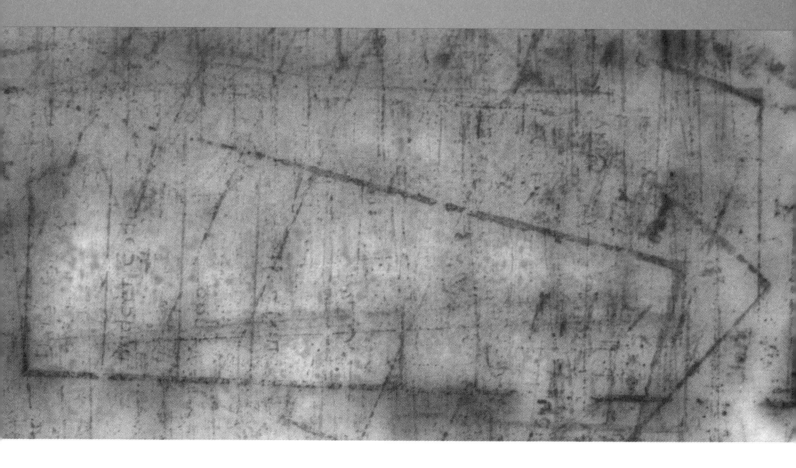

## CHAPTER CONTENTS

# CHAPTER 22
# MENTAL HEALTH CONCERNS REGARDING ADOLESCENTS

Áine Horgan

## EXPECTED LEARNING OUTCOMES

**After completing this chapter, the student will be able to:**

1. Discuss the major concepts associated with adolescent development.

2. Identify normative versus non-normative behavioral patterns in terms of developmental milestones for an adolescent.

3. Describe the major areas to address when assessing an adolescent.

4. Identify the common mental health problems found in the adolescent population.

5. Apply the nursing process from an interpersonal perspective that addresses the care of adolescents with mental health problems.

## KEY TERMS

Binge drinking

Compulsions

Obsessions

Adolescence is characterized by a period of transition from childhood through puberty and on into adulthood. This transition brings with it physical and emotional challenges and is part of normal growth and development. During this period, the social world begins to have a greater influence and the importance of peers becomes evident. This transition period is taking longer than it did 50 years ago, with some suggesting that adolescence now extends into the mid or late 20s (Briggs, 2008). When problems occur in adolescence, particularly mental health problems, they often can be dismissed as part of normal development. Thus, appropriate intervention may not be offered. There is a perception that time will heal mental health problems in adolescents and they will "grow out" of the problem as they proceed into adulthood. However, it is important to highlight that many difficulties experienced by adolescents transcend into adulthood without appropriate intervention.

In the United States, up to 20% of children and adolescents are experiencing a mental illness (Demyttenaere et al., 2004). Furthermore, studies reveal that approximately 58.1% of those between the ages of 12 and 17 years in the United States had screened positive for at least one cluster of symptoms related to a psychiatric disorder (Chen et al., 2005). Adolescents in other countries are also at high risk for mental health problems. For example, in Australia the prevalence of mental health problems is greater among 16 to 24 year olds than any other group across the lifespan (Australian Bureau of Statistics, 2007).

When problems in adolescence are not identified and treated, lifelong problems that may have serious consequences often result (WHO, 2003). In addition, stigma still surrounds the issue of mental health. This is particularly evident in adolescents, as they are searching for self-identity and trying to feel accepted by their peers. This commonly results in many adolescents failing to seek professional help.

This chapter reviews adolescent growth and development, including the important role of peer relationships, and describes important areas to be included in the assessment. The chapter addresses the most common disorders associated with this population and concludes with a discussion of the nursing process from an interpersonal perspective related to the care of an adolescent with a mental health problem.

## ADOLESCENT DEVELOPMENT

The beginning of adolescence is unclear; however, it is generally associated with the onset of puberty. Adolescence is characterized emotionally as a period of searching for self-identity, finding meaning in life, and forming a unique personality separate from those of one's parents. It is a time of external conflict with those in authority and internal conflict with the adolescent struggling with life meaning. Adolescence is a time where confidence and self-esteem can develop or diminish. Conflict with parents is common and often centers on authority, autonomy, and responsibility. This conflict, however, is necessary to prepare adolescents for conflict resolution in later life.

Many theories and models attempt to explain the stages of development experienced by individuals. (See Chapter 21 for additional information on theories of growth and development.) One of the most common theories is that of Erik Erikson (1968), in which he describes the identity crisis that adolescents face. During this crisis, adolescents attempt to discern who they are as they are faced with new feelings, a new body, and a new attitude. Their self-identity is built out of their perceptions of themselves and their relationships with others. Erikson argues that if they do not develop their own self-identity, then role confusion results.

## Puberty and Self-Esteem

One of the major changes experienced by adolescents is puberty. Puberty is characterized by change and development in bodily functions. It usually begins around the age of 10, initially signaled with a growth spurt that continues into the late teenage years. During this time, young people compare themselves to others in terms of appearance and intellect. Sexual awareness also develops, which is often associated with increased self-awareness, which can affect self-esteem.

Self-esteem is important to overall well-being and has been associated with mental health problems in later life. Indeed, low self-esteem is associated with depression, eating disorders, and anxiety problems in adolescents. Levels of self-esteem change during adolescence, with it usually increasing with sexual maturity, but with the multitude of changes that happen during this period, healthy self-esteem may not develop until young adulthood.

## Peer Relationships

Peer relationships develop in young children and play a significant role in overall development. As children become older and transition into adolescence, they spend more and more time with their peers. These relationships strongly influence an adolescent's development. Peer group membership can have a negative effect. For example, lack of acceptance by a peer group can lead to low self-esteem, a decrease in academic performance, and social rejection (Veronneau et al., 2010). In addition, peer group influence can lead adolescents to engage in delinquency and anti-social behaviors (Gifford-Smith et al., 2005). Moreover, the absence of supportive peer relationships can lead to young people living in a state of anxiety or fear, depression, or isolation. Research studies addressing peer relationships in adolescence suggest that stable peer relationships are related to high self-esteem (Black & McCartney, 1997) and that peer attachment may predict life satisfaction in adolescence (Ma & Huebner, 2008). Peer support was reported as protective against depressive symptoms if parental support was also present (Young et al., 2005), whereas peer rejection predicted the onset of depressive symptoms (Witvliet et al., 2010).

Today, peer relationships are becoming more and more important related to the decline in the traditional family system. The numbers of single-parent families and mothers working outside the home have increased. Thus, adolescents are spending increased time with their peers. In addition, technological advances have led to more young people spending more time on computers and less time interacting face to face with their peers. This lack of physical interaction may lead to isolation from the community, resulting in adolescents failing to receive the necessary support to cope with the turbulence of this time of life. Adolescent participation in using social networking websites has dramatically increased, leading more and more young people to communicate previously on the internet. The long-term effects of this are unknown. However, early studies have indicated that it may affect self-esteem, both positively and negatively (Valkenburg et al., 2006). This increased use also has raised growing concern about adolescents being targeted by sexual predators online (Ybarra & Mitchell, 2008).

> *The development of self-esteem and identity are important developmental tasks in adolescence. Peer relationships play a major role in achieving these tasks.*

## ADOLESCENT ASSESSMENT

Assessment, essential to any patient and plan of care, must consider the needs of both the individual adolescent and his or her family. More than one meeting may be needed to fully assess the adolescent's needs and gain an accurate understanding of the problems.

While the involvement of family is essential, assessing the adolescent, individually and by him- or herself, is important because there may be difficulties within the family. As a result, the adolescent may feel uncomfortable sharing information with the family present. In addition, meeting the adolescent alone can help foster the nurse-patient relationship and build trust. Many adolescents may be ambivalent about the difficulties they are facing or fear becoming stigmatized. Or they may be unable to articulate their problems or have issues with authoritative figures. Therefore, sensitivity is a major consideration.

When interviewing the adolescent individually, use appropriate language, remembering that the adolescent is neither a young child nor an adult. The adolescent is the primary concern and development of a therapeutic relationship is needed. Throughout the assessment, listen to the adolescent's view of the problem and try to understand the problem from his or her frame of reference. Direct the questions to obtain information about how the difficulties are interfering with his or her life and how he or she is coping in school (if attending). Ascertain the quality of the relationships with peers and family members. In addition, determine the adolescent's support system, the history of the difficulties, and any drug and alcohol use. To help focus the assessment, use the following questions as a guide:

- *How is he/she engaging with the assessment; are they forthcoming*: "How are you feeling about these questions?"
- *What makes him/her feel anxious, happy, sad*: "What types of things make you happy? Sad? Upset?"
- *What is his/her perception of their family*: "How do you view your family?"
- *How does he/she use leisure time*: "What do you do for fun? For relaxation?"
- *How does he/she view him-/herself*: "How do you picture yourself?"
- *Can he/she easily express his/her feelings*: "How do you express your feelings? Do you talk about things? Do you keep things to yourself?"
- *Does he/she want things to change*: "When you look at your life, is there anything that you would like to change?"
- *How does he/she want things to change*: "You mentioned wanting to change_____. How would you go about changing this?"

Assessment of the adolescent must include a family history addressing information on pregnancy, birth and early health history, medical history, school history, and family health problems. In conducting a family assessment, keep in mind that each family is different and has its own set of norms and internal dynamics. Identify the parenting style of the family (authoritative, coercive, ambivalent, or abusive) and determine if and how it may be influencing the adolescent's behavior or mood.

Using the information from the assessment helps to identify what the adolescent's strengths are, if the adolescent meets the diagnostic criteria for a clinical syndrome, and what intervention may be necessary.

> *Assessment of an adolescent requires sensitivity and use of appropriate language to determine the adolescent's view of the problem from his or her frame of reference.*

## COMMON MENTAL HEALTH PROBLEMS IN ADOLESCENCE

Adolescents can experience many of the mental health problems experienced by adults. However, some are more common, including depression, mania, self-harm, suicidal ideation, alcohol and drug use, eating disorders, and anxiety disorders such as obsessive compulsive disorder. These disorders will be addressed briefly here. (Refer to Chapters 12, 15, 19, and 13, respectively, for more in-depth discussions.)

Some adolescent mental health problems are classified in the *Diagnostic and Statistical Manual of Mental Disorder*, *4th edition, Text Revision* (*DSM-IV-TR*, American Psychiatric Association [APA], 2000) and the *International Classification of Diseases, 10th edition* (*ICD 10*, World Health Organization [WHO],1992). However, adult classifications are used for most illnesses. While both manuals have a section on problems in childhood and adolescence, the focus is on childhood and, in particular, on conduct and behavioral disorders. Although the *DSM-IV-TR* states that it outlines illnesses that are usually first diagnosed in infancy, childhood, and adolescence, it argues that it is not suggesting that there is a clear difference between childhood and adult problems.

Many factors can influence the development of adolescent mental health problems, including adolescent pregnancy, socioeconomic disadvantage, bullying, and abuse and neglect. **Box 22-1** highlights some of the common forms of abuse. These difficulties can lead to a variety of emotional problems manifested by similar signs and symptoms. Therefore, avoiding assumptions and recognizing the signs are of the utmost importance.

> *Adolescents often experience mental health disorders that are the same as those in adults. Depression, mania, self-harm, suicidal ideation, alcohol and drug use, eating disorders, and anxiety disorders, such as obsessive compulsive disorder, are common in adolescence.*

### BOX 22-1: ADOLESCENT ABUSE: SIGNS AND SYMPTOMS

Abuse in adolescence may take several forms. It can range from bullying in school and by peer groups to sexual and physical abuse at home and by significant others.

- *Bullying:* Adolescents are usually bullied due to appearance or social status. Cyber bullying is becoming very common, with almost 50% of middle school and high school students reporting being bullied in this way (Mishna, et. al., 2010). Signs of bullying may include: fear, anxiety, depression, social withdrawal, decreased self-esteem, and talk of revenge.
- *Sexual abuse:* Signs of sexual abuse in adolescents may include: decreased self-esteem, social withdrawal, nightmares, changes in school performance, violence toward others, shame, guilt, and alcohol and drug use.
- *Physical abuse:* Signs of physical abuse may include: aggression, deviancy, fear of adults, disruptive behavior, going to school early and leaving late, fearlessness, risk taking, being described as "accident prone," low academic achievement, wearing clothes that cover most of the body, decreased maturity, regression, and dislike of physical contact.

## Depression

Depressive disorders are widely recognized as one of the priority disorders in adolescence resulting in significant psychological impairment (WHO, 2003). Reports vary as to the prevalence of depression. However, it is believed that 3%–8% of adolescents will experience a depressive disorder prior to entering adulthood (Zalsman, Brent, & Weersing, 2006). In addition, children of parents with depressive disorders are at greater risk for developing depression. A combination of environment and genetic factors are believed to cause depression in adolescents. Little evidence exists to support a molecular link.

The classification of depressive disorders has been described in Chapter 12. In contrast to adults, adolescents often experience a higher co-morbidity with other disorders, such as anxiety disorders, conduct disorders, and substance misuse. In addition, depression is not to be confused with feelings of sadness in adolescents. The turbulence of adolescence commonly causes feelings of sadness and despondence. These feelings are often short-lived and do not necessarily indicate the presence of a depressive illness.

Possible precipitating and predisposing factors for adolescent depression are varied, but may include (MacPhee & Andrews, 2006; Aslund, Nilsson, Starrin, & Sjoberg, 2007):

- Low self-esteem
- Relationship difficulties/break-up
- Academic difficulties, such as examination failure
- Abuse (sexual, emotional, physical)
- Familial relationship problems/parental divorce
- Parental depression
- Parental rejection
- Bereavement
- Peer rejection
- Conduct problems

The major symptoms of depression in adolescents are similar to those in adults and may include: low mood, lack of energy, loss of pleasure, decreased self-esteem and confidence, guilt, feelings of worthlessness, decreased concentration, sleep difficulties, hopelessness, and tearfulness. However, depression may manifest itself a bit differently. For example, the adolescent may present with behavioral problems, such as poor school performance, running away from home, and aggression. These behavioral problems are commonly noted in younger adolescents. Depression also may present as physical pains, often as complaints of headaches.

Treatment of adolescent depression depends on the nature of the problems identified. Treatment should focus on relieving the depressive symptoms, promoting emotional and social functioning, and working with the family. Supportive therapy can be helpful for mild depression, whereas more structured therapeutic approaches are needed for severe depression. Whatever approach is adopted, the adolescent needs to be the central decision maker about his or her care. In some instances, psychopharmacology with antidepressants has been used. Currently, antidepressant medications are recommended only as a last resort because they have been shown to increase the risk of suicidal behavior in adolescents (Richmond & Rosen, 2005). Assessment of suicidal ideation is essential. If it is present, it must be addressed and may require inpatient treatment.

## Mania

Mania is often seen as part of bipolar disorder (see Chapter 12 for more information). It more commonly develops in later adolescence. Mania is characterized by:

- Elevated mood
- Increased energy
- Increased activity
- Restlessness
- Rapid speech
- Flight of ideas

Treatment usually involves a combination of structured therapy, family therapy, and psychopharmacology. According to the American Academy of Child and Adolescent Psychiatry (2007), mood stabilizing agents such as lithium, carbamazepine, and valproic acid may be used. In addition, antipsychotic agents such as risperidone (Risperdol) may be prescribed during an acute manic phase. If the adolescent is prescribed lithium, careful monitoring is needed because lithium can be lethal if taken in an overdose. As a result, it may not be suitable if the adolescent lacks family support to supervise adherence. In addition, there is a lack of controlled trials on the use of antipsychotic medication with adolescents (Schapiro, 2005).

## Self-Harm

The incidence of self-harm is very high in adolescents, conservatively estimated as affecting 5% to 8% of adolescents (Skegg, 2005). However further studies have reported rates as high as 17% with a mean onset age of 15 years (Nixon, et al., 2008). It is most common in young females. Self-harm is often associated with suicide. However, it also can occur without suicidal intent. Thus, a distinction is needed so appropriate intervention can be offered.

Self-harm without suicidal intent often manifests itself as superficial cuts to the body, minor burns, head banging, and inserting foreign objects into the body. The reasons for this type of behavior are often multifaceted and not merely attempts to seek attention as many believe. Indeed, self-harm is often conducted in private without knowledge of family, friends, or health care practitioners. This further adds to the unclear incidence rates, as it is often underreported.

The reasons an adolescent engages in self-harm are numerous. Some of the more common ones include:
- Relief of emotional pain
- Self-punishment
- Stress relief
- Desire to feel physical pain
- Anger expression
- Need to feel in control

Self-harm is believed to be a coping mechanism that an individual may use when experiencing distress. The distress is often related to certain triggers. These triggers are highly variable but may include: bullying or peer rejection; sexual, emotional, or physical abuse or violence in the home; feelings of worthlessness, powerlessness, or loneliness; substance misuse; bereavement; or parental divorce. For some, self-harming behavior can become addictive and, subsequently, difficult to control or stop. Therefore, the focus is on working with the adolescent in trying to find alternative coping strategies through problem solving.

> *An adolescent who engages in self-harm behaviors may or may not be experiencing suicidal ideation. Self-harm behaviors without suicidal intent result from a multitude of reasons and are not attempts to gain attention.*

## Suicide

Suicide is becoming increasingly common in adolescence, particularly in older adolescence. Reports show that of the 4 million suicide attempts around the world each year, 90,000 of those are completed by adolescents (Greydanus & Shek, 2009). Suicide is among the leading causes of death for adolescents worldwide and is ranked as the second-highest cause in the United States. Suicide

attempts need to be taken seriously and require immediate intervention. Four out of five adolescents show warning signs prior to a suicide attempt. Box 22-2 identifies some of the more common signs.

If suicidal signs are present, further assessment is warranted and needs to focus on the following:
- The lethality of the method proposed or used if an attempt was made
- The place where the attempt took place, the likelihood of discovery and precautions taken to avoid discovery
- Motives
- The presence of suicidal communication such as a suicide note or blog entry
- Previous attempts made
- Evidence of a psychiatric disorder
- The continued wish to die

Information gathered about these issues will give an indication of the seriousness of the attempt and the likelihood that a future attempt may be made. Often, alcohol use is associated with suicide attempts and thus should be explored.

The causes of adolescent suicide attempts are often multi-faceted and often a depressive illness is present. Many of the issues discussed as precipitating factors for depression and self-harm may also be present and thus should be explored during the assessment process. One of the most important features present in suicidal individuals is hopelessness and thus any treatment should focus on inspiring hope. The approach should be nonjudgmental and work should be conducted to develop a person's

---

**BOX 22-2: SUICIDE WARNING SIGNS IN ADOLESCENTS**

- No longer interested in activities previously found enjoyable
- Problems at school
- Alcohol or drug use
- Withdrawal
- Acting out behavior
- Self-neglect
- Risk-taking behavior
- Stating "I want to die" or "I want to kill myself"
- Stating "I won't bother you or trouble you anymore"
- Stating "Nobody cares about me"
- Giving away possessions
- Signs of cheerfulness after a period of depression

coping strategies and problem-solving techniques. In patient treatment may be necessary. A range of supportive therapies can be offered.

> *Typically, warning signs of suicide are present before an adolescent attempts suicide. Assessment focuses on the lethality of the method, location, motive, evidence of suicidal communication, previous attempts, and information related to a continued wish to die.*

**BOX 22-3: RISK FACTORS FOR SUBSTANCE USE AND MISUSE**

- Poor school performance
- Early behavioral problems
- Aggression
- Risk-taking behavior
- Low self-esteem
- Peer substance use
- Disadvantaged social environment
- Family history of substance misuse
- Lack of parental involvement, supervision, or discipline
- History of anti-social behavior

## Eating Disorders

Anorexia nervosa and bulimia nervosa are frequently seen in adolescents, particularly in girls (Merikangas et al., 2010). Issues with identity formation and physical growth are common. Both anorexia nervosa and bulimia nervosa involve a preoccupation with food, weight, and body image. Anorexia nervosa has the highest death rate of all psychiatric illnesses, with mortality rates of up to 10% being reported (Huas, 2011). (Refer to Chapter 19 for a complete discussion of these disorders.)

## Substance Misuse and Abuse

The use by adolescents of substances such as alcohol and illicit drugs is growing, with some research suggesting that up to 72.5% of high school students have engaged in drinking alcohol and 36.8% have used marijuana (CDC, 2010). However, decreases in these rates have been noted since 1999. Most adolescents who experiment with alcohol and drugs do not develop a problem with their use. However, this is dependent on the age of onset and the frequency of use.

The reasons for alcohol and drug use by adolescents is multi-faceted and may relate to their personal circumstances, where substances may be used to mask a more deep-rooted problem or may be due to peer group pressure. Additionally, young people may use substances simply because they are available and find it exciting to do so. The exact cause for substance use and misuse is not known. However, several risks factors have been identified. These are highlighted in **Box 22-3**.

The most common mood-altering drug used by adolescents is alcohol, a central nervous system depressant.

Numerous reasons may account for this increased use. Alcohol is more generally accepted because it is a legal drug. Also, alcohol promotes relaxation in social situations, making it appealing to an adolescent who is searching for identity. In recent years, society has changed its response to alcohol use. Its social acceptability and availability has increased due to peer pressure and family and media exposure. Research has reported a strong link between alcohol advertising and the uptake of drinking among young people (Anderson et al., 2009).

Of special interest and growing concern in developing countries is **BINGE DRINKING** by adolescents. The CDC (2010) reported that 24% of high school students engage in binge drinking. Binge drinking occurs when copious amounts of alcohol are consumed over a short period of time. The effects on the adolescent can be fatal, resulting in a wide range of symptoms from complete loss of control to alcohol poisoning. Along with this loss of control comes impaired judgment. Thus, a person may engage in behavior that he or she would normally avoid, such as drunk driving, inappropriate sexual behavior, petty crime, vandalism, or social misconduct (McKay et al., 2006). Physically, this type of behavior damages a number of systems in the body and can lead to long-term alcohol dependence.

Illicit drugs are also commonly used by adolescents, the most common of which include cannabis resin and amphetamines. Cocaine use in adolescents also is on the rise. It is estimated that 3% of high school students have used cocaine (CDC, 2010). These drugs can have a detrimental effect on adolescents because their bodies and minds are still developing.

It is important when working with adolescents to determine if their alcohol or drug use is experimental, recreational, or involves dependence. Alcohol and drugs often may be used to mask another mental health problem.

Therefore, it is important to assess for other mental health issues.

Primary prevention measures have been used to educate adolescents on alcohol and drug use, on making safe decisions, and on problem solving without resorting to alcohol or drug use. The use of alcohol by young people is receiving an increased amount of attention. Mothers Against Drunk Driving (MADD) is a program that works to reduce the social and retail availability of alcohol and supports the enforcement of underage drinking laws. Other initiatives include the Too Smart to Start initiative by the Substance Abuse and Mental Health Services Administration and the Drug Abuse Resistance Education (D.A.R.E.) organization. These programs work to teach young people to avoid drugs. Unfortunately, most programs of this nature have had limited success, as it remains "cool" to use alcohol and drugs.

When assessing an adolescent for drug and alcohol, abuse, some common signs may be observed. These include problems at school, such as truancy, a drop in academic performance, discipline problems, secrecy, withdrawal from family activities, and cigarette smoking. These signs may be a result of other problems; therefore, assessment for any other underlying mental health problems such as depression is necessary.

When an adolescent is using drugs experimentally or recreationally, the focus is on preventing dependency by highlighting the risks, offering real case examples, and trying to encourage the individual to abstain from the drug. When adolescents become dependent, the initial aim is to reduce harm to the individual.

When an adolescent is abusing or is dependent on alcohol or drugs, a family-centered approach is used. In addition, the adolescent's motivation to abstain from using the substance must be established. A period of detoxification may be necessary. (See Chapter 15 for a more in-depth discussion of substance disorders.)

> *Alcohol is the most common mood-altering drug used by adolescents. Cannabis and amphetamines are the most common illicit substances used.*

## Attention Deficit Hyperactivity Disorder

Attention deficit hyperactivity disorder (ADHD) is characterized by hyperactivity, impulsiveness, and inability to focus attention, inconsistent to the age of the individual. It develops in childhood and persists into adolescence and quite often into adulthood. (See Chapter 21 for additional information about ADHD in children.)

Working with an adolescent with ADHD involves a family-centered approach. Often, much of the work is conducted with the parents to assist them in understanding the difficulties and frustration the young person is experiencing. There is increasing evidence that the standard American adolescent diet may be harmful to a person with ADHD (Lavoie, 2009). Providing adolescents and their families with advice on nutrition is essential. It is recommended that protein be included in every meal and that omega-3 fatty acids, vitamin C, and vitamin B12 intake be increased. It is also recommended that consumption of processed, starch-based, and junk foods be decreased or eliminated.

Additional areas to address include helping the adolescent develop his or her social skills and coping strategies and to deal with any anger and frustration that may be associated with the problem. Communication with the adolescent's school is important because this is often where ADHD may first present. The adolescent may have difficulty in paying attention or sitting still in class and teachers may have reported problems. Communication is important to ensure that a comprehensive plan is in place to deal with the difficulties and to ensure there is continuity in the approach at home and at school.

Behavioral techniques have been helpful for the adolescent with ADHD. These include:

- Identifying the problem behavior with the family
- Exploring the antecedents and consequences of the behavior
- Identifying what behavior would be more appropriate in the circumstance
- Working on rewards for appropriate behaviors while avoiding punishment for inappropriate behaviors

Medication also has been successful with individuals with ADHD; however, it needs to be carefully monitored and controlled. Some current medications used include methylphenidate (Ritalin), dexamphetamine (Dexedrine), and lisdexamfetamine dimesylate (Vyvanse). If the symptoms of ADHD are not severe, a medication-free period may be recommended, for example, during school holidays, to determine if the medication is still needed.

## Conduct Disorders

Adolescent-onset conduct disorder is diagnosed when there have been no conduct problems before the age of 10 years. The disorder is usually classified as mild, moderate, or severe, depending on the number and intensity of symptoms present. (See Chapter 21 for a discussion of the signs and symptoms of conduct disorder.)

Conduct disorder must be differentiated from normal adolescent behavior. Adolescents will push boundaries as part of their development. Typically, conduct disorder involves more extreme behavior that violates the norms.

Several situations are associated with the development of conduct disorder. Inconsistent parenting is common in adolescents with conduct disorder; the family system requires enormous support when dealing with this type of behavior. Often the adolescent lacks self-esteem, which is reinforced by punishing parenting styles. Conduct disorders are also frequently seen in adolescents from disadvantaged areas that involve a wide range of social issues.

Treatment can involve a combination of parent training, family therapy, problem-solving therapy, cognitive therapy, and/or medication such as those used in the treatment of ADHD. Group therapy is usually not used because of the potential for copycat behavior to occur. Prognosis for recovery in adolescent onset of conduct disorder is better than in childhood onset.

## Obsessive-Compulsive Disorder

Obsessive-compulsive disorder (OCD) is an anxiety disorder. The first symptoms usually appear in adolescence. **OBSESSIONS** are recurring intrusive thoughts that the person finds distressing. Often, obsessions focus on fear of death, contamination, or harm to others. **COMPULSIONS** are physical repetitive acts that are carried out in an attempt to eliminate the obsession. For example, if the obsession is the fear of contamination, then the compulsion may be to wash the body excessively. Carrying out the compulsion usually reduces the anxiety in the adolescent and thus reinforces the behavior.

OCD in adolescents can have an enormous impact on the family. The family is commonly drawn into the compulsive behaviors of the adolescent to help alleviate his or her anxiety. OCD is treatable, with cognitive behavioral therapy being effective. Some anti-depressants from the SSRI group, such as fluoxetine (Prozac) and sertraline (Zoloft), have been somewhat effective. However, this therapy should be used as a last resort in adolescents due to the increased risk for suicide.

## Social Phobia

Social phobia is common in adolescents. For many, it will diminish naturally as the adolescent develops confidence and self-esteem. It is characterized by a fear of social situations that results from a fear of embarrassment or humiliation. (See Chapter 13 for a more in-depth discussion.) The fear of the social situation is not merely with adults; it is also with their peers. Thus, the adolescent may avoid social situations that will require interaction with others. As a result, the adolescent's development and maturation is impacted, leading to the development of poor social skills and low self-esteem. Social phobia is very treatable but it can become progressively worse and continue into adulthood if not treated appropriately. Cognitive and behavior therapies often are used.

> *Social phobia can lead to the development of poor social skills and low self-esteem, thus affecting the adolescent's development.*

## TREATMENT OPTIONS

Various treatment options are available for the adolescent with mental health problems. These treatment strategies are the same as those used for adults. Several options are addressed here in relation to the adolescent as the patient.

## Cognitive Behavioral Therapy

Cognitive behavioral therapy (CBT) has been identified as a useful approach when working with adolescents with a number of different mental health problems, including depression and eating disorders. As the name implies, concepts include those of cognitive theorists and techniques of behavioral therapy and client-centered psychotherapy. CBT works best when combined with other therapies such as family therapy.

CBT assumes that core beliefs and assumptions that individuals develop in their early childhood are critical to understanding later perceptions of events. The premise is that if the adolescent has learned maladaptive behavior and coping strategies, then they can unlearn them. The practitioner and adolescent work together to identify and understand problems and the relationship between thoughts, feelings, and behaviors. CBT is designed to challenge negative beliefs. The focus is the here and now as individualized, usually time-limited, therapy goals are formulated. Various cognitive and behavioral interventions, such as role play and modeling, are used to target symptoms, reduce distress, reevaluate thinking, and promote helpful behavioral responses. As the adolescent is supported to tackle problems, he or she begins to acquire psychological and practical skills to deal with them. The emphasis on putting what was learned into practice helps to promote change.

## Family Therapy

Typically, many adolescents live within the family system. Thus, the problems and their solutions often involve the family. Family therapy examines what is going on within the family unit, its dynamics, and the types of interactions, both at the current time and in the past. It explores how family interactions affect the everyday lives of the members. (See Chapter 9 for a more in-depth discussion of family therapy.)

Each family is unique and has its own set of norms, interaction patterns, and connections. Patterns of behavior, beliefs, and communication develop over time and may be both the cause of the adolescent's problem and provide the solution for the problem. A combination of approaches such as problem solving, and behavioral, and cognitive techniques can be used. The practitioner works with the family to identify any difficulties that may be present, helps the family to understand the adolescent's problems, and assests in changing any dynamics that are deemed unhelpful.

## Parent Training

Parent training programs may be particularly helpful with parents or guardians of adolescents with ADHD or conduct disorders. However, they are more commonly used with parents of younger children. A number of approaches may be used including:

- *Psychoeducation*: The parent(s) receive instruction on the nature of the adolescent's problems
- *Behavioral approach*: Focus is on the behavior of the parents and adolescent
- *Support counseling-type approach*: Support provided to the parents to help them come to terms with their adolescent's problems; identification of positive and negative parenting styles with reinforcement of those that work well
- *Group work*: Parents of several adolescents coming together to share common experiences and decrease their sense of isolation

## Group Work

Group work can be an important part of holistic care for adolescents with mental health problems. For the adolescent population, groups are important to develop a positive identity and normalize experiences. Group work is a useful means of exploring thoughts, feelings, and beliefs and developing interpersonal skills.

To engage in group work, a careful assessment of the adolescent and his or her ability to interact in a group environment must occur. Additionally, the adolescent's suitability for the group needs serious consideration. Some adolescents may experience increased anxiety when interacting in a group, potentially worsening their mental health problems.

Another consideration is the level of the group member's functioning. This level may be influenced by age, maturity, and severity of mental health problems. For a group to work through the stages of group development, the level of functioning of all members must be similar. Additionally, as with facilitating any group, the timing and the skills of the facilitator need to be considered. Where possible, the groups should be time limited and closed, meaning that the group begins and ends on a specific date and no new members can join the group after it has begun.

Adolescents with mental health problems can be difficult to work with in a group environment. Therefore, it is essential to establish ground rules, such as respect for other members, from the outset. From there, each group will take on its own set of norms and progress in its own way.

The type of group used varies depending on the setting. For example, some groups may be illness focused, such as a group for adolescents with depression or ADHD. Others may be issue focused, such as a group learning to develop positive coping strategies. Still others may be activity focused, such as a group practicing social skills. Regardless of the type of group, a common goal must be identified for the members. (See Chapter 9 for additional information on group therapy.)

> *Ability to interact in a group environment, suitability for a group, and level of group functioning must be considered when determining if group work would be appropriate for an adolescent.*

## Inpatient Care

Ideally, an individual should be cared for in his or her own environment. Thus, adolescents should be cared for in the community setting as much as possible. However, when this is not feasible because of safety or the need for more intensive treatment, inpatient care may be required. The most common reasons for inpatient admission include: the severity of the mental health problem; the family is no longer able to cope; the risk of suicide or threat of violence to others.

Inpatient care, although more restrictive than community care, can be advantageous because it:

- Provides ample opportunity for a thorough assessment over a period of time with careful observation and close supervision for changes in mood and behavior throughout the day, which is especially important for the adolescent at risk to him- or herself or others.
- Permits close monitoring for effectiveness of the therapy as well as for potential side effects if psychopharmacology is being initiated.
- Allows the adolescent to meet other young people who may be experiencing similar difficulties, thus helping to normalize the experience and help reduce the stigma associated with mental health problems.
- Creates separation from family and/or friends in situations where these individuals are adding to the adolescent's stress or contributing to the mental health problems.

Inpatient care also has disadvantages. It can further exacerbate mental health problems. Evidence suggests that copycat behaviors can occur in adolescent units. This occurs when a young person may imitate or copy abnormal behaviors exhibited by another young person, such as cutting themselves and noncompliance. These copycat behaviors add to the adolescent's current problems. As with adult inpatient care, the adolescent may become disempowered and become increasingly reliant on hospital support, finding it more and more difficult to integrate back into society upon discharge. This may, in turn, have an effect on their normal development of independence and maturity.

## Psychopharmacology

The use of medication to treat adolescents with mental health disorders is controversial. Although many medications have claimed to be safe for use in adolescents, critics argue that there are insufficient trials in certain areas to support this claim (Schapiro, 2005; Lader, 2007). The prescription of psychiatric medications for adolescents

*Psychopharmacology is considered only as a last resort when treating adolescents because of the increased risk for suicide.*

needs to be carefully considered and only used as a last resort if other treatment options have not worked. In addition, they should only be used as part of a comprehensive treatment plan wherein other interventions are also offered. Clear explanations of how the medication works and its potential side effects must be provided to both the adolescent and their parent or guardian. **Patient and Family Education 22-1** provides an example of information to include when teaching an adolescent about prescribed medications.

### PATIENT AND FAMILY EDUCATION 22-1: TEACHING AN ADOLESCENT ABOUT ANTIDEPRESSANTS

- Take the medication exactly as your doctor has prescribed it.

- Be aware that it might take several weeks before you notice any changes in your symptoms. Continue to take the medication even if your symptoms do not subside.

- If you miss a dose, do not double up on the next dose.

- Do not stop the drug suddenly, because you might experience withdrawal symptoms.

- Use sugarless hard candy or gum or frequent sips of water you if experience dry mouth.

- Avoid activities that require you to be alert, such as driving, because you may experience drowsiness or dizziness.

- Check with your physician before taking any other medications, including over-the-counter medications and herbal preparations.

- Be alert for signs of worsening depression or suicide. Call your prescriber immediately if you experience any of these.

## APPLYING THE NURSING PROCESS FROM AN INTERPERSONAL PERSPECTIVE

Adolescents experiencing mental health problems may be seen in a variety of settings, such as acute care settings, day hospitalization programs, community and outpatient facilities, as well as general medical facilities, emergency departments, and specialty clinics. Therefore, nurses need a firm understanding of the nursing process that integrates the interpersonal process when caring for adolescents with mental health disorders. In addition, nurses need to remain cognizant of adolescent development to provide an individualized plan of care. (See Chapter 21 for an example of a plan of care that can be adapted to the adolescent.)

> *Therapeutic communication skills including active listening are essential to the development of the therapeutic relationship with an adolescent. The adolescent needs to be treated as an individual whose input is valued.*

### Strategies for Optimal Assessment: Therapeutic Use of Self

The development of a therapeutic relationship with an adolescent is the key to assessment. The nurse spends considerable time with the adolescent and occupies a unique position, communicating with and getting to know the adolescent. The therapeutic use of self allows the nurse to work with the adolescent collaboratively in exploring and understanding the lived experience of the adolescent's distress. During the assessment, this supportive therapeutic alliance is initiated by the nurse being genuine, honest, respectful, empathetic, and flexible. As the adolescent begins to trust the nurse, open and honest communication can occur, allowing the nurse to understand the problem from the adolescent's frame of reference.

Communicating with adolescents can be challenging. Although they are generally considered to be minors and decision making often will be made in conjunction with their parents or guardian, a person-centered approach is essential. The nurse needs to treat the adolescent as an individual, demonstrating that his or her input is valued. The nurse also needs to display an attitude that

demonstrates that he or she is listening to the adolescent. It is easy to be dismissive, believing that as minors, adolescents know little about the world and life. However, only the adolescent truly understands how and what he or she is feeling and experiencing. Through the use of therapeutic communication skills, most importantly, active listening, the nurse can develop an understanding of the adolescent's difficulties. As a result, the nurse can be in a better position to work with the adolescent in resolving these difficulties. **Therapeutic Interaction 22-1** provides a sample interaction with an adolescent. Reciprocity, mutuality, and trust are essential components to the relationship.

### Diagnosing and Planning Appropriate Interventions: Meeting the Adolescent's Focused Needs

After completing the assessment, the nurse and adolescent develop a plan of care with mutual goals and expectations for outcomes. Through the continuing development of the therapeutic relationship, the nurse will work with the adolescent to help identify his or her needs. Outcomes and goals should be realistic and time-oriented, being identified and developed through open negotiation.

When working with the adolescent, the plan needs to be family centered, that is, it must consider the family's ideas and beliefs and address the strengths and weaknesses of the adolescent and family. Throughout the process, the nurse needs to listen carefully to the adolescent and be sensitive to his or her feelings and those of the family, thereby helping the adolescent to focus on recovery.

### Implementing Effective Interventions: Timing and Pacing

A number of potentially effective interventions can be used with adolescents and their families. These include supportive counseling, cognitive behavioral therapy, group work, and family counseling. However, additional research is needed to determine the true effectiveness of these therapies with adolescents.

The exact method for how the plan of care will be delivered and achieved is highly variable and must be individualized to the adolescent. This individualization will determine when and how interventions are implemented. The nurse works collaboratively with the adolescent in a creative and flexible way to promote personal growth and self-awareness. The nurse inspires hope and optimism by maintaining the belief that everyone has the ability to grow

**THERAPEUTIC INTERACTION 22-1:**
**ACTIVE LISTENING WITH AN ADOLESCENT**

The nurse is meeting with Jess, a 15-year-old, for the first time. Jess has reported experiencing depressive symptoms for the past six months. The nurse is trying to determine if there were any precipitating factors.

| INTERACTION | RATIONALE |
| --- | --- |
| **Nurse:** "How did all this begin for you?" (establishes eye contact and sits at the patient's level) | Initiating the interaction using an open-ended question, that allows the patient to direct the interaction.<br><br>Eye contact and positioning on the same level, demonstrates interest in the patient. |
| **Jess:** "I suppose I began to feel bad about 6 months ago when I went back to school after my summer vacation." | Responds to open communication and interest of nurse |
| **Nurse:** "Did anything in particular happen during that time?" (leans forward toward the patient) | Seeking clarification about the connection between the symptoms and school; demonstrates interest in patient's response; leaning forward indicates interest in what patient has to say |
| **Jess:** "Not really; just the usual, you know, you go back to school and you haven't seen people in a while and everybody looks different from last term and people comment on each other. Like if you've put on weight, or lost weight, or got spots, or got taller, people notice. I just hate listening to all that stuff, it's so superficial, and everyone judges you by the way you look." | Beginning to open up about his feelings |
| **Nurse:** "So your classmates were passing comment on other classmates and judging them?" | Validating the patient's statement; demonstrating empathy, showing concern and interest for the patient. |
| **Jess:** "Yeah." | Confirming previous communication |
| **Nurse:** "Do you feel they were judging you?" | Further exploration to gather information about patient's feelings; encouraging patient to share information. |
| **Jess:** "Of course, I mean they do it to everyone." | Expressing distress with classmates' behavior |

*(cont.)*

**THERAPEUTIC INTERACTION 22-1: (*CONT.*)
ACTIVE LISTENING WITH AN ADOLESCENT**

| INTERACTION | RATIONALE |
|---|---|
| **Nurse:** "Sounds like that would be tough. How did that make you feel?" | Acknowledging the patient's feelings, encouraging the patient to describe his feelings further. |
| **Jess:** "I became paranoid, well Mom said I was paranoid anyway. I didn't hear what they said but I know I put on a little weight over the summer so I'd say they were talking about that. I could see them looking and sneering. It's horrible to be looked at like that, it made me so angry, how dare they." | Expressing feelings; opening up to nurse |
| **Nurse:** "That sounds like it must have been difficult. Ok, so what you're telling me is that you think this began when you went back to school after the summer vacation. When you felt that some of your classmates were talking about you and sneering at you because you put on some weight over vaction and this has made you angry. Is that right?" | Summarizing what patient has been saying and seeking clarification to ensure accurate interpretation. |

and foster a positive idea of the future and by remaining grounded in understanding the current problem experienced by the adolescent. In addition, the nurse needs to focus on the adolescent's potential and his or her strengths. Throughout, continued mutual respect is necessary.

Failures and setbacks may occur during this stage. The nurse understands that these events may occur and works to accept them. The nurse also needs to be mindful of the affect that any failures or setbacks may have on the adolescent. The adolescent may experience a loss of confidence or self-esteem. Thus, the nurse continues to work with the adolescent, helping him or her to move past the difficulties and return to the path of recovery.

## Evaluating: Objective Critique of Interventions and Self-Reflection

Evaluation, an ongoing process, addresses the adolescent's goal achievement. Throughout, the nurse encourages the adolescent to reflect on his or her own progress and identify achievements. The nurse can highlight the positives to the adolescent and his or her family and include a plan for aftercare as appropriate.

The nurse also needs to engage in self-reflection during this time, reflecting on the approach to care adopted and the interactions with the adolescent. The nurse explores his or her own thoughts and feelings, what was done well, and what needs to improve. Additionally, the nurse identifies any problems within the therapeutic relationship that may have impacted the care. For example, if an adolescent refuses to engage with the nurse or becomes angry, the nurse should reflect on why this may have happened, and try to understand it from the adolescent's perspective. The nurse can then explore how to approach the situation differently. These actions will help the nurse develop competence and a greater understanding of how to work with this population.

Developing strong therapeutic alliances can be draining on the nurse and burnout can occur without appropriate supports. The nurse needs to learn how to be self-supportive and seek the support of colleagues. Advanced practice nurses work in a variety of settings with adolescents and can be an invaluable source of support for beginning nurses working with this population.

Evaluation is also part of the termination of the nurse-patient relationship. Many times a patient will have a setback due to feelings of loss of this relationship. Termination is accomplished in a stepwise fashion, with the adolescent gradually decreasing his or her dependence on the nurse. The nurse helps the patient to explore his or her feelings and ease this transition while maintaining boundaries (Peplau, 1991).

---

 **SUMMARY POINTS**

- Mental health problems, when they occur in adolescence, can often be dismissed as part of normal development. The perception is that adolescents will "grow out" of the problem as they reach adulthood.

- Adolescence is a period characterized by a search for identity, finding meaning in life, and forming unique personalities separate from the parents. Peer relationships play a significant role in an adolescent's overall development.

- An adolescent should be assessed in private because he or she may be ambivalent about the difficulties being experienced, fearful of becoming stigmatized, unable to articulate the problems, or have issues with authority figures.

- Adolescents experience many of the same mental health problems experienced by adults. Common mental health disorders include depression, self-harm, suicidal ideation, alcohol and drug use, eating disorders, and anxiety disorders.

- Depression in adolescents should not be confused with the typical short-lived feelings of sadness during this stage.

- Self-harm is believed to be a coping mechanism used for distress in response to certain triggers, such as bullying, peer rejection, abuse, feelings of worthlessness, substance misuse, or parental divorce.

- One of the most important features associated with suicidal ideation in adolescents is a feeling of hopelessness.

- Binge drinking is a growing concern among adolescence, the results of which can be fatal.

- Adolescents with ADHD who are prescribed stimulants should periodically undergo a medication-free period to determine if the medication is still necessary.

- Treatment options are similar to those used with adults including cognitive behavioral therapy, family therapy, parent training, group work, and inpatient care.

- Communicating with an adolescent can be challenging. The nurse needs to treat the adolescent as an individual and demonstrate that his or her input is valued and respected.

## NCLEX-PREP*

1. A nurse is preparing a presentation for a local community group about adolescence and mental health problems. Which of the following would the nurse expect to include?

   a. Time typically heals any problems that adolescents experience.
   b. Problems in adolescence can continue into adulthood if not addressed.
   c. Adolescents primarily experience disorders that are uncommon in adults.
   d. The stigma associated with mental disorders is seen less frequently with adolescents.

2. A nurse is interviewing an adolescent for indications of suicidal ideation. Which patient statement would be a cause for concern?

   a. "Don't worry, I'm not going to be bothering anyone anymore."
   b. "Sometimes I feel like my parents are dictators."
   c. "I used to like to draw, but I've found music is more relaxing."
   d. "School is okay but I'd much rather play sports."

3. A group of nursing students are reviewing information about substance abuse in adolescence. The students demonstrate an understanding of the information when they identify which of the following as the most commonly abused substance in adolescence?

   a. Cocaine
   b. Cannabis
   c. Alcohol
   d. Amphetamines

4. The nurse is assessing a female adolescent who engages in self-harming behavior. Which of the following would the nurse identify as a possible trigger? Select all that apply.

   a. Rejection by friends
   b. Substance misuse
   c. Feelings of power
   d. Worthlessness
   e. Parental divorce

5. When applying the therapeutic use of self during assessment, which of the following would be important for the nurse to demonstrate? Select all that apply.

   a. Genuineness
   b. Respect
   c. Empathy
   d. Adherence to rigid rules
   e. Honesty

*Answers to these questions appear on page 639.

## REFERENCES

American Academy of Child and Adolescent Psychiatry. (2007). Practice parameters for the assessment and treatment of children and adolescents with bipolar disorder. *Journal of the American Academy of Adolescent Psychiatry, 4691*, 107–125.

American Psychiatric Association. (2000). *Diagnostic and Statistical Manual of Mental Disorders IV-TR.* Virginia: Author.

Anderson, P., deBruijn, A., Angus, K., Gordon, R., Hastings, G. (2009). Impact of alcohol advertising and media exposure on adolescent alcohol use: a systematic review of longitudinal studies. *Alcohol and Alcoholism, 44*(3), 229–243.

Aslund, C., Nilsson, K., Starrin, B. & Sjoberg, R. (2007). Shaming experiences and the association between adolescent depression and psychosocial risk factors. *European Child and Adolescent, 16*(5), 298–304.

Australian Bureau of Statistics (2007). *National Survey of Mental Health and Wellbeing, Summary of Results.* Australian Bureau of Statistics.

Black, K.A., & McCartney, K. (1997). Adolescent females' security with parents predicts the quality of peer interactions. *Social Development, 6*, 91–110.

Briggs, S. (2008). *Working with adolescents and young adults.* 2nd Edition. New York: Palgrave Macmillan.

Erikson, E. (1968). *Identity: Youth and crisis.* London: Faber and Faber.

Centers for Disease Control and Prevention. (2010). Youth Risk Behavior Surveillance, United States. *MMWR, 59* (SS-5), 1–142.

Chen, K., Killeya-Jones, L.,Vega, W. (2005). Prevalence and co-occurrence of psychiatric symptom clusters in the U.S. adolescent population using DISC predictive scales. *Clinical Practice and Epidemiology in Mental Health, 1,* 22.

Copeland, W., Shanahan, L., Miller, S., Costello, E., Angold, A., Maughan, B. (2010). Outcomes of early pubertal timing in young women: a prospective population based study. *American Journal of Psychiatry, 167*(10), 1218–1225.

Demyttenaere, K., Bruffaerts, R., Posada-Villa, J., Gasquet, I., Kovess, V., Lepine, J. (2004). WHO World Mental Health Survey Consortium. Prevalence, severity and unmet need for treatment of mental disorders in the World Health Organization World Mental Health Surveys. *JAMA, 291*(21), 2581–2590.

Gifford-Smith, M., Dodge, K., Dishon, T., McCord, J. (2005). Peer influence in children and adolescents: crossing the bridge from developmental to intervention science. *Journal of Abnormal Child Psychology, 33*(3), 255–265.

Greydanus, D., Shek, D. (2009). Deliberate self harm and suicide in adolescents. *The Keoi Journal of Medicine, 58*(3), 144–151.

Huas, C., Caille, A., Godart, N., Foulon, C., Pham-Scottez, A., Divac, S., et al (2011). Factors predictive of ten-year mortality in severe anorexia nervosa patients. *Acta Psychiatrica Scandinavica, 123*(1), 62–70.

Lader, M. (2007). Antidepressants and suicidality. *Clinical Risk, 13,* 85–88.

Lavoie, T. (2009). Holistic treatment approaches to ADHD: Nutrition, sleep and exercise. *EP Magazine,* April, 46–47.

Ma, C., & Huebner, S. (2008). Attachment relationships and adolescents' life satisfaction: some relationships matter more to girls than boys. *Psychology in the Schools, 45*(2), 177–190.

MacPhee, A., & Andrews, J. (2006). Risk factors for depression in early adolescence. *Adolescence, 41*(163), 435–466.

McKay, D., Hatton, T., McDougall, T. (2006). Substance misuse, young people and nursing. In T. McDougall (Ed). *Child and Adolescent Mental Health Nursing.* Oxford: Blackwell, pp. 188–206.

Mishna, F., Cook, C., Gadalla, T., Daciuk, J., Solomon, S. (2010). Cyber bullying behaviors among middle and high school students. *The American Journal of Orthopsychiatry, 80*(3), 362–374.

Merikangas, et al (2010). Lifetime prevalence of mental disorders in US adolescents: results from the National Co-morbidity Study. Adolescent supplement (NCS-A). *Journal of the American Academy of Child and Adolescent Psychiatry, 49*(10), 980–989.

Nixon, M., Cloutier, P., Jansson, S. (2008). Nonsuicidal self harm in youth: a population based survey. *CMAJ, 178,* 306–312.

Palmonari, A., Pombeni, M., & Kirchler, E. (1990). Adolescents and their peer groups: a study on the significance of peers, social categorization processes and coping with developmental tasks. *Social Behavior, 5,* 33–48.

Peplau, H.E. (1991). *Interpersonal relations in nursing: A conceptual frame of reference for psychodynamic nursing.* New York: Springer Publishing Company.

Richmond, T.K., & Rosen D.S. (2005). The treatment of adolescent depression in the era of the black box warning. *Current Opinion in Paediatrics, 17*(4), 1466–72.

Samaritans and Centre for Suicide Research (2003). *Youth and self-harm: perspectives.* Surrey: The Samaritans.

Schapiro, N. (2005). Bipolar Disorder in Children and Adolescents. *Jounral of Pediatric Health Care, 19*(3), 131–140.

Skegg, K. (2005). Self harm. *Lancet, 366,* 1471–1483.

Valkenburg, P., Peter, J., & Schouten, A. (2006). Friend networking sites and their relationship to adolescents' well-being and social self-esteem. *Cyberpsychology and Behaviour, 9*(5), 584–90.

Veronneau, M., Vitaro, F., Brendgen, M., Dishion, T., & Tremblay, R. (2010). Transactional analysis of the reciprocal links between peer experiences and academic achievement from middle childhood to early adolescence. *Developmental Psychology, 46*(4), 773–790.

Witvliet, M., Brendgen, M., Van Lier, P., Koct, H., & Vitavo, F. (2010). Early adolescent depressive symptoms: prediction from clique isolation, loneliness and perceived social acceptance. *Journal of Abnormal Child Psychology, 38*(8), 1045–1056.

World Health Organization. (2000). *World Health Report.* Geneva: Author.

World Health Organization. (2003). *Caring for children and adolescents with mental disorders.* Geneva: Author.

Ybarra, M., & Mitchell, K. (2008). How risky are social networking sites? A comparison of places online where youth sexual solicitation and harassment occurs. *Pediatrics, 121*(2), e350–357.

Young, J., Berenson, K., Cohen, P., & Garcia, J. (2005). The role of parent and peer support in predicting adolescent depression: a longitudinal community study. *Journal of Research on Adolescence, 15*(4), 17.

Zalsman, G., Brent D.A., & Weersing, V.R. (2006). Depressive disorders in childhood and adolescence: an overview: epidemiology, clinical manifestation and risk factors. *Child and Adolescent Psychiatric Clinics in North America, 15*(4):827–41.

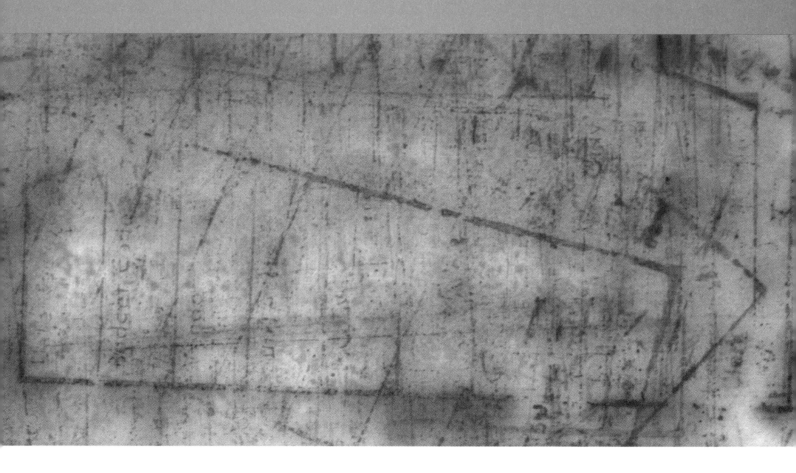

## CHAPTER CONTENTS

## CHAPTER 23

# ISSUES SPECIFIC TO THE ELDERLY

Kimberly S. McClane

## EXPECTED LEARNING OUTCOMES

**After completing this chapter, the student will be able to:**

1. Describe the current demographics of the elderly population.
2. Identify the impact of physical, emotional, and sociocultural issues influencing the mental health of the elderly patient.
3. Discuss the most common mental health disorders associated with the elderly.
4. Identify trends affecting mental health services provided to the elderly.
5. Apply the nursing process from an interpersonal perspective for the care of an elderly patient with a mental health disorder.

## KEY TERMS

Activities of daily living

Emotional loneliness

Geropsychiatry

Insomnia

Loneliness

Polypharmacy

Quality of life

Social loneliness

The elderly are considered to be individuals over the age of 65 years. In 2007, 37.9 million Americans were over the age of 65 years, reflecting an increase of 11.2% since the late 1990s. In the next decade, a further increase in growth of 38% is projected to occur. The current life expectancy in the United States is predicted to be 85.3 years for women and 82.4 years for men. In looking at the entire U.S. population, approximately 12.6% of individuals are 65 years of age or older and the numbers continue to rise. For the first time in history, there will be more individuals over the age of 65 than in any other age group. Additionally, there will be more elderly Americans than there will be Americans in the workforce (Administration on Aging [AoAna], 2010).

This chapter addresses the mental health issues related to the elderly. It describes some of the current statistics related to the elderly population and factors impacting the mental health of the elderly. The chapter reviews the most common mental health disorders affecting the elderly population and trends affecting care delivery. The chapter concludes by applying the nursing process from an interpersonal perspective to the care of an elderly patient with a mental health disorder.

## OVERVIEW OF THE ELDERLY POPULATION

The elderly population, as stated, is increasing. Overall, 39.0% of the aging population believes they are in very good to excellent health and actively access and participate in their health and health behaviors (AoAna, 2010). However, reports suggest that at least 52% of individuals over the age of 65 years will be diagnosed with at least one disability including a sensory, physical, or mental disability. A greater number of elderly report "poor health" (65%) with a diagnosis of at least one chronic illness. Additionally, at least 29% of the elderly reported the need for assistance in completing their **ACTIVITIES OF DAILY LIVING**. These activities include personal hygiene, dressing, eating, mobility, and toileting. Within this population, the risk for mental or behavioral issues also is increased.

### Quality of Life

Another frequent indicator that is used to measure the aging individual's mental and physical health is **QUALITY OF LIFE**. Quality of life, used as an indicator of health by the World Health Organization (WHO), is defined as "a state of complete physical, mental, and social well-being and not the absence of disease or infirmity" (WHO, 2003, p.1). This reflects the strong association of physical and mental health

in the aging individual. Mental health as a component of overall health needs to be as recognized and treated as aggressively as any physical diagnosis in the aging individual. Health care providers are incorporating mental health concepts with chronic disease management and prevention in the aging population. Research development continues for providing appropriate treatment options and services to promote mental health of the aging population.

> *Quality of life is a key indicator of an individual's overall health, but especially the overall health of an elderly individual.*

### Medicare

Providing adequate care to those over the age of 65 years requires identification of funding sources for mental health issues. The primary health insurance provider for many aging Americans is Medicare (Medicare, n.d.). Medicare consists of three components for reimbursement. They are:

- *Medicare Part A:* This covers partial reimbursement to the patient during hospitalization including room, services, and treatments.
- *Medicare Part B:* This segment of the plan covers outpatient treatment, supplies, or other services. Some of these services include: psychiatrist or other doctor; clinical psychologist, social worker, or nurse specialist; nurse practitioner; physician's assistant; group or individual therapy; counseling services; medication; and diagnostic services.
- *Medicare Part D:* This section is the drug reimbursement portion of the plan, that is based on a frequently updated national formulary.

Medicare was never intended to be a 100% reimbursement insurance plan for the elderly and it is strongly advised that each individual have a supplementary plan. It is also necessary to identify health care providers who accept Medicare reimbursement for the provision of health care services (Medicare, n.d.).

## FACTORS INFLUENCING MENTAL HEALTH IN THE AGING POPULATION

Although any individual's mental health can be affected by numerous factors, the older adult population faces multiple variables that can impact their mental health. Often one or more of these variables are present simultaneously.

These variables involve physical, environmental, emotional, and social issues. Factors specific to the aging population are addressed here.

## Physical Changes

Multiple physical changes can impair the mental health of the aging individual. These changes include:

- Acid-based imbalances
- Dehydration
- Electrolyte changes
- Hypothermia or hyperthermia
- Hypothyroidism
- Hypoxia
- Impaired mobility
- Incontinence
- Infection and sepsis
- Medications
- Sensory changes (Gallo, Bogner, Fulmer, & Paveza, 2006)

These changes can be identified and corrected, thus diminishing their long-term effect on the patient.

In many instances, individuals who are over the age of 65 years accept these physical changes as normal changes related to the aging process. However, these age-related changes, even if corrected, can negatively influence the individual's quality of life. For example, a loss of physical function and mobility can lead to a loss of independence. This loss of independence can lead to social withdrawal, self-isolation, and anxiety or depression (Gagliardi, 2006).

> *Typically, physical changes in the elderly are dismissed as normal, age-related changes. However, they can significantly impact the person's mental health, leading to social isolation, anxiety, and depression.*

## Chronic Illness

Estimates reveal that at least 80% of individuals over the age of 65 years have at least one chronic illness. The most common include hypertension, heart disease, lung disease, diabetes, stroke, cancer, and bone and joint disorders. In addition, 52% of aging Americans reported varying levels of disability (sensory, physical, or mental). There is a strong association between chronic illness and mental health, with chronic illnesses often leading to depression and other mental health problems (Chowdhury & Rasani, 2008).

Patients and family need education about the risk for depression or altered mental health with chronic illness. The illness itself may lead to problems, for example, decreased mobility leading to social isolation, withdrawal, and depression or cognitive changes interfering with the patient's ability to function independently. Ultimately, these changes can impact the patient's coping ability and self-esteem. Additionally, prescribed or over-the-counter medications and herbs may produce side effects, such as confusion and disorientation, or interact with one another, predisposing the patient to an increased risk for mental health problems, such as depression or anxiety. The patient and family also need to be aware that a physical illness may exacerbate a previous mental health disorder and that a previous mental health disorder may worsen a physical illness. Thus, if a patient and family have adequate knowledge and understanding of the signs or changes that can be associated with mental health disorders, early interventions can be implemented, thereby diminishing the overall impact (Kramer, Beaudin, & Thrush, 2005).

## Pain

Pain has been designated as the fifth vital sign (in addition to the four vital signs of temperature, pulse, respirations, and blood pressure). The estimated prevalence of pain ranges from 36% to 88% for those in the age group of 65 years and above. Pain related to bone and joint problems, chronic pain related to chronic illness or trauma experienced prior to age 65, or acute illnesses are frequently under diagnosed and under treated. Self-reporting of pain may be viewed as drug-seeking behavior or minimized by the aging individual (Pratt et al., 2007).

Studies related to chronic pain reveal an association with social isolation, decreased physical function, and depression with an increased incidence of suicide. Additionally, the increased cost of health care, decreased quality of life, and possible early retirement that could negatively influence finances are other concerns associated with pain. Moreover, chronic, unresolved pain has been associated with an increased risk of a mental health disorder such as depression, suicide, or anxiety (Blay, Andreoli, Dewey, & Gastal, 2007).

When pain occurs, medication, such as acetaminophen and non-steroidal anti-inflammatory drugs (NSAIDs) are commonly used. However, these medications place the aging adult at risk for adverse drug reactions, or drug-drug interactions. Opioids, commonly prescribed for pain relief, are not first-line choices for aging patients because of the potential for diminished cognition, mood disturbances, insomnia, and addiction.

The ultimate goal is to maximize pain relief with a minimum of side effects. For the elderly, treatment should include physical therapy or the addition of complementary and alternative therapies. Both patient and caregivers need education about pain management and how it might impact the older adult. Studies have shown a strong link among pain, aging, depression, and insomnia, necessitating that all these should be addressed simultaneously (Merck & Co., 2006).

> *The presence of pain, its effect on functioning, and the associated treatment can predispose the elderly patient to mental health problems such as changes in cognition, mood, and sleep patterns.*

## Insomnia

INSOMNIA (difficulty initiating or maintaining sleep) is classified as: transient or short-term (occurring once to twice a week for four to six weeks); intermittent (varying over time without a pattern); or chronic (occurring two or more times per week for more than one month). The aging individual may exhibit signs and symptoms of insomnia such as sleeping for short periods during the night, sleeping during times of normal social activities, arising early in the morning while others sleep, and daytime sleepiness. Other indicators may include increased irritability, decreased mental function, changes in short-term memory, and the need for frequent and lengthy naps during the day (Ancoli-Israel & Cooke, 2005).

Insomnia in the aging adult can be caused by several factors that can occur concomitantly. Examples of causes of chronic insomnia issues are highlighted in **Box 23-1**.

Medications, such as antidepressants, antihistamines, antihypertensive agents, nasal decongestants, chemotherapeutic agents, and opioids can lead to insomnia. In addition, decreased melatonin, poor sleep hygiene, and lack of sunlight are other causes. Sunlight has been associated with insomnia in institutionalized populations who are not exposed to sunlight (Merck & Co., 2006; Medical News Today, 2005).

Measures to combat insomnia include establishing a consistent bedtime and discontinuing or limiting napping during the day, increasing daily activity levels, limiting

---

### BOX 23-1: CAUSES OF CHRONIC INSOMNIA

**ILLNESSES**

- Depression (the most common cause)
- Chronic pain
- Arthritis
- Kidney disease
- Restless legs syndrome
- Heart failure
- Parkinson's disease
- Sleep apnea
- Asthma
- Dementias

**BEHAVIORAL ISSUES**

- Anxiety about not being able to sleep
- Consuming alcohol before bedtime
- Consuming excessive amounts of caffeine
- Smoking cigarettes before bedtime
- Excessive napping in the afternoon or evening

---

caffeine or other stimulants, using the bed for only sex and sleep, avoiding large meals close to bedtime, and not obsessing about falling asleep. If the individual does not fall asleep with one-half hour, meditation or other relaxing activities should be considered. Depending on the individual's physical health status, a sleep apnea study may be warranted (Merck & Co., 2006).

Often, insomnia is treated with medication, such as sedatives and hypnotics or anti-anxiety agents, before bedtime. Unfortunately, these drugs pose a risk for older adults and for people with breathing problems because they suppress the areas of the brain that control breathing. In addition, prescription insomnia medications are often habit forming, although their degree of addiction varies from person to person (Fetveit, 2009). In addition, herbal remedies may be used. Valerian root and melatonin are two common ones.

As with any medications used by older adults, the chronic use of drugs to promote sleep can produce undesirable side effects including impaired memory and alertness, incontinence, daytime sleepiness, and alter metabolic or electrolyte imbalances. These side effects can exacerbate the patient's existing problems or create new ones.

Skilled nursing facilities frequently provide sleeping medications for their residents. Studies show that the use of sleeping medications increases the risk of falls. In addition, insomnia is increased in skilled nursing facilities due to the need for lights to be on at various locations and a louder-than-normal environment at night. Recent studies have shown that there is a decrease in insomnia in many of these residents if they are exposed to short periods of sunlight several times a week (Gobert & D'hoore, 2005). This exposure to natural light helps in the production of the necessary vitamins and chemoreceptors that enhance sleep.

## Disabilities and Handicaps

Pre-existing health issues are often present before the age of 65 years. The aging person will bring their life's health histories, behaviors, and/or handicaps and disabilities to their need for health care. These co-morbid conditions can be very significant in the quality of life and mental health of the elderly. Thus, the many changes that occur with aging and the pre-existing conditions together can significantly influence the overall health of the older person.

## Stress and Change

Many individuals who are retiring have made plans for their finances, residence, activities, and social and community connections and resources. However, as one ages, major stresses may arise leading to altered mental health, especially depression or anxiety. Research has shown that increased stress in an aging individual increases the physical and mental aging processes. In addition, studies have shown that prolonged stress has been associated with decreased immune function and altered health status (Maryland Coalition on Mental Health and Aging, n.d.; McClane, 2005).

Some of the identified situations associated with stress include:
- Caregiving for another person
- Retirement
- Increased leisure or unstructured time
- Health changes
- Reliance on others
- Social adjustments
- Financial changes
- Loss of loved ones
- Pain or disability
- Relocation or housing changes
- Negotiating new systems (i.e., health care benefits)
- Medication use
- Sensory decline (hearing, vision)

- Mobility restrictions
- Change in appearance
- Cultural emphasis on the value of youth

Two of the most common indicators of increased stress in the aging include social isolation and depression, viewed as an inability to manage stress in changed life circumstances. The aging individual may exhibit physical signs and symptoms such as fatigue, headaches, cold feet and hands, neck or back pain, and altered gastrointestinal functions. Many would consider these normal when experiencing stress. However, if these are present more than two to four weeks, further evaluation is necessary.

## Loss

Loss is a major influence on the mental health of the older adults. The loss of a spouse is considered a major risk factor for depression in the elderly. Other losses exerting an influence include loss of siblings, friends, or family pets. This loss can coexist with a change in living arrangements or increased health problems. Moreover, the older adult may be experiencing a loss of mobility, loss of sensory function, or loss of bladder control (incontinence), leading to feelings of decreased self-worth and depression. (Chen & Fu, 2008). Any single loss or combination of losses can lead to social isolation and subsequently depression.

> *Elderly individuals experience a wide range of losses, both physical and emotional, that can occur as single or multiple events, placing them at risk for decreased self-esteem and depression.*

## Family Coping

The relationship, or lack thereof, with family is a factor that influences the quality of an elder's mental health. Factors such as loss of communication, lack of understanding between the elder and family members, an increased need for care of the elder that is not easily available, or lack of knowledge about conditions affecting the elderly can contribute to mental health problems. Historically, the eldest daughter or female relative assumed the caregiving responsibility for aging family members. However, today, with many families depending on dual incomes, the care responsibilities may fall on adolescents or ancillary family members. This situation, coupled with the factors mentioned, can negatively influence the mental health of the elder as well as cause disruptions in the household and the family unit itself (Ron, 2008).

Caregiver stress with associated depression or anxiety often occurs when a family member, often a partner, provides care for a spouse or significant other. Aside from the impact of the stress of the disorder on the patient's functioning, this caring role also takes a physical toll on the caregiver. The lack of access to care, underutilization of available resources, social isolation, or fear of separation can result in significant strain on the caregiver. Additionally, the caregiver may be unable to fully or safely provide care for the patient, creating a dangerous physical environment for both the patient and caregiver (Son, Erno, Feemia, Zarit, & Stephens, 2007).

## Loneliness

Peplau defined LONELINESS as "an unnoticed inability to do anything while alone" (1988, p. 256). The prevalence of loneliness in individuals over the age of 65 years has been estimated to range from 5% to 26%. Loneliness is an individual response to unfulfilled needs for intimacy or social contacts. Two forms of loneliness have been defined. The first, SOCIAL LONELINESS, is related to a loss of contact with peers, friends, or groups that have shared and supported the needs of the elderly individual. The second, EMOTIONAL LONELINESS, is associated with loss of intimacy with a partner, family member, or friend who can no longer support the emotional needs of the elder. Both of these classifications can be experienced alone or in conjunction with one another. There is no defining period for how long loneliness will last.

Social loneliness has been associated with a loss of connectedness to friends, peers, family, or social activities within groups that supported the elder in his or her declining age in many facets of life. A major risk for social loneliness includes relocation of the person's residence, either geographically or to a new housing environment. Individuals who have relocated to assisted living or skilled nursing facilities often face this issue. Although they may have increased contact with other residents, this contact does not translate into the quality of relationships previously experienced (Drageset, 2002).

Emotional loneliness is experienced when an individual or group who provided intimacy and support to the elder no longer does so. As one ages, the loss of a partner, friends, or family increases while the ability to create new relationships decreases. The loss of these bonds and support systems negatively impact the elder. One specific group of elders that has reported slowly but increasing

perceptions of loneliness are caregivers. The need to care for a partner or family member causes a loss of opportunities for socialization, creating social isolation, while the declining health of the individual in need of care may also reflect a decline in emotional support, creating emotional loneliness (Drageset, 2002).

Loneliness has a strong correlation with declining mental health of the aging individual, most commonly depression. Depression is a mental state associated with loneliness. However, not all elders experiencing depression have associated feelings of loneliness. One study reported that the risk for mortality was 2.1 times higher for those experiencing loneliness with depression (Stek et al., 2005). This study also identified other health risks as being associated with loneliness and depression including: increased cognitive impairment, insomnia, impaired nutrition, hypertension, and other cardiac risk factors. An earlier study (Weeks, Michela, Peplau, & Bragg, 1990) correlated a relationship between loneliness and depression. However, this study defined both as separate mental health issues. More recently, O'Luanaigh and Lawlor (2008) discussed the connection between mental health and loneliness in the elderly, exploring physical responses to loneliness, including hypertension, insomnia, abnormal stress responses, and altered nutrition. Thus the issue of loneliness in the elderly can have an associated morbidity to other elder health issues.

The assessment of loneliness as depression is often misdiagnosed, causing decreased quality of life for the patient. Assessment can be confirmed by self-reporting and use of multiple assessment tools designed to improve the recognition of loneliness. The UCLA Loneliness Scale is one of the most common tools used. A knowledge base in assessing and then following through and providing resources for the lonely elder is important (Cornell & Waite, 2009).

Treatment for loneliness is often based on other mental health symptoms such as anxiety or depression. A primary intervention for loneliness in the elderly is to expand contacts and relationships with family and close friends (Petigrew & Roberts, 2008). It was noted that quality of social interactions rather than the quantity of interactions is important (Magai et al., 2008). Improved life satisfaction also occurred in aging individuals with loneliness when they were introduced to the Internet (Patel, 2007). Electronic communication, especially with distant family and friends, has been associated with decreased levels of loneliness. Access to a computer may be a challenge, but many senior citizen centers and public libraries provide opportunities for electronic communication. In addition, psychotherapy, especially group therapy, seems to have some success, but many elders have limited access.

> *Loneliness, an individual response to unfulfilled needs for intimacy or social contacts, occurs in two forms: social loneliness, which is related to a loss of contact with peers, friends, or groups that have shared and supported the elderly individual's social needs; and emotional loneliness, which is associated with the loss of intimacy with a partner, family member, or friend who can no longer support the elderly individual's emotional needs.*

## Abuse and Neglect

Abuse and neglect can be inflicted on an aging individual or be self-imposed. The abuse patterns may involve a family member or caregiver who has some influence in the elder's daily life. Control is the overall issue, that can lead to depression, anxiety, and potentially life-threatening physical injuries. Table 23-1 summarizes the four classifications of abuse that significantly impact the aging individual's mental health. However, all forms of elder abuse can be very threatening and frightening to the abused (Merck & Co., 2006). (See Chapter 24 for a more in-depth discussion about elder abuse.)

## Culture and Spirituality

Culture and spirituality, often closely related, provide a sense of purpose and view of the person's life and accomplishments. These two components play a variety of roles in the lives and activities of the elderly. Many people, as they age, find comfort and purpose by remaining closely affiliated with their beliefs. Others who may have earlier shed their cultural and spiritual beliefs find comfort and solace by returning to their roots. To others, with increasing physical and mental health issues, facing losses in their lives, and with diminished personal energies reject their earlier beliefs and practices to become more isolated individuals in relation to family and community. Each individual will find the answer when challenged with aging and its personal challenges (Trask, Hepp, Settles, & Shabo, 2009).

## COMMON MENTAL HEALTH PROBLEMS ASSOCIATED WITH THE ELDERLY

The elderly experience mental health problems similar to those experienced by adults in their younger years. However, several disorders require specific discussion because of their significant impact on the older adult.

### Depression in the Elderly

Depression in the elderly is reaching epidemic proportions, with some estimates revealing that one in five individuals over the age of 65 years suffers from mild or major depression. In addition, at least six million aging Americans are experiencing depression, with less than 10% of them receiving treatment for the disorder. Depression has also been estimated to be the underlying factor associated with increased health care costs of the elderly. As both life expectancy increases and the overall population over age 65 increases, the expected number of depressed elderly may more than double.

Depression must be differentiated from delirium and dementia. Together, these disorders are often referred to as the 3 Ds of GEROPSYCHIATRY (the study of psychiatric and mental illness in the aging population). These conditions are difficult to diagnose correctly in the elderly because their symptoms can be confused and more than one of the illnesses can be present in the same patient. Table 23-2 summarizes the major aspects for each disorder.

The inability to correctly diagnose the condition can lead to increased length of hospital stays, inappropriate medications, further impairing cognitive function, missed opportunities for treatment, and an overall diminished quality of life. In their most acute forms, these syndromes are associated with 10% to 20% of acute hospitalizations of the elderly (Ski & O'Connell, 2005). One study proposed that the actual cases of delirium occurring in medical-surgical patients 65 years of age and older may be as high as 70% (van Zyl & Seitz, 2006). Projections also reveal that up to 60% of this population will be discharged with and continue to exhibit signs of cognitive impairment.

In 2003, the elderly comprised 12% of the population of the United States but accounted for 16% of all reported suicides. In 2004, 14.3% of every 100,000 people age 65 or older died by suicide. The suicide rates for men rise with age, most significantly after age 65. The rate for men is seven times that for females who are 65 years of age and older. In addition, about 60% of elderly patients who take their own lives see their primary care physician within a

**TABLE 23-1: CLASSIFICATIONS OF ABUSE IN THE ELDERLY**

| TYPE OF ABUSE | DESCRIPTION | IMPLICATIONS FOR THE AGING INDIVIDUAL |
|---|---|---|
| Physical | Result of physical force and violence leading to physical illness or trauma in the elder.<br><br>Includes bodily injury and pain, physical impairment or inappropriate restraints (chemical or physical). | No clear indicator of an elder being more or less at risk for this type of abuse.<br><br>Perpetrators often associated with unmarried family members or caregivers living with the victim and relying on the elder's home and financial support; frequently substance abuse problem involved.<br><br>Careful assessment of elderly patients for signs of unexplained injury or scars, frequent visits to the urgent care or emergency department. |
| Sexual abuse | Any physical contact to which an individual does not consent.<br><br>Includes rape, molestation, insertion of foreign objects, or any other unwanted sexual contact.<br><br>Domestic violence if occurring between marital partners. | Those at risk: aging women, individuals unable to provide consent due to mental impairment, individuals who have poor social skills or are socially isolated, individuals residing in skilled care facilities (often at a higher risk for sexual abuse than those residing in family residences) (Edwards, 2005).<br><br>Assessment of potential victims for any signs of bruises, injuries, or bleeding from the genitalia, inner thighs, or breast area; inability to walk or sit comfortably; frequent urinary tract infections or sexually transmitted diseases (NCPEA, 2008). |
| Psychological abuse | Intentional infliction of mental or emotional anguish because of threats, humiliations, or other verbal or non-verbal conduct. | Perpetrators similar to those of physical abuse, as they may rely heavily on the resources of the aged.<br><br>Indicators difficult to identify as they may result in a more rapid decline in the elder, such as weight loss, insomnia, or other indicators of stress. |
| Neglect | Failure of an individual to receive their daily needs and security.<br><br>*Active* neglect is purposeful and calculated. *Passive* neglect is the result of the inability of the caregiver to provide the daily needs; possibly related to knowledge deficit, personal illness or disability, stress, or lack of resources. | Victim is dependent on assistance because of mental or physical disabilities; individuals requiring a high level of care.<br><br>Possible substance abuse.<br><br>Key indicators: poor nutrition; dehydration; unclean, disheveled appearance; and unhealed lesions or decubiti ulcers (NCPEA, 2008). |
| Self-neglect | Individual as the victim. | Socially isolated, living in an unkempt environment, possibly affecting members of the surrounding community.<br><br>Indicators: hoarding; keeping large volumes of paper, food items, or large numbers of domestic animals.<br><br>Refusal of assistance from family and outside agencies.<br><br>Social services often are required to remove elder from personal environment—the last alternative for the elder, as reports have shown a very low survival rate of six months following the change (Dong et al., 2009). |

| TABLE 23-2: COMPARING DELIRIUM, DEMENTIA, AND DEPRESSION | | | |
|---|---|---|---|
| | **DELIRIUM** | **DEMENTIA** | **DEPRESSION** |
| **Definition** | Rapid and often fluctuating levels of consciousness and disorganized cognitive processes that are temporary in duration<br>Reversal of condition in approximately 10% to 30% of hospitalized elderly | A slowly progressive change in cognitive abilities including short-term memory loss, diminished language skills, and inability to perform activities of daily living | A moderate to rapid change in an individual's behavior or mood that can be related to loss of interest in normally satisfying activities that can also reflect short-term memory loss, altered communication patterns, or inability to perform activities of daily living for at least 14 days |
| **Symptoms** | Onset can be from hours or a few days<br>Cognitive symptoms vary in the day, but may become worse during the night or on awakening<br>Orientation is usually limited to person<br>Behaviors can range from agitated and aggressive to confusion and lethargy<br>Inability to focus on or remain focused on the present<br>Altered perceptions including vivid illusions and hallucinations | A measurable impairment in two or more of the following:<br>• Memory<br>• Language<br>• Personality<br>• Emotional behaviors<br>• Cognitive skills<br>• Visual/spatial perceptions | Cognitive changes can be associated with altered mood<br>May deny sadness/depression but report an increase of somatic disorders that may include:<br>• Increased levels of pain that interfere with normal activities<br>• Altered sleep patterns<br>• Alteration in eating patterns /weight loss<br>• Poor personal hygiene<br>• Cognitive confusion related to specific rather than global activities<br>• Mood alterations, from increased irritability to lethargy<br>• Substance abuse |
| **Thinking** | Alterations in alertness, cognition, thinking patterns, perceptions | Cognitive impairment related to memory and one or more of the following:<br>• Aphasia<br>• Apraxia<br>• Agnosia<br>• Executive functioning | Reduced memory, level of consciousness, and thinking; and low self-esteem |
| **Sleep** | Disturbed without a pattern, changes nightly | Disturbed with a specific pattern | Disturbed with early morning awakening or hypersomnia |
| **Causes** | Underlying physical conditions including:<br>• Urinary tract infections or retention<br>• Cardiovascular events<br>• Constipation<br>• Viral or bacterial infections<br>• Altered metabolic or endocrine states<br>• Renal failure<br>• Medications | Irreversible neurodegenerative diseases including:<br>• Alzheimer's disease (60–75%)<br>• Lewy body dementia<br>• Frontal lobe atrophy<br>• Multi-infarct cerebral vascular accident<br>• Substance-related atrophy<br>• HIV/AIDS | Major causes of depression in the elderly can be related to:<br>• Loss of spouse or significant others<br>• Loneliness and isolation<br>• Chronic illness or health-related issues<br>• Medications<br>• Substance abuse<br>• Stress<br>• Financial circumstances<br>• Uncontrolled environmental issues |

*(cont.)*

**TABLE 23-2: COMPARING DELIRIUM, DEMENTIA, AND DEPRESSION (*CONT.*)**

| | DELIRIUM | DEMENTIA | DEPRESSION |
|---|---|---|---|
| Screening tools | Confusion Assessment Method Algorithm (CAM) "I WATCH DEATH" causes of delirium | Folstein Mini Mental Exam with Clock Drawing Mini-Cog Dementia Screen Cohen-Mansfield Agitation Inventory | Geriatric Depression Scale (GDS 4 Short Form) Cornell Scale for Depression SIG E CAPS (*DSM-IV* criteria) Assessment of Suicide Risk in the Older Adult |

*From Gagliardi, J. P. (2006). Differentiating among depression, delirium, and dementia in elderly patients. American Medical Association Journal of Ethics/personal mentor.org. Retrieved from http://virtualmentor.ama-assn.org/2008/06/cprl1-0806.html; Toronto Best Practice in LTC Initiative. (2007). 3Ds:Assessment tools at your fingertips. Retrieved from http://www.opadd.on.ca/Local%20Projects/documents/LocalProject-Educ.Training-3Dsassessmentguide.pdf*

few months of their death. Depression and chronic unrelieved pain are two significant issues related to suicide in the elderly (American Foundation for Suicide Prevention, 2011). Other contributory factors include chronic or terminal illnesses, social isolation, and access to the means of committing suicide (i.e., firearms in the home).

Once an elderly patient is diagnosed with depression, the potential for suicide needs to be recognized. This is a major health risk for the aging population who disproportionately have limited access or funding to mental health services (Harris, Cook, Victor, Dewilde, & Beighton, 2006).

Another major factor related to depression is the morbidity related to chronic illnesses. Depression is commonly associated with numerous medical diagnoses such as heart attack, Parkinson's disease, multiple sclerosis, diabetes, cancer, and arthritis. In addition, depression can result from other situations that the elderly may experience, such as being a victim of a crime, a change in residence, death of a spouse or family member, poverty, and loneliness (Merck & Co., 2006).

The signs and symptoms of depression in the elderly are as unique as each individual. The primary characteristics of depression in the elderly are frequently related to a chronic illness rather than a mental health disorder. Primary health care providers not trained in evaluating depression in the elderly often focus the treatment on the symptoms. As a result, the patient experiences a diminished quality of life that could lead to an increased risk of suicide. Often the complaints of unexplained or aggravated aches and pains or insomnia are sometimes associated with drug-seeking behaviors rather than a component of the more serious diagnosis of depression.

Treatment of the elderly with depression commonly includes psychopharmacology, nonpharmacologic approaches, and electroconvulsive therapy (Kennedy, 2000; Kneisl, Wilson, & Trigoboff, 2004). (See Chapter 12 for additional information about depression and its treatment.)

Antidepressants are the first line of therapy used on the elderly with depression. Elderly patients typically respond well to the first medication used. In addition, psychotherapy, such as interpersonal psychotherapy and cognitive behavioral therapy are used for aging individuals with depression. The patient may be referred to physical therapy to promote enhanced functioning and mobility and to occupational therapy to help promote feelings of self-worth, personal pride, and independence in activities of daily living.

Reminiscence therapy may be of benefit to the elderly patient with depression. Several studies conducted in Taiwan (Hsu & Wang, 2009; Huang, Li, Yang, & Chen, 2009; Chao, Wu, Jin, Chu, & Clark, 2006) identified the use of reminiscence therapy in institutionalized elders as part of a group therapy structure. This therapy was used primarily with individuals who had both depression and dementia. Success on an individualized basis has not been established with large populations (Bohlmeijer, Smit, Onrust, & van Marwijk, 2009). However, the potential for reminiscence therapy cannot be diminished because it is a cost-effective treatment.

Electroconvulsive therapy (ECT) plays a major role in the treatment of depression in the elderly. Patients selected to receive ECT are those elders who demonstrate a poor or lack of response to multiple medications, have had a psychotic element to their depression, have severe malnutrition, or are at imminent risk for suicide. With increased age and declining cardiovascular function, not all elders are candidates for these procedures. There is also temporary cognitive impairment immediately following the treatment, complicating the recovery process. Usually ECT is given twice weekly for eight to twelve sessions.

> *Depression in the elderly is reaching epidemic proportions, with estimates indicating depression as the major underlying cause for the increased cost of health care in this population.*

## Generalized Anxiety Disorder in the Elderly

The prevalence of generalized anxiety disorder (GAD) is estimated to range from 3% to 10% of individuals over the age of 65 years. (See Chapter 13 for additional information about anxiety disorders.) Studies in the United States and Europe have noted that GAD more commonly appears between the ages of 20 to 50 years, with only 3% of those over age 65 developing GAD. Approximately 32% of adults with GAD demonstrate a genetic predisposition to the disorder.

The symptoms of GAD also fluctuate in response to physical, mental, environmental, social, or other stresses. In comparison to depression, GAD in the elderly is more frequently associated with physical symptoms and less frequently with emotional disturbances. There is some indication that depression can be a component of GAD. For example, Golde et al. (2009) identified a relationship between GAD and loneliness in the community-dwelling elder. As the elder withdraws from social or personal relationships with increasing depression, loneliness can cause further loss of quality of life, self-esteem, and mood changes. Studies also reveal an increased level of anxiety in elders with mild cognitive impairments (Rozzini et al., 2009).

Anxiety is frequently seen in individuals with mild to moderate cognitive impairment. Anxiety in the elderly can also be manifested as a new phobia or a phobia previously experienced in the elderly person may intensify.

Various assessment tools can be used to diagnose anxiety in the elderly: the Generalized Anxiety Disorder Severity Scale, Geriatric Anxiety Inventory, and Anxiety Status Inventory (Weiss et al., 2009). Depending on the onset and severity of GAD in an elderly patient, a computed tomography (CT) scan or magnetic resonance imaging (MRI) scan may be done (Merck & Co., 2006).

Currently there are two schools of thought regarding the treatment of the elder with GAD. One involves psychotherapy as the treatment of choice, with the incorporation of medication. The other promotes the use of cognitive behavioral therapy as the first choice, followed by medication if the therapy is not successful.

Due to the significant physical component to GAD, a complete physical should be done to identify any health issues that can be causing the anxiety. In an elder with limited comorbidity, medications alone may provide relief for the patient (Rangari & Pelissolo, 2006; Flint, 2005).

Four antidepressants have been approved by the Food & Drug Administration (FDA) for use in the elderly. They include the selective serotonin reuptake inhibitors escitalopram (Lexapro) and paroxetine (Paxil) and the serotonin norepinephrine reuptake inhibitors (SNRIs) duloxetine (Cymbalta) and venlafazine (Effexor). These medications have been associated with minimal side effects and interactions with other medications, and limited sedation in the elderly with GAD. Some individuals do, however, discontinue the medication.

Benzodiazepines, both long-acting agents such as diazepam (Valium) and clonazepam (Klonopin) and short-acting agents such as lorazepam (Ativan) and oxapam (Serax), may be used with the elderly. Benzodiazepines achieve a rapid response and may be used with other anxiolytic agents. These are also often affordable to elders on low incomes. Unfortunately, these agents, which classified as anxiolytics, are associated with side effects including drug-dependence, memory loss, impaired movement that can increase the risk of falls, and incontinence. These agents, if used in high doses and for prolonged periods, have been shown to worsen depression and also cause addiction. There have also been reports of accelerated cognitive impairment in patients with associated dementias.

Buspiron (Buspar) is another agent that may be used in the elderly. It has fewer side effects and less interaction with other medications. However, it is not as effective in treating GAD in the elderly as other medications are.

Cognitive behavioral therapy is a major treatment modality for anxiety in the elderly. Other therapy may include alternative or complementary treatments such as chiropractic treatment; holistic treatments to treat the mind, body, and spirit; homeopathy; and the use of food supplements, vitamins, and herbs. Patients need to check with their health care provider before adding any of these modalities to their lifestyle (Flint, 2005).

> *Treatment of generalized anxiety disorder in the elderly typically involves psychotherapy with psychopharmacology, or cognitive behavioral therapy followed by psychopharmacology if not successful.*

## Mood Disorders in the Elderly

Mood disorders in the elderly share the characteristics of those in a younger population. These disorders may have been present prior to the age of 65 years, or may develop after that age. These disorders often include: manic episodes with sustained excitement, euphoria, and hyperactivity; alterations of elations and depressions reflected as bipolar disorders; and major depression that may increase and extend for long periods of time. (See Chapter 12 for an in-depth discussion of these disorders.)

Although the elderly have disproportionately increased incidences of depression and increased risk of paranoia, there are no reports of a higher incidence of mood disorders in this population as compared to the younger population. Treatments for these disorders in the elderly mirror those used with a younger population. However, there are added concerns related to psychopharmocolgic interactions and side effects.

## Substance Use and Abuse and the Elderly

Estimates on the frequency of substance abuse among the elderly have been reported to be as low as 2% or as high as 38% for individuals over the age of 65 years. Research found that prescription drug abuse among the elderly may be as high as 12% to 15% in those seeking health care (Meyer, 2005). It is projected that this number will grow as the aging population increases. The most commonly abused substances in the elderly include alcohol, anxiolytics, nicotine, opioids, sedatives, and polysubstances. As the individual ages, the illegal substance consumption tends to decrease, being replaced by alcohol and prescription medications, especially opioids. The highest rates of substance abuse involve alcohol and nicotine, both of which are related to increased morbidity and mortality including cancer, chronic lung disease, and renal and liver disease. Substance abuse can also be associated with an increased risk for suicide. Studies reveal that unless there are major factors of safety to self or community, substance abuse problems in the elderly are frequently ignored (Benshoff, Harrawood, & Koch, 2003).

One major area of substance use in the elderly is related to **POLYPHARMACY**, defined as the use of multiple medications beyond the clinically identified needs of the individual (University of Chicago, n.d.). This includes prescribed, over-the-counter medications and herbal and homeopathic products. Elderly individuals account for 30% or more of prescribed medications without including other potential products. Often the prime candidate for polypharmacy is the patient who is taking more than one medication from a physician and not getting the response expected. Typically polypharmacy is related to unresolved pain and depression or anxiety. In response, the elder may go to more than one physician for more than one prescription and have the medication filled at different pharmacies. In addition, drug-seeking behaviors identified in younger individuals may also be seen in the older adult. The use of multiple drugs places the elder at increased risk for side effects and addiction.

Beyond monitoring the elderly patient for medication use, drug interaction, or signs and symptoms of alcohol or substance abuse, assessment tools are available that can assist in the diagnosis. **Table 23-3** highlights some of these tools.

> *Polypharmacy is a major problem with the elderly population with the use of multiple medications commonly used to treat unresolved pain, depression, or anxiety.*

# PALLIATIVE AND END-OF-LIFE ISSUES WITH MENTALLY IMPAIRED ELDERS

The majority of deaths in the United States occur in the population of those who are 65 years of age and older. Causes are numerous and can be related to chronic illness, falls or trauma, and dementias. The passage of the Patient Self-Determination Act of 1991 emphasized the right of patients to participate in treatment and health care decisions and the use of advance directives for end-of-life care decisions. An advance directive such as a living will or durable power of attorney is essential for an individual with dementia, cognitive impairment, or chronic diseases. It provides health care providers with guidance as to what level of care the patient is seeking. The directive also includes the provision for palliative or hospice care.

| TABLE 23-3: ASSESSMENT TOOLS FOR SUBSTANCE ABUSE IN THE ELDERLY | |
| --- | --- |
| ALCOHOL CONSUMPTION | |
| Alcohol Problem-Related Survey (ARPS) | 60 self-administered questions including medical and psychiatric conditions |
| Alcohol Use Disorder Identification Test (AUDIT) | Brief, structured interview of 10 questions from the World Health Organization that can be incorporated into an assessment/history |
| Cut-down, Annoyed, Guilty and Eye-opener (CAGE) Questionnaire | 4 specific questions; can be modified for the assessment of chemical abuse |
| Michigan Alcohol Screening Test–Geriatrics (MAST-G) | 24 (yes/no) questions to be completed by the patient; can be modified for the assessment of chemical abuse |
| CHEMICAL/DRUG ABUSE | |
| Drug Use Questionnaire | 20 questions relating to previous 12 month's experiences from the Lawyers Assistance Program; British Columbia |
| Beer's List | National guidelines of the criteria for prescribing and use of medication in the elderly |
| Medication Appropriateness Index | National guidelines of the criteria for prescribing and use of medication in the elderly (computerized) |

Especially with the early diagnosis of dementia and associated depression, the aging patient needs to be educated and encouraged to draw up advanced directives, including a living will and durable power of medical attorney. These decisions need to be made within the family unit with agreement of all participating members. Braun, Beyth, Ford, & McCullough (2008) reported that end-of-life decisions by a surrogate, especially without advanced directives, increases the burdens and anxiety in the decision-making individual.

Another area involved with end-of-life issues is hospice care. In 2004, it was estimated that more than one million individuals use hospice and supportive care (McCasland, 2007). Approximately 1 in 17 elders were diagnosed with a variety of mental health issues including dementias, mood disorders, and depression. As many as 54,000 individuals received hospice care with a primary or associated mental illness. Due to the decreased cognitive ability of many over the age of 65 years, patients and families need to be educated about this treatment option.

## TRENDS IN MENTAL HEALTH CARE FOR THE ELDERLY

Symptoms of depression, anxiety disorders, and other mental health problems often are manifest when older adults are admitted to an acute care unit for medical or surgical interventions. Thus, all nurses need to be able to assess and intervene with these individuals through the development of therapeutic relationships. In addition, there is an increased need for advanced practice nurses with geropsychiatric preparation to assist with and provide appropriate care.

## Acute Care

It has been estimated that up to 30% of hospital admissions of individuals over the age of 65 years are associated with depression or suicide attempt, substance abuse, or other mental health disorder. Identification of a co-mental health condition provides for more immediate and appropriate interventions, can decrease the length of stay, and can allow the elder to receive necessary post-discharge treatments (National Institute of Mental Health, 2009).

It has been estimated that over two-thirds of hospital beds are occupied by those over the age of 65 years, and that 30% to 60% will have a mental health disorder while hospitalized. The most frequently observed conditions are depression, delirium, and dementia. Due to the dual needs of this population, specialized units, such as the Acute Care for Elders (ACE) units, have been developed. These units include patient-centered nursing, regular review of medical and psychiatric care, a multidisciplinary task force, and discharge planning on an individual level to provide for the best quality of life for the elderly patient. On evaluation, these units have discharged patients earlier, have maintained as much independence and activities of daily living as possible, and decreased admission to skilled nursing facilities. There has also been a decrease in impaired cognitive functions. These specialty units are not designed as a one-time admission, but are available for the elders as often as necessary (Hanna, Woolley, Brown, & Kesavan, 2008).

Additionally, there has been a demonstrated need for geropsychiatric practitioners in acute psychiatric facilities. This need was based on a comparison of the acute psychiatric admission of a patient over the age of 65 years with that of a younger patient. Areas reviewed related to participation in activities, lengths of stay, and admission to an acute care facility requiring care for other physical conditions. The future of geriatric mental health can be guided by specialty acute care and psychiatric units, but all support the need for mental health care following discharge.

## Outpatient Services

The access to outpatient-based mental health care has been historically limited. Several factors affect the elderly seeking or receiving mental health services in the community (Chowdhury & Rasani, 2008). Four significant factors that have impacted this issue are related to (1) personal belief in and desire for mental health care services; (2) the ability to meet the costs of services; (3) physical access to the services; and (4) patient care to meet the changing needs of the aging population.

> *Factors influencing the elderly individual's use of mental health services in the community include: the person's belief in and desire for the services, the ability to pay for the services, the ability to physically access the services, and the availability of programs to meet the changing needs of the elderly.*

### Personal Belief and Desire for Mental Health Care Services

Mental health and the need for care have been stigmatized in the health care environment. This can create a lack

in seeking out of services because of personal or family beliefs. Culture also is a major component in whether an individual seeks out mental health services. The primary focus in overcoming these obstacles is education to create an increased awareness in both the public and health care arenas, emphasizing that mental health issues are experienced by all individuals, all cultures, and that mental health is a major component for both health and quality of life. Helping to fuel this educational process is the internet, which offers explanations, signs and symptoms, and resources to all. Professional education is addressing the frequency and morbidity of mental health issues, fostering provision of the appropriate health care institution at the primary level of health care.

### Ability to Meet the Costs of Services

As discussed, Medicare provides minimal reimbursement coverage (approximately 50%) for mental health services. This same limited coverage is also reflected in Medicare supplemental insurance policies. However, the treatment of mental health issues at the primary care level and medications covered by insurance are showing dramatic increases but still do not offer the coverage provided for general health care. A new and different form of coverage has been developed and evaluated. Although primarily available to individuals not on Medicare, the *Carve-out Managed Behavioral Health Care Organizations* (MBHOs) are showing revenue savings that may be extended to individuals receiving Medicare supplements (American Association of Geriatric Psychiatry Online, 2004). This program removes mental health care from existing insurance policies and assigns it to a separate agency or vendor who uses programs, providers, and services different from the original policy. Reflecting cost savings and diminished duplication of services, this program is currently under review.

### Physical Access to Mental Health Services

It has been identified that many elderly in need of mental health services lack physical access to the services in the community setting. This may be related to living in rural areas, lack of transportation, or services not available at a community level. Several alternatives have been identified to meet these needs. A variety of programs have been developed to reach the needy and to incorporate nurse-patient relationships for continuity of care.

One program is On Lok, an new program in San Francisco. It has 10 centers in California and was the foundation of the *Program of All-inclusive Care for the Elderly* (PACE*)*. These centers offer health care services, social interaction, and activities for both the elder and the family based on the concept of maintaining the elder in the home to facilitate quality of life and safety. The PACE program is offered in 29 states with 61 programs (National PACE Association, 2002).

Another program, the *Psychogeriatric Assessment and Treatment in City Housing Program* has been offered in Baltimore, Maryland, for the last 20 years. This project, based on the premise of community health care, provides mobile psychiatric treatment to elders unable to access other programs (Blass et al., 2006). A third program was developed that uses the all-inclusive care unit as a model to diminish functional loss in the acute care setting. The Indiana University for Aging Research spearheaded the development of the *Geriatric Resources for the Assessment and Care of Elders* (GRACE) to slow the physical and cognitive functional status of low-income elders. This program has also decreased acute health care admissions by focusing on maintaining the elderly in their homes rather than using nursing home placement (Counsell, Callahan, Buttar, Clark, & Frank, 2006). Another program, *ElderLynk*, developed in 1999, provides mental health care to rural elders. This community-based program has demonstrated a significant improvement of reported mental health function, reported levels of depression, and reported life satisfaction despite declines of mental status, activities of daily living, and overall health issues (McGovern, Lee, Johnson, & Morton, 2008).

Last, Veterans Affairs (VA) has designed and continues to research a *telepsychology* program (also referred to as telepsychiatry or telemental Health) (Egede et al., 2009). The concepts of this program are based on the ability to reach elderly patients in rural areas, decrease stigmatization associated with traditional mental health services, and decrease issues of mobilization and transportation of individuals with a variety of physical limitations.

## Programs to Meet the Needs of the Elder Population

A variety of *elder day care centers* are available in many regions to provide for daily or respite care to the families of aging individuals. They provide care to the cognitively impaired, frail, or physically impaired elder so the family is able to function as needed. This may include the ability to work away from home, maintain the elder in the home environment, or provide for personal needs. Residential services also have expanded from independent living through extended care for the elderly. Some community, religious-based, or privately owned facilities provide guaranteed care from independence through skilled nursing services in one setting. These arrangements are often chosen by the elders themselves. And geriatric case management services, which offer a variety of services and levels of care, have been developed to assure elders and their families that the care and safety of the elder is maintained through observation and use of resources, often convenient for geographically separated families. The types and costs of these services are highly variable.

## APPLYING THE NURSING PROCESS FROM AN INTERPERSONAL PERSPECTIVE

The nursing process in mental health nursing, as stated throughout this text, is a dynamic, interactive, and problem-solving process that is both systematic and individualized for the patient. The patient is an active participant in his or her plan of care. However, this participation can be a difficult process for the aging individual, especially when the individual is experiencing cognitive changes, such as memory loss or dementia or other problems that can impact his or her functional status or decision-making ability. When this occurs, the focus shifts to include the patient, the caregiver, and the family.

The elderly patient may be seen in a variety of settings, such as acute care, day care centers, community and outpatient centers, and long-term care facilities, including assisted living communities and skilled nursing facilities. Many of the patients will have co-morbidities that may predispose the patient to mental health problems. Or the patient may have a mental health problem that increases the patient's risk for a medical condition or exacerbates a current medical condition or chronic illness. (See Chapter 8 for additional information about the interface of mental health problems and medical illnesses.) Therefore, nurses need a firm understanding of the nursing process that integrates the interpersonal process when caring for elderly patients. (Refer to the specific chapters on the disorders for related plans of care).

## Strategies for Optimal Assessment: The Therapeutic Use of Self

Assessment begins as soon as possible, often with the first meeting of the patient. The nurse collects subjective data directly from the patient if possible. In some cases, the individual may be unable to communicate his or her feelings or personal needs and will need to rely on a family member or other individual to provide the necessary information. The nurse also can gain additional data from previous medical records and any diagnostic testing. This information is especially important if there is concern about any metabolic or physiological changes in the patient such as oxygenation, altered serum electrolytes, glucose levels, and metabolic acidosis/alkalosis that may be impacting his or her abilities.

Objective data are gathered as the nurse carefully observes the communication and behavior of the patient. When a specific behavior is the focus, the nurse must identify the triggering behaviors, situations, or thought processes experienced by the elder.

Often, a more global assessment of the elderly patient's mental status is completed by using a measurement instrument to assess the quality of life. One of the most commonly used assessment tools is the *Medical Outcomes Study – Short Form 36* (SF-36v2). This reliable and valid tool is applicable to individuals over the age of 12 years and is available in over 40 languages. Eight domains are measured by this tool and include: physical functioning, role functioning, bodily pain, general health, vitality, social functioning, emotional role, and mental health. This one-page, self-administered test can provide health care providers with information on actual or potential issues influencing the mental, emotional, and physical status of the elder. This tool can be used initially to establish a baseline and then repeated weekly to monitor the patient's progress (Rand, n.d.).

Another assessment tool specifically for individuals over age 65 was developed by De Leo et al. (1998) in conjunction with the Eastern European Branch of WHO. This tool was specifically designed to provide a more comprehensive evaluation of the elder individual (McClane, 2005). It has been translated in over a dozen languages and consists of 49 self-administered questions. The information obtained from this assessment includes: physical functioning, self-care, depression and anxiety, cognitive and social functioning, sexual functioning, and life satisfaction. The tool allows evaluation of the elder's quality of life, providing an accurate identification of actual or potential concerns. Ideally, it is suggested that this tool be used with each individual seeking health care when turning age 65, and then annually or when a problem is suspected to aid in providing insight into the care of the elderly.

Throughout the initial assessment and interaction with the patient during this orientation phase, the nurse-patient relationship is beginning to form. Information needs to be collected during this time, but the nurse must not remain isolated in doing so. Although the nurse and patient are strangers at this time, it is necessary for the nurse to interact with the patient on a humanistic level to

begin forming the basis of trust between these two individuals (Peplau, 1994). Denying the elder the opportunity to interact with the nurse as self at this early period can negatively affect the therapeutic relationship.

Providing a safe, comfortable environment with minimal external stimulation is necessary to establish an atmosphere of trust. Minimizing stimulation and external stressors also are key to preventing the patient from becoming overwhelmed. If the patient is being admitted to an inpatient facility or acute care facility, investigate with the family about any objects or clothing that can be brought into the therapeutic environment of the aging patient to promote a familiar environment and adaptation to the new surroundings.

The nurse also fosters an atmosphere whereby the patient feels there is genuine interest, acceptance, and positive regard. This is accomplished primarily through therapeutic communication techniques including restating, reflecting, and clarifying. (See Chapter 3 for more information on therapeutic communication.) In addition, when communicating with the patient, speak clearly and distinctly, and allow ample time for the patient to answer. If necessary, break up the assessment into small chunks to avoid overwhelming the patient. With persistence and creativity, the nurse enhances the elder's ability to understand his or her needs for help and altered mental health status, thereby expanding the newly formed therapeutic relationship as they move forward. **Therapeutic Interaction 23-1** highlights an interaction between a nurse and an elderly patient who is depressed.

> *When assessing the elderly individual, the nurse interacts with the patient on a humanistic level to promote trust and foster an atmosphere of genuine interest, acceptance, and positive regard.*

## Diagnosing and Planning Appropriate Interventions: Meeting the Patient's Focused Needs

Once a full assessment is completed the nurse, patient, and family proceed to develop a plan of care with mutual goals and expectations for outcomes. The nurse collaborates with the patient and family to identify their needs and specific problems and then begin a plan for care (Peplau,

> ### THERAPEUTIC INTERACTION 23-1:
> ### WORKING WITH AN ELDER ADULT WHO IS DEPRESSED
>
> Mr. B. has been a patient in the gero psychiatric inpatient unit for 24 hours. He was admitted by his family members who indicated that he was wandering outdoors without a sweater or coat in very frigid weather. He had a history of wandering; the family reported cognitive decline over the past 2 months as well as a lack of verbal interaction—he would often sit for hours in front of the TV. He also refused meals and/or ate very little.

| | |
|---|---|
| **Nurse:** "Mr. B., I am the nurse who will be with you today." | Introduces self and begins development of interpersonal relationship; clearly communicates role |
| **Mr. B.:** (no verbal or nonverbal response; staring into space; has not touched breakfast tray that was delivered to his room) | Not communicative |
| **Nurse:** "Mr. B., I am here to help you with your care. First, I would like to help you with your breakfast. I will stay with you and help you." | Building on the relationship, the nurse reinforces his or her role<br>Prepares breakfast tray for patient |
| **Mr. B.:** (silence continues; still no verbal communication; takes a bite of toast). | Begins to show responsiveness to nurse's contact |
| **Nurse:** "Mr. B., (continues to stay with patient), can I help you prepare your tea?" | The nurse continues to develop therapeutic relationship and focuses on helping the patient accomplish small tasks |
| **Mr. B.:** "I am tired now. I would like to sleep." | Expresses fatigue and desire to avoid interaction |
| **Nurse:** "I will let you rest now. I will come back in 30 minutes to take you to the activity room." | Respects the patient's expressed need, but indicates time frame when the nurse will return to continue relationship |

1991). Focusing on the patient's strengths that were identified in the assessment stage is key when planning interventions. Doing so will also allow for an increased sense of collaboration on the part of the patient and family. Patient care needs are addressed in order of priority and realistic, achievable, measurable, and individualized goals and outcomes are established. Both short- and long-term goals are important.

Due to the wide range of assessment findings noted and multiple problems faced by patients with cognitive disorders, numerous nursing diagnoses would apply. Examples of possible nursing diagnoses would include:
• Acute confusion related to cognitive impairment
• Chronic confusion related to cognitive impairment
• Disturbed sleep pattern related to restlessness
• Risk for injury related to environmental changes, wandering behavior
• Impaired memory related to cognitive impairment
• Caregiver role strain related to lack of support systems

- Compromised family coping related to lack of available resources and support
- Ineffective role performance related to caregiver fatigue
- Self-care deficit (bathing, dressing, feeding, toileting) related to cognitive impairment

These nursing diagnoses also will vary based on the acuity of the patient's illness, co-morbidities, current treatment regimen, and sources of support. Based on the identified nursing diagnoses, the nurse and patient collaboratively would determine the outcomes to be achieved. For example, to address the self-care deficit related to performing activities of daily living, the outcome would be to gradually increase the patient's participation in activities through collaboration.

## Implementing Effective Interventions: Timing and Pacing

During implementation, the nurse continues to monitor the patient and maintain an ongoing assessment of the patient's behavior as interventions designed to promote a specific behavior or response in the patient, are carried out. Above all, patient safety is the priority in maintaining and promoting the patient's optimal mental and physical health.

Depending on the cognitive ability and overall health of the elderly patient, interventions are implemented in a manner that allows for maximum effectiveness. Through the therapeutic use of self and the nurse-patient relationship, the nurse determines the appropriate timing and pacing of the interventions, keeping the patient's safety in the forefront. For example, if a patient is experiencing periods of confusion, the nurse would implement teaching at a time when the patient is more alert. If the patient is experiencing significant anxiety, the nurse would institute measures to reduce the patient's anxiety, such as administering prescribed medications and reducing external stimulation before attempting to engage the patient in a conversation about what is triggering the anxiety. Through the therapeutic use of self, the nurse maintains his or her presence with the patient to demonstrate trust and support.

During this time, as interventions are effective, the patient's role changes to one of greater independence, seeking out the nurse as teacher and socializing agent. For this to be successful, the nurse must be a willing and active participant and resource for the patient.

## Evaluating: Objective Critique of Interventions and Self-Reflection

Evaluation is a very important process in the care of elderly patients. It occurs as a continuous, cyclical, dynamic, and ongoing process involving changes in the patient's status over time. It occurs throughout the phases of the nursing process as the nurse gathers new data, reevaluates nursing interventions, and modifies the plan of care.

During this phase, the nurse reviews all activities of the previous phases and determines whether outcomes identified with and for the patient have been met. Self-reflection is an important tool at this point. Questions such as, "Have I provided the best nursing practice for my patient?" and "Is my patient better after the planned care?" are helpful in determining the effectiveness of the care.

The outcome of evaluation is the resolution phase in which the nurse-patient relationship comes to an end (Peplau, 1994). Many times patients will have a setback due to their feeling of loss of this relationship. The nurse's role is to help them explore their feelings and ease this transition while maintaining boundaries (Peplau, 1994). Ultimately, the goal is for the nurse to provide closure to terminate the relationship.

 **SUMMARY POINTS**

- With the increasing population of elderly individuals, quality of life and the provision of adequate funding sources are important issues impacting the mental health of this population.

- An elderly individual's mental health can be affected by numerous physical, environmental, emotional, and social issues that may occur independently of each other or in combination with each other, which increase the risk for mental health problems.

- Physical changes in the elderly individual are often viewed as normal changes related to aging. However, these changes—even if corrected—can influence the person's mental health.

*(cont.)*

## SUMMARY POINTS (*CONT.*)

- Increased stress in an aging individual can increase the physical and mental aging processes. Prolonged stress also may lead to decreased immune function and altered health status.

- The majority of elderly individuals with depression seek treatment from a primary health care provider, often with complaints related to a chronic illness rather than a mental health problem.

- A major area related to substance use and abuse in the elderly is polypharmacy in which the individual uses multiple medications beyond those that are clinically needed.

- Elderly individuals typically do not seek out or use mental health services for various reasons: personal and family beliefs related to the stigma associated with mental health, limited reimbursement for services by Medicare, inability to physically access services, and availability of programs to meet the changing needs.

- The nurse must demonstrate respect, honesty, genuineness, empathy, interest, and positive regard when developing the therapeutic nurse-patient relationship with an elderly patient to promote the patient's ability to understand his or her needs for help and to develop an individualized realistic plan of care.

## NCLEX-PREP*

1. An elderly patient comes to the clinic complaining of difficulty sleeping, stating, "It just started about a week or so ago." When obtaining the patient's history, which of the following would the nurse identify as potentially contributing to the patient's complaint?

   a. Hypertensive agent added to his medications
   b. History of arthritis
   c. Dinner usually consumed at 5:30 p.m.
   d. Routine bedtime at 11:00 p.m.

2. A nurse is preparing a presentation for a senior citizen group about stresses that may affect their physical and mental health. Which of the following would the nurse least likely include as an effect of stress?

   a. Increased physiologic aging
   b. Enhanced immune function
   c. Slowing of normal mental changes
   d. Increased risk for depression

3. An elderly patient is experiencing social loneliness. Which of the following most likely would be involved?

   a. Loss of contact
   b. Loss of intimacy
   c. Loss of independence
   d. Loss of support

4. An older adult patient is admitted to the acute care facility for treatment of bacterial pneumonia for which the patient is receiving oxygen therapy and antibiotics. When assessing the patient, the nurse notes that the patient has suddenly become confused and agitated and is having increasing difficulty staying focused. The nurse suspects which of the following?

   a. Depression
   b. Dementia
   c. Delirium
   d. Generalized anxiety disorder

*(cont.)*

**NCLEX-PREP\*** (*CONT.*)

5. A group of students are reviewing medications used to treat depression in the older adult. The students demonstrate a need for additional study when they identify which agent as approved for use in the elderly?

    a. Escitalopram
    b. Paroxetine
    c. Duloxetine
    d. Aripiprazole

6. A nurse is preparing a presentation about polypharmacy to a local church group of seniors. Which of the following would the nurse least likely include as a common unresolved issue contributing to this problem?

    a. Depression
    b. Fear
    c. Anxiety
    d. Pain

\*Answers to these questions appear on page 639.

## REFERENCES

Administration on Aging ([AoAna] 2010) Department of Health and Human Services. Retrieved January 24, 2010, from http://www.aoa.gov/AoARoot/Aging_Statistics/index.aspx

American Association of Geriatric Psychiatry Online. (2004). *Demographics of the elderly population.* Retrieved from http://www.aagpgpa.org/

American Foundation for Suicide Prevention. (2011). *Figures and Facts: National Statistics.* Retrieved from http://www.afsp.org/index.cfm?fuseaction=home.viewpage&page_id=050fea9f-b064–4092-b1135c3a70de1fda

American Nurses Association. (1991). Postion Statement on Patient Self-Determination Act. Retrieved from http://www.nursingworld.org/MainMenuCategories/EthicsStandards/Ethics-Position-Statements/prtetsdet14455.aspx

American Psychiatric Association. (2009). *DSM-IV-TR: The current manual.* Retrieved November 28, 2009, from http://www.psych.org/mainmenu/research/dsmiv/dsmivtr.aspx

Ancoli-Israel, S., & Cooke, J. R. (2005). Prevalence and comorbidity of insomnia and effect on functioning in elderly populations. *Journal of the American Geriatric Society, 53,* S264–S271.

Astin, J. R., Pelletier, K. R., Marie, A., & Haskell, W. L. (2000). Complementary and alternative medicine use among elderly persons: One-year analysis of a Blue Shield Medicare supplement. *The Journals of Gerontology. Series A, Biological Sciences and Medical Sciences, 55*(1), M4–9.

Benshoff, J. J., Harrawood, L. K., & Koch, D. S. (2003). Substance abuse and the elderly: unique issues and concerns. *Journal of Rehabilitation, 69*(2), 43–48.

Blass, D. M., Rye, R. M., Robbins, B. M., Miner, M. M., Handel, S., Carroll, J. L., & Rabins, P. V. (2006). Ethical issues in the mobile psychiatric treatment with homebound elderly patients: The psychogeriatric Assessment and treatment in city housing experience. *Journal of the American Geriatric Society, 34,* 843–848.

Blay, S. L., Andreoli, S. B., Dewey, M. E., & Gastal, F. L. (2007). Co-occurrence of chronic physical pain and psychiatric morbidity in a community sample of older people. *International Journal of Geriatric Psychiatry, 22,* 902–908.

Bohlmeijer, E., Smit, F., Onrust, S., & van Marwijk, H. (2009). The effects of integrative reminiscence therapy on depressive symptomology and mastery of older adults. *Community Mental Health Journal, Sept. 24.* Retrieved from http://preview.ncbi.nlm.nih.gov/pubmed/19777348?itool=EntrezSystem2.PEntrez.Pubmed.Pubmed_ResultsPanel.Pubmed_RVDocSum&ordinalpos=2

Braun, U., Beyth, R., Ford, M. E., & McCullough, L. B. (2008). Voices of African-American, Caucasian, and Hispanic surrogates on the burden of making end-of-life decisions. *Journal of Internal Medicine, 23*(3), 267–274.

Chao, S. Y., Wu, C. Y., Jin, S. F., Chu, T. L., & Clark, M. J. (2006). The effects of group reminiscence therapy on depression, self-esteem, and life satisfaction of elderly nursing home residents. *Journal of Nursing Research, 14*(1), 36–45.

Chen, S., & Fu, Y. (2008). Leisure participation and enjoyment among the elderly: individual characteristics and sociability. *Educational Gerontology, 34*(10), 871–89.

Chowdhury, A., & Rasania, S.K. (2008). A community based study of psychiatric disorders among the elderly living in Delhi. *The Internet Journal of Health*, Volume 7, Number 1. Available at: http://www.ispub.com/journal/the_internet_journal_of_health/volume_7_number_1_5/article/a_community_based_study_of_psychiatric_disorders_among_the_elderly_living_in_delhi.html

Christopher, E. J. (2003). Electroconvulsive therapy in the medically ill. *Current Psychiatry Reports, 5*(3), 225–230.

Cornell, E. Y., & Waite, L. T. (2009). Measuring social isolation among older adults using multiple indicators from the NSHAP study. *Journals of Gerontology Series B: Psychological Sciences & Social Sciences, 64*(Supp 1), i38–46.

Counsell, S. R., Callahan, C. M., Buttar, A. B., Clark, D. O., & Frank, K. I. (2006). Geriatric resources for assessment and care of elders (GRACE): A new model of primary care for low-income seniors. *Journal of the American Geriatric Society, 34*, 1136–1141.

De Leo, D., Diekstra, R., Lonnqvist, J., Trabucchi, M., Cleirin, M., Frisoni, G. B., Sampaio-Faria, J. (1998). LEIPAD, an internationally applicable instrument to assess quality of life in the elderly. *Behavioral Medicine, 24*(1), 17–27.

Dearman, S. P., Waheed, W., Nathoo, V., & Baldwin, R. C. (2006). Management strategies in geriatric depression by primary care physicians and factors associated with the use of psychiatric services: A naturalistic study. *Aging & Mental Health, 10*(5), 521–524.

Dong, X., Simon, M., Mendes De Leon, C., Fulmer, T., Beck, T., Heibert, L., & Evans, D. (2009). Elder self-neglect and abuse and mortality risk in a community-dwelling population. *JAMA: Journal of the American Medical Association, 302*(5), 517–526.

Drageset, J. (2002). Loneliness at nursing homes—does a network have any importance for loneliness among nursing home occupants? *Journal of Nursing Research and Clinical Studies, 22*(2), 9–14.

Edwards, D. E. (2005). Thinking about the unthinkable: Staff sexual abuse of residents. *Nursing Homes Long-Term Care Management, 54*(6), 44–47.

Egede, L. E., Frueth, C. B., Richardson, L. K., Acierno, R., Maudlin, P. D., Knapp, R. G., Lejuez, C. (2009). Rationale and design: Telepsychology service delivery for depressed elderly veterans. *Trails, 10*, 22.

Fetveit, A. (2009). Late life insomnia: A review. *Geriatrics & Gerontology International, 99*(3), 220–234.

Fick, D., & Foreman, M. (2000). Consequences of not recognizing delirium superimposed on dementia in hospitalized elderly individuals. *Journal of Gerontology, 26*(1), 30–40.

Flint, A.J. (2005). Generalized anxiety disorder in elderly patients: epidemiology, diagnosis and treatment options. *Drugs & Aging, 22*(2), 101–114.

Forchuk, C. (1992). The orientation phase of the nurse client relationship: How long does it take? *Perspectives in Psychiatric Care, 28*(4), 7–10.

Forchuk, C., Martin, M. L., Chan, Y. L., & Jensen, E. (2005). Therapeutic relationships: From psychiatric hospital to the community. *Journal of Psychiatric and Mental Health Nursing, 12*, 556–564.

Furukawa, Y., Odawara, T., Yamada, Y., Fujita, J., & Hirayasu, Y. (2006). Features of the elderly patient admitted to a general hospital psychiatric unit. *Psychogeriatrics, 6*, 55–59.

Gagliardi, J. P. (2006). Differentiating among depression, delirium, and dementia in elderly patients *American Medical Association Journal of ethics/personal mentor.org*. Retrieved November 22, 2009, from http://virtualmentor.ama-assn.org/2008/06/cprl1–0806.html

Gallo, J. J. & Bogner, H. R. (2006). The context of geriatric care. In J.J. Gallo, H.R. Bogner, T. Fulmer, & G.J. Paveza (Eds.), *Handbook of Geriatric Assessment* (4th ed., pp. 3–12). Boston: Jones and Barrlett.

Gallop, R., & O'Brien, L. (2003). Re-establishing psychodynamic theory as foundational knowledge for psychiatric/mental health nursing. *Issues in Mental Health Nursing, 24*, 213–227.

Gobert, M., & D'hoore, W. (2005). Prevalence of psychotropic drug use in nursing homes for the aged in Quebec and in the French-speaking area of Switzerland. *International Journal of Geriatric Psychiatry, 20*, 712–720.

Golde, J., Conroy, R. M., Denihan, A., Greene, E., Kirby, M., & Lawler, B. A. (2009). Loneliness, social support networks, mood and well-being in community-dwelling elders. *International Journal of Geriatrics, 24*(7), 694–700.

Hanna, S. J., Woolley, R., Brown, L., & Kesavan, S. (2008). The coming of age of a joint elderly medicine-psychiatric ward: 18 years' experience. *Clinical Practice, 62*(1), 148–151.

Harris, T., Cook, D. G., Victor, C., Dewilde, W., & Beighton, C. (2006). Onset and persistence of depression in older people—results from a 2-year community follow-up study. *Age & Aging, 35*(1), 25–32.

Hsu, Y. C., & Wang, J. J. (2009). Physical, effective, and behavioral effects of group reminiscence on depressed institutionalized elders in Taiwan. *Nursing Research, 58*(4), 294–299.

Huang, S. L., Li, C. M., Yang, C. Y., & Chen, J. J. (2009). Application of reminiscence treatment on older people with dementia: A case study in Pingtung, Taiwan. *Journal of Nursing Research, 17*(3), 112–118.

Kapo, J., Morrison, L. J., & Liao, S. (2007). Palliative care for the older adult. *Journal of Palliative Medicine, 10*(1), 185–209.

Kendler, K. S., Meyers, J., & Zisook, S. (2008). Does bereavement-related major depression differ from major depression associated with other stressful life events? *American Journal of Psychiatry, 165*(11), 1449–55.

Kennedy, G. J. (2000). *Geriatric mental health*. New York: The Guilford Press.

Kneisl, C. R., Wilson, H. S., & Trigoboff, E. (2004). Elders. In *Contemporary psychiatric-mental health nursing* (pp. 638–659). Upper Saddle River, N.J.: Pearson, Prentice Hall.

Kramer, T., Beaudin, C. L., & Thrush, C. R. (2005). Evaluation and treatment of depression (part I): Benefits for patients, providers, and payers. *Disease Management & Health Outcomes, 13*(5), 295–306.

Lee, A. G., Beaver, H. A., Jogerst, G., & Daly, J. M. (2009). Screening elderly patient in an outpatient ophthalmology clinic for dementia, depression, and functional impairment. *Ophthalmology, 110*(4), 651–657.

Lyness, J. M., Qin, Y., Wan, T., Xin, T., & Cornwell, Y. (2009). Risks for depression set in primary care elderly patients: Potential targets for preventative interventions. *American Journal of Psychiatry, 166*(12), 0375–1383.

Magai, C., Consedine, N. S., Fiori, K. L., & King, A. R. (2008). Sharing the good, sharing the bad: The benefits of emotional self-disclosure among middle-aged and older adults. *Journal of Aging Health, 21*(2), 286–313.

Maryland Coalition on Mental Health and Aging. (n.d.). *Stress and change*. Retrieved November 25, 2009, from http://www.mhamd.org/aging/agingconsiderations/stresschange.htm

McCasland, L. A. (2007). Providing hospice and palliative care to the seriously and persistently mentally ill. *Journal of Hospice and Palliative Nursing, 9*(6), 305–313.

McClane, K. S. (2005). A screening instrument for use in a complete geriatric assessment. *Clinical Nurse Specialist, 20*(4), 201–207.

McGovern, R. J., Lee, M. M., Johnson, J. C., & Morton, B. (2008). Elderlynk: A community outreach model for the integrated treatment of mental health problems in the rural elderly. *Aging International, 32*, 43–53.

McNaughton, D. B. (2005). A naturalistic test of Peplau's theory in home visiting. *Public Health Nursing, 22*(5), 429–438.

Medical News Today. (10). *Medicalnewstoday.com.* Can sunlight help elderly nursing home residents sleep better? Retrieved November 22, 2009, from http://www.medicalnewstoday.com/articles/22592.php

Medicare. (n.d.). *Medicare.* Retrieved from http://www.medicare.gov/

Merck & Co (2008). Insomnia and excessive daytime sleepiness. In K. Doghramji (Ed.), *Merck Manual of Patient Symptoms* (18th ed.). Philadelphia: Author.

Merck & Co. (2006). Chapter 15: Social Issues. In M. H. Beers (Ed.), *Merck Manual of Geriatrics* (3rd ed., pp. 149–155). Philadelphia: Author.

Merck & Co. (2006). Chapter 33: Depression. In M.H. Beers (Ed.), *Merck Manual of Geriatrics* (3rd ed., pp. 310–322). Philadelphia: Author.

Merck & Co. (2006). Chapter 34: Anxiety and Anxiety Disorders. In M. H. Beers (Ed.), *Merck Manual of Geriatrics* (3rd ed., pp. 322–327). Philadelphia: Author.

Merck & Co. (2006). Chapter 43: Pain. In M. H. Beers (Ed.), *Merck Manual of Geriatrics* (3rd ed., pp. 383–396). Philadelphia: Author.

Merck & Co. (2006). Chapter 47: Sleep Disorders. In M. H. Beers (Ed.), *Merck Manual of Geriatrics* (3rd ed., pp. 452–457). Philadelphia: Author.

Meyer, C. (18). *Prescription drug abuse in the elderly.* Retrieved November 22, 2009, from http://www.associatedcontent.com/article/5731/prescription_drug_abuse_in_the_elderly.html?cat=5

National Committee for the Prevention of Elder Abuse. (2008). *Elder abuse: What are the indicators?* www.preventelderabuse.org. Retrieved November 20, 2009, from http://www.preventelderabuse.org/

National Institute of Mental Health. (2009). *Suicide in the United States: Statistics and prevention.* Retrieved November 30, 2009, from http://www.nimh.nih.gov/health/publications/suicide-in-the-us-statistics-and-prevention/index.shtml

National PACE Association. (2002). *NPA Shared Services Programs.* Retrieved December 3, 2009, from http://www.npaonline.org/website/article.asp?id=4

O'Luanaigh, C., & Lawlor, B. A. (2008). Loneliness and the health of older people. *International Journal of Geriatric Psychiatry, 23*, 1213–1221.

Patel, J. M. (2007). Loneliness and life—satisfaction among the elderly. *Indian Journal of Gerontology, 20*(4), 405–416.

Peplau, H. (1952). *Interpersonal relations in nursing.* New York: G.P. Putnam.

Peplau, H. (1994). Psychiatric mental health nursing: Challenge and change. *Journal of Psychiatric and Mental Health Nursing, 1*, 3–7.

Peplau, H. E. (1988). *Interpersonal relationships in nursing.* London: Palgrave Macmillan.

Peplau, H. E. (1991). *Interpersonal relationships in nursing: A conceptual framework of references for psychodynamic nursing.* New York: Springer.

Petigrew, S., & Roberts, M. (2008). Addressing loneliness in later life. *Aging and Mental Health, 13*(3), 302–309.

Prakash, O., Gupta, L. N., Singh, V. B., Singhal, A. K., & Verma, K. K. (2007). Profile of psychiatric disorders and life events in medically ill elderly: Experiences from a geriatric clinic in Northern India. *International Journal of Geriatric Psychiatry, 22*, 1101–1105.

Pratt, S. I., Kelly, S. M., Mueser, K. T., Patterson, T. L., Goldman, S., & Bishop-Horton, S. (2007). Reliability and validity of a performance-based measure of skills for communicating with doctors for older people with serious mental illness. *Journal of Mental Health, 16*(5), 569–579.

Purnell, L. (2005). The Purnell Model of cultural competence. *Journal of Multicultural Nursing & Health,* Summer, 20–33.

Rand, J.E. (n.d.). *SF-36 health survey update.* Retrieved December 12, 2009, from http://www.sf-36.org/tools/sf36.shtml

Rangari, J., & Pelissolo, A. (2006). Anxiety disorders in the elderly: Clinical and therapeutic aspects. *Psychological Neuropsychiatry Veill, 4*(3), 179–187.

Ron, P. (2008). Offspring caring for their elderly parents: the effect of social support and gender-role orientation on these caregivers' well-being. *Illness, Crisis & Loss, 16*(3), 183–201.

Rozzini, L., Chilovi, B. V., Peli, M., Conti, M., Rozzini, R., Trabucchi, M., Padovovani, A. (2009). Anxiety symptoms in mild cognitive impairment. *International Journal of Geriatric Psychiatry, 24*, 300–305.

Ski, C., & O'Connell, B. (2005). Mismanagement of delirium places patients at risk. *Australian Journal of Advanced Nursing, 23*(3), 42–46.

Son, J., Erno, A., Feemia, E. E., Zarit, S. H., & Stephens, M. A. (2007). The caregiver stress process and health outcomes. *Journal of Aging and Health, 19*(6), 871–887.

Stek, M. L., Vinkers, D. J., Gussekaloo, J., Beekman, A. T., van der Mast, R. C., & Westendorp, R. G. (2005). Brief report: Is depression in old age fatal only when people feel lonely. *American Journal of Psychiatry, 162*, 178–180.

Stockmann, C. (2005). A literature review of the progress of the psychiatric nurse-patient relationship as described by Peplau. *Issues in Mental Health Nursing, 26*, 911–919.

Tadros, G., & Salib, E. (2007). Elderly suicide in primary care. *International Journal of Geriatric Psychiatry, 22*, 750–756.

Toronto Best Practice In LTC Initiative. (2007). *3D's: Assessment tools at your fingertips.* Retrieved November 22, 2009, from http://www.opadd.on.ca/Local%20Projects/documents/LocalProject-Educ.Training-3Dsassessmentguide.pdf

Trask, B. S., Hepp, B. W., Settles, B., & Shabo, L. (2009). Culturally diverse elders and their families: Examining the need for culturally competent services. *Journal of Comparative Family Studies, 40*(2), 293–303.

U.S. Census Bureau. (2001). *Population profile of the United States: the elderly profile.* Retrieved December 3, 2009, from http://www.census.gov/population/www/pop-profile/elder-pop.html

University of Chicago. (n.d.). *Polypharmacy in Older Patients.* Retrieved November 22, 2009, from http://.bsd.uchicago.edu/Polypharmacy/index.html

van Zyl, L.T, & Seitz D.P. (2006) Delirium concisely: condition is associated with increased morbidity, mortality, and length of hospitalization. *Geriatrics,* 61(3): 18–21.

Weeks, D. G., Michela, J. L., Peplau, L. A., & Bragg, M. E. (1990). Relation between loneliness and depression: A structural equation. *Journal of Personality and Social Psychology, 39*(6), 1238–1244.

Weiss, B. J., Calleo, J., Rhoades, H. M., Novy, D. M., Kunik, M. E., Lenze, E. J., Stanley, M. A. (2009). The utility of the generalized anxiety disorder severity scale (GADSS) with older adults in primary care. *Depression and Anxiety, 26,* E10-E15.

World Health Organization. (2003). *WHO definition of health.* Retrieved from http://www.who.int/about/definition/en/print.html

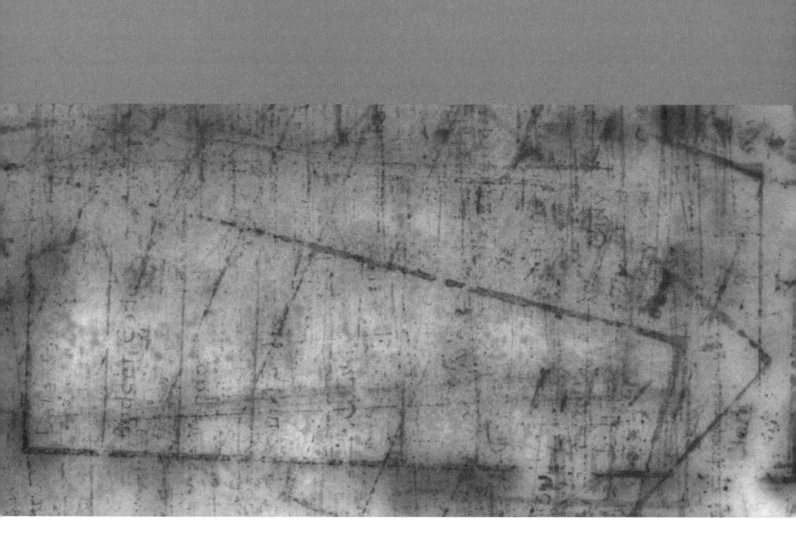

## CHAPTER CONTENTS

## EXPECTED LEARNING OUTCOMES

**After completing this chapter, the student will be able to:**

1. Identify the various types of abuse.
2. Discuss the historical perspectives and epidemiology related to abuse.
3. Explain the psychodynamics influencing the victims as well as the abusers, across the life span.
4. Describe the signs and symptoms indicative of abuse and neglect.
5. Describe the models used to explain abuse, including the Cycle of Violence Wheel and the Power and Control Wheel.

## CHAPTER 24

# VICTIMS AND VICTIMIZERS

Loraine Fleming

Betty Jane Kohal

6. Identify possible barriers faced by the nurse during the assessment process, especially those related to emotional responses that may be experienced when working with victims of abuse as well as with the abusers.

7. Describe the legal and ethical responsibilities of the nurse in reporting suspected abuse or neglect.

## KEY TERMS

Abuse

Battering

Domestic violence

Honor killings

Intimate partner violence

Statutory rape

Although definitions may vary, the Centers for Disease Control and Prevention (CDC) is making efforts to standardize definitions and currently refers to ABUSE as acts of commission or omission that result in harm, potential for harm, or threat of harm (Leeb, Paulozzi, Melanson, Simon, & Arias, 2007). Abusive behavior is used to gain or maintain power and control over another person and is the hallmark of DOMESTIC VIOLENCE. Domestic violence can be defined as:

- Causing or attempting to cause physical or mental harm to a family or household member
- Placing a family or household member in fear of physical or mental harm
- Causing or attempting to cause a family or household member to engage in involuntary sexual activity by force, threat of force, or duress
- Engaging in activity toward a family or household member that would cause a reasonable person to feel terrorized, frightened, intimidated, threatened, harassed, or molested (Child Welfare Information Gateway, 2008, p. 1)

Violence among spouses or domestic partners is referred to as INTIMATE PARTNER VIOLENCE and is included under the umbrella term of domestic violence. Violence is demonstrated through physical, sexual, economic, or psychological abuse, or a combination of methods. The abuse is used to dominate the person. The control can be manifested directly through use of force, or less directly through manipulation, humiliation, or guilt. Even threats can be used as a way to control others and are considered part of the pattern of abuse.

This chapter focuses on abuse and violence across the life span. It describes the types of abuse and provides an overview of the historical aspects and epidemiology related to abuse and violence. The chapter discusses the etiology related to abuse across the lifespan and describes the major models used to explain this behavior. The chapter concludes with a discussion of the nursing responsibilities from an interpersonal perspective when caring for victims of abuse and their victimizers.

> *Abuse reflects a means for exerting power and control over another person.*

## TYPES OF ABUSE

Abuse can come in many forms. It can be physical, emotional, sexual, or economic. Frequently the abuser will use more than one method to achieve his or her goal of power and domination. The abuser may begin by using verbal criticism or emotional abuse and gradually move to physical abuse. The physical abuse may also begin with less injurious acts, such as slapping or pushing, and move on to more serious injuries, including infliction of fatal injuries.

### Physical Abuse

Physical abuse involves an act of aggressive behavior that results in bodily injury, pain, or impairment to another. These actions or behaviors include: hitting, BATTERING (striking someone repeatedly with violent blows), slapping, kicking, pushing, choking, pinching, hair pulling, or any other action that can cause bodily harm. Although it may involve use of an object or weapon, this is not required for physical abuse. It can also entail inflicting burn injuries such as using cigarettes or caustic chemicals. Typically the physical abuse will become a pattern of interactions between the abuser and the victim, and the severity will increase over time.

Physical neglect is another type of physical abuse. However, it is considered a nonviolent form of physical abuse. It involves withholding necessities from the victim, such as denying adequate food, clothing, or medical care and attention.

### Sexual Abuse

Sexual abuse is also used as a way of gaining control over the victim. It can include any type of sexual activity inflicted on a person without his or her consent. Sexual abuse encompasses forcible intercourse, sadistic sexual acts against the victim aimed at causing humiliation, or other forms of sexual assault or molestation including inappropriate touching.

### Emotional or Psychological Abuse

Emotional or psychological abuse involves verbal or nonverbal behaviors that are intended to demean or belittle a person, or cause anguish or distress. Examples of emotional or psychological abuse include insults or constant criticism directed at the person as a way of diminishing his or her self-esteem and self-worth. It can also include threats, intimidation, or harassment that the abuser uses to control the victim. For example, in a same-sex relationship, emotional abuse would be threatening to expose the other's sexual orientation if that fact is hidden. Isolating a victim from his or her family or friends is another way an abuse can inflict emotional distress. Although emotional or psychological abuse does not usually involve physical violence on the part of the abuser, it may involve violence directed at inanimate objects or pets as a way of demonstrating power or dominance and invoking fear. The abuser may also threaten to harm the victim or someone the victim cares for as a way of exerting power without ever actually committing a violent act. Finally, the abuser may blame the victim for the consequences of the abuse, thereby causing guilt or shame and leaving the victim feeling responsible for the situation. Emotional and psychological abuse is extremely effective in reducing the victim's confidence and sense of autonomy, and enhancing the power and control of the abuser.

## Economic Abuse

Economic abuse is another method of gaining authority or dominance over someone. Economic abuse is a tactic used to control a victim's finances, thereby preventing the victim from leaving the relationship. Sometimes the abuser will not permit the victim to work or to maintain control of his or her earnings, thus ensuring dependency upon the abuser. The abuser may also interfere with, or prevent the victim from pursing an education, getting job training, or establishing his or her own credit. Sometimes the abuser will take actions that jeopardize the victim's employment or credit status, causing them to lose a job or suffer financial losses. Lack of income is a common reason victims cite for staying in abusive relationships (Benson & Fox, 2001). Confidence crimes, fraud, and scams for financial gain are examples of economic or financial abuse found in the elderly population (Reed, 2005).

> *The four types of abuse are physical, emotional or psychological, sexual, and economic (or financial) abuse.*

## HISTORICAL PERSPECTIVES

In many cultures throughout history, the value and rights of women and children were limited or nonexistent. During Roman times, the "paterfamilias," or male head of the household had absolute power over his household and children. If his children angered him, he had the legal right to disown them, sell them into slavery, or even kill them. The head of the household also had power over his wife and her property and possessions (Fustel des Coulanges & Numa Denis, 1980). This was also true in many Asian cultures, where women were dominated by the male head of the family and had limited legal rights (Nguyen, 2004).

In North America during Colonial times, the courts typically followed English common law. These laws stipulated that a married woman's property and possessions became her husband's after her marriage (Kerber & De Hart, 1995). Children were often viewed as part of this property and parents could do whatever they wished to their children.

The use of corporal punishment against children can be traced back to biblical times. The St. James version of the Bible states, "Spare the rod, spoil the child." This particular biblical passage has given many persons the "right" to physically hit the child.

American women in the 21st century are no longer legally limited by patriarchal views. However, many personal, religious, and cultural beliefs still influence the role of women and children and how they are treated in the home. Frequently they are relegated to subservient or submissive positions. Over the years, women have frequently been referred to as the "weaker" sex, being considered physically and intellectually inferior to men.

These continuing attitudes have had an impact on the behaviors of some men, leading them to believe that they have the right to control their spouse or partner as well as to use corporal punishment with their children. In addition, historically, domestic violence has not been treated the same way other violent crimes were treated by law enforcement. Many people, including law enforcement personnel, viewed spousal abuse as a private matter. Until the 1950s, written police policies in many jurisdictions actually directed officers to "recognize the sanctity of the home" and to end the disturbance "without making an arrest" (Finesmith, 1983). A husband could even have sex with his wife against her will without being charged with rape.

Over the years, greater understanding of domestic violence created more pressure on law enforcement to change. Yet the violence was still not considered criminal behavior. The abusers were seldom arrested and were rarely tried in court (Finesmith, 1983). It was not until 1994 that increasing public pressure to recognize domestic violence as a crime rather than a family problem resulted in the passage of the federal Violence Against Women Act (VAWA). This Act, and the 1996 additions to the Act, recognize that domestic violence is a national crime. In 1994 and 1996, Congress also passed changes to the Gun Control Act making it a federal crime in certain situations for domestic abusers to possess guns.

Domestic violence is not just a female issue. Men can also be the victims of domestic violence. However, the number of reported cases is small in comparison to those reported by women (Bair-Merritt, 2010). This may be due in part to these traditional ideas about roles such that men are viewed as more powerful. Additionally, little has been done to foster a climate for reporting abuse and little research has been done to address the issues involved with violence against men. As a result, males may feel ashamed or experience fear that no one will believe them. These gender stereotypes may be to blame for the failure of men to report violence they experience in domestic relationships (Domestic Violence.org handbook).

> *Domestic abuse historically was viewed as a family problem. However, increasing public pressure has led to legislation, recognizing domestic violence as a crime.*

## EPIDEMIOLOGY

Abuse crosses all races, genders, socioeconomic status, religions, marital status, ages, and cultures. Anyone can be a victim of abuse or a victimizer. Abuse is a pervasive problem in society (Klein, 2009). Interventions are required at primary as well as secondary and tertiary levels:

- Primary interventions focus on efforts to prevent abuse from ever occurring.
- Secondary interventions focus on identifying risk factors and providing early involvement to reduce negative consequences.
- Tertiary interventions focus on repairing the consequences of abuse.

A recent Cochrane Review of advocacy interventions and approaches to reduce the violence and promote health and well-being looked at secondary and tertiary interventions. The review assessed the results of ten trials with over 1,500 participants and determined that intensive advocacy efforts have some effect on reducing physical abuse one to two years after the intervention but do not clearly demonstrate a beneficial effect on quality of life and mental health (Ramsay, Carter, Davidson, Dunne, Eldridge, Hegarty, Rivas, Taft Warburton, & Feder, 2009). There is certainly a need for further evaluation and review to assist in determining the best course of action when working with victims of domestic violence.

Anyone can be the victim of domestic violence. However, most often, the victims are female and the victimizers are male (Falsetti, 2007). Many victims suffer physical injuries ranging from cuts and bruises to death. However, not all abuse cases involve physical abuse. Domestic abuse can cause serious emotional and psychological harm. The stress that victims feel may also lead to depression and other psychiatric disorders. Some victims even consider and/or commit suicide.

The effects of abuse are far reaching and impact the entire family, not just the designated victim. Abuse leads to increased incidence of health problems, substance abuse, school truancy, and more violence (CDC, 2005). The Adverse Childhood Experiences (ACE) Study conducted in 1998 is one of the largest investigations ever conducted on the links between childhood maltreatment and later-life health and well-being. The findings suggest that adverse childhood experiences are major risk factors for the leading causes of illness and death (Brown, Anda, Tiemeier, Felitti, Edwards, Croft, & Giles, 2009).

## Child Abuse

Child abuse refers to the physical, emotional, and/or sexual abuse of persons under the age of 18 years. Abuse against children occurs most frequently between the ages of 3 and 5, a time when a child is most vulnerable and expects to be protected by the parent and/or caregiver. Most children perceive the victimization as their fault and are often told that by the perpetrator.

The most frequently identified abuser of children between the ages of three and five is someone the child knows, often the stepfather of the child. Victimized children are told "not to tell" or bad things will happen if they disclose their "secret." Numerous studies of adults who are survivors of child abuse reveal that they never disclosed their childhood trauma for fear that no one would believe them, or if they did disclose it their mothers, did not believe them. The result of the child not being trusted to have disclosed the truth is a revictimization of the child.

Physical neglect of children is defined as not providing those things children need to survive the elements, nourish their bodies, prevent disease, and treat illness when it occurs, and to educate them so they will be able to perform self-care. Parents neglect their children either as a mechanism to punish them or due to lack of resources or lack of knowledge.

Almost 3,500 children under the age of 15 die from maltreatment (physical abuse and neglect) every year in the industrialized world. According to data collected from

30 industrialized nations, the risk of death by maltreatment is approximately three times greater for children under the age of 1 year than for those between the ages of 1 and 4 years. In turn, those between the ages of 1 and 4 years face double the risk of those between the ages of 5 and 14. Thus, the risk for abuse is greater in younger children. However, these statistics provide only a partial picture about the extent of the problem because these countries produce about two-thirds of the world's goods and services. Thus, information about an entire one-third of the world is missing.

The risk of fatal maltreatment for children varies by location. The highest homicide rates for children under 5 years are found in Africa—17.9 per 100,000 for boys and 12.7 per 100,000 for girls. However, many child deaths are not investigated. The physical and emotional scars of abuse and neglect linger for generations (UNICEF, 2003).

## Intimate Partner Violence

Domestic violence remains the leading cause of injury to women between the ages of 15 and 44 years, more common than muggings, motor vehicle crashes, and cancer deaths combined. The Federal Bureau of Investigation (FBI) estimates that a domestic violence crime is committed about once every 15 seconds.

In 2000, intimate partner homicides accounted for 34% of the murders of women in the United States. It was the seventh leading cause of premature death for women and the number one cause of death for African American women between the ages of 15 and 34 years in the United States (U.S. Bureau of Justice Statistics, 2003).

Nearly 25% of women in the United States have been raped and/or physically assaulted by an intimate partner at some point in their lives (Catalano, 2007). Almost one-half of this group experienced physical injuries resulting from the violence.

Females account for the majority of victims of family violence. Approximately 84% of spouse abuse victims were female and approximately 86% of victims of abuse at the hands of a boyfriend or girlfriend were female. While about three-fourths of the victims of family violence were female, about three-fourths of the persons who committed family violence were male.

In addition, domestic violence-related police calls have been found to constitute the single largest category of calls received by police. These calls are estimated to account for more than 50% of all calls in certain precincts (Friday, Lord, Exum, & Hartman, 2006). These statistics represent reports filed; unfortunately, studies indicate that only a percentage of domestic violence is reported. Approximately 75–80% of the assaults and rapes of domestic partners go unreported (Gracia, 2004). The same is true for cases of violence against male partners in relationships. Studies indicate that only 10% of male victims of nonfatal partner violence on average contact an outside agency for assistance (U.S. Bureau of Justice Statistics, 2006.)

## Elder Abuse

For the elderly, abuse is often manifested through neglect, which involves failure to provide for the needs of the person, including basic needs of food and shelter as well as medical needs. It is estimated that up to 2 million Americans 65 years of age or older have been injured, exploited, or otherwise mistreated by someone on whom they depend for care or protection (National Research Council, 2003). However, it is felt that for every case of elder abuse, neglect, exploitation, or self-neglect that is reported, five more go unreported (Purcell, 2004). (See Chapter 23 for additional information on elder abuse as a factor for mental health problems.)

> *Anyone can be a victim or perpetrator of abuse. However, victims most often are females and victimizers are most often males.*

## ETIOLOGY

Most experts believe that domestic violence is a learned behavior that is more common for individuals who have grown up in violent homes. It can also be reinforced by cultural beliefs that sanction the use of violence such as those that permit so called HONOR KILLINGS. Honor killings are based on the belief that women are the property of male relatives and embody the honor of the men to whom they "belong." The concepts of male status and family status are of particular importance in cultures where "honor killings" occur. If a woman or girl is accused or suspected of engaging in behaviors that could taint male and/or family status, it is the male's duty to maintain the family honor. The male will kill the alleged offender to maintain the family honor (Coomaraswamy, 2002). Honor killings, although generally not officially sanctioned, continue to occur in many countries (Mayell, 2002). Once example is karo-kari, that is, honor killings that claimed the lives of more than 2,000 women between 1998 and 2003 in Pakistan (United Nations, 2006).

> *The common belief surrounding abuse is that it is a learned behavior, occurring most commonly in households where individuals have grown up being exposed to violence.*

## Child Abuse

Adults who abuse children are often adult survivors of child abuse themselves. Commonly, adult survivors of abuse report never having dealt with the emotions surrounding their trauma. In many instances, the trauma has been repressed so they have no conscious awareness of the experience. Behavioral indicators of unresolved childhood trauma include: self-destructive behavior, failure to complete tasks, unsatisfying intimate relationships, as well as being abusive to their own children. **Box 24-1** summarizes the types of abuse seen in children.

## Intimate Partner Violence

Intimate partner violence (IPV) involves abuse by a current or former intimate partner or spouse. This type of violence can occur among heterosexual or same-sex couples. Current theories regarding domestic violence and IPV agree that it is not specifically caused by illness, genetics, substance abuse, anger, stress, or the behavior of the victim, although these factors may increase the risk of domestic violence (Schewe, Riger, Howard, Staggs, & Mason, 2006).

---

### BOX 24-1: ABUSE IN CHILDREN

*Child Physical Abuse*

- Bringing physical harm to a child with the intent of having power and control over the child
- *Examples*: Fractures, contusions, lacerations, concussions, burn marks from ropes and straps, bite marks

*Child Neglect*

- Both physical and emotional
- *Examples*: Not providing appropriate nourishment; not taking the child to a health care provider when ill; not ensuring the child attends school or, if truant, doing nothing to facilitate the child's attendance; not providing weather-appropriate clothing; leaving the child alone without a caregiver when the child is under the age of 12

*Emotional Abuse*

- Occurs every time physical abuse is experienced
- *Examples*: Failing to provide the child with love and affection; not telling the child he or she is loved or cared for; and not providing appropriate touch
- *Other examples*: Talking to the child in a threatening manner; calling the child demeaning names; exposing the child to profanity

*Child Sexual Abuse*

- Inappropriate touching of the genitals/breasts of a person under the age of 12
- **STATUTORY RAPE**, i.e., sexual intercourse with an adolescent between the ages of 13 and 18
- *Examples*: Inserting things into the vagina or penile penetration of the vagina; having oral or anal sex; having a child perform masturbation either on him/herself or the perpetrator; exposing children to sexually explicit pictures or sexual acts

Additional risk factors include:

- Seeing or being a victim of violence as a child
- Unemployment or work-related stressors
- Poverty
- Personality disorders
- Stress disorders

## Elder Abuse

Some cases of elder abuse involve IPV, but many cases also involve abuse by an adult child of the victim. Abusers may be dependent on their victims for financial assistance due to personal issues, substance abuse issues, or psychiatric problems. The risk for the victim is higher when the abuser lives with the victim. Other factors that have been postulated to contribute to elder abuse include: caregiver strain, the relationship between the caregiver and the patient, and the type of dependency experienced (the more difficult it is to provide care for the patient due to their disturbed behavior, dementia, character disorder, or the extensive nature of their care needs, the higher the risk of abuse). However, research thus far regarding the etiology of elder abuse has not demonstrated consistent findings related to the factors precipitating elder abuse (Nerenberg, 2002).

## PATTERNS OF VIOLENCE

A number of paradigms have been constructed to help describe the phenomenon of domestic violence. Three of these models are described here.

## The Cycle of Violence

The Cycle of Violence was introduced in 1979 by L. Walker based on research she conducted with battered women. Walker concluded that there were three distinct phases involved in the pattern of domestic abuse. **Figure 24-1** illustrates this cycle.

The first phase is referred to as the tension-building phase. During this period, the abuser becomes increasingly hostile and agitated and more and more critical toward the victim. Victims frequently describes feeling as if they are "walking on eggshells" during the period. No matter what they try, they are unable to reduce the tension and appease the abuser. This phase is followed by the acute-battering phase or explosive phase, which involves an actual attack. At first the attack may be only verbal, but it usually progresses to physical violence. The final phase of the cycle is the honeymoon phase or the loving-contrition period. During this phase the abuser tries to make

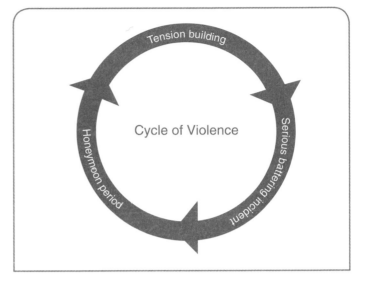

Figure 24-1 *The cycle of violence.*

amends, typically becoming affectionate and solicitous of the victim, often promising that the violence will "never happen again" (Walker, 2009). **Table 24-1** summarizes the behaviors of this cycle.

> *The cycle of violence consists of three phases: tension-building phase, acute battering (or explosive) phase, and the honeymoon (or love-contrition) phase.*

Certain advocacy groups have raised concern that Walker's model may reinforce the concept of "blaming the victim" because in this model, had the victim been able to alleviate the tension, the event would not have happened. There is also concern that the model implies that the "tension" is precipitated by something, which can be misinterpreted as providing an "excuse" for the abuser.

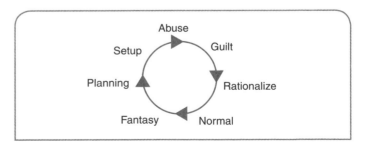

Figure 24-2 *Cycle of abuse.*

| TABLE 24-1: BEHAVIORS IN THE CYCLE OF VIOLENCE | | |
|---|---|---|
| **TENSION BUILDING** | **SERIOUS BATTERING INCIDENT** | **HONEYMOON PERIOD** |
| • Stress increases<br>• Abuser becomes more and more agitated<br>• Victim becomes fearful<br>• Victim makes efforts to appease abuser | • Abuser becomes violent, either verbally or physically<br>• Victim feels trapped and helpless<br>• Victim is traumatized<br>• Abuser blames victim for event | • Abuser become apologetic, loving, and solicitous<br>• Victim feels ambivalent and responsible<br>• Abuser promises it will never happen again<br>• Victim minimizes event |

## Cycle of Abuse

In 1983, the anti-violence movement in Salem, Oregon, proposed another model for the cycle of domestic violence (Mid-Valley Women's Crisis Service). This is illustrated in **Figure 24-2**. The model defines six distinct phases in the cycle.

In the initial phases, the abuser fantasizes and plans the abuse, imagining all the things the victim has done wrong, and plans how to make the victim pay for these actions. The abuser will then "set up" the scenario to perpetrate the abuse. Again, the abuse may be physical, emotional, economic, or sexual. Once the abusive episode is over, the perpetrator may experience guilt but it is postulated that the guilt is not guilt due to the harm caused the victims; rather, the guilt is caused by concerns regarding the consequences of the action. The abuser will become apologetic and solicitous to avoid any repercussions. The abuser will then rationalize the actions and blame the victim for creating the situation that precipitated the violence. The abuser will then return to life as "normal," as if nothing transpired.

> *The Power and Control Wheel emphasizes the responsibility of the individual abuser and the community for controlling the abuser.*

## The Power and Control Wheel

The Power and Control Wheel is another paradigm that helps explain the cycle of violence. It was developed by the Domestic Abuse Intervention Project (DAIP). **Figure 24-3** illustrates this model.

This model asserts that the primary responsibility of placing controls on abusers belongs to the community and the individual abuser, not the victim of abuse. Additionally:

- Battering is a form of domestic violence that entails a patterned use of coercion, intimidation, including violence, and other related forms of abuse, whether legal or illegal (see the Power and Control Wheel). To be successful, initiatives must distinguish between and respond differently to domestic violence that constitutes battering and cases that do not and adjust those interventions to the severity of the violence.
- Interventions must account for the economic, cultural, and personal histories of the individuals who become abuse cases in the system.
- Both the victims and offenders are members of the community. While they must each act to change the conditions of their lives, the community must treat both with respect and dignity recognizing the social causes of their personal circumstances (DAIP, 2008).

The Power and Control Wheel delineates nine behaviors used by an abuser to control the victim. These are described in **Box 24-2**.

## NURSING RESPONSIBILITIES FROM AN INTERPERSONAL PERSPECTIVE

All health care providers need to be aware of the indicators of trauma and abuse so they can be identified and safety can be provided. Recognizing early warning signs is an important part of derailing the cycle of abuse. Therefore, public education efforts are essential. In addition, the nurse must be aware of the legal mandates for reporting each type of abuse.

When dealing with victims of abuse, nurses need to be aware of their own feelings about abuse, victims, and victimizers to prevent these feelings from interfering with the patient's care. The nurse needs to remain nonjudgmental

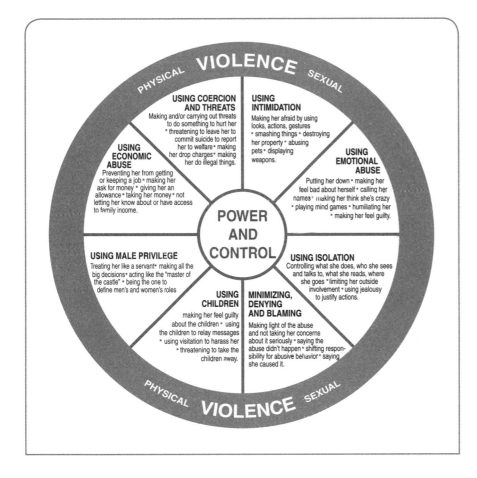

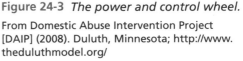

**Figure 24-3** *The power and control wheel.*
From Domestic Abuse Intervention Project
[DAIP] (2008). Duluth, Minnesota; http://www.
theduluthmodel.org/

and employ the therapeutic use of self to establish trust and rapport with the patient.

Although providing care to victims of abuse is similar, the nurse's responsibilities are presented for the specific population affected. Nurses need to keep in mind that victims of abuse may be encountered at any point along the health care continuum.

> *Nurses typically provide care for both the victims of abuse and their victimizers. Therefore, self-awareness of feelings and responses for victims of abuse and victimizers is crucial to ensuring the development of a therapeutic relationship.*

## Child Abuse

The nurse needs to be alert for possible indicators of child abuse. Early warning signs of possible abuse of children may include frequent physical injuries, including fractures, multiple somatic complaints, behavior problems such as aggressiveness, lying, or stealing, or extreme shyness, sexualized behavior on the part of young children, and excessive school absences. Once the abuse is identified, the child's safety is paramount.

Nurses and physicians are required by law to report suspected child abuse. Regulatory agencies generally require that reports of suspected abuse be filed within 24 hours or the clinician can risk losing his or her professional license. Nurses must familiarize themselves with all regulatory requirements in their region.

When abuse is suspected, the child should be examined outside the presence of the parents or caregiver because the child may fear consequences if he or she discloses the trauma. The nurse not only listens to what the child says, but carefully observes nonverbal communication because it can provide valuable information. For example, some possible nonverbal indicators of sexual abuse include: child being unable to sit without pain; or evidence of bloody underclothing, or a positive pregnancy test. A complete physical exam of the child, which may include photographs to document physical or sexual abuse, is required. Often further diagnostic studies including x-rays and laboratory tests are done to rule out the possibility of medical conditions causing the physical findings noted

### BOX 24-2: BEHAVIORS ON THE POWER AND CONTROL WHEEL

*Coercion and threats:*

- Making and/or carrying out threats to do something to hurt the victim
- Threatening to leave, commit suicide, or report the victim to welfare
- Making the victim drop charges
- Making the victim do illegal things

*Intimidation:*

- Making the victim afraid by using looks, actions, and gestures
- Smashing things
- Destroying property, abusing pets, displaying weapons

*Emotional abuse:*

- Putting the victim down
- Making the victim feel bad about him- or herself
- Calling the victim names
- Making the victim think he or she is crazy
- Playing mind games
- Humiliating the victim
- Making the victim feel guilty

*Isolation:*

- Controlling what the victim does, sees and talks to, reads, and goes
- Limiting the victim's outside involvement
- Using jealousy to justify actions

*Minimizing, denying, and blaming:*

- Making light of the abuse and not taking concerns about it seriously
- Saying the abuse didn't happen
- Shifting responsibility for abusive behavior
- Saying the victim caused it

*Using children:*

- Making the victim feel guilty about the children
- Using the children to relay messages
- Using visitation to harass the victim
- Threatening to take the children away

*Economic abuse:*

- Preventing the victim from getting or keeping a job
- Making the victim ask for money
- Giving the victim an allowance
- Taking the victim's money
- Not letting the victim know about or have access to family income

*Male privilege:*

- Treating the woman like a servant
- Making all the big decisions, acting like the "master of the castle," being the one to define men's and women's roles (DAIP, 2008)

during the examination. A complete eye examination is indicated in all infants to evaluate for retinal hemorrhages associated with the shaken baby syndrome.

> *Nurses are legally mandated to report suspicions of child abuse, usually within 24 hours.*

If the nurse suspects that the child is being abused in the home, he or she is responsible to provide for the safety of the child. Therefore, the nurse will not be able to release the child to return home. In these cases, the nurse must contact the local child protective services to provide emergency shelter while an investigation is completed. Planning for the immediate safety of the child is the priority.

When speaking with the child, questions need to be clear and simple. Reassure the child that no one has a right to hurt him or her. If a child has been victimized, he or she may talk in a very low voice and possibly demonstrate an exaggerated startle response when approached.

All children who are victims of trauma will need supportive psychotherapy to help them cope with the anger and rage that can stem from victimization. Treatment approaches will depend on the relationship of the child to the victimizer; the social and emotional support the child experiences within the family system; the mental status of the victim; and the availability of emotional resources within the family system. The time it takes to recover or heal from victimization may be protracted. The more frequent the episodes of victimization are, the longer it takes to heal.

If healing does not occur, victims may engage in many forms of self-destructive behavior, including self-mutilation and substance abuse. They may also experience difficulty establishing healthy interpersonal relationships throughout their lives. In addition, there is significant risk that they will perpetuate the abusive behavior with their own children. A child who has a successful response to treatment will demonstrate resiliency and the ability to form healthy relationships, thus refraining from becoming an abuser.

## Intimate Partner Violence

Since the prevalence of domestic abuse is high, it is essential that the nurse always screens for abuse. The assessment of the possible victim should be a standard component of the patient interview. During the screening process, the nurse looks for indicators of possible intimate partner violence. These indicators may be verbalized specifically by the patient or implied by the victim's statements. Some of the early indicators that may signal potential domestic abuse include: an intense whirlwind romance with the future abuser becoming very possessive and jealous early in the relationship; a relationship that is intentionally kept exclusive, with efforts to isolate the possible victim from family, friends, and social interactions with others; sensitivity on the part of the impending abuser to what is perceived as a lack of interest or attention on the part of the other, thus, needing to be the focal point of their attention; and finally, the latent abuser being unable to accept responsibility for his or her actions or feelings, blaming others for causing the jealousy, or not providing enough attention or affection, thereby demonstrating infidelity or lack of love. It is very common for the abuser to appear very caring and charismatic at the beginning of a relationship. Eventually, however, the need to control and dominate will be manifested through behaviors that are aimed at isolating the victim to diminish any external support network making the potential victim dependent on the abuser. The abuser will also begin to focus fault and blame on the victim for all issues. The abuser will excuse all of his or her own negative actions as justified responses to what is described as the provocative actions of the victim.

Initially, victims frequently accept the responsibility placed on them by abusers. They will feel that they may deserve the criticism and will make efforts to meet the abusers' expectations. Since domestic abuse is not due to interpersonal conflicts, no efforts the victim makes can achieve the goal of reducing domestic violence. Therefore the victim may voice feelings of failure, demonstrating low self-worth and poor self-esteem. The diminished sense of self will reinforce the victim's lack of confidence and fear of leaving the relationship, fostering dependence on the abuser.

While assessing a victim of suspected intimate partner violence, nurses needs to be aware of the possible discomfort the patient might experience in revealing abuse. Nurses should also be aware of any feelings they may have related to domestic violence since these feelings could interfere with establishing a therapeutic relationship with the patient. Help the victim describe the experience as specifically as possible. Offering examples of behaviors and situations may be helpful to reduce the discomfort the victim is experiencing in providing descriptions. Avoid using terms that may evoke strong emotional responses such as rape because these may inhibit the victim from further discussion of the events. Research indicates that victims are three times more likely to reveal abuse when questioned by a health care provider as compared to completing information on a form (McFarlane, Christoffel, Bateman, Miller, & Bullock, 1991). Therefore, the interview is an essential element of the assessment process.

When conducting the assessment, interview the victim and the abuser separately to help reduce the victim's fears. Avoid any judgmental remarks about the possible abuser since this may increase the victim's reluctance to provide information. As discussed, the victim frequently feels responsible for the abuse and still loving toward the abuser, making it difficult to be critical of the abuser. **Therapeutic Interaction 24–1** provides an example of an assessment interview with a victim of violence.

Use the same nonjudgmental, open approach when interviewing the abuser. It is not unusual for the nurse in this situation to experience his or her own feelings regarding both the victim and the abuser. The nurse may find it frustrating to hear the victim excuse the abuser or try to rationalize the event. The nurse may feel antagonism toward the abuser. Therefore, the nurse needs to be self-aware and confront his or her own reactions to ensure that they do not interfere with the therapeutic relationship.

> *When assessing a victim of intimate partner violence, the nurse interviews the victim separately from the victimizer.*

Documentation of the assessment must include an exact description of the patient's account of how an injury happened. Since many victims are seen in the emergency department, the assessment should include a complete physical exam with a detailed description of injuries, and a specific body map indicating site, size, and character of injuries. If possible, photographs should be taken to provide helpful visual documentation of the injuries.

Many victims of abuse may deny abuse. Therefore, it is appropriate to document any inconsistency between the injury and the patient's explanation of how it happened using the patient's exact words. Also important is assessing for the patient's safety prior to discharge, including any suicidal and homicidal ideation since there is an increased risk of both. Also address other safety risks such as the presence of weapons in the home or the use or abuse of alcohol or drugs. Throughout the assessment, the nurse needs to remain cognizant of the impact of the patient's culture on the situation, the victim's potential experience of shame or embarrassment, and the fact that victims frequently minimize their experiences during the assessment process.

For the victim of intimate partner violence the decision to seek help and leave the abusive relationship may not happen even if the victim has experienced repeated episodes of abuse. The victim of abuse may be reluctant to leave because she is hopeful the person may change, or she continues to feel committed to the relationship (Walker, 2009). Even after a decision is made, the victim may change her mind and return to the abusive situation. The decision to end an abusive relationship must be made by the victim when completely ready. Leaving an abusive relationship, along with pregnancy, are two factors that actually increase the risk of further, and at times more serious, abuse.

Finally, if children are in the home, assessment should also include an evaluation of possible child abuse. Obtain information about the children's behavior at home, including signs of problems, such as bedwetting or truancy, as well as any involvement with child protective services. If there is any suspicion of child abuse, mandatory reporting laws must be followed. Although mandatory reporting requirements vary in each jurisdiction, it is generally not mandatory or advisable to report injuries sustained by competent adults without their consent. If a person plans to return to the abusive partner, the report may enrage the abuser and actually lead to further abuse of the victim. However, since regulations vary, nurses should be familiar with the statutory regulations governing their region.

Once the assessment is completed, the nurse determines if the patient is at imminent risk of harm, either from the abuser or self-directed. If there is evidence to support this risk of harm, the nurse must work with the patient to provide immediate safety. If no immediate danger is assessed, the nurse may identify fear and anxiety related to the threat of harm.

Next, the nurse focuses on helping the patient identify relevant concerns and develop a safety plan. The safety plan involves very practical matters the victim should consider. For example, the victim should be advised to avoid being trapped in a room without an exit if a violent episode arises. In addition, the patient needs to be warned to avoid the kitchen and bath due to the presence of potential weapons in these rooms. Emphasize the need to try to access a phone and call 911.

## THERAPEUTIC INTERACTION 24-1:
### INTERVIEWING A VICTIM OF ABUSE

Mrs. L. is a 32-year-old married female who presents to the emergency department with a broken arm and multiple bruises. She is accompanied by her husband who appears extremely anxious and overly concerned about his wife. The nurse is considering the possibility of spousal abuse during the assessment.

| | |
|---|---|
| **Nurse:** "Mrs. L., I'll be performing an assessment now so I need to ask your family to step out." | Begins the process of assessment and provides for a private, safe environment to collect data |
| **Mrs. L.:** "That's OK. He wants to stay." | She is possibly deferring to husband regarding decisions that pertain to control of information |
| **Nurse:** "I still need to have him step out. If I need to clarify anything with him I will do so later." | Establishes control of the situation by stating what the protocol is in a matter-of-fact manner |
| **Mrs. L.:** (very nervous) "OK, but this shouldn't take long should it? I feel better with him here." | Is scared of the new structure of being away from husband and feels vulnerable |
| **Nurse:** "Each case is different; we will take only as long as needed to best determine how to help you." | Provides support and reassurance yet still sticks to the structure of maintaining control of the situation |
| **Nurse:** (after husband goes to the waiting room, nurse pulls up a chair and sits by the patient) "Can you tell me how you got these injuries?" | Provides opportunity for patient to share her story |
| **Mrs. L.:** "I fell down the basement stairs; I am so clumsy, always bumping into things." | Possibly protecting husband and denying the abusive relationship |
| **Nurse:** "Some of these bruises are old. Others look more like blunt trauma injuries, such as being struck with something." | States the findings of her assessment in a matter-of-fact manner |
| **Mrs. L.:** "Like I told you I am always running into things." | Still protecting husband |
| **Nurse:** "Mrs. Long, I need to tell you that in my experience, I feel your injuries are consistent with injuries in victims of spousal abuse." | Provides psychoeducation and opportunity for client to discuss the abuse |

*(cont.)*

**THERAPEUTIC INTERACTION 24-1: (*CONT.*)**
**INTERVIEWING A VICTIM OF ABUSE**

| | |
|---|---|
| **Mrs. L.:** (seems more anxious) "What are you saying? He would never intentionally hurt me." | Is feeling more vulnerable |
| **Nurse:** "Our conversation is strictly confidential. I am asking you, based on my assessment, are you the victim of spousal abuse?" | Assures her of the confidentiality and again presents her with an opportunity to discuss the potential abuse |
| **Mrs. L:** "No." | Possibly in denial |
| **Nurse:** "Before we move forward with treating these wounds, I would like to give you a phone number and a website you can go to for more information regarding my concern." | Accepts that the patient is not yet ready to seek help Offers information for her to consider later |
| **Mrs. L.:** "I guess so." | Accepts offer, possibly to bring to the conversation to a close |
| **Nurse:** "This is the number of the local domestic violence shelter; this is their website for more information. Please put these in a private place and look into them at the next opportunity." | Provides instruction on how to access services and stresses privacy knowing that if she is the victim of domestic violence, she could be at higher risk if the abuser learns of this conversation |

The internet also provides many resources for victims of domestic violence. The National Center on Domestic and Sexual Violence also provides a site with examples of personal safety plans to assist victims when they are preparing to leave an abusive situation (http://www.ncdsv.org/publications_safetyplans.html).

Victims need a safety plan that will provide protection; the protection must encompass more than just being safe from further physical abuse. It must take into consideration other aspects of the victim's life that have been threatened: for instance, financial stability; the well-being and safety of children, pets, and other loved ones; social status; psychological health; and the sense of self-worth and hope for the future that may be in jeopardy (Hamby & Bible, 2009). **Patient and Family Education 24-1** highlights some of the important information to include in a safety plan.

The victim should also be counseled to make certain preparations in advance so that if he or she does decide to leave, he or she will be better equipped to manage the change. When assisting the victim in developing a personalized safety plan, be sure that the victim includes: arrangements for a place to stay that will be safe from the abuser, a list of people who would be able to provide assistance, and information regarding counseling services available in the community. To provide effective assistance, the nurse working in this area must have a thorough knowledge of community resources, including contact information or referrals for shelters for victims of domestic violence, as well as an understanding of the risks associated with a victim leaving an abusive relationship. In addition, the nurse needs a thorough knowledge and understanding of the cultural considerations related to both the victim and the abuser and the risks and obstacles the victim will face

### PATIENT AND FAMILY EDUCATION 24-1: MAKING A SAFETY PLAN IN PREPARATION FOR LEAVING

- Begin to save money

- Copy important documents such as
  - Identification forms such as birth certificates and passports
  - Insurance information
  - Financial information such as bank accounts, mortgages, and loans
  - Legal documents that may be relevant such as custody or divorce papers
  - Court documents
  - Medical records

- Prepare a list of important phone numbers and addresses, including area shelters

- Identify a destination once you make the decision to leave

- Arrange travel plans

- Pack important items such as a child's favorite toy or family jewelry

- Do not take property that belongs to the abuser—this can lead to legal issues for you

> *A nurse must never force or coerce a victim of intimate partner violence to leave an abusive relationship. This decision is entirely the victim's choice.*

if he or she decides to leave the relationship. The nurse is responsible for educating the victim about this information, the patterns of abuse, the inherent dangers the victim may face, and the available resources in the community.

Although it may seem in the victim's best interest to leave an abusive relationship, it is never appropriate to pressure the victim to leave. The victim must make the decision to leave independently and must understand that the risk of violence increases after leaving the abusive situation. Nonjudgmental and empathic support is needed throughout the process to enhance the victim's sense of self-worth and autonomy and promote improved self-esteem. The nurse working with the victims of abuse needs to be aware of the myriad reasons that victims stay in abusive relationships. These can include real or perceived dependence on the abuser, both financial and emotional, fear, love, or shame (Walker, 2009).

Frequently, victims of domestic violence will also pursue legal protection through the courts. They may obtain emergency protective orders, or temporary or permanent restraining orders that direct the abuser to avoid contact with the victim. If the abuser does not adhere to the conditions of the order, he or she risks legal consequences.

After a victim of domestic violence leaves the abusive situation, it is not uncommon to experience ambivalence regarding the decision. Limited financial resources, lack of support from family and friends, as well as low self-esteem contribute to the victim's concern that leaving is a mistake. The fact that extended exposure to an abusive relationship also diminishes the victim's confidence and self-image will only reinforce this ambivalence. For those who have endured abuse over an extended period, the risk for posttraumatic stress disorder is increased. The increased fear, anxiety, and depression associated with this disorder may negatively impact the victim's ability to successfully cope with newly achieved autonomy.

The victim needs support during this period, including mental health counseling and services necessary to avoid self-harm and to develop the coping skills necessary to sustain independence. The role of the nurse will include education regarding what a victim can realistically expect to experience, including the social, financial, and emotional responses that frequently accompany abuse and its aftermath. The nurse will also provide counseling regarding health maintenance and self-care activities, as well as stress reduction and assertiveness.

For victims experiencing PTSD, cognitive behavioral therapy may be used to achieve symptom resolution. Other programs for victims of abuse also may be available. For example, Walker (2009), in collaboration with a team of researchers, has developed a formal program specifically for abused women. It is called the Survivor Therapy Empowerment Program (STEP). The program consists of twelve units, each containing an educational, discussion, and skills-building component to foster increased knowledge regarding domestic violence, to recognize its impact

## EVIDENCE-BASED PRACTICE 24-1: ELDER ABUSE

### STUDY

Sandmoe, A., & Kirkevold, M. (2010). Nurses' clinical assessments of older clients who are suspected victims of abuse: An exploratory study in community care in Norway. *Journal of Clinical Nursing, 20,* 94–102.

### SUMMARY

This study was designed to investigate the assessment process used by nurses in the community when dealing with the potential for abuse of the older adult. Ten nurses, selected because of their clinical experience and expertise, were interviewed in-depth about their understanding of abuse, their assessment techniques, including reporting of the abuse and management of the problem, such as dealing with the problem, collaborating with others, and obtaining support to lessen the difficulty of the situation. The study revealed that nurses' opportunities to identify the older patient who is being abused might fail unless certain conditions are present that facilitate the clinical assessment. One condition identified as important was the involvement of the nurse's supervisor or manager. Additionally, family members' support and the presence of alliances in the assessment process seem also to be important for the nurse to feel comfortable in proceeding in following through with their "hunches." Results indicated that a systematic framework for assessment is needed to help ease the difficulty in working with elderly patients experiencing abuse. In addition, the researchers felt that such a framework was important for delivering of quality care to these patients.

### APPLICATION TO PRACTICE

Nurses are in unique opportunities both in the emergency department and in community settings, often being the first front line personnel to detect elder abuse. This study emphasized the need for a structured framework to help facilitate the systematic clinical assessment of suspected older, abused patients in community care. Such a framework might ensure a more consistent frequency of assessment and quality of the service provided to victims of abuse.

### QUESTIONS TO PONDER

1. *While working at a community health setting during a blood pressure screening day, an elderly patient comes to your table. As she rolls up her sleeve to have her blood pressure taken, you notice multiple bruises on her arm. How would the information gained from this study help you to proceed?*
2. *A home health care aide at the agency where you work comes to you and says that she believes one of her elderly patients is being abused by their son and asks you to come with her on the next visit to assess for yourself. Which factors identified by the study would be important? What would your first response be to this aide?*

on victims' lives, and to increase their ability to effectively manage the consequences (Walker, 2009).

Interventions for the perpetrators of abuse frequently involve legally mandated participation in intervention programs focused on changing the attitudes, beliefs, and behaviors of the abuser. It is generally accepted that domestic violence is not reduced through family and couples therapy.

Ultimately, the desired outcomes for the victim focus on:

- Ending the cycle of abuse
- Promoting recovery from physical aspects of abuse
- Developing a positive self-image without guilt or self-blame
- Becoming financially self-sufficient
- Achieving a supportive social network
- Being able to engage in non-abusive relationships

For the abuser, the desired outcome is completion of a batterer intervention program that will lead to acceptance of responsibility for the violence, a significant change in his or her attitudes, and an elimination of violent and abusive behaviors.

## Elder Abuse

As with other forms of abuse, recognition of potential indicators is important. Look for any indication that the victim has not received adequate care. Some obvious physical signs include poor physical hygiene, uncombed hair, dirty clothes, urine smell, signs of malnourishment, dehydration or bruises, scratches, burns, or pinch marks. The victim may also appear withdrawn, confused, or frightened. Take note of caregivers who restrict the elder's social contacts or who do not allow the elder to speak freely. If financial abuse is a possibility, try to ascertain changes in spending patterns, numerous unpaid bills, or unusual bank account activity (California Office of Attorney General, 2002).

When assessing the elderly patient, ask direct and simple questions in a nonjudgmental or nonthreatening manner. Conduct a portion of the interview with the patient in the presence of the caregiver to evaluate the nature of the patient-caregiver interaction. Also conduct a portion with the patient and caregiver individually to detect inconsistencies and to provide the elderly patient an opportunity to discuss possible abuse. Be sure to allow adequate time and privacy so that the patient feels comfortable and safe. **Evidence-Based Practice 24-1** highlights a research study underscoring the importance of this assessment.

A thorough physical examination is completed, including an evaluation of evidence of old injuries and/or pressure ulcers. During the physical examination, note the size, shape, and location of all injuries. Incorporate the use of body maps or diagrams when extensive injuries are present. If appropriate, photograph the injuries.

A key aspect of the plan of care for a victim of elder abuse is ensuring the patient's safety. Contacting adult protective services may be necessary. In addition, be knowledgeable about state and local reporting requirements. In many jurisdictions, suspected elder abuse requires that the clinician report it to local authorities. However, although federal laws on child abuse and domestic violence fund services and shelters for victims, there is no comparable federal law on elder abuse. The Federal Older Americans Act of 1965 provides federal funds for the National Center on Elder Abuse (NCEA). This center is directed by the U.S. Administration on Aging and provides for certain elder abuse awareness and coordination activities in states and local communities. However, the center does not provide funds for shelters or victim services. The 2009 U.S. Congress has been working on a number of bills regarding elder abuse and neglect to provide a greater level of protection, but these federal bills are yet to be enacted.

The nurse also works to make provisions to ensure that the elder's ongoing biopsychosocial and spiritual needs are met. This would include coordinating services with other providers, such as home care services, alternative residential placement, and respite care, based on the particular needs of the individual.

### SUMMARY POINTS

- Abuse is an act designed to obtain and maintain power and control over another. It may be physical, emotional, sexual, or economic.

- Domestic violence is now considered a national crime due to enactment of the Violence Against Women Act of 1994 and its additions in 1996. In certain situations, it

*(cont.)*

## SUMMARY POINTS (*CONT.*)

is against the law for a domestic abuser to have guns.

- Children between the ages of 3 and 5 are most commonly abused; most children view the abuse as their fault. Domestic violence remains the leading cause of injury to women between the ages of 15 to 44 years. The majority of family violence victims are female while approximately ¾ of the perpetrators are male. Elderly abuse is commonly manifested as neglect and often underreported.

- Various models have been developed to describe abuse and violence. The Cycle of Violence Model consists of three phases depicting the pattern of domestic abuse. The Cycle of Abuse Model consists of six phases. The Power and Control Wheel identifies nine specific behaviors used by an abuser.

- A nurse is responsible for reporting suspicions of abuse based on local and state laws. All nurses are mandated to report suspicions of child abuse within 24 hours. The nurse is also responsible for conducting a thorough assessment and for documenting findings clearly, often using body maps and possibly photographs.

- When caring for a victim of intimate partner violence, the nurse should assist the victim in developing a personalized safety plan should the victim decides to leave the relationship.

- As with any victim of abuse, safety, especially for the elderly abuse victim, is a priority. Adult protective services may need to be contacted.

## NCLEX-PREP*

1. A nurse is preparing a presentation for a local community group about abuse and violence. Which of the following would the nurse most likely include?

   a. Abuse is primarily seen in lower socioeconomic areas where poverty is rampant.
   b. Children typically are around the ages of 8 to 10 when they suffer abuse.
   c. Abuse indicates an underlying mental health disorder that is out of control.
   d. An abuser frequently uses more than one method to achieve the goal.

2. A woman is brought by her husband to the emergency department. The woman has significant swelling surrounding her right eye and bruising over the right side of her face. She is also holding her right upper arm that is covering a large bruised area. The nurse suspects intimate partner violence. When interviewing the woman, which statement would indicate that the woman is in the honeymoon phase of the cycle of violence?

   a. "I feel like I'm walking on eggshells."
   b. "He said he was sorry and wouldn't do it again."
   c. "I need to make sure I don't make him angry."
   d. "It was my fault because I didn't have dinner ready on time."

(*cont.*)

3. When applying the Power and Control Wheel to evaluate a victimizer's behavior, which of the following would indicate intimidation?

   a. Calling the victim names

   b. Making the victim feel guilty

   c. Destroying property

   d. Controlling who the victim talks to

4. The following are phases identified by the model proposed by the anti-violence movement in Oregon. Place them in the proper sequence from beginning to end.

   _3_ a. Setup

   _1_ b. Fantasy

   _2_ c. Planning

   _4_ d. Abuse

   _6_ e. Rationalize

   _5_ f. Guilt

   _7_ g. Normal

5. When assessing an older adult for suspected abuse, the nurse interviews the victim together with the caregiver based on which rationale?

   a. To evaluate the patient and caregiver relationship

   b. To identify inconsistencies in their statements

   c. To confirm the patient's level of alertness

   d. To determine the need for adult protective services

6. A nurse is working in the community and is preparing a presentation for a local group of parents about child abuse. Which of the following would the nurse most likely include in this presentation?

   a. Physicians are the individuals responsible for reporting suspected child abuse.

   b. Child abuse primarily involves emotional and sexual abuse.

   c. The perpetrator is commonly someone the child knows.

   d. When children do reveal abuse, they experience revictimization.

*Answers to these questions appear on page 639.

## REFERENCES

Bair-Merritt, M. H. (2010). Intimate partner violence. *Pediatrics in Review, 31*(4), 145–150. Retrieved from: https://phstwlp1.partners.org:2443/login?url=http://ovidsp.ovid.com/ovidweb.cgi?T=JS&CSC=Y&NEWS=N&PAGE=fulltext&D=medl&AN=20360408

Benson, M.L., & Fox, G.L. (2001). *Economic distress, community context and intimate violence: an application and extension of social disorganization theory, final report.* U.S. Dept of Justice, National Institute of Justice Police Foundation.

Brown, D. W., Anda, R. F., Tiemeier, H., Felitti, V. J., Edwards, V. J., Croft, J. B., & Giles, W. H. (2009). Adverse childhood experiences and the risk of premature mortality. *American Journal of Preventive Medicine, 37*(5), 389–396. doi:DOI: 10.1016/j.amepre.2009.06.021

Bureau of Justice Statistics. (2003). U.S. Department of Justice. Retrieved from http://bjs.ojp.usdoj.gov/content/intimate/ipv.cfm

California Office of the Attorney General. *2002 Citizen's guide to preventing & reporting elder abuse.* Retrieved from http://ag.ca.gov/bmfea/publications.php

Catalano, S. (2007). *Intimate partner violence in the United States.* Washington, DC: Bureau of Justice Statistics, U.S. Department of Justice.

Child Welfare Information Gateway (2008). Definitions of domestic violence: Summary of state laws. Children's Bureau/ACYF Washington, DC: U.S. Department of Health and Human Services. Retrieved from: www.childwelfare.gov/systemwide/laws_policies/statutes/defdomvio.cfm

Coomaraswamy, R. (2002) *Integration of the human rights of women and the gender perspective violence against women. Report of the Special Rapporteur on violence against women, its causes and consequences.* Commission on Human Rights, Fifty-eighth session, UN Economic and Social Council.

Domestic Abuse Intervention Project [DAIP] (2008). Duluth, Minnesota. Retrieved from http://www.theduluthmodel.org/

Falsetti, S. A. (2007). Screening and responding to family and intimate partner violence in the primary care setting. *Primary Care; Clinics in Office Practice, 34*(3), 641–657. Retrieved from https://phstwlp1.partners.org:2443/login?url=http://ovidsp.ovid.com/ovidweb.cgi?T=JS&CSC=Y&NEWS=N&PAGE=fulltext&D=medl&AN=17868764 http://www.domesticviolence.org/who-are-the-victims/

Fellitti, Vincent J, Anda, Robert F, et. al .(1998) *Relationship of childhood abuse and household dysfunction to many of the leading causes of death in adults: The Adverse Childhood Experiences (ACE) Study.* American Journal of Preventive Medicine. Volume 14, Issue 4. pages 245–258. Retrieved from: http://www.ajpm-online.net/article/PIIS0749379798000178/fulltext

Finesmith. (1983). *Police response to battered women: a critique and proposal for reform.* 14 Seton Hall Law. Rev. 74, 79.

Friday, P., Lord, V., Exum, M., & Hartman, J. (2006). *Evaluating the impact of a specialized domestic violence police unit. Final report for National Institute of Justice,* NCJ215916.

Washington, DC: National Institute of Justice, U.S. Department of Justice. Retrieved from http://www.ncjrs.gov/App/Publications/abstract.aspx?ID=237505

Fustel des Coulanges, & Numa Denis. (1980*). The ancient city: A study of the religion, laws, and institutions of Greece and Rome.* Baltimore: The Johns Hopkins University Press.

Ganley, A.L., & Schecter, S. (1996). *Domestic violence: A national curriculum for children's protective services.* San Francisco: Family Violence Prevention Fund.

Gracia, E. (2004). Unreported cases of domestic violence against women: towards an epidemiology of social silence, tolerance, and inhibition. *J Epidemiol Community Health 58,* 536–537. doi: 10.1136/jech.2003.019604

Hamby, S., & Bible, A. (2009). *Battered women's protective strategies.* Harrisburg, PA: VAWnet, a project of the National Resource Center on Domestic Violence/Pennsylvania Coalition Against Domestic Violence. Retrieved from: http://www.vawnet.org

Kerber, L.K., & De Hart, J.S., Editors (1995). *Women's America: refocusing the past.* New York: Oxford University Press.

Klein, A. (2009) .*Practical implications of current domestic violence research: for law enforcement, prosecutors and judges.* U.S. DOJ Office of Justice Programs, National Institute of Justice Special Report.

Leeb, R.T., Paulozzi L., Melanson, C., Simon, T., & Arias, I. (2007). Child maltreatment surveillance: uniform definitions for public health and recommended data elements, version 1.0. Atlanta (GA): Centers for Disease Control and Prevention, National Center for Injury Prevention and Control; Retrieved from: http://www.cdc.gov/ViolencePrevention/pub/CMP-Surveillance.html

Mayell, H. (2002) Thousands of women killed for family "honor." *National Geographic News.*

McFarlane, J., Christoffe, K., Bateman, L., Miller, V., & Bullock, L. (1991). Assessing for abuse: self-report versus nurse interview. *Public Health Nurse,* Dec; *8*(4):245–50.

Mid-Valley Women's Crisis Service Salem Oregon. Retrieved from http://www.mvwcs.com

National Elder Abuse Incidence Study. (1998). *Fact sheet.* Washington, DC: National Center on Elder Abuse at American Public Human Services Association.

National Research Council Panel to Review Risk and Prevalence of Elder Abuse and Neglect. (2003). *Elder mistreatment: abuse, neglect and exploitation in an aging America.* Washington, DC.

Nerenberg, L. (1999). *Forgotten victims of elder financial crime and abuse: a report and recommendations.* Produced by the Goldman Institute on Aging for the National Center on Aging (NCEA), Volume 12 Number 2 (2000) of the Journal of Elder Abuse & Neglect.

Nerenberg, L. (2002) *Caregiver stress and elder abuse,* Washington, DC NCEA National Center on Elder Abuse. San Francisco, California Produced by the Institute on Aging (formerly Goldman Institute on Aging).

Nguyen, T.D. (2004). *Vietnamese women and domestic violence: A qualitative examination. the qualitative report, 9*(3), 435–448. Retrieved from http://www.nova.edu/ssss/QR/QR9-3/nguyen.pdf

Orloff, L.E. (1996). Effective advocacy for domestic violence victims: Role of the nurse-midwife. *Journal of Nurse Midwifery, 41*(6): 473–494, November/December.

Purcell, B. (2004) Too many elder abuse cases go unreported. Report on Elder Abuse Global Action on Aging, NY. Retrieved from: http://www.globalaging.org/elderrights/us/2004/toomany.htm

Reed, K. (2005). When elders lose their cents: Financial abuse of the elderly. *Clinics in Geriatric Medicine, 21*(2), 365–382. Retrieved from https://phstwlp1.partners.org:2443/login?url=http://phstwlp1.partners.org:2057/ovidweb.cgi?T=JS&CSC=Y&NEWS=N&PAGE=fulltext&D=med4&AN=15804556

Ramsay, J., Carter Y, Davidson, L., Dunne, D., Eldridge, S., Feder, G., Hegarty, K., Rivas, C., Taft, A., & Warburton, A. (2009). Advocacy interventions to reduce or eliminate violence and promote the physical and psychosocial well-being of women who experience intimate partner abuse. Cochrane Database of Systematic Reviews 2009, Issue 3. Art. No.: CD005043. DOI: 10.1002/14651858.CD005043.pub2

Sandmoe, A., & Kirkevold, M. (2010) Nurses' clinical assessments of older clients who are suspected victims of abuse: an exploratory study in community care in Norway, *Journal of Clinical Nursing,* 20, 94–102.

Schewe, P., Riger, S., Howard, A., Staggs, S., & Mason, G. (2006). Factors associated with domestic violence and sexual assault victimization. *Journal of Family Violence, 21*(7), 469–475. Retrieved from http://search.ebscohost.com/login.aspx?direct=true&db=jlh&AN=2009373467&site=ehost-live

Tjaden, P., & Thoennes, N. (2000). *Extent, nature and consequences of intimate partner violence: findings from the national violence against women survey*: National Institute of Justice and the Centers of Disease Control and Prevention, U.S. Retrieved from http://bjs.ojp.usdoj.gov/index.cfm?ty=smp

UNICEF. (2003). *A league table of child maltreatment deaths in rich nations*, Innocenti Report Card No.5. UNICEF Innocenti Research Centre, Florence.

United Nations. (2006). In-depth study on all forms of violence against women Report of the Secretary-General, Sixty-first session United Nations A/61/122/ General Assembly. Retrieved from: http://www.un.org/ga/search/view_doc.asp?symbol=A/61/122/Add.1

U.S. Centers for Disease Control and Prevention. (2008). Adverse health conditions and health risk behaviors associated with intimate partner violence. *Morbidity and Mortality Weekly Report (MMWR)* 57(5), 113–117. Retrieved from http://www.cdc.gov/mmwR/preview/mmwrhtml/mm5705a1.htm

Walker, L. (2009) *The battered woman syndrome*, New York: Springer Publishing Company.

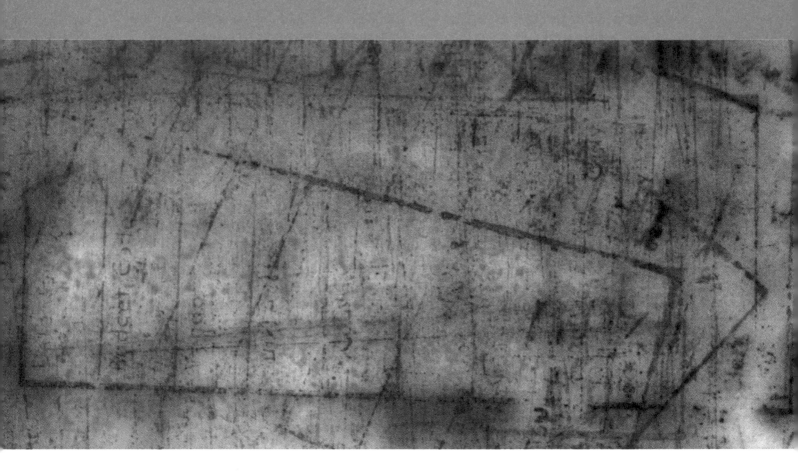

## CHAPTER CONTENTS

## CHAPTER 25
# PSYCHIATRIC-MENTAL HEALTH NURSING ACROSS THE CONTINUUM OF CARE

Patricia Smythe Matos

Lori A. Neushotz

## EXPECTED LEARNING OUTCOMES

**After completing this chapter, the student will be able to:**

1. Define the continuum of care.

2. Describe available treatment options and community-based resources for psychiatric-mental health patients.

3. Correlate the adequacy of care settings as they relate to patient acuity and needs.

4. Explain how the psychiatric-mental health nurse (PMHN) applies the nursing process throughout the diverse settings within continuum of care.

5. Discuss the specialized roles that PMHNs may assume within the continuum of care.

## KEY TERMS

Continuum of care

Forensic nursing

Least restrictive environment

Telehealth

Therapeutic milieu

Psychiatric mental health nursing is a specialized area of nursing practice committed to promoting mental health through the assessment, diagnosis, and treatment of patients presenting with mental health problems and psychiatric disorders along a CONTINUUM OF CARE (an integrated system of settings, services, health care clinicians, and care levels spanning illness to wellness states [Boyd, 2008]) in a variety of health care settings (American Nurses Association [ANA] et al., 2007). The practice of psychiatric-mental health nursing is based on the nursing process and operationalized through the scope and standards outlined by the American Nurses Association, the American Psychiatric Nurses Association, and the International Society of Psychiatric-Mental Health Nurses (2007; see Chapter 1 for a description of the scope and standards of practice). These standards provide a firm basis for psychiatric-mental health nursing practice across all levels of care and span diverse settings, including inpatient units and community mental health clinics.

This chapter describes the various levels of care in which the psychiatric-mental health nurse (PMHN) practices and the principles of practice appropriate for each level of care. It also integrates the nursing process as the primary method for PMHNs in providing care to patients. The chapter concludes with a discussion of some of the specialized roles for PMHNs along the continuum of care.

## PSYCHIATRIC-MENTAL HEALTH NURSING ACROSS THE CONTINUUM OF CARE

As stated above, the continuum of care spans from illness to wellness. It maximizes the coordination of care and services including nursing, medical, psychological, and social services. This coordination ensures that patients receive all appropriate services necessary for optimal health.

Psychiatric-mental health nursing employs the purposeful use of self as its art, based on Peplau's theory (1991). The science is based in nursing, psychosocial, and neurobiological theories and research evidence. PMHNs promote and provide the delivery of holistic, patient-centered, interpersonal, and comprehensive primary mental health services to patients and families within their communities. The nurse always remains cognizant of the need to practice evidence-based care, thereby avoiding the use of untested alternative therapies. The advanced practice nurse should not recommend or prescribe treatments that are not grounded in solid research.

The PMHN's role is diverse and encompassing. For example, PMHNs provide care in hospitals, outpatient clinics, and day treatment programs. They also develop health and wellness promotion programs addressing mental health issues, advocate for the prevention of mental health problems, and provide direct care and treatment to persons with psychiatric disorders. In addition, PMHNs may be employed in research, act as expert consultants, be self-employed and practice autonomously, or within a group practice.

PMHNs integrate the interpersonal process, incorporating the therapeutic use of self and the collaborative partnership between the nurse and patient (Peplau, 1991), and the nursing process to develop a plan of care for the patient with a psychiatric-mental health problem. In doing so, the PMHN is able to assist patients, their families, and their communities at all levels on the continuum of care, from the acutely unstable to the chronic, long-term care patient.

> *The continuum of care covers the range from illness to wellness and requires coordination of care and services for the patient to achieve optimal health.*

## Goal of the Least Restrictive Environment

The continuum of care is designed to ensure that treatment provided to a patient is one that allows the patient the highest level of functioning in the LEAST RESTRICTIVE ENVIRONMENT, that is, in the safest environment with the minimum restrictions on personal liberty necessary to maintain the safety of the patient and the public, and to allow the patient to achieve independence in daily living as much as possible. Least restrictive environments respect the individual's personal needs for dignity and privacy while enhancing personal autonomy. In 1999, with the Olmstead decision, the Supreme Court affirmed that the unjustified institutionalization of a person with disabilities is discriminatory. The decision also affirmed that such an action violates the Americans with Disabilities Act. As a result, psychiatric-mental health treatment is more often delivered in community settings rather than in highly restrictive inpatient hospital settings (ANA, 2007).

## Consultation-Liaison Services

When a patient requires psychiatric-mental health care in a setting other than a psychiatric service setting, such as a medical hospital unit, nursing home, and rehabilitation facility, a PMHN, typically at the advanced level of practice, may be called upon to provide consultation-liaison services. In this role, the nurse assesses the patient's mental health needs and makes recommendations for nursing interventions in the setting in which the patient is being treated. These recommendations are carried out by the staff in that medical setting. The consultation-liaison nurse also provides education for the staff as needed, provides follow-up visits to assess the patient's response to the nursing intervention, and/or makes recommendations to modify the interventions based on this evaluation.

## LEVELS OF CARE

Care is provided in a variety of different settings along the continuum of care and ranges from acute emergency treatment to long-term chronic care. Many factors, including current research findings, cost effectiveness, level of reimbursement, social factors, and the availability of pharmacological treatments, influence which level of care is appropriate for the patient.

## Psychiatric Emergency Care

Psychiatric emergency care is similar to medical emergency care. Both often involve life and death situations. Patients may be a danger to themselves or others. Their thinking or judgment may be so impaired that they cannot safely care for themselves.

If a patient is receiving individual treatment with an advanced practice nurse such as nurse practitioner or other mental health practitioner, the first step is to ensure that the patient and those around him are safe. The nurse assesses the patient for suicidal or homicidal ideation and for the ability to maintain control. Once the nurse has identified the problems, he or she must then decide which setting is most appropriate and develop a plan for providing that level of care. Some communities have mobile crisis teams that come to the setting and provide emergency treatment to the patient in crisis. These teams also may transport the patient to a safer setting. Other communities may depend on 911 or police emergency systems. The nurse considers the urgency of the situation as well as community resources in developing the plan.

Communicating pertinent clinical information (diagnosis, psychiatric history, current medications, current concern/risk, etc.) to the providers at the next level of care is essential, especially in an emergency situation. In addition, the nurse remains available to those providers throughout the patient's care and discharge. Following

any patient emergency, the nurse reviews the case with the collaborating physician and/or treatment team to evaluate the treatment plan and develop new interventions if needed upon the patient's return to outpatient care.

> *Like medical emergency care, psychiatric emergency care, often involves life and death situations. The safety of the patient and those around him or her is the priority.*

## Acute Inpatient Care

Inpatient care for the psychiatric-mental health patient is most often acute and short-term. The inpatient unit may be in a general medical hospital or psychiatric hospital. The goal of inpatient care is stabilization of symptoms and discharge to a safe and therapeutic living environment with the appropriate level of outpatient treatment. Inpatient treatment is reserved for patients who cannot be safely treated outside of the hospital setting and require 24-hour nursing supervision and care.

Upon admission, the nurse completes a full assessment of the patient. Assessment tools, although variable from facility to facility, generally incorporate medical, nursing, and social assessments. Based on these assessments, an interdisciplinary treatment plan is developed and shared with the patient. Behavioral outcomes that are clear and measurable are included.

The PMHN develops a plan of care that includes interventions addressing the biological, psychosocial, and spiritual needs of the patient. Patient and family education about the diagnosis, treatment, and strategies to improve and maintain health are an essential part of this plan.

Typically, a THERAPEUTIC MILIEU is created on the inpatient unit. A therapeutic milieu involves a focus on creating a climate and environment that is therapeutic and conducive to psychiatric healing within a structured group setting that encompasses the elements of trust, safety, peer support, and repetition of recovery psychoeducation to enable patients to work through psychological issues. This milieu is designed to promote healing for all of the patients on that unit. The nurse is responsible for providing the structure necessary to maintain this environment. In collaboration with other health care providers, families, and patients, groups and activities are prescribed based on the patient's assessment and cultural background. The nurse provides orientation and education for expected behaviors and interpersonal relationships. The nurse also ensures that safety for all is maintained in the least restrictive environment.

The PMHN continuously communicates an evaluation of the patient's response to treatment and progress toward goals to other members of the interdisciplinary team. This communication is a collaborative process and is ongoing throughout the patient's inpatient stay. Changes in treatment and interventions are based on the patient's response and are used to develop appropriate discharge plans.

When a patient is admitted to an acute inpatient facility, discharge planning begins on admission. Collaboration occurs among all parties involved, such as the patient, family, interdisciplinary team, and outpatient provider. The nurse is a leader in the discharge planning process and coordinates the care needed to ensure that the patient is discharged to a safe living environment and has adequate resources for care and support.

## Intermediate/Long-Term Inpatient Care

Intermediate or long-term inpatient care is required for patients who cannot be stabilized in an acute setting; for example, patients who are chronically self-destructive, psychotic, or unsafe to others in the community. These patients may spend many months or years in a chronic care facility such as a state hospital. However, over the past 20 years, the trend has been toward discharging these patients to the community. In some cases, patients may require a specialized treatment program, such as drug or alcohol rehabilitation, necessitating a longer length of stay (typically 28 days but it may be up to six months), or an eating disorder program. While the length of stay may be different than acute inpatient hospitalization, application of the nursing process, the interpersonal process, and standards of practice remain the same.

## Partial Hospitalization/Day Treatment

Partial hospitalization is an intense, ambulatory mental health program for patients who require a structured treatment program during the day, but are stable enough to return to their living environment at night. These programs can be designed for treatment ranging from three to five days per week. The time frame for the program can be for a full or halfday. Patients appropriate for this setting generally cannot function autonomously on a daily basis. However, with the structure and support of this type of

program, the patient is deemed safe to be in treatment outside of an inpatient setting. Partial hospitalization may be used as an alternative to inpatient admission or as a transition from inpatient to outpatient care. Treatment provided includes individual and group therapy, psychopharmacologic treatment as needed, and education. Individualized plans are developed by the interdisciplinary treatment team and may include social skills groups, illness and relapse prevention education, time management classes, and expressive and supportive psychotherapy. The nurse implements the nursing process for each patient, incorporating it into the interdisciplinary treatment plan.

The PMHN is involved in discharge planning and coordination of care, ensuring that the patient's medical, financial, and housing needs are met. He or she also provides education to the family or nighttime caregiver as needed. Discharge to a less intensive level of care, such as an outpatient mental health clinic or private practitioner, is usually the goal. Unfortunately, some patients may require inpatient treatment if symptoms worsen or the living environment becomes unstable.

> *A partial hospitalization program provides a structured treatment program during the day, with the patient returning to his or her living environment at night.*

## Residential Services

The search for non-hospital-based options for psychiatric patients requiring acute care has become a focus in light of current efforts to control medical costs. Residential facilities combine and provide mental health treatment and residential care to the seriously and persistently mentally ill population who may be diagnosed with persistent and unremitting psychotic and mood disorders and/or substance use disorders. These facilities may be publicly or privately owned and funded. Intensive residential services provide patients with a place to stay in conjunction with supervised care over a 24-hour period. Length of stay may be brief (ranging from days to weeks) or extended (ranging from months to years). Medical, nursing, psychosocial, recreational, and other support services are available. In addition, assistance with vocational training and activities of daily living training are provided.

The PMHN is in a unique position and plays an important role in the care of persons with severe and persistent mental illness who require residential services. The Scope and Standards of Psychiatric Mental Health Nursing provides a guide for nurses in the delivery of patient care in this setting (American Nurses Association, 2007). PMHNs assess and provide supportive services to patients and provide psychoeducation about diagnosis, symptom management, anger management, and prescribed medication. PMHN also assess the patient's level of motivation to treatment and tailor appropriate interventions while emphasizing the importance and benefit of adherence to treatment. Supervised self-administration and management of medication also is provided.

Rehabilitation is often a goal for residential treatment facilities. A return to independent living and work life with psychosocial supports in place has been achieved for many persons diagnosed with mental illness.

> *Residential services are used for patients experiencing seriously persistent mental illness, such as persistent and unremitting psychotic or mood disorders.*

## Community-Based Care

Community-based psychiatric-mental health care covers a wide range of services. PMHNs provide care in partnership with patients within the community as an effective method of responding to the mental health needs of individuals, families, and groups. Care may be delivered in the patient's home, on the worksite, or at a school mental health clinic. Community mental health care is also provided in clinics, health maintenance organizations (HMOs), day treatment programs, homeless shelters, crisis centers, senior centers, group homes, and churches. Regardless of where the community mental health care is delivered, it is provided in a manner that respects the cultural and spiritual diversity of the patient and the community.

The PMHN assumes various roles within community-based care. In general, PMHNs identify and assess the mental health needs of the group and design programs and educational health and wellness outreach activities to target vulnerable populations. In the school setting, PMHNs engage in primary prevention and early intervention to promote good future health. They provide psychoeducation to students, parents, and teachers; assess and evaluate students for mental health difficulties; and

provide psychiatric services, such as therapy and psychopharmacologic interventions to students.

## Psychiatric Rehabilitation Programs

Psychiatric rehabilitation, also known as psychosocial rehabilitation or psych rehab is a collaborative, patient-centered approach that promotes individual empowerment, community integration, and improved quality of life for patients diagnosed with mental health conditions. Recovery is a critical component of outpatient and psychiatric rehabilitation treatment programs and focuses on helping individuals develop the skills to assist them in sustaining relationships, employment, and housing (Anthony, Cohen, Farkas, & Cagne, 2002). Services provided include psychopharmacological management, social skills, and vocational training, and access to leisure activities. Physicians, nurse practitioners, social workers, nurses, and other mental health workers work collaboratively with patients toward, the goals of empowerment, social inclusion, decreased stigma, and psychosocial recovery. The roles of the PMHN in these programs include psychopharmacological management, psychoeducation, group facilitation, and case management.

## Assertive Community Treatment

Assertive community treatment (ACT) offers services that are customized to the individual needs of the consumer, delivered by a team of practitioners to the patients where they live, and are available 24 hours a day. The goal of ACT is to prevent hospitalization and to develop skills for living in the community. The constant availability of practitioners provides support and assistance to patients and families whenever a crisis arises. Patients are provided emergency contact numbers; when a crisis occurs, mobile treatment teams provide outreach crisis prevention services. Linkage to appropriate services are negotiated and arranged. ACT teams have been effective in reducing service costs and decreasing inpatient hospital admissions (Kane & Blank, 2004).

## Clubhouse Model

The clubhouse model was created in 1947 by a group of patients recovering from mental illness. They believed that they could support each other through recovery and return to productive lives in society. This group, "We Are Not Alone" or WANA, eventually developed and became the Fountain House in Manhattan (www.fountainhouse.org). The clubhouse model differs from day treatment programs in that it is primarily a self-help model. The members hire the professional staff and partner with them to provide daily structure and support services as needed. The role of the PMHN in this setting differs from other health care settings in that the nurse does not direct care, but rather partners with the patients to encourage utilization of coping techniques and interpersonal skills. The PMHN assists the patient to develop independent skills for problem solving and provides health care teaching as needed. Patients are considered club members and share chores and duties. They may join work units within the clubhouse. As they become more skilled and socially adept, the members may transition to paid employment. There is no time limit on membership (Clubhouse model, n.d.).

## Respite Care

Respite care is available to families who are the primary caregivers of a person with a psychiatric-mental illness, and who endure high levels of stress in the caregiving role. It provides short-term relief to families by supplying short-term housing for the patient. This type of service can dramatically lower stress for the family. PMHNs act as family advocates, assisting families in connecting with available services and providing psychological support. Unfortunately, accessing respite care can be problematic due to several obstacles, such as expense, a shortage of trained providers and quality programs, restrictive eligibility, and fragmented, duplicative systems.

## Nursing Homes

Downsizing of psychiatric institutions in the 1970s combined with the aging of the United States population have resulted in increased numbers of patients with psychiatric-mental health disorders residing in nursing homes. After deinstitutionalization, many psychiatric-mental health patients were unable to live independently. Thus, they were discharged from state hospital facilities to intermediate and skilled-care nursing facilities. Nursing homes and equivalent settings have become an increasingly common residence for patients with mental illness in the later stages of life.

Facilities primarily engaged in the assessment, diagnosis, treatment, and care of mental health disorders are designated by the federal government as an institution of mental disease (IMD). The state must assume financial responsibility for funding IMDs, because they do not qualify for matching federal Medicaid dollars (CMMS 2002).

The holistic care and treatment of patients in intermediate and skilled nursing facilities incorporates the physical, emotional, social, and spiritual aspects of patient care. Generalist PMHNs working in these settings are in a unique position to advocate for patients in need of increased services for psychiatric-mental health issues. Advanced practice PMHNs assess, diagnose, and provide psychopharmacological and psychotherapeutic treatments to psychiatric-mental health residents in intermediate and skilled nursing facilities.

## Outpatient Care

Along the continuum of care, patients discharged from inpatient settings are generally referred for outpatient follow-up. Outpatient services promote optimal symptom management and patient functioning while integrating the patient back into the community. This follow-up care and treatment, which may be intensive, daily, weekly, or monthly, involves supportive services including individual and/or group psychotherapy, medication management, substance abuse treatment, and skills training. In addition, many outpatient programs have developed specific tracts to address diagnostic and symptom-specific problems such as depression, anxiety, post-traumatic stress disorder, and substance abuse.

> *With outpatient care, the patient's symptoms are managed as he or she is integrated back into the community.*

Outpatient therapy affords the PMHN time not available during the course of time-limited inpatient hospitalization to employ the nursing process. Advanced practice PMHNs assess, diagnose, and provide psychotherapeutic treatments to outpatients in the clinic setting often for a prolonged period of time. A variety of psychotherapies may be implemented to address specific mental disorders; for example, cognitive behavioral therapy or interpersonal therapy for depression, dialectical behavior therapy for borderline personality disorder, and cognitive rehabilitation for schizophrenia. Advanced practice PMHNs also collaborate with the physician and prescribe medications (based on the prescriptive privileges of the state in which they are practicing).

Research confirms that psychiatric patients have an increased risk of medical co-morbidities including obesity, hypertension, and diabetes (Marder et al., 2004). Due to the unique trusting therapeutic relationship developed with patients and the need for all patients receiving psychopharmacologic therapy to have frequent metabolic monitoring, advanced practice PMHNs often monitor the necessary lab tests and collaborate with primary care colleagues in managing the patients' medical conditions.

Moreover, advanced practice PMHNs often assume the case manager role in the outpatient setting, acting as leaders, resources, teachers, surrogates, counselors, and technical experts in advocating for and assisting patients in negotiating the sometimes complex tasks of obtaining benefits, resolving legal issues, and arranging medical appointments and transportation.

At times, a patient may present as a danger to self or others. Therefore the level of care needs to be increased. In such situations, many advanced practice PMHNs working in the outpatient setting have also established liaisons with emergency services and inpatient psychiatric facilities to assist with hospitalization in the event of a crisis situation or decompensation in a patient's condition.

## Home Care

Patients unable to attend outpatient services due to debilitating physical or psychiatric conditions are treated at home. Programs such as Visiting Nurse Service address the assessment, diagnosis, and treatment management of home care patients. PMHNs provide case management services to assess and address needs for psychiatric stabilization, medical follow-up, and medication management, and compliance.

## Primary Care

Simple uncomplicated cases of depression, anxiety, and substance abuse are more often treated in primary care settings due to recent changes in the health care system, stigma related to behavioral health treatment and fiscal concerns (Olfson, et al., 2002). The role of the PMHN, at the basic or advanced level of practice, is one of expert collaboration and consultation. Primary care providers often request consultation or referral for challenging and complex cases. Many practice sites employ basic and advanced practice PMHNs as providers of direct mental health care within the primary care setting to provide psychoeducation about mental health issues, symptom management, and relaxation techniques via individual and/or group modality.

> *Primary care is often used to treat uncomplicated cases of depression, anxiety, and substance abuse.*

## HOUSING SERVICES

A stable living environment is an important factor in the ongoing recovery process of the psychiatric-mental health patient. Homelessness increases stress on the individual, contributes to a decline in physical health and non-compliance with psychiatric-mental health treatment, and increases the risk of substance abuse, illegal activity, and arrest (Boyd, 2008). A large percentage of homeless people have been identified as mentally ill. Successful reintegration into the community necessitates appropriate living situations for patients with psychiatric-mental health disabilities. The importance of adequate living situations was emphasized by the Substance Abuse and Mental Health Services Administration (SAMHSA) in 2003. SAMHSA issued a report documenting the following findings regarding homeless populations:

- 38% report alcohol use problems
- 26% report other drug use problems
- 39% report some form of mental health problem, and 20% to 25% meet criteria for serious mental illnesses
- 66% report substance use and/or mental health problems
- Their symptoms are often active and untreated, making it extremely difficult for them to meet basic needs for food, shelter, and safety
- These individuals are impoverished, and many are not receiving benefits for which they may be eligible
- Up to 50% have co-occurring mental illness and substance use disorders
- People with serious mental illnesses have greater difficulty exiting homelessness than others. They are homeless more often and for longer periods of time than other homeless populations. Many have been on the streets for years.

Assessment of the patient's living situation is a key responsibility of the PMHN at any level of care. Appropriate referral for services and advocacy for individuals without stable housing must be part of the nurse's practice. The PMHN, in collaboration with other mental health professionals such as social workers, assesses the patient's need for housing and makes referrals to the appropriate level of care. Although not usually employed in alternative housing settings, the nurse would be responsible for maintaining communication and collaborating with the staff of these settings to ensure that the patient is receiving optimum care and services.

## Personal Care Homes

Personal care homes are residences that provide shelter, meals, supervision, and assistance with personal care tasks. These residences typically accept the elderly, individuals with physical or mental disabilities, or those who for other reasons cannot care for themselves but do not require medical or nursing home care. While most of these homes are licensed by the state, this varies from area to area.

## Supervised Apartments

This form of housing is appropriate for patients who are fairly independent with activities of daily living. The patient, or the patient and a roommate, live in an apartment and have regular visits from a supervisor who offers support as needed.

## Therapeutic Foster Care

In this living situation, specially trained families take children or adults with psychiatric-mental health disorders into their homes and provide a stable, family-oriented living environment. The patient is expected to contribute to completion of daily chores. In most cases, he or she is also involved in some form of treatment program. Family members are trained to deal with medication supervision and crisis management.

## Halfway House/Sober House

A halfway house is similar to a group home but generally has more staff supervision and an active treatment program running throughout the day. Residents receive intensive individual and group counseling. Halfway houses designed solely for the treatment of substance abuse issues are generally referred to as sober houses. Again, there is an active rehabilitation program in place while the patient secures new employment, housing, and a support network. **How Would You Respond?** 25-1 provides an example for this type of housing situation.

> *Personal care homes are most often used for patients who are elderly, have physical or mental disabilities, or cannot care for themselves but would not require medical or nursing home care.*

## THE CONTUNUUM OF AMBULATORY BEHAVIORAL HEALTH SERVICES

The Association for Ambulatory Behavioral Health care (AABH) has developed a model for the movement of patients along the continuum of available services to the most clinically appropriate and cost effective level of care. The model addresses variables related to services and to patients. These variables are explained in **Table 25-1**. According to the AABH model, ambulatory services are classified into three levels based on the variables related to services and the patient.

Ambulatory Level 1 services are inclusive of partial hospital programs and other intensive hospital diversion services, including home-based crisis intervention or stabilization services (ACT Teams, Mobile Crisis Teams). Patients appropriate for this level of care demonstrate disabling to severe symptoms resulting from either an acute illness or exacerbation of a chronic illness. The goal of treatment is to stabilize the crisis and reduce acute symptoms. This level may also include a less intensive residential component such as the family treatment home for children. **Table 25-2** summarizes the service and patient variables for the three levels of ambulatory behavioral health care.

Ambulatory Level 2 services are characterized by active treatment with rehabilitation and transitional services that incorporate a stable, staff-supported milieu extending beyond the treatment setting and into the patient's community. Level 2 patients may function adequately in other structured settings, such as school or work. Milieu-based intensive outpatient programs, day treatment programs, and vocational training programs in which patients are guided to achieve work goals and given the opportunity to work in a community setting are examples of Level 2 services.

Ambulatory Level 3 services are offered under the direction of a coordinated treatment plan. However, these services do not necessarily include a stable patient community or structured program activities. This level also represents a step up from outpatient care for individuals who may need a more intensive array of services. Level 3 services are differentiated from outpatient care by the number of hours of daily and weekly involvement, the multi-modal approach, and the availability of specified crisis intervention services 24 hours per day. Patients treated at this level of care either maintain their role functioning in several areas or have adequate family and/or community support such that they do not require a sense of community solely from treatment.

> *Behavioral ambulatory care is classified into three levels, with Level 1 being appropriate for patients experiencing disabling to severe symptoms.*

## SPECIALIZED ROLES OF PMHNS WITHIN THE CONTINUUM OF CARE

PMHNs assume a wide variety of roles within the continuum of care. Some of the more specialized roles are described here.

## Self-Employment

The practice of self-employed advanced practice PMHNs is governed by the individual state's licensing and/or health and public safety laws. The requirements and scope of practice for all advanced practice nurses are further defined in these statutes. Differences among state statutes result in differences in the level of independent practice, presence or absence of prescription privileges, and legislative authorization for reimbursement.

Advanced practice PMHNs provide direct patient mental health services, including psychotherapy and psychopharmacological treatments to individuals, families, and groups. When in private practice, these nurses treat self-pay patients and contract with insurance companies, managed care companies, home care agencies, and

---

### HOW WOULD YOU RESPOND? 25-1:
### A PATIENT'S EXPERIENCE ALONG THE CONTINUUM OF CARE

The patient is a 34-year-old single male with a history of paranoid schizophrenia diagnosed shortly after leaving home to attend college when he was 20 years old. While living away from home for the first time, the patient became increasingly suspicious of his dormmates. He gradually became delusional that they were plotting against him and became too fearful to leave his dorm room. Campus counseling services evaluated him and he was hospitalized for the first time. He did not return to college. He returned to live with his mother who is described as "odd" and extremely controlling. She discourages the patient from having social relationships and demands that he stay at home with her.

She does not believe in medication and has encouraged the patient to stop taking his antipsychotic medication on several occasions. He was hospitalized three more times over the years, related to stopping his medication and becoming psychotic and homebound.

The patient is currently hospitalized on an inpatient, general psychiatric unit. He presented with the same symptoms and medication non-compliance. He has been amenable to education about his illness and medications and states that he feels "better" when taking medication. He expressed fear that if he returns to live with his mother, he will decompensate again. He describes feeling lonely, isolated, and "useless." His current aftercare plan includes returning home and seeing a therapist twice a month.

As his nurse, you are attending a discharge planning meeting regarding this patient. In addition to you, the meeting will include his physician, social worker, and psychiatric rehabilitation therapist. How would you respond?

### CRITICAL THINKING QUESTIONS

1. *What concerns will you share with the team?*

2. *Will you recommend any changes to his discharge plan?*

3. *Would you recommend a meeting to involve the patient's mother? Anyone else?*

**APPLYING THE CONCEPTS**

As his nurse, you need to present a coherent assessment of the patient and the problems that must be addressed in the discharge plan. These problems include: continuing isolation, lack of meaningful life goals, inability to cope with mother's demands/influence, and medication non-compliance. Based on the failure of similar aftercare plans and subsequent re-hospitalizations, you will need to suggest alternative discharge plans.

Ideally, the patient should be referred to a halfway house. This would allow the patient to separate from his mother, but unlike his attempt at college, he would have intense support in terms of individual and group counseling. In addition, he would be less isolated with the opportunity to develop social relationships. Because halfway houses also incorporate active rehabilitation programs, the patient could develop skills that would lead to employment. This might also help the patient achieve meaningful life goals.

The major obstacle to healthy functioning identified by the patient is his mother. Any plans for the patient not including the mother are likely to fail. The patient must be reassured that the mother has participated in the planning and supports it. If the mother is resistant, you and the team must make all efforts to support the patient's decision. In addition to the mother, the patient's current therapist must be included in the planning. The therapist can serve as an ally and advocate for the patient after discharge.

Finally, as his nurse, you should plan on making at least two post-discharge phone calls to the patient. The purpose of these calls is therapeutic, not social, and this should be clarified with the patient prior to discharge. The purpose of the calls is to complete the nursing process stage of evaluation. You will want to find out how the plan is working, if the interventions succeeded, and if there any adjustments needed to the plan. Your assessment of the plan should be shared with the patient's current treatment team.

Employee Assistance Program (EAP) services. In addition, nurse entrepreneurs form nurse-owned corporations providing mental health service contracts to industries and employers.

Applying the nursing process, the self-employed advanced practice PMHN performs a thorough assessment of the patient based on interviews, behavioral observations, and corroborative information provided by the patient's family, employers, and/or friends. A diagnosis is formulated based on current classifications of mental disorders outlined the *Diagnostic and Statistical Manual of Mental Disorders, 4th edition, Text Revision (DSM-IV-TR)* of the American Psychiatric Association (APA, 2000), diagnostic classifications of the North American Nursing Diagnosis Association (NANDA, 2008), and the International Classification of Diseases ([ICD-10];WHO, 1993). The nurse and patient validate the diagnosis and develop a treatment plan which is then implemented. Periodic evaluation and revision of the plan of care and patient response to treatment is essential to achieve and sustain optimal patient outcomes.

## Telehealth

**TELEHEALTH** refers to psychiatric intervention via telecommunications such as phone or video conferencing. It provides an expanded means of communication that promotes access to health care for patients living in rural communities or communities without adequate mental health services. Problems with access to care may be related to numerous factors, such as clinician shortages, lack of transportation, or poverty. Access to psychiatric-mental health services can be improved and the reach of clinicians can extend beyond the walls of a traditional psychiatric facility, thus expanding continuity of care. A wide variety of assessment and treatment interventions, including tools to assess and manage symptoms, medication adherence checks, and the provision of support and psychoeducation can be delivered to patients using remote monitoring systems.

The PMHN may use electronic means of communication such as telephone consultation, computers, mail, and interactive video sessions to establish and maintain

## TABLE 25-1: PATIENT AND SERVICE VARIABLES ACROSS THE CONTINUUM

| SERVICE VARIABLE | DEFINITION |
|---|---|
| Service function | Specific patient care mission of the services |
| Scheduled programming | Planned hours of treatment |
| Crisis backup availability | Crisis intervention and emergency services describing the blanket of protective services that cover the patient during non-treatment hours |
| Medical involvement | Degree of responsibility and participation assumed by medical and nursing personnel |
| Accessibility | Mechanisms by which a new patient makes contact and is able to begin treatment; intake and admission procedures |
| Milieu | Cohesive, consistent, therapeutic environment created either within a program or community or through coordination of people, space, materials, equipment, and activities |
| Structure | Routines, scheduled activities, expectations, and special treatment procedures integral to non-hospital-based services |
| Responsibility and control | Role of treating professionals in providing a safety net for the patient |

| PATIENT VARIABLE | DEFINITION |
|---|---|
| Level of functioning | The patient's ability to perform the various tasks of daily living |
| Psychiatric signs and symptoms | Patient's presenting problems and requisite assessment of suicidal or homicidal tendencies, thought processes, and orientation |
| Risk/dangerousness | The degree of jeopardy present secondary to the patient's psychiatric illnesses, including dangerousness to self and others, need for confinement, and potential for escalation of symptoms |
| Commitment to treatment/ follow through | The patient's ability to comprehend and accomplish the tasks necessary to benefit from treatment at a specified level of care |
| Social support system | Patient's ability to ask for, use, and accept assistance provided by family members or community supports |

*From the Association for Ambulatory Behavioral Healthcare (AABH) (2010). A position paper. Available at: http://www.aabh.org/content/continuum-ambulatory-behavioral-health-services.*

a therapeutic relationship with patients by creating an alternative sense of nursing presence, a way of continuing to be present in the patient's life when actual physical presence is not an option (ANA, 2009). For example, research suggests that telephone intervention after discharge may increase community survival in patients with schizophrenia who are discharged from psychiatric inpatient settings (Beebe, 2001). **Evidence-Based Practice 25–1** highlights this study. Additional research shows that telephone intervention helps improve the verbal responses in patients with schizophrenia after discharge (Beebe & Tian, 2004). **Evidence-Based Practice 25-2** highlights this study.

Telehealth needs to be differentiated from telemedicine. Telemedicine often refers only to the provision of clinical services while the term telehealth can refer to clinical and nonclinical on-line services including education, administration, and research. Issues related to confidentiality may arise with telehealth encounters. PMHNs need to be aware of state, federal, and international regulations about this issue when engaging in telehealth services, and take measures to ensure patient confidentiality and the integrity of all transmitted documentation.

> *Telehealth includes services provided by telephone, computers, email, and interactive video sessions.*

## Case Management

Case management is the coordination of integrated care that may be provided to individuals, families, and specific populations who require health care services. The goal of

**TABLE 25-2: SERVICE AND PATIENT VARIABLES FOR THE LEVELS OF AMBULATORY CARE**

| SERVICE VARIABLE | AMBULATORY LEVEL 1 | AMBULATORY LEVEL 2 | AMBULATORY LEVEL 3 |
|---|---|---|---|
| Service function | Crisis stabilization and acute symptom reduction; serves as alternative to and prevention of hospitalization. | Stabilization, symptom reduction, and prevention of relapse. | Coordinated treatment for prevention of decline in functioning where outpatient services cannot adequately meet patient need. |
| Scheduled programming | Minimum of 4 hours per day scheduled and intensive treatment over 4–7 days. | Minimum of 3–4 hours per day, at least 2–3 days per week. | A minimum of 4 hours per week. |
| Crisis backup availability | An organized and integrated system of 24-hour crisis backup with immediate access to current clinical and treatment information. | A 24-hour crisis and consultation service. | A 24-hour crisis and consultation service. |
| Medical involvement | Medical supervision. | Medical consultation. | Medical consultation available. |
| Accessibility | Capable of admitting within 24 hours. | Capable of admitting within 48 hours. | Capable of admitting within 72 hours. |
| Milieu | Preplanned, consistent, and therapeutic; primarily within treatment setting. | Active therapeutic within both treatment setting and home and community. | Active therapeutic; primarily within home and community. |
| Structure | High degree of structure and scheduling. | Regularly scheduled, individualized. | Individualized and coordinated. |
| Responsibility and control | Staff aggressively monitors and supports patient and family. | Monitoring and support shared with patient family and support system. | Monitoring and support placed primarily with patient family and support system. |
| Service examples | Partial hospitalization programs; day treatment programs; intensive in-home crisis intervention; outpatient detoxification services | Psycho-social rehabilitation; intensive outpatient programs; behavioral aids; assertive community treatment; 23-hour observation beds | 23-Hour respite beds; multi-modal outpatient services; aftercare; clubhouse programs; in-home services |
| Level of functioning | Severe impairment in multiple areas of daily life. | Marked impairment in at least one area of daily life. | Moderate impairment in at least one area of daily life. |
| Psychiatric signs and symptoms | Severe to disabling symptoms related to acute condition or exacerbation of severe/persistent disorder. | Moderate to severe symptoms related to acute condition or exacerbation of severe/persistent disorder. | Moderate symptoms related to acute condition or exacerbation of severe/persistent disorder. |
| Risk/dangerousness | Marked instability and/or dangerousness with high risk of confinement. | Moderate instability and/or dangerousness with some risk of confinement. | Mild instability with limited dangerousness and low risk for confinement. |
| Commitment to treatment/ follow-through | Inability to form more than initial treatment contract requires close monitoring and support. | Limited ability to form extended treatment contract requires frequent monitoring and support. | Ability to sustain treatment contract with intermittent monitoring and support. |
| Social support system | Impaired ability to access or use caretaker, family, or community support. | Limited ability to form relationships or seek support. | Ability to form and maintain relationships outside of treatment. |

*From Association for Ambulatory Behavioral Healthcare (AABH) (2010). A position paper. Available at: http://www.aabh.org/content/continuum-ambulatory-behavioral-health-services.*

**EVIDENCE-BASED PRACTICE 25-1:**
**TELEPHONE SUPPORT TO PROMOTE SURVIVAL IN THE COMMUNITY**

STUDY

Beebe, L.H. (2001). Community nursing support for clients with schizophrenia. *Archives of Psychiatric Nursing, 15*(5): 214–222.

SUMMARY

The researcher used a true experimental, posttest only, control group design to determine the effectiveness of a telephone nursing intervention in assisting patients with schizophrenia to remain in the community. The study was based on the vulnerability framework. The researcher proposed that the telephone intervention would reduce the effects of stress on individuals diagnosed with schizophrenia after discharge.

Individuals in the experimental group received the telephone intervention every week for a period of 3 months. Those in the control group received informational type telephone calls at 6 and 12 weeks. Findings revealed that the readmission rate for the experimental group was 13%, whereas it was 23% for the control group. Additionally, when compared to the control group, the experimental group experienced a 4% increase in community survival and a 27% reduction in length of stay if readmission occurred.

APPLICATION TO PRACTICE

The findings suggest that telephone intervention, an intervention that is more than just providing information, can increase community survival in persons with schizophrenia. Future studies should focus on increasing sample size, refining the intervention, and applying the research question in other psychiatric populations, for example, patients with depression or mood disorders. Several inpatient psychiatric treatment centers have instituted telephone follow-up calls post-discharge to ensure patients understand and have followed through with their discharge plan and are maintaining progress toward their treatment goals.

QUESTIONS TO PONDER

1. *What is the vulnerability framework mentioned in this research?*
2. *What other vulnerable patient populations may also benefit from telephone therapy?*

---

case management is to decrease fragmentation of care and ensure access to appropriate, individualized, and cost-effective treatment along the continuum of care.

PMHN case managers utilize a holistic approach in treating individuals, families, and communities that is cognizant and respectful of cultural and spiritual norms and values.

To operate complex case management systems effectively, team leaders must be experienced, trained mental health professionals (Rapp, 1998). PMHNs have been identified as a key ingredient for achieving positive patient outcomes in case management teams (McGrew & Bond, 1995), with a knowledge of systems and an ability to work between systems, connecting patients to services, and

> **EVIDENCE-BASED PRACTICE 25-2:**
> **TELEPHONE HELP FOR SCHIZOPHRENIA AND IMPROVED VERBAL RESPONSES**

### STUDY

Beebe, L.H., & Tian, L. (2004). TIPS. Telephone intervention-problem solving for persons with schizophrenia. *Issues in Mental Health Nursing, 25,* 317–329.

### SUMMARY

The researchers used a prospective experimental design to evaluate if face-to-face meetings with patients diagnosed with schizophrenia had an effect on their verbal responses when following up with the patients at a later time using a telephone intervention for problem solving (TIPS). The researchers defined verbal responsiveness as the length of the telephone conversation, number of feeling statements expressed, and number of one-word responses. Participants were placed into one of two groups: an experimental group and a control group. The experimental participants met with individual who would be conducting the follow-up telephone calls twice while hospitalized; the participants in the control group did not. All participants received weekly telephone calls from a psychiatric nurse for six weeks after hospital discharge. Findings revealed that the experimental participants engaged in longer conversations at every measurement point. Their conversations also were significantly longer during the first three weeks. In addition, the experimental participants were approximately twice as likely to make a feeling statement as those in the control group.

### APPLICATION TO PRACTICE

The findings from this study suggest that establishing a connection and rapport prior to initiating telephone follow-up is important. The study also suggests that two face-to-face meetings should be conducted to establish rapport when using TIPS to assist patients in the community. Moreover, the study helps to underscore the importance of establishing rapport in the therapeutic nurse-patient relationship.

### QUESTIONS TO PONDER

1. *How might the feeling statements of the experimental participants influence subsequent care?*
2. *What other factors may have influenced the results obtained from the control group?*

serving as an important safety net in the event of service gaps (ANA, 2007).

PMHN case managers may function as direct care providers and/or may co-ordinate care delivered by others. They locate providers, coordinate primary care and mental health appointments, and ensure that the patient receives the treatment and care necessary to maintain optimum health. These points of connection between agencies are vital to the realization of individualized recovery plans (SAMSHA, 2005). Barriers to care may be identified, addressed, and overcome to maximize patient outcomes. In addition, the PMHN case manager must be highly proficient and knowledgeable about psychopathology, group and individual psychotherapies, family systems theory, psychopharmacology, community resources, and crisis intervention.

A form of case management, called intensive case management, is available to adults and children requiring care for serious mental illness and emotional disturbances. The seriously and persistently mentally ill may require this type of service. PMHN intensive case managers generally have a lesser case load and higher levels of proficiency with this population. See Chapter 7 for an in-depth discussion of psychiatric-mental health case management.

## Disaster Response

Psychiatric mental health nurses have mobilized and responded to recent man-made and environmental disasters, including 9/11, the Haitian earthquake, and Hurricane Katrina in New Orleans. Both basic and advanced practice PMHNs provided mental health counseling, debriefing, and support services to survivors, families, and emergency workers.

## Forensic Nursing

**FORENSIC NURSING** refers to specialty practice that provides services to the legal and criminal system. Research confirms a high rate of psychiatric-mental health disorders in the prison population (Fazel & Damesh, 2002). Forensic PMHNs at the basic and advanced practice level provide mental health services within the prison system by assessing, diagnosing, and treating the forensic population. Forensic nurses may become certified by the American Nurses Credentialing Center (ANCC). As in all other psychiatric-mental health settings, advanced practice PMHNs provide psychiatric treatment, including therapy and psychopharmacological interventions. PMHNs, both at the generalist and advanced practice level, provide education to prison staff about psychiatric-mental health issues. (See Chapter 26 for additional discussion of forensic nursing.)

## SUMMARY POINTS

- The continuum of care involves a system of integrated settings, services, health care clinicians, and care levels covering the range from illness to wellness.

- The least restrictive environment is the guiding principle underlying the concept of the continuum of care.

- The level of care is influenced by factors such as current research findings, cost-effectiveness, reimbursement levels, social factors, and the availability of pharmacological interventions.

- Acute inpatient care is typically short-term, with the goal of stabilizing the patient's symptoms for discharge to a safe and therapeutic living environment with an appropriate level of outpatient treatment. The therapeutic milieu is the key component of acute inpatient care.

- Community-based care is provided in various settings, such as in the patient's home,

worksite, school, clinics, health maintenance organizations, homeless shelter, senior centers, group homes, and churches.

- Assertive community treatment offers customized services for an individual via a team of practitioners who are available 24 hours a day.

- The clubhouse model is primarily a self-help model in which members hire the professional staff and partner with them to provide daily structure and support services.

- Examples of housing services include: personal care homes, supervised apartments, and halfway houses.

- Ambulatory behavioral health services are categorized into three levels based on service and patient variables.

- Nurses can assume specialized roles along the continuum of care, including self-employment, telehealth, case management, disaster response, and forensic nursing.

## NCLEX-PREP*

1. A group of students are reviewing information related to the variables associated with the levels of ambulatory behavioral care. The students demonstrate understanding when they identify which of the following as a service variable?

   a. Risk/dangerousness
   b. Social system support
   c. Level of functioning
   d. Milieu

2. A patient is being referred for a Level 2 ambulatory behavioral health care service. Which of the following might the nurse expect to be used?

   a. Partial hospitalization program
   b. Assertive community treatment
   c. Day treatment program
   d. Clubhouse program

3. A PMHN is working with patients with psychiatric-mental health disorders who are incarcerated. The nurse is engaging in which of the following?

   a. Forensic nursing
   b. Disaster response
   c. Case management
   d. Telehealth

4. A patient who is exhibiting acute psychotic symptoms is determined to be of threat to himself. Which level of care would be most appropriate for the patient to receive?

   a. Acute inpatient care
   b. Partial hospitalization
   c. Psychiatric emergency care
   d. Residential services

5. After teaching a group of students about housing services along the continuum of care, the instructor determines that the students need additional teaching when they identify which of the following as an example?

   a. Halfway house
   b. Psychiatric home care
   c. Supervised apartment
   d. Therapeutic foster care

*Answers to these questions appear on page 639.

## REFERENCES

American Nurses Association, American Psychiatric Nurses Association and International Society of Psychiatric-Mental Health Nursing Practice (2007). *Psychiatric-mental health nursing: scope and standards practice.* Silver Spring, MD. Nursebooks. org. American Nurses Publishing.

American Psychiatric Association (2000). *Diagnostic and statistical manual of mental disorders;* Fourth Edition, Text Revision. Washington, D.C.: Author.

Anthony, W., Cohen, M., Farkas, M., & Cagne, C. (2002). *Psychiatric Rehabilitation.* 2nd ed., Boston: Center for Psychiatric rehabilitation.

Association for Ambulatory Behavioral Healthcare. (2010). A position paper from the Association for Ambulatory Behavioral Healthcare. Available at: http://www.aabh.org/content/continuum-ambulatory-behavioral-health-services. Retrieved April 11, 2011.

Beebe, L.H. (2001). Community nursing support for clients with schizophrenia. *Archives of Psychiatric Nursing, 15*(5), 214–222.

Beebe, L.H., & Tian, L. (2004). TIPS. Telephone intervention-problem solving for persons with schizophrenia. *Issues in Mental Health Nursing, 25,* 317–329.

Boyd, M.A. (2005). *Psychiatric Nursing Contemporary Practice, 4th edition.* Philadelphia: Lippincott Williams & Wilkins.

Centers for Medicaid and Medicare Services (2002). *Institutions for mental disease.* Baltimore, MD. Retrieved 10/1/2009 from www. cms..hhs.gov http://mentalhealth.samhsa.gov/publications/all-pubs/SMA03–3830/content03.asp

Clubhouse model of service for adults with mental illness. Available at http://www.the kentcenter.org/ClubhourseModel.doc. Retrieved April 10, 2010.

Fazel, S., & Damesh, J. (2002). Serious mental disorders in 23,000 prisoners: A systematic review of 62 surveys. *Lancet. 359,* 645–650.

Kane, C.F., & Blank, M.B. (2004). NPACT: enhancing programs of assertive community treatment for the seriously mentally ill. *Community Mental Health Journal, 40* (6), 549–559.

Kiser, L., Lefkowitz, P., Kennedy, L., Knight, M. (2010) The Continuum of Ambulatory Behavioral Healthcare Services. *A position paper from the Association for Ambulatory Behavioral*

*Healthcare.* Retrieved from http://aabh.org/about-aabh/continuum

Marder, S., Essock, S., Miller, A., Buchanan, R., Casey, D.M.D., Davis, J., et al. (2004). Physical health monitoring of patients with schizophrenia. *Am J Psychiatry, 161,* 1334–1349, August 2004.

McGrew, J.H., & Bond, G.R. (1995). Critical ingredients of assertive community treatmentudgements of the experts. *Journal of Mental Health Administration, 22,* 113–125.

North American Nursing Diagnosis Association. (2008). *Nursing Diagnoses: Definitions and Classifications 2009–2011.* Retrieved April 10, 2010. from www.nanda.org

Olfson, M., Tobin, J.N., Cassels, A., & Weissman, M. (2002). Improving the detection of drug abuse, alcohol abuse and depression in community mental health centers. *J. Health Care Poor Underserved, 14* (3), 386–402.

Rapp, C.A. (1998) The active ingredients of case management: A research synthesis. *Community Mental Health Journal,43,* 363–380.

Substance Abuse and Mental Health Services Administration (SAMHSA) (2003). Homelessness-provision of substance abuse and mental health services. DHHS Pub No. SMA-05-4060. Rockville, Md; SAMHSA. Retrieved September 12, 2009 from http://mentalhealth.samhsa.gov/publications/allpubs/sma06–4195/Chapter21.asp

U.S. Department of Health and Human Services. (2003). Blueprint for change: ending chronic homelessness for persons with serious mental illness and co-occurring substance use disorders. Retrieved October 10, 2009, from: http://mentalhealth.samhsa.gov/publications/allpubs/SMA04–3870/chapter2.asp#C2TocIndividualRisk

Walter, G., & Rey, J.M. (1999). The relevance of herbal treatments for psychiatric practice. *Australian and New Zealand Journal of Psychiatry, 33(4),* 482–489.

World Health Organization (1993). *The ICD-10 classification of mental and behavioural disorders. Diagnostic criteria for research.* World Health Organization.Geneva, Switzerland.

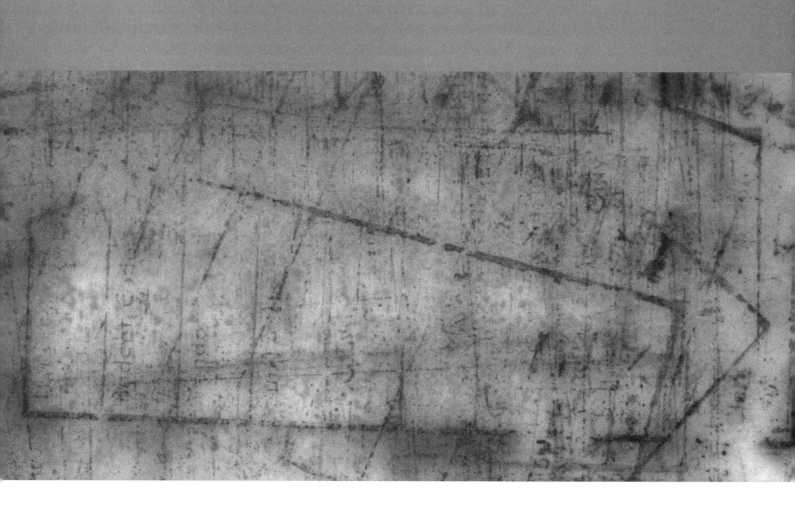

## CHAPTER CONTENTS

## CHAPTER 26

# VULNERABLE POPULATIONS AND THE ROLE OF THE FORENSIC NURSE

Melanie S. Lint

## EXPECTED LEARNING OUTCOMES

**After completing this chapter, the student will be able to:**

1. Identify certain populations as being legally classified as vulnerable.
2. Describe the role of nurses in working with these populations.
3. Demonstrate understanding of the challenges experienced by vulnerable populations related to care access and provision.
4. Explain the specialty practice of forensic nursing.

## KEY TERMS

Developmental disability

Disparity

Forensic nursing

Intellectual disability

Transinstitutionalization

Vulnerable populations

VULNERABLE POPULATIONS are those groups typically defined by race/ethnicity, socio-economic status, geography (urban or rural), gender, age, disability status, and risk status related to sex and gender. These populations are highly visible throughout society and include, but are not limited to the children, elderly, minority groups, those with intellectual disabilities, the homeless, and those who are incarcerated. The demographics of these populations highlighted in **Box 26-1** are constantly changing and it is difficult to determine at any point in time which group consists of the largest numbers. For example, the numbers of homeless individuals actually may be higher than that for minority groups, but due to lack of reporting about the homeless population, minority groups may be identified as being larger. Regardless of the numbers, vulnerable populations experience DISPARITY, or lack of equality, when it comes to health and health care.

According to Healthy People 2020, the term "disparities" often refers to racial or ethnic disparities. However, disparities can result from additional conditions such as age, socioeconomic status, geographic location, cognitive, sensory or physical disability, religion, mental health, sexual identity, and gender. According to the U.S. Department of Health and Human Services (2010), "if a health outcome is seen in a greater or lesser extent between populations, there is disparity."

Vulnerable populations and health disparities were addressed in the plan for transforming the mental health care system by the President's New Freedom Commission on Mental Health (2003). One of the major goals identified was to eliminate disparities in mental health care. Specifically, the report identified concerns about the involvement of people with mental disorders in the criminal justice system and about the homelessness among those with mental disorders as national priorities (McNeil, Binder, & Robinson, 2005). In addition, various governmental agencies such as the Office of Minority Health (OMHD) and the Centers for Disease Control and Prevention (CDC) are working to eliminate health disparities for vulnerable populations in the hopes of reducing the impact of these disparities on the overall health of the United States population.

All nurses, in all areas of practice and all settings, are ethically bound to provide care to patients regardless of their level of functioning, age, race, or status in life. When working with vulnerable populations, the nurse plays a major role in advocating for vulnerable patients because they may be unable to do so themselves. When the patient can do for him- or herself, the nurse allows him or her to do so. When the patient has physical or mental limitations, the nurse helps the patient with what he or she needs and assumes the responsibility to protect those who cannot protect themselves.

Psychiatric-mental health nurses (PMHNs), at the basic or advanced practice level, frequently interact with patients belonging to vulnerable populations groups. One example of an advanced practice role in working with a vulnerable population is that of the forensic nurse. The forensic nurse most commonly works with individuals involved with the criminal justice system and their families.

This chapter describes the vulnerable populations most often encountered by PMHNs. It addresses the major mental health issues commonly involved and the nurse's role when working with each of these populations. The chapter also explores the specialty practice of forensic nursing, describing the requirements for practice and the forensic nurse's roles and functions.

> *When working with vulnerable populations, nurses function as advocates for those populations and work to ensure the safety of all involved.*

## CHILDREN AND MENTAL HEALTH AND ILLNESS

Children are vulnerable because they often are not old enough to advocate for themselves. In some cases, they may grow up in foster care settings without one or both biological parents able to care and advocate for them. They may be born to homeless parents or live with parents who become homeless due to illness, loss of jobs, or loss of housing. Mental health care services may be inadequate and/or inaccessible for lower income families or those who lack any income. Children may not receive mental health services due to the stigma of mental illness. Sometimes,

---

**BOX 26-1: SELECTED VULNERABLE POPULATIONS**

- Children
- Elderly
- Minority groups
- Individuals with intellectual disabilities
- Homeless individuals
- Individuals who are incarcerated

youth are not diagnosed and treated for mental health issues until they enter the criminal justice system. In addition, many states have a shortage of psychiatrists and advanced practice PMHNs who specialize in treatment of children and adolescents. Often their mental health concerns go untreated. Unfortunately, psychiatric conditions can become chronic and recur if they go untreated.

Attention deficit hyperactivity disorder (ADHD) is a disorder that often comes to mind when thinking about mental health issues in children. However, children also suffer from anxiety disorders, depression, conduct disorders, and intellectual and developmental disabilities. Children are also victims of physical, emotional, and sexual abuse. Adolescents are increasingly more likely to become involved with substance use and abuse.

## Nurse's Role When Working With Children

The nurse works to gather information about the child, the child's family, and his or her functioning ability in school if the child is old enough for school. In addition, the nurse gathers information about the child's social relationships. For example, how does the child get along with his or her peers? Is the child's behavior appropriate for his chronological and developmental age? Does the child shrink, retreat, or appear frightened when adults approach? Also, information about the child's growth and development is important. Has the child reached his or her appropriate milestones? Has the child shown any regression in development? For example, a child who was previously toilet-trained begins wetting the bed. This information may provide clues to possible abuse. School nurses as well as teachers are excellent resources because they are often in a position to observe a child's functioning in school and with their peers. If abuse is suspected, nurses are ethically and legally bound to report suspected child abuse. (See Chapters 21 and 22 for an in-depth discussion of mental health issues related to children and adolescents.)

## AGING INDIVIDUALS AND MENTAL HEALTH AND ILLNESS

Another vulnerable population that nurses in all areas of practice will encounter is the elderly. People aged 65 and older are at the highest risk for completed suicide. In 2002, older adults accounted for 25% of completed suicides, yet only accounted for 12% of the U.S. population. White men older than 85 year of age have an especially high rate of suicide (59 per 100,000; Ellson, 2007).

Older Asian American women have the highest suicide rate of all women over age 65 in the United States (Office of Minority Health, U.S. Department of Health and Human Services). Possible risk factors for higher suicide rates in later life include: older age; male gender; living alone; mental illness; access to firearms; social isolation; loneliness; depression; recently widowed, divorced, or separated; multiple chronic illnesses; alcohol or substance abuse; hoarding of medications; need for multiple medications; feelings of hopelessness and worthlessness (Ellson, 2007). In addition, older adults are more vulnerable to abuse because of social isolation and mental impairment such as dementia or Alzheimer's disease. Elder abuse can affect people of all ethnic backgrounds and social status and affect both men and women. Family members are more often the abusers than any other group. Spouses and adult children are the most common abusers of family members. Elder abuse is a family issue. (See Chapter 23 for an in-depth discussion of issues related to the elderly; Chapter 24 for additional information on elder abuse; and Chapter 16 for an in-depth discussion of cognitive disorders such as dementia of the Alzheimer's type.)

## Nurse's Role When Working With the Elderly

The role of the nurse when working with the elderly is diverse. It may involve helping to improve the patient's overall health and mental health wellbeing. Activities may include conducting depression screening or screening for dementia and for suicide risk at a nearby senior center or assisted living community, possibly in conjunction with other screening programs, such as hypertension and diabetes screening. Nurses visiting elderly patients in the home assess for depression and suicidal thoughts. They can also teach patients and families about the signs and symptoms that need to be identified. This is important as "older adults with depression have a high suicide attempt and success rate" (Shawler, 2010). Psychiatric-mental health nurses might be involved in individual, group, and family therapies to assist patients who are struggling with symptoms of anxiety and/or depression. They may help patients set up weekly medication boxes to ensure that they are more likely to remember to take their medications.

The PMHN also is ever vigilant in assessing for possible abuse. If abuse is suspected, laws in most states require health care providers to report suspected abuse or neglect to appropriate law enforcement agencies and adult protective services. (See Chapter 24 for more information about the nurse's role in elder abuse.)

Specialized educational opportunities are available for registered nurses who provide direct care to vulnerable older adults in various settings. One course developed by the International Association of Forensic Nurses (IAFN) provides nurses with the essential knowledge and skills for responding appropriately to elder mistreatment. More information for those interested can be obtained from the IAFN website, http://www.iafn.org.

> *Populations at the opposite ends of the age spectrum, that is, children and the elderly, are considered vulnerable.*

## MINORITY GROUPS AND MENTAL HEALTH AND ILLNESS

Racial and ethnic minority groups are identified based on federal categories. These categories include: African Americans (Blacks), American Indians and Alaska Natives, Asian Americans and Pacific Islanders, and white Americans (Whites). Hispanic American (Latino) is an ethnicity and may apply to a person of any race.

According to the Mental Health: Culture, Race, and Ethnicity supplement to Mental Health: A Report of the Surgeon General, minorities have less access to and availability of mental health services (U.S. Department of Health and Human Services, 1999). In addition, minorities in treatment often receive a poorer quality of mental health care. For example, errors in diagnoses are made more often for African Americans than Whites for certain disorders such as schizophrenia and mood disorders. Moreover, minorities are underrepresented in mental health research.

The African American Community Mental Health Fact Sheet published by the National Alliance on Mental Illness ([NAMI], www.nami.org) states that "African Americans in the United States are less likely to receive diagnoses and treatments for their mental illnesses than Caucasian Americans." Reasons cited for this disparity include stigma and misunderstanding about mental illness in the African American community; cultural biases against health care and mental health care professionals by African Americans; reliance on family, religious, and social communities for social support rather than health care professionals; and lack of health insurance for both medical and mental health care in this population.

The NAMI (2004) also cites that some mental illnesses are more prevalent in the African American population when compared to other cultures in the United States. For example, in a study investigating suicide rates over a 15-year period, the rate of suicide for African Americans was dramatically increased when compared to that of White Americans for the same age group. The suicide rate increased 233% for African Americans (NAMI, 2004). The study also showed that African Americans somaticize or manifest physical illness related to mental health problems more often than White Americans. Moreover, some studies suggest that African Americans metabolize medications more slowly than White Americans but they often receive higher doses of psychotropic medications, which may result in an increase in side effects and a decrease in medication compliance (NAMI, 2004). Genetic variation, exposure to different diets and environments, and other medications in use contribute to ethnic differences in metabolism of psychotropic medications and the effects of drugs on target organs (Flaskerud, 2000).

Data for other minority groups also reveal disparities. For example, American Indian/Alaska Natives are five times more likely to die of alcohol-related causes than are Whites. The suicide rate in this population is 50% higher than the national rate.

The availability of mental health services is severely limited by the rural, isolated location of many of these communities.

Nearly half of Asian Americans and Pacific Islanders has problems with availability of mental health services because of limited English proficiency and lack of providers with appropriate language skills. Refugees from Southeast Asian countries are at risk for posttraumatic stress disorder (PTSD) as a result of trauma and terror preceding their immigration to the United States. Because of the difference in their rates of drug metabolism, some Asian Americans and Pacific Islanders may require lower doses of certain drugs than those prescribed for Whites.

Moreover, Hispanic American youth are at significantly higher risk for poor mental health than White youth by virtue of higher rates of depressive and anxiety symptoms, as well as higher rates of suicidal ideation and suicide attempts (U.S. Department of Health and Human Services, 1999).

> *Access to and availability of mental health services is limited for many minority groups.*

## Nurse's Role When Working With Minority Groups

One of the recommendations of the President's New Freedom Commission on Mental Health is to help provide better access to mental health services for members of minority groups and people in rural areas and to provide culturally competent care (President's New Freedom Commission on Mental Health, 2003). When working with members of minority groups, the nurse must be sensitive to the traditions and customs of people of that minority group, especially related to health care in general as well as mental health care. According to Hill (2006), cultural differences between the professional nurse and their patients increase the complexity of providing care within the health care environment. Thus, to improve the health status of ethnic minority populations, nurses must first reflect on their own beliefs and values to assist them to respect the individuality of their patients and to provide culturally competent care (Hill, 2006).

## INDIVIDUALS WITH INTELLECTUAL DISABILITIES AND MENTAL HEALTH AND ILLNESS

**INTELLECTUAL DISABILITY**, known as mental retardation, is a term used when a person's ability to learn at an expected level and function in daily life are limited. Mental retardation is classified in the *Diagnostic and Statistical Manual of Mental Disorders, 4th edition, Text Revision* with specific criteria.

Intellectual disabilities are caused by a problem that begins prior to birth up until the child turns 18. The cause is unknown in many children. However, intellectual disabilities may result from injury, disease, or a problem in the brain. Examples of common causes of intellectual disability include Down's syndrome, fetal alcohol syndrome, genetic conditions, and infections which happen before birth (Centers for Disease Control and Prevention [CDC], 2005). The level of intellectual disability can vary greatly from a problem that is very severe to one that is slight. Individuals may have trouble taking care of themselves and letting others know their wants and needs. Sometimes the disabilities co-exist with physical illnesses as well.

Intellectual disabilities are a type of **DEVELOPMENTAL DISABILITY**, a diverse group of severe chronic conditions that are due to physical and/or mental impairments. Individuals with developmental disabilities have problems with major activities of daily living such as mobility, learning, language, self-help, and independent living. These disabilities begin at any time, from development through 22 years of age. They often last a lifetime (CDC, 2004).

## Nurse's Role When Working With Individuals With Intellectual Disabilities

Nurses may provide care for children or adults with developmental and intellectual disabilities in settings such as group homes, adult care homes, home health care, hospitals, sheltered workshops, or jails or prisons, among other places. Some individuals have triple diagnoses of serious mental illness, substance abuse, and intellectual disabilities. It is essential for nurses to help protect the rights of these vulnerable individuals who may easily be victimized by others.

*Individuals with intellectual disabilities vary in their functional ability. Regardless of the severity of the disability, the nurse advocates for the individual and works to protect the rights of the individual.*

## THE HOMELESS AND MENTAL HEALTH AND ILLNESS

A **HOMELESS PERSON**, first identified by Public Law 100-77 (more commonly known as the "McKinney Act"), is described as one who lacks a fixed, regular, and adequate nighttime residence; that is, a supervised publicly or privately operated shelter, a temporary residence for individuals intended to be institutionalized, or a public or private place not ordinarily used as a regular sleeping accommodation for human beings (National Coalition for Homeless Veterans, 2009). The numbers on the homeless are staggering. Box 26-2 highlights some of the general statistics.

The correlation between homelessness and mental health problems is significant. Approximately 22% of the American population suffers from mental illness. A small percentage of the 44 million people who have a serious mental illness are homeless at any given point in time (National Coalition for Homeless, 2008). Additionally, an average of 16% of the single adult

**BOX 26-2: DATA ON HOMELESSNESS**

- Estimated that 800,000 persons are homeless every day; 200,000 of these individuals are children.
- As many as 2.3 to 3.5 million persons are homeless at some point during an average year; of these, 33% are represented by families with children (Amerson, 2008)
- Hunger and homelessness are among the most pressing issues faced by U.S. cities
- The number of people experiencing homelessness in major U.S. cities increased by an average of 2% in 2010 (City Mayors, 2011)

homeless population suffers from some form of severe and persistent mental illness.

A significant portion of the homeless population is veterans, accounting for approximately 26% of the homeless population; about 33% of the male homeless population is veterans (National Coalition for Homeless Veterans, 2009). Due to the nature of homelessness, accurate numbers of homeless veterans based on specific community reports are not available. However, the Department of Veterans Affairs (VA) estimates nearly 196,000 veterans are homeless on any given night. According to the Community Homelessness Assessment, Local Education and Networking Groups (VA CHALENG) Report, approximately 400,000 veterans experience homelessness during the year (National Coalition for Homeless Veterans, 2009).

## Impact on Mental Health

The homeless population is affected by a complex set of factors that impact the overall health of the individuals who are homeless. According to the National Coalition for the Homeless (2009), a number of factors contribute to homelessness, including:

- Foreclosures on homes
- Poverty
- Eroding work opportunities
- Decline in public assistance
- Lack of affordable housing and limited scale of housing assistance programs
- Lack of affordable health care
- Domestic violence, addiction disorders, and mental illness

Homelessness is a problem that is experienced by some individuals with severe mental illness. For example, individuals with serious mental illnesses sometimes have difficulty carrying out basic activities of daily living such as self-care and household management, such as paying bills on time and keeping a house or apartment clean. Also, they may have difficulty forming and maintaining relationships with family, friends, and caregivers who might be able to provide support so that the individual might be able to live independently. Or the mentally ill person may have worn out his or her welcome with various family members who no longer want the individual to live with them. Sometimes suspiciousness, paranoia, and irrational thinking contribute to the individual losing his or her housing.

Moreover, those who have serious mental illnesses may often neglect their physical health. It may have been years since the individual has seen a dentist or had his vision examined. Medications can often contribute to weight gain, elevated cholesterol, and elevated blood sugar, in combination with patients' already poor eating habits. They may choose high calorie foods such as sweets, fried snack foods, hamburgers and french fries, and super-sized drinks that are loaded with sugar and caffeine. Those individuals who are mentally ill and homeless and living in close quarters with others may be more likely to develop skin infections, or respiratory illnesses, and have exposure to HIV or tuberculosis (National Coalition for the Homeless, 2009). Inadequate hygiene in the homeless is also a contributing factor. Individuals who are homeless and mentally ill often suffer from drug and alcohol abuse or dependence as well. Use of street drugs by mentally ill individuals in an attempt to self-medicate can lead to disease transmission from use of unclean needles. In addition, a large number of displaced and at-risk veterans live with the lingering effects of posttraumatic stress disorder.

*Veterans account for a significant number of homeless individuals. These veterans often experience the effects of posttraumatic stress disorder.*

## Nurse's Role When Working With the Homeless Population

When working with the homeless population, as with any patient population, a caring, nonjudgmental approach is necessary. PMHNs care for homeless patients in varied settings, such as homeless shelters, outreach vans from mental health agencies, and meeting the patient on his or her own turf, wherever there might be groupings of homeless individuals living in tents, abandoned buildings, or in cardboard boxes under freeway overpasses. PMHNs also may encounter homeless individuals when working in free health care clinics run by churches or local health departments staffed by doctors and nurses from local hospital systems. Homeless patients may be admitted to psychiatric or general hospitals. If the nurse works with individuals who have recently been released from jail or prison for re-entry into the community, some of these individuals could be homeless.

Although the PMHN might be focused primarily on providing mental health care to homeless individuals (such as giving a patient a long-acting antipsychotic injection), patients who are homeless are likely to have a number of untreated medical illnesses such as high blood pressure, diabetes, or skin or foot problems as well. Thus the PMHN addresses these needs, and may play a role in helping the patient explain his or her current symptoms to an emergency department staff member or clinic physician.

Issues involving medication are prevalent for patients who are homeless. Although a physician orders the appropriate medication for the patient's mental health or physical health issues, the patient may have no way to pay for the prescriptions. Therefore, nurses working in outpatient settings may be in a position to assist the patient who has no medical insurance to apply for patient assistance programs that may be available for certain mental health medications. These programs are available through various pharmaceutical companies, often helping the patient to obtain the medication at no cost.

# INDIVIDUALS WHO ARE INCARCERATED AND MENTAL HEALTH AND ILLNESS

Individuals who are incarcerated have been involved with the criminal justice system, which includes jails, prisons, juvenile detention centers, substance abuse treatment facilities, and other facilities (American Nurses Association [ANA], 2007). Jails, prisons, correctional centers, and juvenile detention facilities house individuals who are among the most vulnerable populations in society—those who are impoverished, marginalized, and subject to discrimination and stigmatization (Peternelj-Taylor, 2003).

Jails and prisons are probably two of the most commonly known facilities associated with incarceration. Although similar, they are different in terms of length of stay, mental health services provided, location, offenses (crimes), and governance. Jails, which are locally governed, typically house individuals for a shorter period time and offer few mental health services. Prisons, which are generally under state or federal jurisdiction, generally house individuals incarcerated for longer time frames, possibly even for life, and access to mental health and social services is somewhat improved. **Table 26-1** highlights these differences.

## Impact of Incarceration on Mental Health

Individuals who are incarcerated experience the stigma associated with being a "criminal." In addition, many individuals who are incarcerated also experience the stigma of mental illness. Estimates indicate that between 10% and 16% of people in state prisons can be considered to have a mental illness (Metraux, 2008). Thus, these individuals suffer a double stigma, further underscoring their vulnerability.

Estimates related to the number of incarcerated individuals experiencing mental illness are based on numbers resulting from deinstitutionalization and **TRANSINSTITU-TIONALIZATION**. Deinstitutionalization of state mental hospitals in 1955 led to 560,000 patients being released into the community. In 2007, this number dropped to 70,000. Transinstitutionalization denotes the transfer of this care to jails and prisons where there are three times more patients with mental health problems than in mental hospitals, and where one in six detainees is diagnosed with a mental illness. For example, due to the numbers in the Los Angeles County jail, it has been hailed as the largest mental health system in the world (Keltner & Vance, 2008).

## Nurse's Role When Working With Incarcerated Patients

Corrections nursing is the practice of nursing and the delivery of patient care within the unique and distinct environment of the criminal justice system. The American Nurses Association (ANA) has developed a Scope and Standards of Practice Guide for Corrections Nursing (2007) that provides guidance to nurses working in this field.

PMHNs often provide group therapy to inmates in prisons and jails. Examples of groups are highlighted in **Table 26-2**.

PMHNs or medical nurses administer psychotropic medications to incarcerated inmates. Advanced practice nurses or psychiatrists evaluate and prescribe psychotropic

**TABLE 26-1: COMPARING JAILS AND PRISONS**

| | JAILS | PRISONS |
|---|---|---|
| Length of stay (sentence) | Shorter stays, usually under 1 year | Sentences generally greater than 1 year to life |
| Institutional community | Little | Organized and stable |
| Mental health services | Few; unsophisticated Custody officers with little mental health training | Better access to mental health, educational and social services |
| Location | Near inmate's community | Usually farther away from inmate's hometown |
| Organized gang presence | Limited | Common and routine |
| Offenses | All types of crimes and allegations | Felonies, although crimes highly variable |
| Danger of patient exploitation | Moderate | Moderate to very high (especially for those with mental illness or intellectual disability) |
| Governance | Local | State or federal |

*From Reid, W. H. (2000). Offenders with special needs. Journal of Psychiatric Practice, 6(5), 280–283; Bell, C. (2005) Correctional Psychiatry. In Sadock, B., and Sadock, V.: Kaplan & Sadock's Comprehensive Textbook of Psychiatry, Volume II, Philadelphia: Lippincott Williams and Wilkins.*

**TABLE 26-2: EXAMPLES OF GROUPS FOR INCARCERATED PATIENTS**

| SKILL BUILDING/INFORMATION | INSIGHT DEVELOPMENT/PEER SUPPORT | DISORDER SPECIFIC |
|---|---|---|
| Anger management Communication skills Problem solving Medication education Life skills/social skills Relaxation and stress management | 12-step meetings such as Alcoholics Anonymous/ Narcotics Anonymous (AA/NA) Victim awareness Family relations (for sex offenders) Grief/bereavement | Coping with schizophrenia Depression management Understanding anxiety disorders Substance abuse programs Bipolar management group |

medications for inmates in jails and prisons. Often, due to budget constraints, medications must be listed on a special formulary or restricted list. Typically, medications that appear on the formulary are those that are available in a generic form.

Some nurses may work in the medical department of a correctional facility. They may be responsible for tasks such as drawing blood; holding nurses sick call each day for inmate's who are experiencing acute physical health problems; following up with inmates who have chronic health problems; distributing medications at prescribed times of the day; treatments such as dressing changes; and providing health teaching on such topics as hepatitis C, HIV, diabetes, hypertension, asthma, and sexually transmitted infections.

Several issues are unique to working with this highly vulnerable population. One is the maintenance of professional boundaries, which is essential in the corrections environment. The nurse needs to act in the best interest of the patient's medical or mental health condition, but must maintain a safe and secure environment at the same time. Nurses who cross professional boundaries place themselves, the patients, other health care workers, and custody staff in a position of compromised personal safety and security (ANA, 2007). Nurses need to treat each patient with dignity and respect, regardless of their circumstances.

A second issue is the therapeutic relationship. In the correctional setting, the therapeutic relationship becomes more complex. It is also important for nurses working in a correction setting to be open-minded, nonjudgmental, and self-aware, particularly when dealing with sex offenders or murderers. Poor nurse-patient relationships are often due to boundary violations, where boundary formation within the relationship is stressed by the patient's likely lifelong patterns of exploitation, intimidation, pathological manipulation, and perverted intimacy (Cashin, 2010). For example, inmates may sometimes report mental health symptoms that they do not really have in order to spend more time with female staff members or in an attempt to get psychotropic medication that will help them sleep or that they can sell to get some other commodity that they need.

Nurses need to be particularly vigilant when working with inmates in jails and prisons, because these individuals can be at high risk for suicide attempts and completed suicides.

Usually inmates are assessed for previous history of suicidal thoughts and suicide attempts as well as current suicidal thoughts, plans, and intents. The initial screening might be done by a corrections officer and/or a nurse. Prior risk of suicide is strongly related to future risk (Hayes, 2007).

> *Medical forensic nurses working in correctional facilities administer psychopharmacology, engage in groups, perform medical functions such as drawing specimens for testing, follow up with individuals with chronic illnesses, perform treatment, and provide education.*

## FORENSIC NURSING

The International Association of Forensic Nurses (IAFN) and the American Nurses Association (ANA) define **FORENSIC NURSING** as "the application of forensic science combined with the biopsychological education of a registered nurse in scientific investigation, evidence collection, preservation, and analysis, and prevention and treatment of trauma and/or death-related medical-legal issues." For example, a forensic nurse may provide care to patients who have experienced abuse or violence. Additionally, integrating his or her specialized knowledge of the legal system, a forensic nurse may be involved in evidence collection, provide medical testimony in court, and/or serve as a consultant to legal authorities.

Forensic nursing practice works with vulnerable populations, most often those involved with the criminal justice system. Subspecialties of forensic nursing include:
- Forensic psychiatric nurses
- Correctional nurses
- Legal nurse consultants
- Forensic sexual assault nursing examiners (SANEs)
- Nurse attorneys
- Nurse coroners
- Forensic nurses trained to work in the area of mass disasters
- Forensic nurses working in the area of elder mistreatment
- Forensic nurse death investigators
- Interpersonal violence specialists who may work in trauma, transplant, emergency, critical care nursing, and primary care clinics

## Educational Preparation

Educational programs for forensic nurses are usually at the graduate level, but certificate programs also are available. Schools may have master's degree programs, specialty programs for forensic clinical nurse specialists or adult nurse practitioners, as well as certificate programs for forensic nursing and legal nurse consulting. Training programs to become a forensic sexual assault nursing examiner (SANE) also are available. Nurses learn about proper care of victims of both physical and sexual assault by recognizing, collecting, and preserving evidence and interviewing the patient. A minimum of 40 hours of classroom training are recommended (www.iafn.org). Other programs require a certain number of clinical hours as well.

> *Forensic nurses typically require a graduate level education and work as forensic psychiatric nurses, correctional nurses, legal nurse consultants, forensic sexual assault nursing examiners, nurse attorneys, nurse coroners, death investigators, and clinical nurse specialists in trauma, transplant, and emergency, and critical care.*

Forensic nurses also may become members of the professional organization, the International Association of Forensic Nurses (IAFN). Canada has a forensic nurses' society (Forensic Nurses Society of Canada [FNSC]), that attempts to bridge the gap between forensic nurses as well as paramedics, physicians, nursing students, legal professionals, social workers, police, and scientists.

## Roles of the Forensic Nurse

As stated previously, forensic nurses work directly with individual patients and their families, most often those of vulnerable populations involved with the criminal justice system. They also work as consultants to other nurses and to medical and legal agencies. They function as expert witnesses providing court testimony related to the adequacy of service delivery, in areas dealing with trauma, and in specialized diagnoses or specific conditions related to nursing (www.iafn.org). In the emergency or trauma setting, forensic nurses work with victims of automobile accidents, suicide attempts, disasters (such as earthquakes or hurricanes), work-related injuries, and traumatic injuries. In addition, they work in the public health and safety arena with food and drug tampering, drug or alcohol abuse, environmental hazards, and tissue or organ donation. In area of interpersonal violence, the forensic nurse may work with victims of domestic violence or sexual assault, child or elder abuse, human trafficking, and physical or psychological abuse. In patient care facilities such as hospitals or nursing homes, they may help investigate accidents, injury, neglect, and inappropriate medication or other treatments.

Forensic nurses may also work in correctional institutions, coming face-to-face with unique challenges in their attempt to deliver nursing care to stigmatized individuals within a custodial environment (Cashin, 2010). In all cases, nurses focus on therapy and caring. In correctional institutions, they also work alongside corrections or custodial officers whose primary focus is on security and maintaining order and discipline. As corrections officers often supervise nursing procedures, interference with professional "caring" can arise. For example, confidentiality and the development of trust necessary for the nurse-patient relationship may be hindered by the need for supervision by corrections and custodial staff. In addition, the correctional environment and surroundings can lead to suspiciousness. Inmates, already feeling isolated because of the incarceration, may fear being further stigmatized by a mental illness. Nurses working in the correctional setting often are suspicious of inmates, which can lead to alienation and burnout among nursing staff (Cashin, 2010).

The practice of forensic nursing is challenging. Often, forensic nurses working in corrections settings are faced with numerous, often emotionally charged issues. In this setting...

*The common experience of caring for and working with this vulnerable population has forced forensic psychiatric nurses to examine the obvious health issues that society has tried to hide behind prison walls—issues such as interpersonal and family violence, childhood sexual abuse, the criminalization of mental illness and substance abuse, poverty, homelessness, lack of education and meaningful employment, and the abandonment of older adults.* (Peternelj-Taylor, 2003)

Thus, forensic nurses need to be ever-vigilant in monitoring personal reactions to these issues.

## SUMMARY POINTS

- Vulnerable populations are defined as groups based on ethnicity/race, socioeconomic status, geography, gender, age, disability status, and risk status secondary to sex and gender. Common vulnerable populations that nurses deal with include the homeless, minorities, the elderly, children, the intellectually disabled, and the incarcerated.

- All nurses are ethically bound to provide care to patients regardless of their level of functioning, age, race, or status in life. Advocacy is a key role.

- Homeless individuals are at risk for mental health issues; individuals with mental health problems, specifically those with serious and persistent disorders, are at risk for homelessness.

*(cont.)*

## SUMMARY POINTS (*CONT.*)

- Minorities have decreased access to and availability of mental health services. Disparities may be the result of stigma, misunderstandings, cultural biases, reliance on family for support, and lack of health insurance.

- Older adults are at increased risk for suicide, abuse, social isolation, and mental impairment.

- The mental health problems of children and adolescents often go untreated, which can lead to chronic and recurrent problems.

- Intellectual disability (mental retardation) is a type of developmental disability. Nurses play a key role in protecting the rights of these individuals because they are easily victimized.

- Two issues associated with working with incarcerated individuals are the maintenance of professional boundaries and the therapeutic relationship.

- Forensic nursing is a specialty area of practice that often involves scientific investigation, evidence collection, preservation, and analysis, and prevention and treatment of trauma and/or death-related medical-legal issues.

- The forensic nurse works directly with individuals (including incarcerated persons), acts as consultant and expert witness, works with victims of emergency or trauma, works in the public health and safety arena, works with victims of interpersonal violence, and acts as investigator in patient care facilities.

## NCLEX-PREP*

1. When describing vulnerable populations to a group of students, which of the following would the nursing instructor include?

    a. They typically experience increased risks for depression.
    b. Advocacy is a primary nursing role.
    c. The patient is usually completely dependent on the nurse.
    d. Children are more vulnerable than the elderly.

2. A nurse is preparing a presentation for a local community group about health care disparities and minorities. The nurse uses the African American population as an example. Which of the following would the nurse include in the presentation?

    a. They are more likely to receive a diagnosis for mental health conditions.
    b. The rates for suicide are lower in this population.
    c. They tend to report physical complaints related to mental illness.
    d. Lower doses of psychotropic medications are commonly prescribed.

3. The nurse is assessing an elderly patient. The nurse determines that the patient is at risk for suicide based on which of the following? Select all that apply.

    a. Female gender
    b. Living alone
    c. History of diabetes, arthritis, and stroke
    d. Polypharmacy
    e. Recent death of spouse

(*cont.*)

**NCLEX-PREP***

4. A nurse is thinking about working in a correctional facility. Which characteristic would be important for the nurse to have?

   a. Self-awareness

   b. Prejudice

   c. Cultural bias

   d. Inflexibility

5. A nurse working at a homeless shelter in a large downtown area should be aware that there are many factors that contribute to homelessness of the mentally ill. Which of the following would the nurse identify as potentially contributing to homelessness? Select all that apply.

   a. Substance abuse

   b. Poverty

   c. Inadequate housing

   d. Low-paying jobs

   e. Rise in public assistance

   f. Affordable health care

*Answers to these questions appear on page 639.

## REFERENCES

American Nurses Association (ANA). 2007. *Corrections Nursing Scope and Standards of Practice*. Silver Springs, MD: Nursebooks.org

Amerson, R. (2008). Mental Illness and Homeless Families. *The Journal for Nurse Practioners, 4*(2), 109–113.

Bell, C. (2005) Correctional Psychiatry. In: Sadock, B. and Sadock, V. Kaplan & Sadock's Comprehensive Textbook of Psychiatry, Volume II, Eighth Edition. Philadelphia: Lippincott Williams and Wilkins.

Cashin, A., Neuman, C., et al. (2010). An Ethnographic Study of forensic nursing culture in an Australian prison hospital. *Journal of Psychiatric and Mental Health Nursing, 17*, 39–45.

Centers for Disease Control (CDC) – Office of Minority & Health Disparities (OHMD), Retrieved from:http://www.cdc.gov/omhd/About/about.htm

Centers for Disease Control (CDC) – Department of Health and Human Services. Intellectual Disability Fact Sheet. http://www.cdc.gov/actearly

Centers for Disease Control (CDC)-Department of Health and Human Services. (2004). Developmental Disabilities. Retrieved from: http://www.cdc.gov/ncbddd/dd/dd1.htm

Centers for Disease Control and Prevention [CDC] (2005). National Center on Birth defects and Developmental Disabilities, 2005, at www.cdc.gov/ncbddd/ddmr2.htm

City mayors: Hunger and homelessness in American cities. Information based on 2010 report Hunger and Homelessness in US Cities by the US Conference of. Available at: http://www.city mayors.com/features/uscity_poverty.html Accessed April 26, 2011.

Ellson, N.W. (2007). Suicide in older adults: A priority concern. *Advance for Nurse Practitioners, 15* (12).

Flaskerud, J. H. (2000) Ethnicity, culture, and neuropsychiatry. *Issues in Mental Health Nursing, 21*(1).

Forensic Nurses' Society of Canada (FNSC) http://www.forensic-nurse.ca

Hayes, L. M. (2007). Guiding principles to suicide prevention in correctional facilities. from website: http://www.nciatnet.org/suicideprevention/publications/guidingprinicples.asp

Hill, D. (2006). Sense of belonging as connectedness, American Indian worldview and mental health. *Archivews of Psychiatric Nursing, 20*(5), 210–216.

International Association of Forensic Nurses (IAFN). Website: http://www.iafn.org

International Association of Forensic Nurses (IAFN). "What is forensic nursing?" Available at: http://www.iafn.org/display-common.cfm?an=1&subarticlenbr=137 Accessed 4/30/2011.

Keltner, N. L., & Vance, D. E. (2008). Biological perspectives incarcerated care and quetiapine abuse. *Perspectives in Psychiatric Care, 44* (3), 202–206.

McNeil, D. E., Binder, R. L., & Robinson, J. C. (2005). Incarceration associated with homelessness, mental disorder, and co-occurring substance abuse. *Psychiatric Services, 56*(7), 840–846.

Metraux, S. (2008). Examining relationships between receiving mental health services in the Pennsylvania prison system and time served. *Psychiatric Services, 59*(7), 800–802.

National Alliance on Mental Illness (NAMI).(2004). African American community mental health fact sheet. Available at: www.nami.org

National Coalition for the Homeless. (July 2009). NCH fact sheet— Mental illness and homelessness. Available at: http://www.nationalhomeless.org/factsheets

National Coalition for the Homeless. (July 2009). NCH fact sheet— Why are people homeless? Available at: http://www.nationalhomeless.org/factsheets

National Coalition for the Homeless (July 2009). NCH fact sheet— How many people experience homelessness? Available at: http://www.nationalhomeless.org/factsheets

National Coalition for the Homeless (July 2009). NCH fact sheet— Who is homeless? Available at: http://www.nationalhomeless.org/factsheets

National Coalition for Homeless Veterans. (2009) Homeless veterans fact sheet. Available at: www.nchv.org

National Committee for the Prevention of Elder Abuse (NCPEA) Website: http://www.preventelderabuse.org

Nies, M.A., & McEwen M., (2007). *Community/Public Health Nursing: Promoting the Health of Populations*. St. Louis, Missouri: Saunders Elsevier.

Ohio Department of Mental Health Coordinating Centers of Excellence. Available at: http://mentalhealthohio.gob/what-we-do/promote/coordinating-centers-of-excellence.shtml Accessed April 21, 2011.

Office of Minority Health, US Department of Health and Human Services. Mental health data/Statistics from a variety of government reports from 2001–2009. Available at: http://minorityhealth.hhs.gov Accessed Apil 26, 2011.

Peternelj-Taylor, C. (2003) Incarceration of vulnerable populations. *Journal of Psychosocial Nursing, 41*(9), 4–5.

President's New Freedom Commission. (2003). Final report to the President. Retrieved from http://www.mentalhealthcommission.gov/ August 1, 2010.

Reid, W. H., M.D. (2000). Offenders with special needs. *Journal of Psychiatric Practice, 6*(5), 280–283.

Substance Abuse and Mental Health Services Administration (SAMHSA). http://www.samhsa.gov/

Shawler, C. (2010). Assessing and maintaining mental health in elderly individuals. Nursing Clinics North America; 45, 635–650.

U.S. Department of Health and Human Services. (1999) *Executive Summary-Mental Health: Culture, Race, and Ethnicity – A Supplement to Mental Health: A report of the Surgeon General.* Rockville, MD. Retrieved February 21, 2010, from http://www.surgeongeneral.gov/library/mental health/cre/execsummary-7.html

U.S. Department of Health and Human Services (2010). Healthy People 2020 Objectives. Available at: http://www.healthypeople.gov/2020/topicsobjectives2020/overview.aspx?topicid=28 Retrieved January 16, 2011.

Williams, C.L., & Tappen, R. M. (1999). Can we create a therapeutic relationship with nursing home residents in the later stages of Alzheimer's Disease? *Journal of Psychosocial Nursing and Mental Health Services, 37*(3), 28–35.

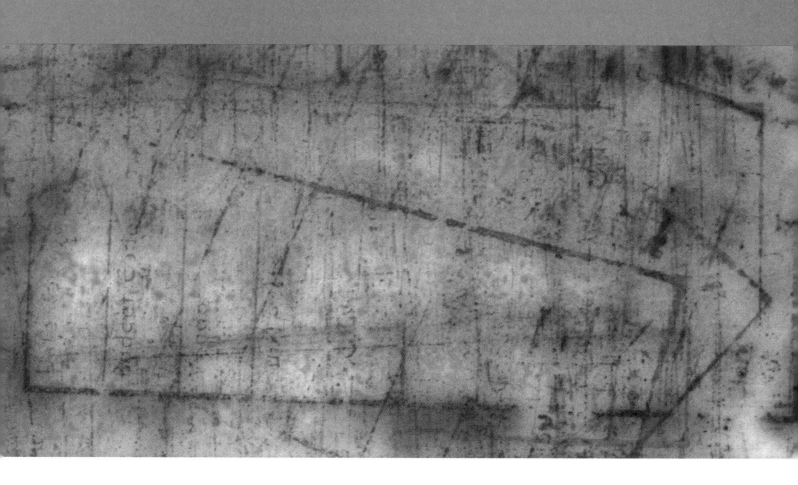

## CHAPTER CONTENTS

## CHAPTER 27
# CULTURAL, ETHNIC, AND SPIRITUAL CONCEPTS

Vicki P. Hines-Martin

## EXPECTED LEARNING OUTCOMES

**After completing this chapter, the student will be able to:**

1. Identify the core concepts associated with culture.
2. Describe the impact of ethnic and cultural factors on the delivery of mental health care.
3. Explain the concept of spirituality as it relates to health, including mental health.
4. Integrate concepts of cultural competence into interpersonal modes of practice.
5. Demonstrate culturally sensitive and congruent care to different patient populations.

## KEY TERMS

Cultural competence

Cultural congruence

Culture

Diversity

Enculturation

Ethnicity

Linguistic competence

Race

Religiosity

Spirituality

The constitution of the World Health Organization (WHO) states that the enjoyment of the highest attainable standard of health is one of the fundamental rights of every human being without distinction of race, religion, political belief, or economic or social condition (WHO, 1948). Over 60 years after this constitution was adopted, wide variations in health still exist. In 2009, WHO stated that

> Globalization is putting the social cohesion of many countries under stress, and health systems, as key constituents of the architecture of contemporary societies, are clearly not performing as well as they could and as they should.... Few would disagree that health systems need to respond better—and faster—to the challenges of a changing (and diverse) world. (WHO, 2009)

Psychiatric-mental health nurses must be cognizant of the impact of globalization on health care and be prepared to intervene appropriately with patients who are culturally, ethnically, and spiritually different. Yet, we must also understand that the process of globalization is blurring the differences between cultures and groups. It is most important to head the words of psychiatrist Harry Stack Sullivan (1947, p. 7) who noted "...we are all more basically human than otherwise." There is a common nature among all human beings and the belief that we are all more alike than different should pervade our mental health understandings and work (Sullivan, 1947).

Within the context of understanding that the similarities are more important than the differences among individuals and cultural groups, this chapter discusses the relationship between culture, ethnicity, spirituality, and health, and identifies the influence these factors have on mental health and illness. It also describes the essential need for nurses to be culturally competent when providing mental health care.

## CORE CONCEPTS

It is important to have an understanding of the key concepts related to culture and diversity. **Box 27-1** presents the definitions for the major concepts. These definitions have been formulated from the current literature and are widely accepted in nursing and health care.

**DIVERSITY** is defined narrowly to include age, race, gender, ethnicity, religion, and sexual orientation. Most comprehensively, diversity is reflected through examination of difference, identity, community, privilege, power, and responsibility. Diversity may be reflected in a broad spectrum of demographic and philosophical differences.

## GLOBALIZATION AND HEALTH CARE DISPARITIES

The world is viewed as a global community, and as part of that global community, the U.S. population has become increasingly diverse. Although some literature indicates significant progress in the U.S. health care system for racial, ethnic, and cultural minority groups (Collins, Hughes, Doty, Ives, Edwards, & Tenney, 2002), evidence exists identifying that the need for equitable health services among racial, ethnic, and cultural groups is still high (Collins, et al., 2002; Smedley, Stith, & Nelson, 2002; Kaiser Family Foundation, 2011).

In addition, the United States is experiencing an increase in people coming from economically developing counties and/or countries experiencing military or political strife. These groups are particularly at risk for poor health care services due to unfamiliarity with the U.S. health care system, lack of health care coverage and/or limited access, and language barriers. Research with a variety of populations, such as African, Arabic, Asian, Australian, British, and Caribbean, have identified that understanding culture, religion, and social and political forces are critical to adequately meet the health care needs of individuals and groups (Kim, Atkinson, & Umemoto, 2001; Morgan et al., 2005; Owen & Khalil, 2006; Steel et al., 2006; Scheffler et al., 2011).

The Health Care Quality Survey study, completed by the Commonwealth Fund in 2001, was done to evaluate health care quality from the perspective of patients who received care. The study found that minority Americans reported a lower level of health care quality when compared to American European counterparts (Collins et al., 2002).

As with other areas of health care, disparities in the provision of mental health care have also been clearly identified (U.S. Department of Health and Human Services [DHHS], 2001). Research in the United States has shown lower rates of mental health service utilization by ethnic, racial, cultural, and social (including religious) minorities. Additionally, when these minority individuals utilize care, it is more likely to be poor in quality (DHHS, 2001). As a result, ethnic, racial, cultural, and social minority groups carry a greater burden from unmet mental health needs. Therefore, it is important to understand how mental health services are provided to meet special sociocultural needs of these identified groups (Snowden & Hu, 1997; Kim, Atkinson, & Umemoto, 2001; Wang, Berglund, & Kessler, 2001; Shin, 2002; Kirmayer, Groleau, Guzder, Blake, & Jarvis, 2003; Woodward et al., 2008; Sorsdahl et al., 2009).

> ### Q BOX 27-1: DEFINITIONS OF IMPORTANT CONCEPTS
>
> **CULTURAL COMPETENCE:** A set of congruent behaviors, attitudes, and policies that come together in a system, agency, or among professionals, and enables that system, agency, or those professionals to work effectively in multicultural situations and with diverse social groups. It emphasizes effectively operating in different cultural/social contexts. It is a developmental process that evolves over an extended period. Both individuals and organizations are at various levels of awareness, knowledge, and skills along the cultural competence continuum.
>
> **ETHNICITY:** Selected cultural characteristics used to classify people into groups or categories considered to be significantly different from others. In some cases, ethnicity involves merely a loose group identity with little or no cultural traditions in common. In contrast, some ethnic groups are coherent subcultures with a shared language and body of tradition. Newly arrived immigrant groups often fit this pattern.
>
> **ENCULTURATION:** Process by which a person learns the requirements of the culture with which he or she is surrounded, and acquires values and behaviors that are appropriate or necessary in that culture. As part of this process, the influences that limit, direct, or shape the individual (whether deliberately or not) include parents, other adults, and peers. If successful, enculturation results in competence in the language, values, and rituals of the culture.
>
> **LINGUISTIC COMPETENCE:** Capacity to communicate effectively, and convey information in a manner that is easily understood by diverse audiences, including persons with limited English proficiency, those who have low literacy skills or are not literate, and individuals with disabilities that impair communication and comprehension.
>
> **RACE:** Biological characteristics and variations within humans, originally consisting of a more or less distinct population with anatomical traits that distinguish it clearly from other races. Increasingly it has been identified that biological differences are limited between populations. In addition, the term race has included the political and social history that impact the collective and individual experiences of people identified as part of that racial group.
>
> **RELIGIOSITY:** Specific behavioral and social characteristics that reflect religious observance within an identified faith.
>
> **SPIRITUALITY:** Cognitions, values, and beliefs that address ultimate questions about the meaning of life, God, and transcendence, which may or may not be associated with formal religious observance.

> *Ethnic, racial, cultural, and social minorities use mental health services to a lesser degree and, when used, the services tend to be poorer in quality.*

## RACE, ETHNICITY, AND CULTURE AND MENTAL HEALTH

Race, ethnicity, and culture are a significant part of the context in which each individual exists. Therefore, they have influence on perceptions of well-being and illness, health care decision making and help-seeking, and health service utilization.

## Racial, Ethnic, and Cultural Diversity

Diversity in race, ethnicity, and culture affect three areas of functioning that influence mental health and mental health care delivery. These three areas are cognitive styles, negotiation strategies, and value systems. **Table 27-1** explains these three areas.

Consider the area of value systems and decision making. Some cultural groups view decision making as a role to be assumed by the designated family head or leader rather than the affected individual. When health decisions

### TABLE 27-1: IMPACT OF CULTURE, RACE, AND ETHNICITY

| | |
|---|---|
| • Cognitive styles | • How we organize and process information |
| • Negotiation strategies | • What we accept as evidence for change |
| • Value systems | • The basis for behavior<br>- Locus of decision making<br>- Sources of anxiety/anxiety reduction<br>- Issues of equality/inequality |

must be made, providers and the patient must include the family leader before any decision is made. Although very different from most experiences in the United States, this process is one that is common in other cultural groups. Awareness of this family dynamic on the part of the nurse is essential in helping individuals to think through a problem, determine what is and is not appropriate or acceptable based upon their value system, and decide on a course of action. Nurses and other health care providers must assess the impact of these influences with each patient, and assist the patient by providing information and support for the decision-making process.

Studies have shown that ethnic and racial groups with histories of inequality and who are experiencing current disadvantaged socioeconomic circumstances are at a higher risk for mental health conditions (Harrell, 2000; Williams & Williams-Morris, 2000). However, despite these risks for emotional distress and mental illness, diverse ethnic, racial, and cultural groups also demonstrate protective factors that mediate risks for mental illness. The literature has identified the role of family, closely held beliefs, group identity, and community and mutual support as external mediators against stress and mental illness.

> *Despite potential increased risks for emotional distress and mental illness among diverse ethnic, racial, and cultural groups, protective factors such as family, group identity, mutual support, and closely held beliefs help to reduce these risks.*

## Language Variations

Variations in language may also influence how mental health and illness are discussed. For example, research has shown that in some racial or ethnic groups such as Iranian, Rwandan, and Eastern Indian, mental and physical health are encompassed into one word or emotional distress is reflected through descriptions of the "body" being sick (Khandelwal, Jhingan, Ramesh, Gupta, & Srivastava, 2004; Summerfield, 2005; Martin, 2009). In addition, studies have identified that cultural and ethnic or racial groups may avoid using the word "mental illness" and use other terms such as "nerves," "feeling down or blue," and "emotional problems." Psychiatric-mental health nurses who become aware of the language that is and is not used by diverse patient groups are better able to respond appropriately when counseling, educating, or referring individuals for treatment. Because there is stigma associated with the term "mental illness," using more culturally or socially acceptable terms may avoid an unintended barrier to mental health care.

## Gender Roles and Expectations

Cultural precepts related to gender roles and expectations differ from culture to culture. Some cultural groups assign specific daily tasks and responsibilities according to whether the person is female or male. Other cultures identify who makes important family decisions based on gender. Although in most Western societies these gender roles and expectations vary and are not as clearly defined, these beliefs can significantly affect mental health within societies that have long held traditions as part of daily living. Consider the Asian culture. Many traditional Asian group values include collectivism, conformity to norms, deference to authority, emotional self-control, family recognition through achievement, filial piety, humility, compliance, and avoidance of shame based on hierarchical relationships (Kim, Atkinson, & Memento, 2001; Cheung, 2009). "Saving face" (*chemyun* in Korean culture) or honor is critically important. Thus, being exposed to circumstances that threaten one's ability to "save face" can affect emotional health.

Increasing evidence reveals that many cultures focus on the family as a collective unit whereby important decisions are made, with all relevant family members engaging in the decision-making process. The emphasis in Western culture is on individual decision making, which may be in stark contrast to other cultural groups and, as a result, possibly act as a barrier to care (Morgan et al., 2005; Shin, 2002; Steel et al., 2006).

> *Differences in language as well as gender roles and expectations can influence how mental health and illness are discussed and how decisions are made in this area.*

## Immigration

Experiences related to refugee and immigrant status add stressors to an individual or group. These stresses may be related to clashes of culture and the process of acculturation into a different society and its accompanying norms; that is, adapting to a culture other than one's own. Research conducted with African, Korean, Mexican, and Yugoslavian immigrant populations have identified a cluster of factors affecting the mental health of those who flee from or leave their country of origin, and now find themselves part of a minority population elsewhere (Borges et al., 2009; Fozdar, 2009; Shin, 2002). **Box 27-2** lists these risk factors.

> *Risk factors for mental illness in immigrant populations include: social exclusion due to low English language proficiency, decreased interaction with the new culture, culture shock, family or social isolation, employment difficulties, prejudice and discrimination, and feelings of persecution due to prior trauma.*

## Mental Health, Mental Illness, and Mental Health Service Use Among Ethnic, Racial, and Cultural Groups

Although the overall incidence of mental health conditions is similar among and between racial and ethnic groups, some variability does exist for different types of disorders. For example, some studies have found higher rates of depressive disorders among Latinos than non-Latino Whites in U.S. population-based studies (Dunlop et al., 2003; Minsky et al., 2003). Mexican nationals who have family members working within the United States

### BOX 27-2: IMMIGRATION AND RISK FACTORS FOR POOR MENTAL HEALTH

- Social distance related to low English proficiency
- Cultural beliefs leading to lack of interface with new culture
- Acculturation stress resulting from culture shock
- Social isolation secondary to family separation and absence of support system
- Unemployment or underemployment
- Experiencing prejudice and discrimination
- Prior trauma or persecution (refugees)

have higher rates of suicidal ideation and are at increased risk for alcohol and substance abuse (Borges et al., 2009). Immigrant Mexican American youth reported significantly higher social anxiety and loneliness than U.S.-born Mexican American youth (Polo & Lopez, 2009).

Approximately 7.5 million African Americans have a diagnosed mental illness. Their risk for depression is higher, in part due to socioeconomic factors such as urban living and risk for exposure to traumatic events. African Americans also are less likely than Whites to use outpatient mental health services and to find antidepressant medication acceptable. In fact, only 32% of African Americans with mental health disorders have been found to use professional services, with 48% of those with severe major depressive symptoms receiving treatment (Williams, 2007). Moreover, African American men are less likely to use mental health services than their female counterparts.

Use of mental health services by minority children and adolescents also varies. The use of crisis care by African American and Native American children and youth is greater than Whites. In addition, studies reveal that Latino and Asian youth used intensive crisis services to a higher degree. However, access to non-crisis services by minority youth is less than that of White youth. Moreover, African American adolescents received less mental health treatment, including outpatient care, than White adolescents, and Latino children received fewer counseling sessions and specialty mental health services than White children (Pumariega & Rothe, 2003; Snowden & Yamada, 2005; Snowden et al., 2008).

Much of the current literature has identified stigma as a critical barrier to seeking mental health services among individuals from minority groups (Shin, 2002; Kim, Atkinson, & Umemoto, 2001). Research on the Asian

**EVIDENCE-BASED PRACTICE 27-1:**
**PATIENT CHOICE AND MENTAL HEALTH CARE**

### STUDY

Hope, T. (2002) Evidence-based patient choice and psychiatry. *Evidence Based Mental Health*, 5, 100–101.

### SUMMARY

The emphasis on "evidence-based practice" (EBP) in nursing and other health care professions to support science-based choices about practice in a variety of specialties, including psychiatric-mental health care, is readily apparent. However, the focus of this EBP has been on decisions from the perspective of the care provider with much less emphasis on the patient's role in the decision-making process. As a result, the use of an "evidence base" for patient choice has emerged as a developing area of the literature since 1996, with much of that literature focusing on patient choice with physical health and end-of-life decisions.

Evidence-based patient choice in psychiatric-mental health care has received very little attention. The author states that:

> Psychiatry is a particularly challenging area of medical practice in which to promote evidence-based patient choice, because mental illness can affect both understanding and decision-making abilities. However, the danger is that [mental health care providers] may too readily assume, in a particular case, that a patient cannot cope with information and choice. As the evidence base in [mental health] increases, so do the opportunities for respecting the autonomy of mentally ill patients. (Hope, 2002, p. 100)

According to the author, evidence-based patient choice results from the provision of evidence-based knowledge to patients to enhance their power, provide science-based knowledge on which they can make a choice congruent with their beliefs and values, and assist in the development of increasingly effective (and congruent) patient-directed mental health care. The author identifies four key elements of evidence-based patient choice in mental health care:

- The issue is important to patients making choices
- The evidence must be of good quality
- Evidence should be in a form that is accessible to patients but with minimum bias
- Information can be used by patients to enhance choice

The article raises issues about patient choice that need to be weighed in relation to the patient's illness and the degree of cognitive impairment.

### APPLICATION TO PRACTICE

Although this article does not involve a research study, it does underscore the need for EBP in the psychiatric-mental health care setting. Psychiatric-mental health nurses can use the information from this article in promoting decision making and choices based on appropriate evidence-based care for their patients. The four key elements identified can be applied to any situation involving psychiatric-mental health patients. Psychiatric-mental health nurses need to remain cognizant of these four elements when promoting patient decision making and consider these elements in conjunction with the patient's condition.

*(cont.)*

> **EVIDENCE-BASED PRACTICE 27-1:** *(CONT.)*
> **PATIENT CHOICE AND MENTAL HEALTH CARE**
>
> QUESTIONS TO PONDER
>
> 1. *What are some of the beliefs and values discussed in this chapter that might be most problematic for the nurse when using evidence-based patient choice?*
> 2. *How might a psychiatric-mental health nurse use the key elements of evidence-based patient choice with a culturally or religiously diverse patient who refuses to accept mental health care for a serious condition?*

culture reveals influences on mental health and illness and accessing mental health care. For example, those who hold traditional Asian values believe that each individual should be able to resolve his or her own mental health problems by using inner resources and willpower (Kim, Atkinson, & Umemoto, 2001). Thus, mental health problems are best addressed through moderating one's emotions and behavior, controlling troublesome thoughts, and seeking inner peace. For some Asians, the need for mental health assistance is a sign of weakness. Asian Americans and Asian immigrants have been shown to underutilize mental health services. In addition, they typically wait longer before accessing treatment than African Americans and White Americans (Shin, 2002).

In Latin American countries, information about mental health is limited (Razzouk et al., 2008). However, in one study examining the Brazilian population, 9% of the population over 16 years of age sought mental health treatment in the previous year. Most of these individuals used public mental health services (de Toledo Piza Peluso, de Araujo, & Blay, 2007). Unfortunately, understanding of mental illness is still poor and most individuals who express having mental health concerns do not seek treatment.

Information about mental health in developing and low- and middle-income countries is lacking (Padmavati, 2005; Patel & Bloch, 2009; Stein & Sedat, 2007). Although conditions such as depression, anxiety, and post-traumatic stress disorder are widespread and have been identified by WHO, research articulating the extent of these conditions and perceptions of mental health is limited. For example, studies from India identify that the prevalence of mental illness ranges from 9.5 per 1000 to 370 per 1000 people within the general population. Among the homeless (beggars) in India, mental illness ranges from 22.6 to 131 per 1000. Most recent estimates

of mental health conditions in India indicate that approximately 12.5% to 18.9% of primary care patients have a mental health condition. Of these conditions, affective disorders, neuroses, and alcohol and drug disorders rank the highest (Khandelwal et al., 2004).

New studies from South Africa indicate that approximately 30% of adults have experienced a mental health disorder in their lifetimes. Anxiety disorders account for 16% of the disorders, mood disorders account for 10%, while substance abuse disorders account for 13% (Stein et al., 2008). In areas where traditional African belief systems predominate, many individuals believe that mental health problems result from bewitchment or current influences exerted on them by their dead ancestors, such as feelings of being cursed, punished, or controlled by them (Abdool & Ziqubu, 2004).

> *Stigma is often an important barrier affecting whether an individual from another racial or ethnic group seeks mental health services.*

## Implications for Psychiatric-Mental Health Nursing

Although each of the diverse populations discussed reflects some differences in relation to mental health beliefs, mental health factors, and mental health service use, they all demonstrate the need for better understanding to address their mental health needs. Disparity exists in circumstances surrounding risks for mental illness and access and use of mental health services. Addressing such disparities requires care strategies that demonstrate compatibility between perceptions, social context, needs, and mental health care services (**Evidence-Based Practice 27-1**).

## SPIRITUALITY, RELIGION, AND MENTAL HEALTH

As with other components of one's culture, spirituality and religion influence mental health. Although the terms religion and spirituality are sometimes used interchangeably, they are different in their focus. Spirituality focuses on the cognitions, values, and beliefs that address ultimate questions about the meaning of life, God, and individual existence. Examples include "Why are we here?" or "Where do we go after this life?," which may or may not be associated with formal religious observance or rituals. Religion encompasses a set of prescribed beliefs concerning the cause, nature, and purpose of the universe, which includes the belief in a supernatural entity or entities from which all life originates. Also, religion usually involves devotional and ritual observances, and often contains a moral code that governs how humans should and should not behave in accordance with their religious beliefs.

The difference between spirituality and religion to a large degree has to do with uncertainty and certainty about life, individual purpose, origins of the universe, and how we should behave. Religion provides more certainty in all those areas for those who hold religious beliefs. Despite these differences, religion and spirituality influence coping, the causes of mental illness, and the symptoms presented.

### Influence on Coping

Use of spirituality and religion has been integrally associated with coping during periods of emotional distress. Both reflect deep-rooted internal aspects of an individual, that can provide a connection to a larger community, a sense of meaning and understanding of one's life and world, and a core foundation offering guidance and a framework for decision making. Studies have found that religiosity can be either a positive or negative coping strategy when individuals and families experience psychological crises (Hackney & Sanders, 2003). Variations in spiritual beliefs and practices come into play as individuals cope with mental illness.

Research on spirituality and religion has identified diverse results related to racial, ethnic, and cultural groups. One study examined religious coping when dealing with stressful situations among African Americans, Caribbean Blacks, and non-Hispanic Whites (Chatters, Taylor, Jackson, & Lincoln, 2008). Results revealed that African Americans and Caribbean Blacks reported higher use of religious coping when compared to non-Hispanic Whites. Another study examined the help-seeking process for Korean immigrants with depression (Shin, 2002). Findings identified the use of multiple steps and four stages:

- Stage 1 included prayer and faith
- Stage 2 involved reliance on family and friends
- Stage 3 included (among other strategies) traditional Asian practitioners and counseling from ministers
- Stage 4 involved consideration of mental health services

In a South African national study that included Blacks, colored (mix-race), Indian/Asian, and White citizens who sought services for mental and physical health conditions, 7% sought assistance from spiritual or religious advisors. Blacks were more likely to seek these services as well as the services of traditional healers (Sorsdahl et al., 2009).

In India, religion plays a major role. The Shaman is a religious healer that may be used to address mental health issues. Hindu priests may be consulted when mental health issues arise because certain Hindu deities are believed to guard against evil powers. Sufi shrines of Islamic saints are visited by many people in India for answers to mental health concerns. In addition, non-religious traditional healers, such as herbalists, witchcraft practitioners, and faith healers may be used to address mental health problems (Khandelwal et al., 2004).

### Influence on the Etiology of Mental Illness

Even as religious beliefs can assist in coping with mental illness, it can also be used to explain the origins of mental illness. For example, in traditional Islam, it is common to hear of a *jinn* (race of beings who can transform and possess others) and *sihr* (magic, sorcery, or witchcraft). These entities can cause lethargy, illness, bad dreams, hearing voices, anger or sadness, and bizarre body movements that are associated with psychosis. Some Christian faiths believe in spiritual possession of the body resulting in bizarre thoughts and behavior. Belief in witchcraft as an influence in mental illness is found in many societies such as in Africa, Asia, the South Pacific, and the Caribbean. The belief that spiritual ailments that manifest themselves as mental illnesses result from spells and possessions are also held in Western societies. Many cultures believe that the "evil eye" or bringing attention to one's self or family in a prideful manner can lead to both physical and mental health disorders (Ally & Laher, 2008; Martin, 2009).

## Influence on Mental Illness Symptomatology

Mental illness presentations are strongly influenced by cultural and religious meanings. Mental health conditions that affect cognition, such as psychotic disorders that result in delusions and hallucinations, may have religious content. For example, religious themes in delusions and hallucination have been reported in all cultures and are influenced by the norms of the group to which the individual belongs. Yamada, Barrio, Morrison, Sewell, & Jest (2006) found no significant differences among African American, Latinos, and Whites with respect to the prevalence of religious content. However, another study found that mental health professionals in the United States gave lower ratings of pathology for individuals who had delusions or hallucinations reflecting Catholic or Mormon beliefs, whereas religious content reflecting the views of the Muslim faith was seen as more pathological by mental health professionals (O'Connor & Vandenberg, 2005).

In Western culture, especially the United States, Christian religious beliefs are more familiar to the general population, including mental health professionals. As a result, these beliefs are perceived as acceptable even when there is an intense focus on these beliefs in the patient's communication within a mental health setting. Adherents to these beliefs are seen as "religious expression" rather than "delusional or pathological content." This disparity in diagnosis supports the need for cultural competence in the provision of equitable mental health care.

> *Religion and spirituality can influence an individual's coping methods, beliefs about the causes of mental illness, and how symptoms are manifested.*

## BARRIERS TO MENTAL HEALTH SERVICES

Regardless of types of professional mental health services that diverse populations seek, barriers exist that need to be overcome. These obstacles occur at the individual, environmental, and institutional levels. Individual obstacles originate from within the individual, such as mistrust and lack of knowledge, which inhibit help seeking. Environmental barriers reflect factors that occur within the milieu of the affected individual and inhibit attempts toward seeking help, such as stigma. When individual and environmental barriers are overcome, institutional obstacles such as health care provider and service barriers provide significant obstacles (DHHS, 2001).

> *Barriers to mental health services occur at three levels: individual, environmental, and institutional.*

## Overcoming Barriers

Access or pathways to mental health care use has been studied in a variety of populations in the United States and world-wide (Morgan, 2005; Steel et al., 2006; Shin, 2002). Most studies focused in this area examine institutional barriers that may impede an individual's entrance into the health care system for mental health care. A smaller but growing number of studies examine individual and environmental barriers involving the choices people make prior to accessing service and when they make initial contact seeking access. The study described here is used to illustrate some of the findings related to the choices made and the experiences and barriers faced by the individuals who are African American. The information from this study is then correlated with similar findings related to other cultures.

### Access and Use of Services

A series of studies were performed to examine the pathway used to access mental health services for first-time African American users. The studies also examined the role that family, community, and mental health services played in that pathway selection (Hines-Martin, 1998, 2003a, 2003b). The results reveal some common patterns of participant behavior. Two groups of experiences and common experiences influenced these patterns.

### *Life of Overload*

The participants described obstacles encountered as part of day-to-day living. These obstacles involve ongoing multiple stressors experienced by participants over an extended period of time. These stressors occur in addition to the participants' mental health problems. Participants reported assuming or experiencing these stressors throughout their lives, coping and adapting with minimal resources. Most participants did receive assistance from family and significant others in dealing with these stressors.

The initial part of the participants' trajectory of the illness also was described, resulting from exposure to the multiple stressors in addition to the already present mental health problems. All participants had periods in which their ability to cope waxed and waned based on changes in their daily lives, resources, and their response to the rising emotional and /or behavioral problems.

### Marginal Living

Most participants also experienced a pattern of behavior in response to an identified problem. The participants' ability to perform work, engage in interpersonal relationships, and participate in daily living changed in a way that was distinctly different from that which was previously experienced. Distress was heightened and illness behaviors increased significantly, leading to an increasing loss of normalcy. As a result, losses multiplied, and risky behaviors, primarily avoidance techniques, increased. Male participants reported more behaviors involving violence and experienced more severe life disruption with loss of family ties.

A significant number of participants experienced multiple episodes in which they fluctuated between a state of marginal living and a higher-level functioning. Factors that influenced these episodes included the participants' knowledge level about mental health services and their beliefs and values about service use. However, the most important influencing factor was the impact of family and significant others. These individuals function as a facilitator for or barrier to seeking mental health services for a solution. Whether the individuals or family members acted as a facilitator or barrier was based on one or more of the following:
- The desire of the participant to be reunited or to improve relations with the significant other
- The significant other's perception of the problem and acceptable solutions
- The significant other's experiences with or knowledge of mental health services and its potential benefit to the participant

### Turning Point

Ultimately, participants made their way to mental health services either on their own or through the intervention of others. They recognized the meaning of past behaviors, illness, and problems and their effect on the current situation. As a result, participants recognized the need for change by accessing recognizable mental health services as a last resort toward improving their life situation. If the individual manifested life-threatening, destructive behavior and/or hopelessness, a family member or significant other intervened and mental health services were identified as the last option. Participants in this situation generally felt coerced into mental health services.

### Pathway Choices

The pathway to mental health services was for the most part lengthy and tortuous for participants in this study. Patterns were revealed, depicting how the participants made the decisions and choices. **Figure 27-1** illustrates the pathways described in the study.

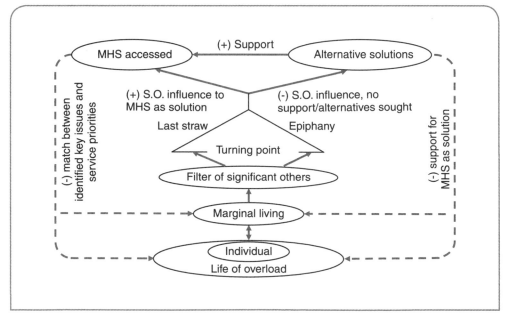

**Figure 27-1** *Patterns and pathways to mental health services.*

*From Hines-Martin V., Brown-Piper A., Kim S., & Malone M. (2003b). Enabling factors of mental health service use among African Americans. Archives of Psychiatric Nursing, 17, 197–204. With permission of Elsevier.*

## Correlation to Other Cultures

Research involving other ethnic and racial groups reveal similar experiences. For example, in the study involving Korean Americans addressing spirituality and religion previously discussed, Shin (2002) identified four stages that occur in identifying mental health problems. Those stages are similar to the behavior patterns described in the research on African Americans (Hines-Martin et al., 1998, 2003a, 2003b). First, the individual takes time to understand what is occurring based on his or her belief system. Next, they use family and social networks to evaluate and seek help to address the problem. Accessing formal mental health services is done only as a last option because doing so is incongruent with their perceptions, culture, and language limitations. Many aspects identified in the studies by Hines-Martin and Shin are also identified in studies in the United Kingdom involving African Caribbean and Black African subjects and in Australia involving Australian, Vietnamese, Chinese, and Arabic subjects. The results all indicate that individual, environmental, and service barriers to care exist and must be addressed (Morgan et al., 2005; Steel et al., 2006).

## Implications for Psychiatric-Mental Health Nursing

These studies underscore the need to address barriers with diverse populations. Therefore, to promote access to services, individual barriers such as beliefs and knowledge, environmental barriers such as family and social networks, and service barriers such as culture and language, must be addressed. Assisting individuals and families to overcome barriers to mental health care can be accomplished in any setting because all health concerns have mental health implications. The following can be used to assist patients and their families to overcome barriers:

- Be aware of potential cultural or religious differences between one's self and the patient
- Recognize signs and symptoms of emotional or mental distress during patient assessments
- Use evidence-based practice to be informed of conditions that may have a high incidence of mental health co-morbidity, such as diabetes and cardiovascular disease, and use that knowledge for a more thorough assessment and patient and family education
- Be knowledgeable of resources that can be used to address mental health needs
- Bring in the cultural expertise of others when needed to encourage and support the patient's access to mental health care using culturally sensitive language

> *Regardless of the population involved, overcoming barriers to accessing mental health care is a priority.*

# CULTURALLY COMPETENT AND CONGRUENT CARE

The globalization of the world and the diversity of populations demonstrate the need for all psychiatric-mental health nurses (PMHNs) to provide culturally competent and congruent mental health care. This need is further emphasized by the U.S. Surgeon General's Report (2001), the World Health Organization, and professional nursing organizations such as the International Society of Psychiatric and Mental Health Nurses and the American Psychiatric Nurses Association. Culturally competent care requires provider competence and organizational competence.

Provider competence is based on understanding the theoretical basis for professional development and the use of resources to better understand the populations for which mental health care is being provided. Nursing has several frameworks on which to base professional development in cultural and linguistic competence. These include Leininger, Giger-Newman and Davidhizer, Purnell and others. Nurses also have additional resources to assist with culturally appropriate assessment of immigrants and refugees (Congress, 1994, 2004). Additional areas for assessment with immigrant and refugee populations include reasons for relocation, legal status, crisis events, and prior trauma, especially with refugees. Developing provider competence does not occur overnight. Rather, it develops over a period of time and requires awareness and knowledge of the various cultures to develop specific skills for each culture.

Organizational competence requires nurses and other providers to work within their service settings to develop mental health services and resources to address the needs of diverse populations using these services. The National Center for Cultural Competence identifies the following principles for service organizations:

- Cultural competence is achieved by identifying and understanding the needs and help-seeking behaviors of individuals and families.
- Culturally competent organizations design and implement services that are tailored or matched to the unique

needs of the individuals, children, families, organizations, and communities served.

• Practice is driven in service delivery systems by the patient's preferred choices, not by culturally blind or culturally free interventions.

• Culturally competent organizations have a service delivery model that recognizes mental health as an integral and inseparable aspect of primary health care (National Center for Cultural Competence, 2009).

Organizations that strive for cultural competence must focus on delivery of services that are culturally congruent. **CULTURAL CONGRUENCE** has been defined as the distance between the cultural competence characteristics of a health care organization and the patient's perception of those same competence characteristics as they relate to the patient's cultural needs (Costantino, Malgady, & Primavera, 2009). In other words, congruence is the degree of match between what the health care setting provides and the patients' perceptions of what they need. In order to establish and maintain appropriate congruence between the health care organization and the patients that they serve, there must be constant growth and development through partnership, with the diverse populations that seek services within that setting. An exemplar illustrating how mental health services can increase cultural congruence is the Nathan Kline Institute (NKI) Center of Excellence in Culturally Competent Mental Health. Information about NKI and the use of EBP to address

the perspectives of specific populations can be viewed at http://ssrdqst.rfmh.org/cecc/sites/ssrdqst.rfmh.org.cecc/Video/NKI-CC1/CC1.html.

> *Provider and organizational cultural competence is necessary to meet the needs of the diverse populations being served.*

Addressing and deceasing mental health service disparities have been identified as goals by the Office of the U.S. Surgeon General, the National Institutes of Health, and the World Health Organization. Accomplishing those goals requires a better understanding of the experience of individuals from diverse ethnic, racial, social, and cultural backgrounds as they seek assistance with mental health concerns. Nurses need to be knowledgeable about the culturally based values and beliefs related to the meaning of mental health and illness, and about help-seeking from the perspective of individuals from diverse groups. This awareness provides a firm knowledge foundation about the pathways used to access services and what and how self-care decisions are made. As a result, nursing care strategies can be tailored to meet the needs of diverse population groups and individuals to achieve optimal mental health outcomes.

## SUMMARY POINTS

• The attainment of the highest level of health is a fundamental right of each person regardless of race, religion, political belief, or economic or social condition. As the population of the United States is becoming increasingly diverse, the need for equitable health care for all is also increasing.

• Race, ethnicity, and culture are significant parts of the context in which an individual lives, influencing the person's perception of well-being and illness, health care decisions, and health services use.

• Differences in ethnicity, race, and culture impact cognitive styles, negotiation strategies, and value systems.

• Many cultures focus on the family as a collective decision-making unit, contrasting Western culture that emphasizes individual decision making.

• Different racial and ethnic groups experience variability in incidence and prevalence rates for different mental health disorders.

• Spiritual or religious advisors, traditional healers, religious healers, priests, and shrines may be sought out by different cultural groups as a means to address mental health concerns. Religious beliefs may be used to explain the causes of mental illness or may be evidenced in symptoms that are manifested.

*(cont.)*

## SUMMARY POINTS (*CONT.*)

- Individual barriers such as mistrust and lack of knowledge, environmental barriers such as attitudes and stigma, and institutional barriers such as health care providers and services can interfere with one's access to mental health services.

- Providing culturally competent and congruent care is essential to meet the needs of the diverse populations being served to promote achievement of optimal outcomes.

## NCLEX-PREP*

1. The nurse is working with group of patients who have immigrated to the United States from several Latin American and South American countries and is reviewing the situation for possible barriers to accessing mental health services. Which of the following would the nurse identify as an environmental barrier?

   a. No translator on staff at the facilities
   b. Knowledge about the mental health problems
   c. Availability of family support
   d. Beliefs of mental illness caused by demon

2. A nurse is interviewing a patient who came to the area after she fled her home country, during a political revolution. When assessing the patient, the nurse notes that the patient has adopted several of the local customs of the area. The nurse identifies this as which of the following?

   a. Ethnicity
   b. Enculturation
   c. Spirituality
   d. Religiosity

3. A nurse is working in an area that has a high concentration of Asian immigrants and is developing a plan to minimize possible risk factors for poor mental health. Which of the following would the nurse least likely address?

   a. Social isolation
   b. Interaction with new culture

   c. Feelings of persecution
   d. Stress of acculturation

4. A nurse is providing an in-service presentation for staff members of a clinic about how the clinic is promoting culturally competent care. Which of the following would the nurse include?

   a. Emphasis on mental health as a separate entity from primary health care
   b. Services that are broad in scope, reflecting general cultural concepts
   c. Services that are focused primarily on the major cultural group
   d. Focus on the help-seeking behaviors of the unique populations being served

5. A group of students are reviewing information about the impact of culture, race, and ethnicity on mental health and mental health care delivery. The students demonstrate understanding when they identify which of the following as reflecting cognitive styles?

   a. Methods for processing information
   b. Information denoting evidence for change
   c. Primary locus of decision making
   d. Sources of anxiety and anxiety reduction

*Answers to these questions appear on page 639.

## REFERENCES

Abdool, K., & Ziqubu-Page, T. (2004). Bridging the gap: Potential for a health care partnership between African traditional healers and biomedical personnel in South Africa: South African Medical Association. Retrieved October 29, 2009 at http://www.samedical.org

Ally, Y., & Laher, S. (2008). South African Muslim faith healers perceptions of mental illness: Understanding, aetiology and treatment. *Journal of Religion and Health, 47,* 45–56.

Borges, G., Breslau, J., Su, M., Miller, M., Medina-Mora, M.E., & Aguilar-Gaxiola, S. (2009). Immigration and suicidal behavior among Mexicans and Mexican Americans. *American Journal of Public Health, 99(4),* 728–733.

Chatters, L.M., Taylor, R.J., Jackson, J.S., & Lincoln, K.D. (2008). Religious coping among African Americans, Caribbean blacks and non-Hispanic Whites. *Journal of Community Psychology, 36(3),* 371–386.

Cheung, M. (2009). Asian male domestic violence victims; services exclusively for men. *Journal of family violence, 24(7),* 447–462.

Collins, K.S., Hughes, D.L., Doty M.M., Ives B.L., Edwards, J.N., & Tenney, K. (2002). Diverse communities, common concerns: Assessing health care quality for minority Americans. New York: The Commonwealth Fund.

Congress, E.P. (1994). The use of culturagrams to assess and empower culturally diverse families. *Families in Society, 75(9),* 531–538.

Congress, C.W. (2004). Cultural and Ethical issues in working with culturally diverse patients and their families: The use of the culturagram to promote cultural competent practice in the health care setting. In Metteri et al. (Eds), *Social Work Visions from Around the Globe: Citizens, Methods and approaches.* Hawthorne, NJ: Hawthorne Press.

Costantino, G., Malgady, R.G., & Primavera L.H. (2009) Congruence between culturally competent treatment and cultural needs of older Latinos. *Journal of Consulting and Clinical Psychology, 77(5),* 941–949.

de Toledo Piza Pelusa, E., deAraujo Peres, C., & Blay, S.L. (2008). Public conceptions of schizophrenia in urban Brazil. *Social Psychiatry and Psychiatric Epidemiology, 43,* 792–799.

Dunlop, D.D, Lyons, J.S., Manheim, L.M.,..... et al. (2003). Racial/ethnic differences in rates of depression among preretirement adults. *American Journal of Public Health, 93*(11), 1945–1952.

Fozdar, F. (2009). "The Golden country": Ex-Yugoslav and African refugee experiences of settlement and "depression." *Journal of Ethnic and Migration Studies, 35*(8), 1335–1352.

Hackney, C.H., & Sanders, G.S. (2003). Religiosity and mental health: A Meta-Analysis of recent studies. *Journal for the Scientific Study of Religion, 42*(1), 43–55.

Harrell, S.P. (2000). A multidimensional conceptualization of racism-related stress: Implications for the well-being of people of color. *America Journal of Orthopsychiatry, 70*(1), 42–57.

Hines-Martin, V. (1998). Environmental context of caregiving for severely mentally ill adults: An African American experience. *Issues in Mental Health Nursing, 19,* 433–451.

Hines-Martin, V., Brown-Piper, A., Kim, S., & Malone, M., (2003b). Enabling factors of mental health service use among African Americans. *Archives of Psychiatric Nursing, 17,* 197–204.

Hines-Martin, V., Malone, M., Kim, S., & Brown-Piper, A. (2003a). Barriers to mental health care access in an African American population. *Issues in Mental Health Nursing, 24*(3), 237–256.

Kaiser Family Foundation. (2011). Kaiser's monthly update on minority health disparities. Available at: http://www.kff.org/minorityhealth/report.cfm Retrieved April 7, 2011.

Khandelwal, S. K., Jhingan, H.P., Ramesh, S., Gupta, R. K., & Srivastava, V. K. (2004). India mental health country profile. *International Review of Psychiatry, 16*(1–2), 126–141.

Kirmayer, L. J., Groleau, D., Guzder, J., Blake, C. & Jarvis, E. (2003). Cultural consultation: A model of mental health service for multicultural societies. *Canadian Journal of Psychiatry, 48*(3), 145–152.

Kim, B.S., Atkinson, D.R. & Umemoto, D. (2001). Asian cultural values and the counseling process: Current knowledge and directions for future research. *The Counseling Psychologist, 29*(4), 570–603.

Martin, S.S. (2009). Health care-seeking behaviors of older Iranian immigrants: Health perceptions and definitions. *Journal of Evidence-Based Social Work, 6,* 58–78.

Minsky, S., Vega, W., Miskimen, T.,..... et al. (2003). Diagnosic patterns in Latino, African American, and European American patients. *Archives of General Psychiatry, 60*(6), 637-644.

Morgan, C., Mallett, R., Hutchinson, G., ... & Leff, J. (2005). Pathways to care and ethnicity. 2: Source of referral and help-seeking. *British Journal of Psychiatry, 186*(2), 290–296.

National Center for Cultural Competence. (2009). Cultural competence in service organizations. Retrieved on November 2, 2009 at http://www.georgetown.edu/research/gucchd/nccc

O'Connor, S., & Vandenberg, B. (2005). Psychosis or Faith? Clinicians' assessment of religious beliefs. *Journal of Consulting and Clinical Psychology, 73,* 610–616.

Owen, S., Khalil, E. (2007). Addressing diversity in mental health care: A review of guidance documents. *International Journal of Nursing Studies, 44,* 467–478.

Padmavati, R. (2005). Community mental health care in India. *International Review of Psychiatry, 17*(2), 103–107.

Patel, V., & Bloch, S. (2009). The ethical imperative to scale up health care services for people with severe mental disorders in low and middle income countries. *Postgraduate Medical Journal, 85,* 509–513.

Polo, A.J., & Lopez, S. R. (2009). Culture, context, and the internalizing distress of Mexican American youth. *Journal of Clinical Child & Adolescent Psychology, 39*(2), 273–285.

Pumariega, A.J., & Rothe, E. (2003). Cultural considerations in child and adolescent psychiatric emergencies and crises. *Child and Adolescent Psychiatric Clinics of North America, 12,* 723–744

Razzouk, D., Gallo, C., Olifson, S., Zorzetto, R., Fiestas, F.,... et al. (2008). Challenges to reduce the "10/90 gap": Mental health research in Latin American and Caribbean countries. *Acta Psychiatrica Scandinavica, 118,* 490–498.

Scheffler, et. al. (2011). Human resources for mental health: low-and middle- income countries. France: WHO.

Shin, J.K. (2002). Help-seeking behaviors by Korean immigrants for depression. *Issues in Mental Health Nursing, 23,* 461–276.

Smedley, B.D., Stith, A.Y., Nelson, A.R. (2002). *Unequal treatment: Confronting racial and ethnic disparities in health care.* Washington, DC: National Academy Press.

Sorsdahl, K., Stein, D.J., Grimsrud, A., Seedat, S., Flisher, A.J., Williams, D.R., & Myer, L. (2009). Traditional Healers in the treatment of common mental disorders in South Africa. *The Journal of Nervous and Mental Disease, 197*(6), 434–441.

Snowden, L., & Hu, T. (1997). Ethnic differences in mental health services use among the severely mentally ill. *Journal of Community Psychology, 25*(3), 235–247.

Snowden, L.R., Masland, M.C., Libby, A.M., Wallace, N., & Fawley, K. (2008). Ethnic minority children's use of psychiatric emergency care in California's public mental health system. *American Journal of Public Health, 98,* 118–124.

Snowden, L.R., & Yamada, A. (2005). Cultural differences in access to care. *Annual Review of Clinical Psychology, 1,* 143–166.

Steel, Z., McDonald, R., Silove, D., Bauman, A., Sandford, P., Herron, J., & Minas, I.H. (2006). Pathways to the first contact with specialist mental health care. *Australian and New Zealand Journal of Psychiatry, 40,* 347–354.

Stein, D.J., & Seedat, S. (2007). From research methods to clinical practice in psychiatry: Challenges and opportunities in the developing world. *International Review of Psychiatry, 19*(5), 573–581.

Stein, D.J., Seedat, S., Herman, A., Moomal, H., Heeringa, S.G., Kessler, R.C., & Williams, D.R. (2008). Lifetime prevalence of psychiatric disorders in South Africa. *British Journal of Psychiatry, 192,* 112–117.

Sullivan, H. S. (1947). *Conceptions of modern psychiatry.* Washington, DC: William Alanson White Psychiatric Foundation.

Summerfield, D. (2005). "My whole body is sick…my life is not good": a Rwandan asylum-seeker attends a psychiatric clinic in London, in Ingleby, D. (ed.) *Forced Migration and mental health: Rethinking the Care of Refugees and Displaced Persons.* New York: Springer Science, 97–114.

The Commonwealth Fund. Health Quality Care Survey. Available at: http://www.cmwf.org. Retrieved on November 8, 2009.

U.S. Department of Health and Human Services. (2001). *Mental health: Culture, race, and ethnicity—a supplement to mental health: A report of the Surgeon General.* Rockville, MD: U.S. Department of Health and Human Services, Substance Abuse and Mental Health Services Administration, Center for Mental Health Services.

Wang, P., Berglund, P., & Kessler, R. (2001). Recent care of common mental disorders in the United States. *Journal of General Internal Medicine, 15*(5): 284–292.

Williams, D.R., Gonzales, H.M., Neighbors, H.W. … (2007). Prevalence and distribution of major depressive disorder among African Americans, Caribbean blacks and non-Hispanic whites: Results from the national survey of American life (SNAL). *Archives of General Psychiatry, 64,* 305–315.

Williams, D.R. & Williams-Morris, R. (2000). Racism and mental health: The African American experience. *Ethnicity and Health, 5,* 243–268.

Woodward, A.T., Taylor, R. J., Bullard, K.M., Neighbors, H.W., Chatters, L.M., & Jackson, J.S. (2008). Use of Professional and informal support by African Americans and Caribbean Blacks with mental disorders. *Psychiatric Services, 59*(11), 1292–1298.

World Health Organization [WHO] (2009). The World Health 2008 Report. Retrieved November 3, 2009 at http://www.who.int/

World Health Organization [WHO] (2001). World Health Report. Geneva, Switzerland: World Health Organization.

Yamada, A.M., Barrio, C., Morrison, S.W., Sewell, D., & Jeste, D.V. (2006). Cross-ethnic evaluation of psychotic symptom content in hospitalized middle-aged and older adults. *General Hospital Psychiatry, 28,* 161–168.

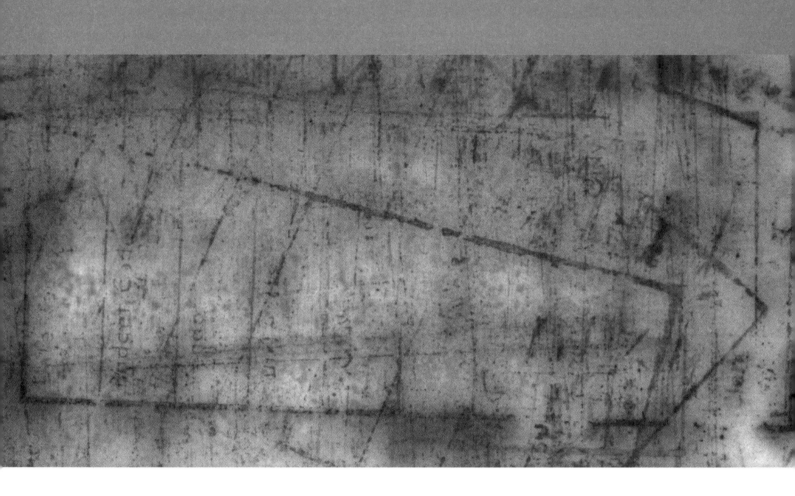

## CHAPTER CONTENTS

Ethics

Legal Issues

Nursing Responsibilities

## EXPECTED LEARNING OUTCOMES

**After completing this chapter, the student will be able to:**

1. Identify ethical theories that may be used when providing care to psychiatric-mental health patients.

2. Analyze the steps of the ethical decision-making process, applying them to nursing processes.

3. Describe the rights and responsibilities of psychiatric-mental health patients across the continuum of care.

4. Compare the similarities and differences between voluntary and involuntary admission for mental health care.

5. Describe the concepts of competency and self-determination as they apply to the psychiatric-mental health patient.

## CHAPTER 28

# ETHICAL AND LEGAL PRINCIPLES

Katherine R. Casale

6. Explain the methods for ensuring patient safety when implementing restraint and seclusion.
7. Discuss the responsibilities of the psychiatric-mental health nurses (PMHNs) in providing ethical and legal nursing care.

## KEY TERMS

Autonomy

Beneficence

Competence

Ethics

Fidelity

Involuntary commitment

Justice

Kantianism

Nonmaleficence

Seclusion

Self-determination

Utilitarianism

Veracity

Voluntary admission

Psychiatric-mental health nurses (PMHNs) make critical decisions about patient care every day. To make the best decisions, they must reflect on principles of good and bad as well as consider which choices benefit the individual as well as the group. Ethical and legal decision-making situations are seldom black or white, and this is especially true in psychiatric-mental health nursing. Therefore, PMHNs need a firm understanding of ethical theories and legal tenets that form the foundation from which to make ethical and legal decisions to protect their patients and themselves.

This chapter discusses the major ethical theories used as a foundation for ethical decision making and presents an example of the process based on the nursing process. The chapter describes the legal issues involved in psychiatric-mental health nursing care and treatment, and addresses the nursing responsibilities necessary to ensure the ethical and legal provision of care.

## ETHICS

ETHICS is a collection of philosophical principles that examine the rightness and wrongness of decisions and conduct as human beings. Ethicists, including nursing scholars and clinical ethics consultants, use various approaches to address practical moral dilemmas (Abma, 2008). Personal moral convictions of PMHNs serve as a foundation to reflect on ethical quandaries that arise in their daily work (Skott, 2003). Nurses who are engaged in providing care to patients with mental illnesses face unique challenges that can test their moral and ethical reasoning. Thus, an understanding of ethical theories and principles is important in determining the proper decision.

The scope of responsibility as well as the rights and standards of practice for professional nurses is clearly delineated in the American Nurses Association (ANA) *Code of Ethics for Nurses with Interpretive Statements* (2001). This code is a written statement of the expected behaviors and practices of every nurse every day. The practice of nursing requires ethical conduct and moral decision making during the care of patients; the Code of Ethics is updated regularly to guide nurses in their daily duties, whether providing direct or indirect care to those patients. In the face of ever-changing technology, nurses encounter increased responsibilities and increased stress. First and foremost, the nurse has a primary responsibility to protect the rights, health, and safety of the patient. However, exactly how does the nurse act ethically to protect the patient? **Evidence-Based Practice 28-1** summarizes two important studies related to doing the right thing and the ethical nursing practice.

> *Ethics involves the principles that address right and wrong.*

## Ethical Theories and Principles

Several ethical theories and principles mold the professional practice of psychiatric-mental health nursing and provide a firm foundation to guide professional decision making.

UTILITARIANISM professes that decisions should be based on producing the best outcome or the greatest happiness for the greatest number of people. Proponents of utilitarianism believe that the end justifies the means, whereas opponents might argue that the interests of the minority and of individuals should not be ignored (Chitty, 2005).

The ethical principle of KANTIANISM is in contrast to utilitarianism. It focuses primarily on performing one's duty rather than the "rightness" or "wrongness" of the outcome. This theory explores the concepts of AUTONOMY (capacity to make decisions and act on them), BENEFICENCE (doing what is best), NONMALEFICENCE (doing no harm), JUSTICE (fair and equal treatment), VERACITY (honesty and truthfulness), and FIDELITY (acting as promised).

Beneficence and nonmaleficence focus on patient advocacy; that is, doing what is best for the patient and not doing anything that will harm him or her. These two principles go hand-in-hand. Beneficence forms the foundation for all care decisions. For example, beneficence is demonstrated by administering antidepressant medications to a patient experiencing depression, providing emotional support to patients experiencing anxiety, and identifying signs that a patient is being abused. Nonmaleficence expands the principle of beneficence and involves actions that are proactive. For example, in the case of abuse, the nurse reports this abuse to reduce the risk for recurrence.

Doing the "right" thing implies that every individual has the ability to make an informed choice (autonomy). However, this concept of autonomy is flawed when one considers the decision-making abilities of certain subpopulations, such as infants and patients who are considered legally incompetent. PMHNs must recognize that individuals with serious, uncontrolled mental illness may not be capable of making an independent choice. In that instance, it is the responsibility of the mental health care team to make certain that the rights of each patient are protected by an appointed representative. At times, to

**EVIDENCE-BASED PRACTICE 28-1:
ETHICAL PRACTICE**

## STUDY

Smith, K.V., & Godfrey, N.S. (2002). Being a good nurse and doing the right thing: A qualitative study. *Nursing Ethics, 9*(1), 301–312.

Catlett, S., & Lovan, C. (2011). Being a good nurse and doing the right thing: A replication study. *Nursing Ethics, 18*(1), 54–63.

## SUMMARY

This qualitative research effort that was undertaken in 2002 and replicated almost a decade later identifies four areas in which nurses are characterized as ethical and good practitioners. Philosophers define ethical behavior as being morally sound with virtuous actions. In nursing, this is translated into caring practice. Both Smith and Godfrey's original research and Catlett and Lovan's re-examination of the topic reinforced the concept of intentional ethical caring as an essential quality of the good nurse. Participants described good nurses who consistently do the right thing in four general areas: "personal traits and attributes, technical skills and management of care, work environment and co-workers, and caring and caring behaviors" (Catlett and Lovan, 2011, p. 58). Organizations can use these findings to hire nurses who demonstrate these skills and can provide continuing education to reinforce and strengthen these essential attributes. Working in an ethical environment improves job satisfaction, strengthens retention, and minimizes job turnover.

## APPLICATION TO PRACTICE

Findings from both studies demonstrate the complexity of training needed to develop ethical, caring nurses. The nurse's ability to perform technical tasks efficiently and safely is only one trait of the good nurse. This knowledge has a significant impact on professional nursing education, as students must focus on developing character traits in addition to clinical competence. Characteristics such as trustworthiness, caring, honesty, and empathy can be learned and reinforced in the classroom. Nursing students can hone and perfect the interpersonal skills that make nurses among the most trusted professionals in the workforce through the use of case studies, simulation, and clinical practice. Students who struggle with making ethical choices can learn to do so by observing peer mentors and faculty.

## QUESTIONS TO PONDER

1. *How has the health care environment changed since the original study was conducted?*
2. *Consider the following: You are one of two registered nurses working nightshift on a mental health unit. A patient on the unit is prescribed diazepam 5 mg every 8 hours as needed for anxiety. You observe that the patient is calm and relaxed in bed at 11:00 p.m. At 11:05 you note that the other registered nurse pulls a dose of diazepam for the patient but does not bring it to the patient's room. How would you handle this situation?*

preserve the safety of the patient and those around him or her, a patient may lose the right of **SELF-DETERMINATION** (freedom to make decisions without consulting others). In addition, PMHNs constantly use critical thinking to ensure a balance between autonomy and beneficence. At times, the difficulty lies in deciding which ethical principle should have the highest priority.

Nursing theorist Hildegard Peplau (1991) proposed that a primary role of the PMHN is that of patient advocate and supporter. She emphasized that nurses should provide education about patients' rights, choices, and access to services.

The concept of justice refers to distributing resources equally to all patients and combating discrimination of any type. The just PMHN treats all patients fairly and equally.

Veracity and fidelity, being honest and faithful, are two similar ethical principles that may be difficult to maintain. Lachman (2008) noted: "Because of cost and access constraints in today's health care environment, the virtues of honesty and integrity are constantly under assault. Integrity can be preserved only if nurses' actions are consistent with the values and ethics of the profession." **Box 28-1** lists the ethical principles and theories and how the PMHN applies them.

## Model for Ethical Decision Making

Throughout the educational experience, nursing students are encouraged to engage in the nursing process for clinical decision making. Peplau, known for her work with the interpersonal process (see Chapter 2) identified four phases of the nurse-patient relationship that have been correlated to the nursing process. Both can be integrated and adapted for use as a guide for ethical decision making in psychiatric-mental health nursing. The following example demonstrates the steps of the decision-making process for a PMHN who encounters an ethical dilemma. It also incorporates several ethical principles that the nurse needs to consider during the process.

> *Ethical theories and principles provide the foundation from which the PMHN integrates the nursing process to make an ethical decision when faced with an ethical dilemma.*

### Orientation/Assessment phase

George is a 22-year-old recent college graduate with a degree in international business. He is in excellent health except for a recent depressed mood. George has $60,000 in unpaid student loans, which are coming due. He has been unable to find a job during the last four months since graduation. He has depleted his meager savings and is sleeping on a friend's couch and eating meals at a homeless shelter. George knows he will need to find new living arrangements soon. He has been diagnosed with situational depression at the local community health clinic and has been taking fluoxetine (Prozac) for two weeks. He is treated by Jamal, a psychiatric advanced practice nurse.

On the Internet, George discovers a private clinic in Mexico that is searching for voluntary organ donors. The advertisement states that the clinic will pay $75,000 for a kidney donated from a person with type AB blood. George has type AB blood and becomes excited about the possibility of selling one of his kidneys. He can pay off his loan and be able to afford to rent and furnish an apartment of his own. He shows the advertisement to Jamal and asks his advice.

### Identification Phase/Nursing Diagnoses and Planning

Based on the assessment, some possible nursing diagnoses might be:

- Ineffective community coping related to deficits in financial resources
- Fear related to financial and potential health stressors
- Powerlessness related to community and financial stressors
- Risk for compromised human dignity related to potential change in body integrity
- Risk for complicated grieving related to lack of job and potential loss of body part
- Risk for infection related to surgery at illegal private clinic
- Anxiety related to psychological conflict and situational depression

George asks Jamal for his professional nursing opinion about the positives and negatives of deciding to travel to another country to sell a kidney. Jamal uses his training in ethical considerations to help George.

First, they consider the ethical principle of utilitarianism, which states that actions are good if they produce happiness and bad if they cause unhappiness. George notes that selling a kidney would bring him happiness because the $75,000 he earns will improve his financial security. Jamal questions his thinking by asking how happy

## BOX 28-1: APPLYING ETHICAL THEORIES AND PRINCIPLES TO PSYCHIATRIC-MENTAL HEALTH NURSING

| | |
|---|---|
| Ethical principle | The nurse adheres to the American Nurses Association Code of Ethics. |
| Utilitarianism | The nurse collaborates with other health professionals and the public in promoting community, national, and international efforts to meet health needs. |
| | The nurse participates in the advancement of the profession through contributions to practice, education, administration, and knowledge development. |
| Kantianism | The nurse participates in establishing, maintaining, and improving health care environments and conditions of employment conducive to the provision of quality health care and consistent with the values of the profession through individual and collective action. |
| Autonomy | The nurse promotes, advocates for, and strives to protect the health, safety, and rights of the patient. |
| Beneficence and nonmaleficence | The profession of nursing, as represented by associations and their members, is responsible for articulating nursing values, for maintaining the integrity of the profession and its practice, and for shaping social policy. |
| Justice | The nurse, in all professional relationships, practices with compassion and respect for the inherent dignity, worth, and uniqueness of every individual, unrestricted by considerations of social or economic status, personal attributes, or the nature of health problems. |
| Veracity | The nurse owes the same duties to self as to others, including the responsibility to preserve integrity and safety, to maintain competence, and to continue personal and professional growth. |
| Fidelity | The nurse's primary commitment is to the patient, whether an individual, family, group, or community. |

*From the American Nurses Association, Code of Ethics for Nurses with Interpretive Statements, Silver Spring, MD: American Nurses Publishing, 2001.*

George would be if the surgery was performed incorrectly and caused renal failure, or if George developed a life-threatening infection after surgery.

Second, they consider the principle of Kantianism, which is centered on making choices based on a sense of duty and morality. Jamal points out that this surgery is technically unlicensed and unregulated, and therefore morally wrong. George argues that it is his kidney and his body, and no one should have the power to tell him what he can do with it, illustrating the principle of autonomy.

The discussion moves on to the ethical concepts of beneficence and nonmaleficence. Jamal, in his role as nurse, advocates for George's best interests. He teaches George about all of the potential complications of a nephrectomy (removal of a kidney), including hemorrhage, infection, pneumothorax, and azotemia, and points out that George may be making the decision based on his current depression. As noted by Peplau, advocacy is an essential role of the nurse (Peplau, 1991).

Using the principle of veracity, which is truthfulness, Jamal expresses his concerns about George making this life-changing decision. George argues that he has been taking antidepressant medications and is no longer depressed. He states that selling a kidney is the only way to move forward in his life without being a burden on society. Jamal explains that the fluoxetine may not have reached peak effectiveness or the dose might need to be increased. He believes that George should make the final decision about how to proceed, but only when his depression is resolved and he has all the facts.

## Exploitation Phase/Implementation

During the next two weeks, George considers Jamal's points. He researches the patient outcomes of organ sellers who have used the private Mexican clinic, and learns that 50% of patients suffered post-operative complications and several have died. As the fluoxetine reaches full therapeutic effectiveness, George's depression lifts and he intensifies his job search. He realizes that he has three options.

First, he can ignore Jamal's concerns and travel to Mexico for the nephrectomy. Choosing this option meets his desire for autonomy. He will benefit financially but risks his health because of the 50% complication rate. He is also negating Jamal's efforts of beneficence and nonmaleficence.

Second, he can elect to take no action, which is an action in itself. In this case, George does not travel to Mexico, so he does not risk his health (nonmaleficence). He does not find employment and is left homeless, which does not lead to utilitarianism (the greatest good).

Third, he can decide to find a new solution to his financial and housing problems. He can move in with his parents, who will offer emotional and financial support, and look for job opportunities in his home town.

## Resolution Phase/Evaluation

George continues to believe in ethical autonomy, that is, individuals should have the right to sell their own body organs if they choose. He notes that in many states, people can sell their blood. George believes that selling one of duplicate organs is an extension of that right.

However, he also believes in respecting moral and ethical laws (Kantianism). He is concerned that the clinic is unlicensed and unregulated. George also questions the outcome of a procedure in which half the participants experience complications. He realizes that the surgery may not be in his best interest and decides to contact his legislators to support a bill that will make the sale of one's own body organs legal within the United States.

Meanwhile, George selects option three. He moves in with his parents, which temporarily relieves his housing and financial dilemmas and enables him to maintain a healthy professional relationship with Jamal. After an extensive job search, George finds an entry-level business position, and is able to build his savings with a long-term plan of buying a home. He is weaned off the antidepressant medication and his health remains excellent, with both kidneys intact.

## LEGAL ISSUES

Like any nurse, PMHNs also are faced with legal issues related to patient care. However, these legal issues take on even greater importance because of the situations involved in caring for patients with mental health disorders, such as competency and involuntary admission.

### Bill of Rights for Mental Health Patients

The Mental Health Systems Act of 1980 outlined a Bill of Rights for Mental Health Patients. The intent of this document was to ensure the rights of patients who might be unable to speak for themselves. **Box 28-2** highlights these rights.

> *The Bill of Rights for Mental Health Patients is designed to protect the rights of any mentally ill patient who is unable to speak for him- or herself. Each patient has the right to the most supportive care in the least restrictive environment.*

### Voluntary and Involuntary Admission

When psychiatric-mental health patients require inpatient treatment, their admission may be either voluntary or involuntary. A **VOLUNTARY ADMISSION** is as the term implies, when the patient agrees or consents to admission. The majority of mental health patients apply for service voluntarily and stay for as long as the treatment team feel it is necessary. In addition, a patient may request treatment at an inpatient psychiatric facility. The facility may accept the person as a voluntary patient if the hospital agrees that the individual needs treatment. The hospital may require the person to sign a written request for hospital treatment. This is called a voluntary paper. When a patient is admitted to the hospital under voluntary status, he or she may ask to leave at any time. If the patient did not sign a voluntary paper, the hospital must release the patient when he or she asks to leave (C.G.S. 17a-5066(b)). If an individual did sign a voluntary paper, his or her request to leave must be made in writing. The hospital can keep a patient for 5 business days after a request to leave (C.G.S. 17a-506(a)). During this time, the hospital may file an application for civil commitment with the probate court.

**Box 28-3**

## BOX 28-2: BILL OF RIGHTS FOR MENTAL HEALTH PATIENTS

1. The right to the most supportive treatment in the least restrictive environment.
2. The right to participate in developing and revising an individualized written plan of care.
3. The right to receive explanations of treatment decisions and process.
4. The right to refuse any treatment except in times of emergency or as indicated by law.
5. The right to refuse to participate in experimental unproven treatment.
6. The right to remain unrestrained and unsecluded except in emergency situations.
7. The right to privacy, humane treatment, and protection from harm.
8. The right to confidentiality of information and written records.
9. The right to access personal medical records, except when access may harm the patient's health.
10. The right to communicate with visitors via mail, telephone, and personal visits, except when such communication would be detrimental to the patient's health.
11. The right to receive clear comprehensible communication of these rights.
12. The right to make a grievance when rights are withdrawn.
13. The right to be referred to other levels of mental health services upon discharge.

*Adapted from Mental Health Systems Act, 1980.*

The hospital may then keep the patient for up to 10 more days if the probate court orders the commitment. The hospital may not continue to hold a patient if the probate judge rules that the patient does not meet the standards for civil commitment.

With involuntary hospitalization, also termed **INVOLUNTARY COMMITMENT** or involuntary admission, the patient is admitted against his or her wishes. In other words, the patient may be sent to a facility even though he or she does not want to go. This can occur via two mechanisms. A medical doctor can sign an emergency certificate if the doctor thinks the patient requires immediate treatment. This is called emergency certification. This patient may also be sent to the facility by a judge

after a hearing in probate court. This is called civil commitment. How long a patient can be kept in a hospital if he or she does not want to be there depends on whether the patient was admitted through voluntary admission, emergency certification, or civil commitment. **Box 28-3** identifies the four situations in which involuntary commitment may occur.

Involuntary commitment is usually initiated by family members, friends, health care providers, police, or firefighters who encounter a patient with ineffective community coping. While involuntary commitment restricts an individual's rights, the referral is made for the protection of the patient. The court oversees the process, ensuring that all decisions are made in the patient's best interest.

*A patient who is admitted voluntarily can ask to leave at any time. Conversely, a patient who is involuntarily admitted cannot. If this admission restricts the patient's rights, the court assumes responsibility to ensure that the patient is protected and decisions made are in his or her best interests.*

## Competency

**COMPETENCE** is determined by the legal system and the definition may vary from state to state. Most health care providers define competence as the degree to which a patient possesses the cognitive ability to understand and process information. A patient may have periods of competence interspersed with episodes of incompetence.

Competence is the underlying theme for consent and the right to self-determination. The American Nurses Association Code of Ethics dictates that patients have the right to self-determination and autonomy. This overarching priority of advocating for patients' rights is echoed in the American Hospital Association's Patients' Bill of Rights, which states that patients have the right to confidentiality, privacy, participation in the plan of care, and to choose or refuse treatment. Simply stated, patients have the right to receive or refuse medical information, treatment, and medications, and should be involved in planning their own health care to the extent possible (nursingworld.org/code/ethics, 2009). This includes the right to informed consent

---

**BOX 28-3: SITUATIONS THAT CAN RESULT IN INVOLUNTARY COMMITMENT**

| | |
|---|---|
| Emergency commitment | • Patient's behavior is dangerous to self or others |
| | • Time limited—usually court hearing within 72 hours |
| | • Court may order involuntary commitment for 7–21 days |
| Mentally ill person in need of treatment | • Patient defined as mentally ill and unable to make health care decisions or manage personal needs |
| | • Likely to harm self or others |
| Involuntary outpatient commitment | • Court-ordered outpatient treatment |
| | • Without treatment patient is likely to deteriorate and require inpatient care |
| | • Severe persistent mental illness limits ability to understand importance of compliance with treatment |
| Gravely disabled patient | • Unable to provide for basic needs (shelter, food, clean clothing) |
| | • Lacks ability to use available community and personal resources |
| | • Court may order guardian or conservator |

---

about anything that will be done to the patient. For example, the effects and side effects of medications should be explained in words that the patient understands. Any prescribed treatments, such as electroconvulsive therapy (ECT), should also be discussed and the patient should have the right to select or reject these interventions. Thus, the PMHN is challenged to uphold the patient's right to autonomy in a complex era of conflicting priorities, fiscal limitations, staffing shortages, and litigation risks.

On December 1, 1991, the federal Patient Self-Determination Act (PSDA) took effect across the United States, requiring health care institutions to ask all adults admitted as inpatients whether they have an advanced directive and to inform them of their right to refuse treatment. The PSDA and advanced directive statutes assume that lay people want, need, and can appreciate information about medical technologic intervention. It further assumes that health professionals and institutions will respect those decisions (Heitman, 1992). For the patient with mental health problems, this means that an individual, when competent, can make health care decisions that will be honored in the event of evolving incompetence, when symptoms impair sound decision making (Chitty, 2005).

> *Consent and the right to self-determination are based on a person's competency.*

## Least Restrictive Environment

It is essential that nurses understand the concept of the right to treatment in the least restrictive environment. In 1975, as an outcome of the legal case of *Dixon v. Weinberger*, a person committed for mental health treatment won the right to receive treatment in the least restrictive environment as well as the right to refuse medications (Substance Abuse and Mental Health Services Administration [SAMHSA], 2010).

Consider the environment of psychiatric-mental health care as mapped along a visual continuum to apply the concept of the least restrictive environment. **Figure 28-1** depicts this continuum. Whenever possible, patients are offered individual or group therapies in a community setting. If that is not feasible, the next level of care is at

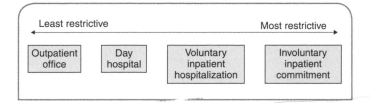

Figure 28-1 *Visualizing the continuum of mental health care.*

outpatient day hospitals or community centers. When appropriate, patients may voluntarily admit themselves for inpatient mental health treatment. The most restrictive level of care is involuntary hospitalization or commitment.

Similarly, the types of treatments offered progress from less to more restrictive. For example, treatment first begins with talk therapy and progresses to behavioral therapy, to involuntary medication interventions, seclusion, and physical restraint. While the goal for most psychiatric-mental health care providers is to attain a restraint-free environment, this must be balanced with protecting the patient, staff, and other patients. On occasion, nurses may be unable to de-escalate a patient's behavior using supportive verbal interventions. Physical restraints and seclusion, when used in a caring and empathetic manner, may maintain safety while protecting the dignity of the patient (Moylan, 2009).

## Restraints and Seclusion

Of the practical moral problems inherent in psychiatric-mental health nursing, one of the most debated is the use of restraints and other restrictions on individual freedom. Restraining a patient presents PMHNs with potential legal and ethical dilemmas. For example, what is reasonable force and when is it appropriate (Abma, 2008)?

During the past decade there has been a concerted movement among mental health practitioners to decrease the use of restraints. Although restricting movement or behavior may violate patients' autonomy, there are circumstances under which it may be legally and ethically appropriate or necessary to protect the safety of the client, fellow patients, and staff.

Restrictions to patient restraint and seclusion were also addressed in the Mental Health Act of 2001, instituted in the United Kingdom. Section 69 of that Act notes that a person may not be bodily restrained or secluded in an isolation room unless it is absolutely necessary to maintain safety and security. Australian mental health providers have instituted national safety priorities with an end goal of reducing or eliminating seclusion and restraint practices (Grigg, 2006).

The Bill of Rights for mental health patients as well as the United States Constitution reinforce the right of individuals to freedom from restraint or seclusion except in emergency situations. Professional judgment is necessary to establish when a patient's behavior has become unsafe and out of control to the point of imminent danger. In these instances, patients may require assistance of chemical or mechanical restraints to regain personal control and safety. Chemical restraints include medications, ordered by the treatment team, that are administered to diminish agitation or assist the patient to regain personal control. Mechanical restraints include straps that are placed on the arms and legs of an agitated patient to protect from injury to self, others, or the environment until the patient is able to regain self-control. Restraints are never to be used as punishment or for staff convenience. **SECLUSION**, which means placing the patient in a safe room alone, may also be used to diminish agitation and external stimulation.

> *Restraints and seclusion are used only when there is an emergency and it is determined that the patient's behavior is unsafe and there is imminent danger.*

Organizations such as Crisis Prevention Institute (CPI) were established to address the need for standardized training in safe, respectful, non-invasive methods for patient restraint. CPI is an international training organization that focuses on prevention through education and empowerment of professionals (CPI, 2011). Training programs teach all levels of mental health caregivers to manage disruptive and assaultive behavior in a manner that is compatible with the staff's duty to provide the best possible care.

When a situation arises, the staff must take prompt action when safety is in jeopardy. Several trained employees converge to safely control the patient as well as to ensure the safety of everyone on the unit. The team approaches in a unified manner, and explains that they are there to help and will not allow the patient to harm anyone. This convergence of several professionals also conveys a message of determination to take control of an uncontrolled situation. On occasion, this action may be sufficient to de-escalate the patient's behavior to a manageable level. If not, the team may restrain the patient at both wrists and ankles to a bed. A waist restraint may be added if needed. Restraints are snug enough so that the patient cannot slip them off, but loose enough so as not to impede circulation. Within one hour of this action, the nurse obtains an order for restraint and a physician will assess the patient in person.

Health care professionals around the world have participated in CPI education to learn these proven strategies for safely resolving situations when confronted by anxious, hostile, or violent behaviors, while still maintaining the therapeutic relationships with those in their care.

Seclusion may also be used to diminish agitation and external stimulation. The room is locked for the safety of the patient, staff, and other patients on the unit. The patient is continuously monitored through a window or video monitor. Any patient who is placed in seclusion or restraints retains basic personal rights. The patient's physical and emotional well-being are carefully monitored. If any injuries were sustained in the take-down, the patient receives prompt first aid. Medications are administered as ordered, and vital signs are taken. Staff members remove the restraints at specified intervals to allow range of motion and change of position. As indicated, patients receive hydration and nutrition, and are given the opportunity for normal elimination.

The Joint Commission (JC), formerly the Joint Commission on Accreditation of Health care Organizations (JCAHO) has established restraint and seclusion standards, and revises them on an ongoing basis. As of July 1, 2009, currents standards include the following:

- A restraint order that is being used for violent or self-destructive behavior has a definite time limit associated with it (see Standard PC.03.05.05, EP4).
- Unless state law is more restrictive, orders for the use of restraint or seclusion for the management of violent or self-destructive behavior that jeopardizes the immediate physical safety of the patient, staff, or others may be renewed within the following limits:
  - 4 hours for adults 18 years of age or older
  - 2 hours for children and adolescents, 9 to 17 years of age
  - 1 hour for children under 9 years of age
  - Orders may be renewed according to the time limits for a maximum of 24 consecutive hours

  The Joint Commission mandates go on to state:
- The physician or licensed independent practitioner evaluates the patient in person within one hour of the initiation of the restraints.
- A registered nurse or a physician assistant may conduct the in-person evaluation within one hour of the initiation of restraint or seclusion if this person is trained in accordance with requirements in Standard PC.03.05.17, EP3.

- If the one-hour face-to-face evaluation is completed by a trained nurse or trained physician assistant, he or she would consult with the attending physician or other licensed independent practitioner responsible for the care of the patient after the evaluation, as determined by hospital policy (PC.03.05.11 EP2).

Some states may have statute or regulation requirements that are more restrictive than the requirements in this standard. PMHNs are required to adhere to the most stringent of the standards. To ensure patient and staff safety, PMHNs should be educated about restraint and seclusion policies and procedures. Ongoing assessment and respectful care throughout its duration, including frequent monitoring of vital signs, cardiorespiratory status, skin status, hydration, elimination, and privacy are essential (Winship, 2006). Patients are visually observed either continuously or every 10 to 15 minutes, per institution policy.

Despite strict regulations, both adults and children can be injured during restraint and seclusion. There are numerous documented instances of injuries and even deaths resulting from inappropriate actions taken by the restrainers and secluders. A Government Accountability Office (GAO) study found:

> ...hundreds of cases of alleged abuse and death related to the use of these methods on school children during the past two decades. Examples of these cases include a 7 year old purportedly dying after being held face down for hours, 5 year olds allegedly being tied to chairs with bungee cords and duct tape and suffering broken arms and bloody noses, and a 13 year old reportedly hanging himself in a seclusion room after prolonged confinement. (GAO-090719T, May 19, 2009)

*If restraints are used, they must be applied so that circulation is not restricted and the patient cannot slip out of them. Ongoing monitoring is necessary to ensure the patient's safety.*

## NURSING RESPONSIBILITIES

Nurses are legally responsible to protect the private health information of all patients through federal laws and through regulations subscribed by the State Board of Examiners for Nursing of the state in which they practice. These laws and rules protect the rights of all patients. Patients with mental health problems and those with substance abuse issues have even more rules to protect their privacy. Thus, PMHNs need to be ever vigilant in providing care that adheres to these ethical and legal principles.

## Confidentiality

As with all patients, confidentiality is a priority. However, because PMHNs communicate with patients in an intensely personal way, maintaining confidentiality of the patient's private thoughts and feelings is essential when establishing a therapeutic nurse-client relationship. Doing so establishes trust and rapport necessary to proceed. The communication is protected by law and also by the ethical concept of non-disclosure. It is an ethical breach of confidentiality to disclose or share patient information without permission. For example, it would be an ethical breach to share medical information with a patient's adult child unless the nurse obtained permission from the patient (Abma, 2008).

The U.S. federal government enacted the Health Insurance Portability and Accountability Act of 1996 (HIPAA). Part of this legislation provides legal protection to privacy and confidentiality of patient information. Patients must give written permission for release of records that deal with psychiatric-mental health treatment. The patient also must agree to exactly what part of the medical record will be released, the purpose for sharing the information, and who will have access to the information.

However, there are also laws that protect members of society from unsafe actions by people with illnesses that affect behavior. Nursing professionals may, in certain instances, be legally required to break confidentiality and disclose information without the patient's permission. An example of this is a patient disclosing to the home-care PMHN about a plan to shoot the mailman when he makes his next delivery. When there are clear threats of other-directed violence, the nurse is legally required to report the threat to authorities. This is sometimes known as a mandate to inform, or the Tarasoff decision. This court case (*Tarasoff vs. Regents of the University of California*) involved a college student who shared his obsession about another student, Tatiana Tarasoff, with a university psychologist. The college student then proceeded to murder Ms. Tarasoff. The ultimate ruling was that mental health professionals are responsible to exercise reasonable care in protecting potential victims of patients' violent intentions (Borum & Reddy, 2001).

> *Maintaining confidentiality is a priority. However, if a patient clearly threatens violence to another, a nurse is legally responsible to report this information.*

## Legal Liability

As with other practice areas, psychiatric-mental health care can pose legal liability for PMHNs. However, PMHNs can avoid legal liability by adhering to standards of nursing practice and by practicing within the appropriate scope of practice. Malpractice, which includes practicing outside the scope and standards of psychiatric-mental health nursing, can result from unprofessional behaviors. Inappropriately sharing confidential patient information can lead to breach of confidentiality or defamation of character lawsuits. If the breach is oral, slander occurs; if the breach is written, libel occurs.

In addition, psychiatric-mental health nursing differs from other forms of nursing in the degree of personal touch between nurse and patient. If a mentally ill patient is touched without his or her permission other than for routine nursing care, the nurse may be charged with medical battery. If the nurse indicates intent to touch the patient without permission, a charge of assault may be made.

The majority of mental health patients voluntarily seek admission and treatment. These individuals sign consents for treatment, which is considered a contract for care for which PMHNs provide an important component. PMHNs can reduce the risk for legal liability by adhering to the highest standards of nursing practice while simultaneously advocating for the patient.

## SUMMARY POINTS

- Ethical theories and principles used in ethical decision making include: utilitarianism, Kantianism, autonomy, beneficence, non-maleficence, justice, veracity, and fidelity.

- When faced with an ethical dilemma, the PMHN applies the ethical principles and theories integrating the nursing process and the therapeutic nurse-patient relationship to arrive at an ethical decision.

- A Bill of Rights for mental health patients has been established to protect the rights of patients who might be unable to speak for themselves.

- Psychiatric-mental health patients may be admitted for inpatient treatment voluntarily or involuntarily (against his or her wishes).

- Competency is a legal determination and typically involves the degree to which a patient has the cognitive abilities to understand and process information. It is essential for consent and the right to self-determination.

- Every psychiatric-mental health patient has the right to treatment in the least restrictive environment.

- When a patient requires restraints, a physician's order must be obtained within one hour of initiating the restraints.

- Communication between a PMHN and a psychiatric-mental health patient is protected by law and the concept of non-disclosure. It is an ethical breach to disclose or share patient information without the patient's permission. However, if there is clear threat of violence to another, the nurse is legally required to breach confidentiality and report the information.

- A PMHN can be charged with medical battery if he or she touches a mentally ill patient without his or permission for other than routine nursing care. He or she may be charged with assault if there is an intent to touch the patient without permission.

## NCLEX-PREP*

1. A group of nursing students are reviewing ethical principles and theories. They demonstrate understanding of the information when they identify utilitarianism as which of the following?

   a. Honesty
   b. Fair and equal treatment
   c. Doing no harm
   d. Greater good

2. A PMHN is engaged in advocacy for patients of a local clinic. The nurse is employing which ethical principle?

   a. Beneficence
   b. Fidelity

   c. Kantianism
   d. Veracity

3. Which of the following patients would be least likely to require involuntary commitment?

   a. Patient convicted of substance abuse required to undergo treatment
   b. Patient who is actively experiencing suicidal ideation
   c. Patient with depression who is in need of treatment
   d. Patient deteriorating from a severe, persistent mental illness

*(cont.)*

## NCLEX-PREP* (*CONT.*)

4. The following are examples of therapy that may be used with a patient experiencing a psychiatric-mental health problem. Place the treatments in the proper order based on the concept of the least restrictive environment.
   a. Talk therapy
   b. Involuntary medication administration
   c. Behavioral therapy
   d. Seclusion

5. A situation with a patient is escalating and the staff determines that restraints are necessary. Which of the following would occur first?
   a. Explaining that the staff is there to help

   b. Approaching the patient slowly as a unit
   c. Taking down the patient to apply the restraints
   d. Obtaining an order for the restraints

6. A nurse breaches a patient's confidentiality and shares this confidential information in writing. The nurse would most likely be charged with which of the following?
   a. Slander
   b. Medical battery
   c. Libel
   d. Assault

*Answers to these questions appear on page 639.

## REFERENCES

Abma, T.A. (2008) Dialogical nursing ethics: the quality of freedom restrictions. *Nursing Ethics* 15(6): 789–802.

American Nurses Association. *Code of Ethics for Nurses with Interpretive Statements.* Silver Spring, MD: American Nurses Publishing, 2001. Available at: http://www.nursingworld.org/MainMenuCategories/EthicsStandards/CodeofEthicsforNurses.aspx

Borum R., & Reddy, M. (2001). Assessing violence risk in Tarasoff situations. *Behavioral Science and the Law, 19:3,* 375–386.

Center for Mental Health Services. (2009). *Advocacy Unlimited, Inc.* Retrieved from http://www.mindlink.org/rights.html. Retrieved February 2, 2010.

Chitty, K. (2005) *Professional Nursing Concepts and Challenges, fourth edition.* St. Louis, MO: Elsevier.

Crisis Prevention Institute. (2011). *Crisisprevention.com.* Retrieved from http://www.crisisprevention.com/About-CPI

Current Nursing. (2009). *Nursing theories: A companion to nursing theories and models.* Retrieved from: http://currentnursing.com/nursing_theory/application_Peplau's_interpersonal_theory.html

Grigg, M. (2009). Eliminating seclusion and restraint in Australia. *International Journal of Mental Helath Nursing, 15,* 224–225.

Heitman, E. (1992) The Patient Self-Determination Act and public assessment of end-of-life technology; International Society of Technology Assessment in Health Care. Meeting. *Abstr Int Soc Technol Assess Health Care Meet.* 1992;10. University of Texas, Health Science Center, Houston 77225 http://icn.ch/ethics.htm. Retrieved April 13, 2009.

Joint Commission. (2010). *National patient safety goals.* Retrieved from: http://www.jointcommission.org/AccreditationPrograms/Hospitals/Standards/09_FAQs/PC/Restraint+_Seclusion+For+Hospitals+That+Use+The+Joint+Commission+For+Deemed+Status+Purposes.htm. Retrieved 12/02/09.

Lachman, V. D. (2008). Ethical choices: Weighing obligations & virtues. *Nursing, 38*(10), 43–46.

Lightner, D.L.(1999). *Asylum prison and poorhouse: The writings and reform work of Dorothea Dix in Illinois.* Carbondale IL: Southern Illinois University Press.

Moylan, L.B. (2009) Physical restraint in acute care psychiatry. *Journal of Psychosocial Nursing, 47,* 41–47.

Partners in Information Access for the Public Health Workforce. (2009). *Mental health and mental disorders.* Retrieved from http://phpartners.org/hp/mentalhealthandmentaldisorders.html

Substance Abuse and Mental Health Services Administration. (2010). Mental Health, United States, 2008. HHS Publication No. (SMA) 10-4590, Rockville, MD: Center for Mental Health Services, Substance Abuse and Mental Health Services Administration.

Skott, C. (2003). Storied ethics: Conversations in nursing care. *Nursing Ethics, 10:* 368–76.

U.S. Department of Health and Human Services. (2000). *Healthy People 2010 (2nd edition).* Washington, DC: U.S. Government Printing Office.

U.S. Department of Health and Human Services. (2010). *Healthy People 2020.* Retrieved from http://www.healthypeople.gov/Document/HTML/Volume2/18Mental.htm# Toc486932690

United States Government Accountability Office. Seclusions and Restraints: Selected Cases of Death and Abuse as Public and Private Schools and Treatment Centers, GAO-09-719T (May 19, 2009). Available at: http://www.gao.gov/products/GAO-09-719T

Winship, G. (2006). Further thoughts on the process of restraint. *Journal of Psychiatric and Mental Health Nursing, 13,* 55–60.

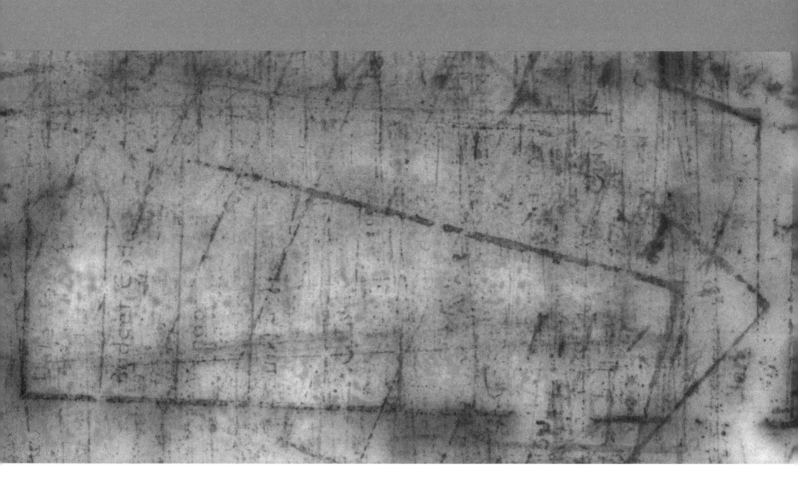

## CHAPTER CONTENTS

## CHAPTER 29

# POLICY, POLICY MAKING, AND POLITICS FOR PROFESSIONAL PSYCHIATRIC NURSES

Shirley A. Smoyak

## EXPECTED LEARNING OUTCOMES

**After completing this chapter, the student will be able to:**

1. Demonstrate understanding of key terms related to political forces affecting health care.
2. Describe how health care policy is made.
3. Identify milestones in policy impacting undergraduate nursing curricula.
4. Delineate current issues affecting psychiatric nursing education.

## KEY TERMS

Lobbying

Policy

Policy making

Political action

Politics

Policy, policy making, politics and politicians are all derived from the Greek word for cities, *polis*, which was used roughly from 800 to 400 B.C. These ancient Greek city-states were organized by individuals who had agreed upon principles and rules by which they wish to be governed. Our modern word—metropolis—has that meaning embedded.

Mason, Leavitt, and Chaffee (2002), in defining "politics" in the introductory chapter to their book *Policy & Politics in Nursing and Health Care*, point out that "Few words elicit the emotional response that the word *politics* does" (p. 9). Politics has become associated with negative images, which have very personal associations. For some, it is synonymous with shady deals, secrecy, favoritism, corruption, buying votes, and paying off debts incurred by prior favors and deals. Yet politics need not have these negative connotations. Seen more neutrally, **POLITICS** simply means the process of influencing the allocation of scarce resources, whether these are time, money, energy, services, and so on.

*Influencing* means using one's persuasive powers. Nurses do the work of influencing as part of their daily tasks. In fact, psychiatric nursing might be defined as influencing people to change their views, consider new options, have new perspectives, and open their minds to new ideas. The essence of psychotherapy is introducing new ideas and options to replace paranoia, delusional thinking, or depression.

*Allocation*, another key word, means making decisions about how resources, particularly when they are scarce or in short supply, should be divided or shared. Organizing one's work, in the short term or for longer periods, requires allocating how personal energy will be spent. People who manage to meet their daily goals usually have spent time making lists of what to do or specifying their priorities. As new demands arise, these lists can be adjusted. Values, personal preferences and beliefs, religious views, and previous experiences all are factored into these decision equations.

## AN OVERVIEW OF HOW POLICY IS MADE

*Policy* can have multiple meanings, depending on the situation. When individuals refer to personal policies, they mean the principles by which they choose to live and work. These personal rules are sometimes difficult to discern because they may not have been articulated. For instance, most people cannot easily say how they learned to be kind, polite, or helpful to babies and elders other than by watching and imitating what others did. Nor can they easily figure out how racism or sexism may have become a part of their "nature." The essence of family therapy is to help all family members bring into awareness what these personal policies are and where they came from. The question that family therapists suggest for persons in their care to contemplate very seriously is: "Who has the right to do what to whom under what circumstances?" Mulling this over, and finding words to express the answer, sheds light on personal policies, which often are in conflict.

**POLICY** in institutions, agencies and governments, is the sets of rules, guidelines, procedures, and processes that allow workers or officials to know how to go about conducting their daily tasks. Policies determine what to do or not to do when allocating scarce resources, when deciding who goes first, when conducting elections for officers, when deciding who or what gets excluded, when making appointments to positions, or when firing someone. Much of the work in governments at any level is policy related, taking the form of statutes or laws.

**POLITICAL ACTION** is accomplished by people organizing themselves into a group to influence others to make changes. **POLICY MAKING** is a broad term, which embodies all the processes in political action. However, policy making may also occur on a smaller level as within a family or a hospital unit.

> *Political action is accomplished by a group of people organizing themselves to influence others to make changes.*

**LOBBYING** is any action undertaken by an individual or group to influence the thinking and decision making (e.g., voting on a bill) of an elected official at any level of government. The term was derived in the early days of this country when activist citizens waited in the *lobby* of Congress to confront the people they had elected to office. The word remained in use through the years. Today *lobbyist* generally refers to a person who is paid by an organization to do lobbying work for them. The best lobbying is done person-to-person, with live interaction. With today's technology, lobbying sometimes is done by email to specific officials, or by posts to blogs or web sites.

Policies, policy making, and politics are generally understood as taking place within larger systems, even entire countries. Yet they can also occur in much smaller systems.

Policy changes can occur in many ways, including taking individual actions on a local level within your own community or within institutions that provide services for you and family members.

A personal story clarifies one way in which I was able to help change hospital policy.

Standing policy at the hospital where my daughter was born dictated that, even if babies were being nursed, they had to be returned to their cribs in a central nursery with all the bottle-fed babies. Rooming-in, allowing mothers to have the babies' cribs in their own rooms, was a relatively new idea and had only been adopted by a few hospitals. Late the second night after my daughter was born I wandered over to the nursery and saw that she had a bottle propped in her mouth. I was furious! I entered the nursery, ignoring the nurses' shouts that I was not allowed there, and moved my baby and her crib to my room. Thus rooming-in came to be at this hospital. The crib could not be returned to the nursery because it was contaminated. Proper policy change took a few more weeks to be put into place.

Another personal example of a policy change took place at a county psychiatric hospital in the early 1970s. I was an instructor on an acute care unit with about 50 male patients; there were 10 undergraduate senior nursing students in my class. My challenge to these students was this: "During this semester, design a plan and carry it to completion with the individual patient to whom you are assigned, or the group with whom you are working." Each student would earn an A if the patient *collaborated* (not cooperated) in the plan and it met with success. Voting in the Presidential election was targeted as the situation for which a plan was to be designed; 7 of the 10 students and their patients collaborated. This idea was generated because of a lecture in which I had explained that being admitted to a mental hospital, even involuntarily, did not remove one's right as a citizen to vote. How "incompetence" was adjudicated was part of the lecture.

During the month of October, each of the 7 students arranged a visit to the municipal records hall of the town in which the patient had resided before admission. The clerk was contacted beforehand to inform him or her of the reason for the visit—to establish residency and therefore voting registration for the patients. In several instances, where the landlord had rented the patients old apartment because the patient had been hospitalized for years, letters had to be written and notarized, attesting to residency. For those patients who had lived with families, their relatives wrote letters. On Election Day, all patients received day passes and I borrowed a 15-passenger university van to transport them to the voting place. As a result, a new hospital policy was adopted: All patients would be reminded of their citizens' rights on admission and by posters displayed on the wards. The students' evaluation of this assignment was that it was well worth the effort, but that they had no idea how complex voting could be.

The following spring, a new group of ten students designed another project that resulted in a policy change. There was a new indoor pool at the county hospital, but patients had yet to use it. A collaborative effort was required to change this situation, including: (1) gaining benefactors to supply bathing trunks and large towels; (2) renewing Red Cross Life Guard certifications; (3) convincing the hospital to "staff" the pool with male aides for at least two hours a day; (4) and convincing the ward staff that we would take measures to ensure no patient would be able to run away. (Male aides were necessary because the students were all women and the patients were all men.)

The result: Patients began using the pool and the students learned the fine art of negotiating beyond the status quo mentality that they had encountered with staff. They also learned how important it was to fully document their plans and outcomes. Several patients also began to work on a "patient governance" committee, whcih would help to identify and resolve obvious issues.

## Theory Building and Policy Generation

Theory building and policy generation are very similar. Both start with an observation of repeated instances or situations that are puzzling or of processes that seem to be wrong or in need of repair. In rare instances, one glaring instance may jump-start a policy, such as in the newborn "rooming-in" example provided earlier.

> *Theory building and policy making are very similar processes.*

After making the observations, questioning begins: How could it be that way? Why is it so? If theory building is the path taken, then the scientist designs a study. Observations are analyzed and taken apart, and re-named as variables, which are then assigned instruments for measurement. Analyses and findings follow. Reports of the conclusions are published. Policymakers, on the other hand, move in the direction of producing rules aimed at fixing the perceived problem. Policymakers in institutions and agencies must convince their boards or trustees that change is needed. Policymakers who are government officials must convince their constituencies. Politicians must convince their party bosses, and ultimately the voters who place them in office.

Professional associations are also in the business of generating policies for their governance and also for the public they serve. In fact, association missions can be seen as policy statements. The American Nurses Association (ANA) exists to serve not only registered nurses, but also the patients for whom they care. Only nurses may be members and some states have different levels of membership. The National League for Nursing (NLN) exists because its mission or policy is to ensure excellent education for nurses. Non-nurses may be members of the NLN. The American Psychiatric Nurses' Association (APNA) exists because the specialty, psychiatric and mental health nursing, was not the chief focus and concern of either the ANA or the NLN. Other specialty nurses' associations for critical care, occupational health, and oncology had already been organized.

## Nursing's Political Roots

Ehrenreich and English (2010) in their classic *Witches, Midwives & Nurses* (2010), eloquently point out that women have been persecuted not because of wrongdoings, errors, malfeasance, meanness, or acts of violence, but because they have done very good things, and in so doing, have frightened men. Women discovered that foxglove was a source of digitalis that could help patients with heart problems. Midwives used natural ergot to prevent post-partum bleeding. In Ehrenreich and English's view, the profit-driven, fragmented, deeply inequitable health care system has evolved because of the relatively powerless status of nursing. Of course, nursing's status has been orchestrated for hundreds of years by men of all professions, eventually primarily medicine. Before male physicians dominated the health care scene, there was a long tradition of female lay healing, with roots in Europe and Africa. Early American lay healers were autonomous and functioned independently. Their positions as healers were often connected to the leadership in their communities. Examples are Harriet Tubman, a healer, who led slaves to freedom via well-hidden underground railroads. Later, Anne Hutchinson, a midwife and a religious dissident, fled Massachusetts and helped to found Rhode Island. Still later, Wilma Scott Heide, a nurse, started the National Organization for Women (NOW). Ehrenreich

and English's straightforward approach to making her points should serve as a guide for new political activists.

Florence Nightingale's lessons on how to institute policy change are well-recognized within the nursing profession. Many nurses do not realize, however, that she was a psychiatric nurse. When visiting the Nightingale Museum at St. Thomas Hospital in London, England, several years ago, the docent asked if there were questions. I asked, "Was Florence Nightingale a psychiatric nurse?" He did not know the answer, but invited me to examine their newly digitized archives. I discovered that "lunatic," "insane," and "idiot" yielded letters and reports she had written, documenting her work with people who were mentally ill. In these cases, she influenced change in the way these individuals were being treated and, in several instances, where they were cared for.

> *Florence Nightingale not only influenced change in hospital systems but also in how the mentally ill were cared for.*

## IDEOLOGIES, FACTS, AND POLITICS

As part of a theory building course I emphasized the idea that facts were simply facts and nothing more. Then I would add that: "To go beyond facts, theories are necessary to give them voices." Next, I would have the students name some facts, choosing ones that were disturbing (e.g., only 2% of RNs are men; minorities represented in nursing do not match the percentage of minorities in the general population). Next students would be challenged to generate testable theories about those facts.

Ideologies are like facts. We need good policies and politics to change these ideologies.

**Fact:** *American health care policy is different from health policy in other industrial nations.*

The reason that the United States has no national health care plan is that self-interest dominates political decision making. In fact, unabashed self-interest is what many foreigners notice first about the U.S. health care system (Monroe, 2005). And although there have been attempts at policy change, these attempts have not met with success because the powerful medical and pharmaceutical industries and their related hospital associations and insurers use millions of dollars to get the votes to elect the legislators to keep the status quo.

**Fact:** *Citizens and politicians in the United States have not generated a consensus on what direction health policy making should take.*

Individuals and political parties do not agree on how much personal versus government responsibility there should be. Should individual people regulate their health behavior in all matters? Who should pay when the outcome is illness caused by smoking, illegal drug use, or obesity? Individual fault versus social causation can be framed as sets of facts, but arguments about policy have not been resolved.

Taking an economic perspective suggests three important questions: (1) How much? (2) Who pays? (3) Who benefits?

**Fact:** *Individual nurses and physicians collaborate well on a daily basis, particularly in relation to the clinical care of patients. Professional politics between the overwhelmingly powerful medical associations and less powerful nursing groups continues.*

As far back as the 1970s, the American Medical Association (AMA) and the American Nurses Association (ANA) attempted to change the domination of medicine and the disparities in positive regard and income encountered by nurses. Their very successful campaigns, conferences, and publications ultimately ceased because the AMA withdrew funding, and no longer supported physicians to attend joint meetings. An instructive history of this National Joint Practice Commission (NJPC) is described thoroughly by Fairman in her 2008 book *Making Room in the Clinic: Nurse Practitioners and the Evolution of Modern Health Care.*

Fairman further captures the history of many attempts by nurses to gain a prominent place in health care, devoting an entire chapter—"Coming Together, Breaking Apart"—on the history and politics of the NJPC. She notes several factors as precipitating causes of a sense of competition felt by physicians, such as the rise of the nurse practitioner movement and the enhanced voice of nurse clinicians.

The NJPC ceased to exist by 1979, joint practice committees at local and state levels were formed and continue to function. An example is the Fairview University Medical Center (FUMC), which established a joint practice committee in 1998. According to Disch and Taranto (2002), its purpose was "to provide an interdisciplinary forum to discuss patient care issues, barriers to change and to recommend policy changes related to those issues which cross departmental and disciplinary lines at FUMC" (p. 340). The last part of this mission statement clearly addresses the systems question: "Who has the right to do what to whom under what circumstances?" (Smoyak, 1990).

**Fact:** *Psychiatric hospitals, both public and private, were managed first by physicians as superintendents and later by professionally trained administrators.*

In the 1970s, administrative practices and policies came under close scrutiny by young lawyers, eager to correct the injustices suffered by involuntarily committed patients who remained on locked wards for decades. Deinstitutionalization had theoretically been put into place by new federal incentives in the prior decade. Yet most psychiatric hospitals were very slow to move their residents either to designated places in the community or simply to release them.

Legal cases such as *Wyatt v. Stickney* (1970) illustrate the manner in which changes can be made through litigation. *Wyatt v. Stickney* is the most well-known case in which a hospital was ordered to release patients unless they were provided with therapy. Many similar cases were brought to state and federal courts in that decade and into the 1980s. Another case, *Doe v. Klein* (Doe for all patients at Greystone Park Psychiatric Hospital in New Jersey and Klein for the Commissioner of Health at the time), lasted the longest, from 1977 until 2009. Here, court-ordered monitors functioned to ensure that the hospital's policies and practices were changed to facilitate improved care and treatment for patients—a dramatic change in the bureaucratic status quo. Monitors included a psychiatric nurse, (Smoyak), a psychologist, a social worker, a former patient, and several community members with family concerns.

## The Politics of Communication

Any dimension of politics, political activism, or policy-making requires communication—verbal, gestural, and written. Direct practice, rather than simulations or listening to lectures or reading articles, is the preferred way to learn the skills in communicating to influence others. The messages and inputs received by students as they learn the interviewing process are the bedrock to improving verbal skills.

It is important to acknowledge that historically women and nurses had been socialized to be deferent to men, and their ways of communicating reflected this. When the Women's Movement gained the attention of nurses in the 1970s, nurses began to recognize how they communicated, and that the ways they communicated with men and women should be re-thought. At the time, after I had done several workshops on confrontation (what it was and how it proceeded), I was invited by the editors of the *American Journal of Nursing* to write an article on the topic. The article states: "...confrontation is known as a tactic in the larger game of power politics, a strategy for conflict resolution" (Smoyak, 1974, p. 1632). Confrontation as a strategy had not been "thinkable" previously by nurses. Steps of the confrontation process involve: (1) doing the homework by getting the facts straight and pre-planning; (2) staying at the system level to state the issue and make compelling points; and (3) strengthening the new perspectives or images presented and repeating the desired messages following the confrontation.

New audiences must be considered as communication strategies are developed. The workplace or classroom is obviously where most encounters happen. However, if becoming more politically active has become a priority, then a new list of places for encounters is needed. Visits to elected officials with specific messages in mind is an important place to begin.

Challenging the normative order goes hand in glove with confrontation. "One cannot be a nurse without being a philosopher and an ethicist at the same time" (Smoyak, 1985). This statement, which appeared in an article titled: "Have You Questioned Authority Today?," does not suggest that authority should be challenged as a routine practice, but rather that nurses should not go along with unfair rules or unsafe practices.

## Federal Legislators, New Laws, and Health Policies

Health policy concerns remain central in state and federal public policy arenas. How responsibility is shifted from the federal level to the states is a topic that analysts have grappled with and written about for more than a half century. During the period of deinstitutionalization in the 1960s, the federal government acted at local levels bypassing state budgets. Funds went directly to local community mental health centers. This money route, which lasted less than a decade, was replaced by block grants, with federal funds allocated to states for their decision making about distribution. This long and involved health policy change was a very political, complex, and emotional process. Imagine the difficulty experienced by administrators and researchers in local mental health facilities as they tried to determine to whom to write grants and how to understand the process of securing funds for programs.

Public opinion polls in the early 1990s documented the American public's frustration and anger with the rising costs of health care, the growing inaccessibility of services, and the simultaneous increase in taxes. The consensus was that the entire health care system was broken and needed to be rebuilt. This was the climate that led then President Clinton in 1993 to propose major health care reform by introducing the Health Care Security Act. The story of the subsequent political and policy battles filled newspapers, journals, and scientific media in economics, political science, and public administration. The outcome was the ultimate rejection of the Clinton plan. Powerful stakeholders, such as business and insurance industries, were still left to face two valid concerns: inadequate access to care by the millions of uninsured and underinsured Americans and the continuing rise of health care costs.

Wakefield, Gardner, and Guillet (2002) note that Congress, while reluctant to embrace any sweeping changes after the political backlash against the Clinton plan, "preferred smaller, politically acceptable changes, including enactment of the Health Insurance Portability and Accountability Act (HIPPA) and the State Children's Health Insurance Plan (S-CHIP)" (p. 421). They go on to say, "Meanwhile, in the vacuum left by the failure of comprehensive national reform, all states enacted legislation that incrementally improved access while containing costs" (p. 421). The unintended consequences of the regulations evolving from HIPAA have been many. For example, HIPAA has impacted not only the domains of privacy within health care establishments, but also in places like banks, who no longer share data within households or family systems.

Continuing health policy issues include areas such as Medicare, genetics, long-term care, the uninsured, and health care quality in general. Our nation's most costly health care programs continue to be Medicare and Medicaid. The fact that this is a general concern of all citizens is documented by almost daily editorials and public opinion pieces warning that federal dollars will not be able to keep up with the rising costs. Demographic trends are noted and quoted repeatedly: "Whereas 9% of the population was 65 and older in 1960 this number will be increased to 20% in 2030" (Wakefield et al., 2002, p. 422) The retirement of baby boom generation, which began in 2010 when the oldest of that cohort reached 65, will continue to swell the demands on Medicare and Medicaid.

Prescription drug benefits are central in the debate about the fair price of drugs and the inability of elders and others on fixed incomes to afford them. Some health care insurance companies have dropped these benefits as part of their plans; others have increased co-pays. Debates about generic versus trade-name drugs continue.

Genetic testing is a relatively new term on the health care scene. It refers to testing or screening for diseases that may be inherited and other diseases to possibly yield an early diagnosis. Some of these diseases may or may not have treatment available. To complete the map of deoxyribonucleic acid (DNA) was a scientific triumph. Yet its success as a technology has not been established. Genetic screening can be done effectively for a very few, rare diseases.

Another highly visible and controversial issue is the matter of stem cells, including embryonic, embryonic germ, and adult cells. Religious values are at the root of this issue, since some religious beliefs are that life begins at the moment of conception. In these religious views the use of embryonic cells, even those that are scheduled for destruction in cell banks because they are outdated, would be equivalent to causing the death of a human being.

Long-term care costs and accessibility of placements are fueled as issues because of the coming of age of the baby boomers. Those with adequate retirement plans have more choices than those living at or below poverty levels. The increasing popularity of assisted living options, for the most part, is available only for those with personal resources.

One of Henry Kissinger's famous quotes is an apt summary to include in this chapter on legislators, laws, and politics: "A frustrating paradox is faced by policymakers: When their scope for action is widest, their knowledge is often minimal, and when their knowledge is greatest, their scope for action has frequently disappeared" (Kissinger, 1998, p. 15).

## LEGISLATION, LAW, AND REGULATIONS

Nurses can only influence legislative and regulatory processes if they understand how the game is played in specific sectors. Becoming involved with the units of state nurses associations who work with legislators to design bills should be a part of every nurse's personal and professional agenda. State nurses associations work with boards of nursing, tracking how nurses and their licenses are monitored. Students in nursing and nurses at all levels should become involved with both state nurses associations and boards of nursing. It is easy to join a state nurses association. Appointments to boards of nursing are usually done by governors of states; most have a public portion during their meetings.

*All nurses, regardless of their preparation, can become politically active and influence legislative and regulatory processes if they understand how the game is played in specific sectors.*

All nurses should know how a bill becomes a law. Also within their knowledge set should be the roles and jurisdictions of the United States president, senators, representatives, and federal Judges as well as the key governing officers at the state and local levels.

Many nurses associations have political action committees that are tuned into the issues on the forefront of health care policy. They are the association fundraisers for political action. Because of the nature of their work—influencing politicians—it is important to understand what networks are developed and how their relationships with politicians are managed.

Among the controversial issues addressed are programs to handle the problems with nurses losing their licenses for substance abuse, including for example, drinking on the job, diverting or stealing drugs, and other such offenses. Another is whether or not nurses should be involved with needle-exchange programs (clean needles for intravenous drug users). States also have enacted laws and regulations about safe practices, such as the number of continuous hours worked by nurses. Advanced practice nurses, who have prescriptive authority, are regulated in many different ways depending on where they practice. Whether or not, and where, nurses can pronounce death is also regulated.

Lorette and Jansto provided a personal vignette, "How Regulations are Shaped: The Rules of the Game," for the book by Mason et al. (2002) that is well-worth reading. Their opening statement summarizes their story: "The successful passage of a piece of legislation is almost always a cause for celebration among those responsible for its development and implementation. A bill becoming law represents the culmination of many months, sometimes years, of intense research, lobbying, fundraising, and grassroots efforts to obtain support for the bill's underlying concept" (p. 467). While the bill's passage is the end of a long and intense effort, it truly is just a beginning. Next comes the hard work of designing regulations and securing funding for the work that has to be done to put life into the law. A law without regulations is like a report that is filed on a shelf, and never read or used. Equally so, the entire business of oversight and regulatory provisions is another political arena.

The New Jersey *Doe v. Klein* court-appointed committee mentioned previously is an example of the judicial system taking over what is normally a health care administrative role. Betts and Keepnews (2002) give further examples of why courts are important for nurses and their work. One of their very important statements is this: "Nurses should not regard the legal system as the exclusive domain of lawyers and judges any more than they regard the legislative process as the exclusive domain of legislators and lobbyists" (p. 471).

The courts are an important forum or arena for nurses to advocate for themselves, as well as their patients. Nurses must learn to be their own advocates, paying attention to how courts will interpret and act on laws passed by the legislative sector. History has shown that no external advocacy body will do this work for nurses; there are no guardian angels or fairy godmothers out there.

The legal and judicial systems are arenas in which people have traditionally sought vindication of their rights. Courts have acted to test, affirm, or invalidate legislative laws and administrative rules stemming from the laws. Courts have ruled about when, where, and how employees can bargain collectively and when they can strike or actively protest within clinical settings. Courts also adjudicate issues with professional licenses, scopes of practice, antitrust laws, and accusations of one profession encroaching on another's jurisdiction.

Nurses should know that the United States has two major parallel court systems, federal and state. The jurisdiction of the federal courts concerns matters that involve the U.S. Constitution, federal legislation, and regulation and rights conferred under federal law. They can also hear cases when the issue has come before the courts in two different states. District courts are the entry point for most federal cases; there are 94 such courts throughout the states and territories. The court of last resort for federal cases is the U.S. Supreme Court (Betts & Keepnews, 2002).

States rights prevail when it comes to court systems, with each state having its own determination of what kinds of cases to hear. Generally, there are trial level and appellate divisions, and a high court, used as a last resort. Within the state system are rules for what types of courts there can be at municipal or county levels, and what kinds of cases they can hear. Within these courts, there are usually family, probate, and drug courts. Other divisions are civil and criminal.

Betts and Keepnews (2002) explain how impact legislation has evolved and resulted in establishing rights by affirming or clarifying rights previously established by the U.S. Constitution or a particular statute. A prominent and well-known impact legislation is *Brown v. Board of Education*. In 1954, the U.S. Supreme Court struck down school segregation and mandated that public schools desegregate their students. This case rested on the Equal Protection Clause of the 14th Amendment to the U.S. Constitution.

Another such case is *Roe v. Wade* (1973) in which the U.S. Supreme Court found that women had a right to the medical procedure of abortion during the first two trimesters of pregnancy. Although *Roe v. Wade* has been modified and narrowed in some respects by subsequent decisions, the basic right remains.

The U.S. Supreme Court has also been asked to convene over matters of assisted suicide and refusal of life-sustaining treatment. There are, as yet, no judicial outcomes at this level, but states' courts have become embroiled in these issues.

At the state level, courts have been used to enforce existing legislation. In 1992, the Alabama State Nurses Association and the Alabama Board of Nursing, with the support of the ANA, and the Emergency Nurses' Association, successfully sued local hospitals that were planning to hire technicians as staff to replace nurses in emergency departments. Nurses alleged that this would violate the existing Alabama Nurse Practice Act, since these technicians were neither educated nor licensed for such work. The nurse plaintiffs won, and the hospitals were forced to end this plan. Unlicensed assistive personnel (UAPs) have been the issue in several states, with the nurse group successfully limiting the UAP practice and having them supervised by nurses.

The fact that states have traditionally and historically guarded their rights has been noted. Specifically, states have maintained their rights to develop and maintain policies about all matters in health care, including how professional people will be licensed, what agencies and institutions will be accredited, and what taxes will be levied. The 50 different state governments are not united in how they regulate the work of advanced practice nurses, including prescriptive authority, how insurance for the poor will be provided, or how to manage home care for elderly and/or disabled persons. Under the era of Roosevelt's New Deal, the federal government exercised much more authority. Since then, a devolution of power has emerged, with states commanding more and more regulatory action.

While states differ regarding their operating rules, they all have a common leadership structure; state nurses' association are familiar with these nuances and differences, and keep track of how the legislative leaders shift and change. All states, except Nebraska, have two houses. Each house has a leader, elected from within the majority party. These leaders or chairs make the appointments to the various committees. The work of developing bills is done largely within these groups. Most states have at least one committee whose domain is largely health care; large states have several. All nurses should know how these health committees work, whether or not being more active is a part of the nurse's professional plans.

## Nurses in Congress

The Honorable Lois Capps is a nurse and a member of Congress. Her path to that seat was a very unusual one. Her husband, Walter Capps, was elected to the House of Representatives in 1996 and she followed him to Washington, D.C. He died of a sudden heart attack in October, 1997, and while she was still in grief and mourning for her husband she was approached to fill his seat (Copps, 2002, p. 534). She lists the many questions she had of herself, and others, and decided to become a member of Congress. She also says: "Nurses have credibility and respect. People trust us. Our professional knowledge enables us to advocate for safe, quality health care; promote education for children; and address other issues on patients' behalf....We need more nurses to become involved" (p. 535).

Another nurse, the Honorable Carolyn McCarthy, also has an unusual story on her route to Congress. She was a suburban Long Island homemaker and licensed practical nurse. In late 1993, her husband and son, riding on the Long Island Rail road returning home from work, were shot by a lone gunman. Her husband was killed and her son wounded. This triggered her interest in rules and regulations about guns and gun control. A complicated personal and political story includes her leaving the Republican party, becoming a Democrat, and winning a seat in Congress (McCarthy, 2002).

As of 2010 there are seven members of Congress who are nurses. Students may also find information regarding the Congressional Nursing Caucus of interest. You should know whether or not your town or your state has nurses as elected officials. This information is available from the state nurses association.

## THE FUTURE OF (PSYCHIATRIC) NURSING

As Editor of the *Journal of Psychosocial Nursing and Mental Health Services,* I wanted our readers to be aware of how our specialty was presented or described in the Institute of Medicine's (IOM) report "The Future of Nursing: Leading Change, Advancing Health" (2010). It reminded me of the 1970s and the National Joint Practice Commission (NJPC) whose mission was to improve collaboration between physicians and nurses and to address expanded practice for nurses. This section is based on key points I made in the journal article (Smoyak, 2011).

There are striking similarities between the IOM Report (2010) and the work of the NJPC. These are: the reluctance of physicians and the medical establishment to allow nurses to practice to their full capacity; the realization that health care would improve with re-aligned roles of physician and nurse; and the lack of adequate attention to the mental health needs of people of all ages and the skills and competencies of psychiatric nurses.

The three primary concerns targeted by health care reform are quality, access, and value. In fact, these concerns are woven into the descriptions of current and projected academic changes and delivery pattern modifications and more drastic re-structuring. No one could argue with the statements made about the need for seamless, coordinated care. The examples and case studies provided in the IOM Report are well done and deliver messages about how change happened in a specific place, with an enlightened provider or network. What is missing, however, is how these examples could become a wider reality, for example, in psychiatric services by psychiatric nurses across the nation.

The key messages in the IOM Report (2010) are highlighted in **Box 29-1**.

There are eight recommendations listed within the IOM Report (2010). These are as follows:

*Recommendation 1: Remove scope-of-practice barriers.* Advanced practice registered nurses should be able to practice to the full extent of their education and training. (p. 279).

*Recommendation 2: Expand opportunities for nurses to lead and diffuse collaborative improvement efforts.* Private and public funders, health care organizations, nursing

---

### BOX 29-1: THE FOUR KEY MESSAGES IN THE IOM (2010)

1. Nurses should practice to the full extent of their education and training.
2. Nurses should achieve higher levels of education and training through an improved education system that promotes seamless academic progression.
3. Nurses should be full partners with physicians and other health professionals in redesigning health care in the United States.
4. Effective workforce planning and policy making require better data collection and an improved information infrastructure.

education programs, and nursing associations should expand opportunities for nurses to lead and manage collaborative efforts with physicians and other members of the health care team to conduct research and to redesign and improve practice environments and health systems. These entities should also provide opportunities for nurses to diffuse successful practices. (p. 279).

*Recommendation 3: Implement nurse residency programs.* State boards of nursing, accrediting bodies, the federal government, and health care organizations should take actions to support nurses' completion of a transition-to-practice program (nurse residency) after they have completed a prelicensure or advanced practice degree program or when they are transitioning into new clinical practice areas. (p. 280).

*Recommendation 4: Increase the proportion of nurses with a baccalaureate degree to 80% by 2020.* Academic nurse leaders across all schools of nursing should work together to increase the proportion of nurses with a baccalaureate degree from 50% to 80% by 2020. These leaders should partner with education accrediting bodies, private and public funders, and employers to ensure funding, monitor progress, and increase the diversity of students to create a workforce prepared to meet the demands of diverse populations across the lifespan. (p. 280).

*Recommendation 5: Double the number of nurses with a doctorate by 2020.* Schools of nursing, with support from private and public funders, academic administrators and university trustees, and accrediting bodies, should double the number of nurses with a doctorate by 2020 to add to the cadre of nurse faculty and researchers, with attention to increasing diversity. (p. 281).

*Recommendation 6: Ensure that nurses engage in lifelong learning.* Accrediting bodies, schools of nursing, health care organizations, and continuing competency educators from multiple health professions should collaborate to ensure that nurses and nursing students and faculty continue their education and engage in lifelong learning to gain the competencies needed to provide care for diverse populations across the lifespan. (p. 282).

*Recommendation 7: Prepare and enable nurses to lead change to advance health.* Nurses, nursing education programs, and nursing associations should prepare the nursing workforce to assume leadership positions across all levels, while public, private, and governmental health care decision makers should ensure that leadership positions are available to and filled by nurses. (p. 283).

*Recommendation 8: Build an infrastructure for the collection and analysis of interprofessional health care workforce data.* The National Health Care Workforce Commission, with oversight from the Government Accountability Office and the Health Resources and Services Administration, should lead a collaborative effort to improve research and the collection and analysis of data on health care workforce requirements. The Workforce Commission and the Health Resources and Services Administration should collaborate with state licensing boards, state nursing workforce centers, and the Department of Labor in this effort to ensure that the data are timely and publicly accessible. (p. 284).

The IOM Report (2010) sets the tone for the gravity of the situation facing all of us in the business of delivering health care. The urgency to make changes quickly is certainly well-stated and repeated often. The plan for the future is that action groups will be constituted at the state level to move the key messages and recommendations to positive outcomes.

## THE FUTURE OF BACCALAUREATE EDUCATION FOR PSYCHIATRIC NURSES

The content of the psychiatric nursing examination questions within NCLEX is determined by sets of experts, many of whom are recent graduates practicing primarily in hospitals. There has been no study of how the various psychiatric nursing curricula in schools of nursing in the United States influence the NCLEX questions or how the examination influences what faculty choose to teach.

The American Association of Colleges of Nursing (AACN) has developed standards for professional nursing curricula (AACN, 2008) titled "The Essentials of Baccalaureate Education for Professional Nursing Practice." Their assumptions regarding the baccalaureate generalist nurse graduate are listed in **Box 29-2**.

Until recently there has not been a group of nurse educators, organized nationally, to address the matter of what should be taught at the baccalaureate level for psychiatric nursing. At the graduate level, however, there has been national interest and also funding. When the National Institute for Mental Health, (NIMH) was put into place by Congress in 1946, funds were allocated for yearly meetings of program directors at the master's

## BOX 29-2: AACN ESSENTIALS OF BACCALAUREATE EDUCATION FOR PROFESSIONAL NURSING

- Practice from a holistic, caring framework
- Practice from an evidence base
- Promote safe, quality patient care
- Use clinical/critical reasoning to address simple to complex situations
- Assume accountability for one's own and delegated nursing care
- Practice in a variety of health care settings
- Care for patients across the health-illness continuum
- Care for patients across the lifespan
- Care for diverse populations
- Engage in care of self in order to care for others
- Engage in continuous professional development

*From American Association of Colleges of Nursing. (October, 2008). The Essentials of Baccalaureate Education for Professional Nursing Practice. Washington, DC.*

level to come together to discuss how their programs were developing, and to share curricula ideas, along with recruitment and retention strategies. When federal funds were no longer available, a group of these directors organized themselves as the Society for Education and Research in Psychiatric Nursing (SERPN), a group that continues today.

There have been many subsequent efforts to determine the necessary content for basic psychiatric nursing practice. It was hoped that undergraduate education for psychiatric nursing would be given more attention when the American Psychiatric Nurses' Association (APNA) was formed 25 years ago. However, the APNA never had a formal infrastructure for educators. The most recent work is the collaboration of several psychiatric nursing groups, and the work is currently in progress, with the American Academy of Nursing (AAN) at the helm (AAN Expert Panel, "Essential Psychiatric, Mental Health and Substance Use Competencies for the Registered Nurse," 2010–2011). This document contains core competencies and related content areas for preparing nurses for basic psychiatric mental health and substance use practice.

## SUMMARY POINTS

- The professional activist nurse considers him- or herself as a professional agent of change (Ehrenreich & English, 2010). Thus, the new professional nurse goes beyond being an expert in clinical practice, and transforms into an activist, an advocate, a risk taker, a confronter, or a challenger of the status quo.

- The roots of theory building and policy generation are very similar. Both start with observation of repeated instances of things that are puzzling or processes that seem to be wrong or in need of repair.

- All nurses should know how a bill becomes a law.

- The four key messages in the IOM Report (2010) are:
  1. Nurses should practice to the full extent of their education and training.
  2. Nurses should achieve higher levels of education and training through an improved education system that promotes seamless academic progression.
  3. Nurses should be full partners with physicians and other health professionals in redesigning health care in the United States.
  4. Effective workforce planning and policy making require better data collection and an improved information infrastructure. (p.4)

- The American Academy of Nursing (AAN) Expert Panels' "Essential Psychiatric, Mental Health and Substance Use Competencies for the Registered Nurse," 2010–2011 contains core competencies and related content areas for preparing nurses for basic psychiatric mental health and substance use practice.

### NCLEX-PREP*

1. A student nursing government organization (SNGO) has become aware of an important issue needing addressed at the college. The SNGO decides that they can address the issue through political action because:

   a. It is a group of people organizing themselves to influence others to make changes.
   b. They can threaten a lawsuit if their demands are not met.
   c. They want to proceed cautiously to avoid upsetting the administration.
   d. They don't want to damage their future careers as nurses.

2. The same SNGO meets to decide on its first approach to taking political action. They agree to lobby select administrators for the changes they feel are important. How would they initially be most effective?

   a. Buy radio time to get their message across.
   b. Put up flyers around the campus.
   c. Meet with the administrators individually.
   d. Send out college wide emails.

3. The three primary concerns targeted by health care reform are:

   a. Source, prevention, and waste
   b. Quality, access, and value

   c. Limitation, categorization, and chronicity
   d. Ageism, comprehensiveness, and expense

4. Influencing means using one's persuasive powers. Psychiatric nurses are well-equipped to participate in the political process because they are skilled at:

   a. Influencing people to change their views, consider new options, have new perspectives and open their minds to new ideas
   b. Developing treatment plans that affect change for the individual
   c. Understanding personalities and personality disorders
   d. Juggling multiple facets of a person's care and tend to think holistically

5. The roots of theory building and policy generation are very similar because:

   a. Both can be a very politically influenced.
   b. There are multiple levels, each with a different implication.
   c. Neither can ever be proven as fact.
   d. Both start with observation of repeated instances of things that are puzzling or processes that seem to be wrong or in need of repair.

*Answers to these questions appear on page 639.

## REFERENCES

American Academy of Nursing Expert Panel. (2010–2011). *Essential psychiatric, mental health and substance use competencies for the registered nurse: 2010–2011*. Washington, DC: Author.

American Association of Colleges of Nursing. (October, 2008). *The essentials of baccalaureate education for professional nursing practice*. Washington, DC: Author.

Betts, V. T., & Keepnews, D. (2002). Nursing and the courts. In D. Mason, J. Leavitt, & M. Chaffee (Eds.), *Policy & politics in nursing and health care* (4th ed., pp. 471–478). St. Louis, MO: Saunders (Elsevier).

Copps, L. (2002). Vignette: The nurse as a member of congress in the workplace. In D. Mason, J. Leavitt, & M. Chaffee (Eds.),

*Policy & politics in nursing and health care* (4th ed., pp. 533–535). St. Louis, MO: Saunders (Elsevier).

Disch, J., & Taranto, K. (2002). Creating change in the workplace. In D. Mason, J. Leavitt, & M. Chaffee (Eds.), *Policy & politics in nursing and health care* (4th ed., pp. 333–345). St. Louis, MO: Saunders (Elsevier).

Ehrenreich, B., & English, D. (2010). *Witches, midwives & nurses: A history of women healers*. New York: Feminist Press at the City of New York.

Fairman, J. (2008). *Making room in the clinic: Nurse practitioners and the evolution of modern health care*. New Brunswick, NJ: Rutgers University Press.

Kissinger, H. (1998). *Knowledge and power: Occasional paper of the council of scholars* (Report No. 6). Washington, DC.

Lorette, J., & Jansto, C. (2002). Vignette: How regulations are shaped: The rules of the game. In D. Mason, J. Leavitt, & M. Chaffee (Eds.), *Policy & politics in nursing and health care* (4th ed., pp. 467–470). St. Louis, MO: Saunders (Elsevier).

Mason, D., Leavitt, J., & Chaffee, M. (Eds.). (2002). *Policy & politics in nursing and health care* (4th ed.). St. Louis, MO: Saunders (Elsevier).

McCarthy, C. (2002). Vignette: I believed I could make a difference. In D. Mason, J. Leavitt, & M. Chaffee (Eds.), (4th ed., pp. 536–538 ). *Policy & politics in nursing and health care.* St. Louis, MO: Saunders (Elsevier).

Monroe, J. (2005). Morality, politics, and health policy. In D. Mechanic, L. Rogut, D. Colby, & J. Knickman. *Policy challenges in modern health care* (pp. 13–25). New Brunswick, NJ: Rutgers University Press.

Smoyak, S. (1974). The confrontation process. *American Journal of Nursing, 74*(9), 1632–1635.

Smoyak, S. (1985). Have you questioned authority today? *Nursing Success Today, 2*(8), 16–19.

Smoyak, S. (1990). General systems model: Principles and general applications. In W. Reynolds & D. Cormack (Eds.). *Psychiatric and mental health nursing: Theory and practice* (pp. 133–152). London: Chapman and Hall.

Smoyak, S. (2011). The future of (psychiatric) nursing. *The Journal of Psychosocial Nursing and Mental Health Services, 49* (8), 35–41.

Wakefield, M., Gardner, D., & Guillett, S. (2002). Contemporary issues in government. In D. Mason, J. Leavitt, & M. Chaffee (Eds.), *Policy & politics in nursing and health care* (4th ed., pp. 421–450). St. Louis, MO: Saunders (Elsevier).

*Wyatt v. Stickney* (1970). Reported by Carr, Lauren, Wyatt v. Stickney: A landmark decision, Alabama Disabilities Advocacy Program, Newsletter, July 2004.

# NANDA-I NURSING DIAGNOSES 2009–2011

Note: In order to make safe and effective judgments using NANDA nursing diagnoses it is essential that nurses refer to definitions and defining characteristics of diagnosis listed in this work.

## Domain 1

### Health Promotion
Ineffective Health Maintenance (00099)
Ineffective Self Health Management (00078)
Impaired Home Maintenance (00098)
Readiness for Enhanced Immunization Status (00186)
Self Neglect (00193)
Readiness for Enhanced Nutrition (00163)
Ineffective Family Therapeutic Regimen Management (00080)
Readiness for Enhanced Self Health Management (00162)

## Domain 2

### Nutrition
Ineffective Infant Feeding Pattern (00107)
Imbalanced Nutrition: Less Than Body Requirements (00002)
Imbalanced Nutrition: More Than Body Requirements (00001)
Risk for Imbalanced Nutrition: More Than Body Requirements (00003)
Impaired Swallowing (00103)
Risk for Unstable Blood Glucose Level (00179) 79
Neonatal Jaundice (00194)

Risk for Impaired Liver Function (00178)
Risk for Electrolyte Imbalance (00195)
Readiness for Enhanced Fluid Balance (00160)
Deficient Fluid Volume (00027)
Excess Fluid Volume (00026)
Risk for Deficient Fluid Volume (00028)
Risk for Imbalanced Fluid Volume (00025)

## Domain 3

### Elimination and Exchange
Functional Urinary Incontinence (00020)
Overflow Urinary Incontinence (00176)
Reflex Urinary Incontinence (00018)
Stress Urinary Incontinence (00017)
Urge Urinary Incontinence (00019)
Risk for Urge Urinary Incontinence (00022)
Impaired Urinary Elimination (00016)
Readiness for Enhanced Urinary Elimination (00166)
Urinary Retention (00023)
Bowel Incontinence (00014)
Constipation (00011)
Perceived Constipation (00012)
Risk for Constipation (00015)
Diarrhea (00013)
Dysfunctional Gastrointestinal Motility (00196)
Risk for Dysfunctional Gastrointestinal Motility (00197)
Impaired Gas Exchange (00030)

## Domain 4

### Activity/Rest
Insomnia (00095)
Disturbed Sleep Pattern (00198)
Sleep Deprivation (00096)
Readiness for Enhanced Sleep (00165)
Risk for Disuse Syndrome (00040)
Deficient Diversional Activity (00097)
Sedentary Lifestyle (00168)
Impaired Bed Mobility (00091)
Impaired Physical Mobility (00085)
Impaired Wheelchair Mobility (00089)
Delayed Surgical Recovery (00100)
Impaired Transfer Ability (00090)
Impaired Walking (00088)
Disturbed Energy Field (00050)
Fatigue (00093)
Activity Intolerance (00092)
Risk for Activity Intolerance (00094)
Risk for Bleeding (00206)
Ineffective Breathing Pattern (00032)
Decreased Cardiac Output (00029)
Ineffective Peripheral Tissue Perfusion (00204)
Risk for Decreased Cardiac Tissue Perfusion (00200)
Risk for Ineffective Cerebral Tissue Perfusion (00201)
Risk for Ineffective Gastrointestinal Perfusion (00202)
Risk for Ineffective Renal Perfusion (00203)
Risk for Shock (00205)
Impaired Spontaneous Ventilation (00033)
Dysfunctional Ventilatory Weaning Response (00034)
Readiness for Enhanced Self-Care (00182)
Bathing Self-Care Deficit (00108)
Dressing Self-Care Deficit (00109)
Feeding Self-Care Deficit (00102)
Toileting Self-Care Deficit (00110)

## Domain 5

### Perception/Cognition
Unilateral Neglect (00123)
Impaired Environmental Interpretation Syndrome (00127)
Wandering (00154)
Disturbed Sensory Perception (Specify: Visual, Auditory, Kinesthetic, Gustatory, Tactile, Olfactory) (00122)
Acute Confusion (00128)
Chronic Confusion (00129)
Risk for Acute Confusion (00173)
Deficient Knowledge (00126)

Readiness for Enhanced Knowledge (00161)
Impaired Memory (00131)
Readiness for Enhanced Decision-Making (00184)
Ineffective Activity Planning (00199)
Impaired Verbal Communication (00051)
Readiness for Enhanced Communication (00157)

## Domain 6

### Self-Perception
Risk for Compromised Human Dignity (00174)
Hopelessness (00124)
Disturbed Personal Identity (00121)
Risk for Loneliness (00054)
Readiness for Enhanced Power (00187)
Powerlessness (00125)
Risk for Powerlessness (00152)
Readiness for Enhanced Self-Concept (00167)
Situational Low Self-Esteem (00120)
Chronic Low Self-Esteem (00119)
Risk for Situational Low Self-Esteem (00153)
Disturbed Body Image (00118)

## Domain 7

### Role Relationships
Caregiver Role Strain (00061)
Risk for Caregiver Role Strain (00062)
Impaired Parenting (00056)
Readiness for Enhanced Parenting (00164)
Risk for Impaired Parenting (00057)
Risk for Impaired Attachment (00058)
Dysfunctional Family Processes (00063)
Interrupted Family Processes (00060)
Readiness for Enhanced Family Processes (00159)
Effective Breastfeeding (00106)
Ineffective Breastfeeding (00104)
Interrupted Breastfeeding (00105)
Parental Role Conflict (00064)
Readiness for Enhanced Relationship (00207)
Ineffective Role Performance (00055)
Impaired Social Interaction (00052)

## Domain 8

### Sexuality
Sexual Dysfunction (00059)
Ineffective Sexuality Pattern (00065)
Readiness for Enhanced Childbearing Process (00208)
Risk for Disturbed Maternal/Fetal Dyad (00209)

## Domain 9

### Coping/Stress Tolerance
Post-Trauma Syndrome (00141)
Risk for Post-Trauma Syndrome (00145)
Rape-Trauma Syndrome (00142)
Relocation Stress Syndrome (00114)
Risk for Relocation Stress Syndrome (00149)
Anxiety (00146)
Death Anxiety (00147)
Risk-Prone Health Behavior (00188)
Compromised Family Coping (00074)
Defensive Coping (00071)
Disabled Family Coping (00073)
Ineffective Coping (00069)
Ineffective Community Coping (00077)
Readiness for Enhanced Coping (00158)
Readiness for Enhanced Community Coping (00076)
Readiness for Enhanced Family Coping (00075)
Ineffective Denial (00072)
Fear (00148)
Grieving (00136)
Complicated Grieving (00135)
Risk for Complicated Grieving (00172)
Impaired Individual Resilience (00210)
Readiness for Enhanced Resilience (00212)
Risk for Compromised Resilience (00211)
Chronic Sorrow (00137)
Stress Overload (00177)
Autonomic Dysreflexia (00009)
Risk for Autonomic Dysreflexia (00010)
Disorganized Infant Behavior (00116)
Risk for Disorganized Infant Behavior (00115)
Readiness for Enhanced Organized Infant Behavior (00117) 286
Decreased Intracranial Adaptive Capacity (00049)

## Domain 10

### Life Principles
Readiness for Enhanced Hope (00185)
Readiness for Enhanced Spiritual Well-Being (00068)
Decisional Conflict (00083)
Moral Distress (00175)
Noncompliance (00079)
Impaired Religiosity (00169)
Readiness for Enhanced Religiosity (00171)
Risk for Impaired Religiosity (00170)
Spiritual Distress (00066)
Risk for Spiritual Distress (00067)

## Domain 11

### Safety/Protection
Risk for Infection (00004)
Ineffective Airway Clearance (00031)
Risk for Aspiration (00039)
Risk for Sudden Infant Death Syndrome (00156)
Impaired Dentition (00048)
Risk for Falls (00155)
Risk for Injury (00035)
Risk for Perioperative-Positioning Injury (00087)
Impaired Oral Mucous Membrane (00045)
Risk for Peripheral Neurovascular Dysfunction (00086)
Ineffective Protection (00043)
Impaired Skin Integrity (00046)
Risk for Impaired Skin Integrity (00047)
Risk for Suffocation (00036)
Impaired Tissue Integrity (00044)
Risk for Trauma (00038)
Risk for Vascular Trauma (00213)
Self-Mutilation (00151)
Risk for Self-Mutilation (00139)
Risk for Suicide (00150)
Risk for Other-Directed Violence (00138)
Risk for Self-Directed Violence (00140)
Contamination (00181)
Risk for Contamination (00180)
Risk for Poisoning (00037)
Latex Allergy Response (00041)
Risk for Latex Allergy Response (00042)
Risk for Imbalanced Body Temperature (00005)
Hyperthermia (00007)
Hypothermia (00006)
Ineffective Thermoregulation (00008)

## Domain 12

### Comfort
Readiness for Enhanced Comfort (00183)
Impaired Comfort (00214)
Nausea (00134)
Acute Pain (00132)
Chronic Pain (00133)
Social Isolation (00053)

## Domain 13

### Growth/Development
Adult Failure to Thrive (00101)
Delayed Growth and Development (00111)

Risk for Disproportionate Growth (00113)
Risk for Delayed Development (00112)
Total Urinary Incontinence
Rape-Trauma Syndrome: Compound Reaction
Rape-Trauma Syndrome: Silent Reaction

Effective Therapeutic Regimen Management
Ineffective Community Therapeutic Regimen
  Management
Disturbed Thought Processes

# GLOSSARY

**ABUSE:** Acts of commission or omission that result in harm, potential for harm, or threat of harm. *See also* Drug Abuse

**ACTIVE LISTENING:** Concentrated effort on the part of the nurse to pay close attention to what the patient is saying, both verbally and nonverbally

**ACTIVITIES OF DAILY LIVING:** Activities that include personal hygiene, dressing, eating, mobility, and toileting

**ADDICTION:** Chronic, relapsing brain disease that is characterized by compulsive drug seeking and use, despite harmful consequences

**AFFECTIVE DISORDER:** A term frequently used interchangeably with depressive or mood disorders; predominantly involves a persistent disturbance in mood

**AFFECTIVE FLATTENING:** Restricted range and intensity of emotion

**AGORAPHOBIA:** Fear of being in a place or situation where escape might be difficult or help unavailable in the event of a panic

**ALOGIA:** Decreased production of speech

**AMBIVALENCE:** A state of conflicting or opposing ideas, attitudes, or emotions

**ANHEDONIA:** Inability to feel pleasure or joy from life

**ANOREXIA NERVOSA:** Refusal or inability to maintain a minimally normal body weight

**ANOSOGNOSIA:** Poor insight

**ANXIETY:** Vague feeling involving some dread, apprehension, or other unknown tension

**ASSISTED SUICIDE:** Providing a person with an available means for death such as pills or weapons, with the knowledge of the person's intent to use those means to die but without acting as the direct agent for the death

**ATTITUDES:** General feelings or that which provides a frame of reference for an individual

**AUTISM:** Literally, "living in self"; inability to relate to people and situations, and failure to learn to speak or convey meaning to others through language

**AUTONOMY:** Capacity to make decisions and act on them

**AVOLITION:** Diminished goal-directed activity

**BAD NEWS:** Any new information that the patient interprets as representing significant loss

**BATTERING:** Striking someone repeatedly with violent blows

**BEHAVIORAL PSYCHOLOGY THEORY:** Scientific approach that limits the study of psychology to measurable or observable behavior

**BELIEFS:** Ideas that an individual holds to be true

**BENEFICENCE:** Ethical principle involving doing what is best

**BINGE DRINKING:** Copious amounts of alcohol consumed over a short period of time

**BINGE EATING DISORDER:** Characterized by episodes of binge eating; i.e., eating in a discrete period of time an amount of food that is larger than most other people would eat in a similar period under comparable circumstances

**BIOFEEDBACK:** Also referred to as *applied psychophysiological feedback;* the process of displaying involuntary or subthreshold physiological processes, usually by electronic instrumentation, and learning to voluntarily influence those processes by making changes in cognition

**BIOLOGICAL PSYCHOLOGY THEORY:** The study of human or animal psychology using a biological approach in order to understand human behavior; involves brain physiology, genetics, and evolution as means for understanding behavior

**BOUNDARIES:** The professional spaces between the nurse's power and the patient's vulnerability

**BOUNDARY CROSSING:** A transient, brief excursion across a professional boundary. The action may be inadvertent, unconscious, or even purposeful and done to meet a specific therapeutic need

**BOUNDARY VIOLATION:** Situation resulting when there is confusion between the needs of the nurse and those of the patient; allows nurse to meet his or her own needs rather than the patient's needs

**BROKER CASE MANAGEMENT:** Case management model in which single individuals (brokering case managers) are responsible for referral, placement, and monitoring of patients

**BULIMIA NERVOSA:** Repeated episodes of binge eating followed by compensatory behaviors

**CASE MANAGEMENT:** An outcome-oriented process that coordinates care and advocates for patients and patient populations across the health care continuum

**CHEMICAL CASTRATION:** A hormone medication that reduces testosterone and therefore sexual urges

**CIRCULAR REACTIONS:** Motor reflexes, such as thumb sucking and hand grasping, that then develop into object manipulation that invokes a response from people or the environment (rattle shaking)

**CLASSICAL CONDITIONING:** The learned associative behavioral stimulus-response discovered by Pavlov

**CLINICAL CASE MANAGEMENT:** A worker-intensive, clinical case management model where the individuals commonly have the greatest need for services

**COGNITIVE DEVELOPMENT:** One's ability to understand the world, including interaction with stimuli and objects in the environment, social interactions related to thinking patterns, and how one receives and stores information

**COGNITIVE DISORDERS:** Group of disorders in which a person experiences a disruption in areas of mental function. These areas include orientation, attention, logic, awareness, memory, intellect, language, abstract thinking, and reasoning

**COGNITIVE DISSONANCE:** The inability of the human mind to contain two disparate, conflicting thoughts or beliefs simultaneously. It also includes the process of how a person will engage in rationalization, change beliefs or behaviors to eliminate the tension or imbalance associated with cognitive dissonance, and restore cognitive or mental balance

**COGNITIVE PSYCHOLOGY THEORY:** The study of higher mental processes such as attention, language use, memory, perception, problem solving, and thinking

**COGNITIVE RESTRUCTURING TECHNIQUES:** Strategy that helps a person recognize how his or her thoughts and feelings are contributing to the behavior and then assists the patient in reshaping this thinking to result in more appropriate behaviors and emotions

**COLORADO MODEL:** Continuum of care model of psychiatric case management that combines focused therapy, assertive community treatment, and family-centered interventions

**COMMUNICATION:** The transmission of information or a message from a sender to a receiver

**COMPASSION FATIGUE:** The emotional and physical burnout that may interfere with caring

**COMPETENCE:** The degree to which a patient possesses the cognitive ability to understand and process information

**COMPULSIONS:** Repetitive behaviors (e.g., hand washing, ordering, checking) or mental acts (e.g., praying, counting, repeating words silently) that a person feels driven to perform in response to an obsession or according to rules that must be applied rigidly

**CONFRONTRATION:** Technique used to help the patient take note of a behavior and then examine it

**CONSERVATION:** The ability to recognize that despite something changing shape, it maintains the characteristics that make it what it is (e.g., clay)

**CONTINUUM OF CARE:** Integrated system of settings, services, health care clinicians, and care levels spanning illness to wellness states

**COUNTERTRANSFERENCE:** Occurrence when the health care professional develops a positive or negative emotional response to the patient's transference

**COURAGEOUS CONVERSATIONS:** Conversations held at certain turning points so that the patient and family are able to successfully navigate the predictable and sometimes not-so-predictable pitfalls that accompany illness journeys

**CRISIS:** A time-limited event, usually lasting no more than 4 to 6 weeks, that results from extended periods of stress unrelieved by adaptive coping mechanisms

**CRISIS INTERVENTION:** A time-limited professional strategy designed to address an immediate problem, resolve acute feelings of distress or panic, and restore independent problem-solving skills

**CRITICAL INCIDENT DEBRIEFING:** A formally recognized program with trained staff that allows staff to vent and process feelings in a structured way after particularly stressful patient contacts

**CRITICAL THINKING:** A purposeful method of reasoning that is systematic, reflective, rational, and outcome-oriented

**CRITICAL THINKING INDICATORS™:** Behaviors that demonstrate the knowledge, characteristics, and skills needed to promote critical thinking for clinical decision making

**CULTURAL COMPETENCE:** A set of congruent behaviors, attitudes, and policies that come together in a system, agency, or among professionals and enables that system, agency or those professionals to work effectively in multicultural situations and with diverse social groups

**CULTURAL CONGRUENCE:** Distance between the cultural competence characteristics of a health care organization and the patient's perception of those same competence characteristics as they relate to the patient's cultural needs

**CULTURE:** An integrated pattern of human behavior that includes thought, communication, actions, customs, beliefs, values, lifestyles, and institutions of racial, ethnic, religious or social groups

**CURATIVE FACTORS:** Common factors operating in all types of groups that describe the patterns of interaction in a therapeutic group

**DEBRIEFING:** Method used following a crisis incident to allow staff to verbalize their feelings and thoughts about the event

**DEINSTITUTIONALIZATION:** Movement of patients in mental health institutions back into the community

**DELIRIUM:** An acute disruption in consciousness and cognitive function

**DELUSION:** Erroneous false, fixed beliefs; a misinterpretation of an experience

**DEMENTIA:** A group of conditions that involve multiple deficits in memory and cognition

**DEPENDENCY:** The final stage of substance use and refers to a maladaptive pattern of behavior characterized by progression, tolerance, withdrawal, preoccupation with the behavior regardless of any consequences, and has the potential to be fatal

**DETOXIFICATION:** Process of managing a patient during withdrawal. Detoxification is composed of three components: evaluation, stabilization, and readiness for treatment

**DEVELOPMENTAL DISABILITY:** A diverse group of severe chronic conditions that are due to physical and/or mental impairments

**DIALECTICAL BEHAVIOR THERAPY (DBT):** A form of cognitive behavioral therapy that helps individuals take responsibility for their own behaviors and problems; teaches individuals how to cope with conflict, negative feelings, and impulsivity, thereby enhancing capabilities and improving motivation, which lead to a decrease in dysfunctional behavior

**DISPARITY:** Lack of equality, usually in reference to health and health care

**DISPOSITIONS:** The way a person approaches life and living

**DIVERSITY:** Reality created by individuals and groups from a broad spectrum of demographic and philosophical differences; narrowly, includes age, race, gender, ethnicity, religion, and sexual orientation

**DOMESTIC VIOLENCE:** Causing or attempting to cause physical or mental harm to a family or household member; placing a family or household member in fear of physical or mental harm; causing or attempting to cause a family or household member to engage in involuntary sexual activity by force, threat of force, or duress; engaging in activity toward a family or household member that would cause a reasonable person to feel terrorized, frightened, intimidated, threatened, harassed, or molested

**DRUG ABUSE:** The initial stage of substance use where the individual may have recurrent substance use that leads to failure to meet obligations, puts the individual in hazardous situations, causes legal problems, or results in social, interpersonal, or professional problems

**EATING DISORDER:** A serious disturbance in behaviors associated with eating

**ECHOLALIA:** Parrot-like repetition of another's words

**ECHOPRAXIA:** Involuntary imitation of another's movements and gestures

**EGO DEFENSE MECHANISMS:** Conscious and unconscious tools used to protect and defend the ego

**EMERGING IDENTITIES:** Phase of Travelbee's model characterized by the nurse and the ill person each perceiving the other as unique individuals. The bond of a relationship is beginning to form

**EMOTIONAL LONELINESS:** Loneliness associated with loss of intimacy with a partner, family member, or friend who can no longer support the emotional needs of the elder

**EMPATHETIC LINKAGES:** The ability to feel in oneself the emotions experienced by another person in the same situation

**EMPATHY:** Phase of Travelbee's model characterized by the ability to share in the other person's experience; putting yourself in the other person's shoes, or seeing the world through the other person's eyes

**ENCULTURATION:** Process by which a person learns the requirements of the culture by which he or she is surrounded, and acquires values and behaviors that are appropriate or necessary in that culture

**ENDORPHINS:** Chemicals in the body that are responsible for increasing the sense of well-being; potent mood elevators

**ENRICHED MODEL OF DEMENTIA:** A model that acknowledges that the primary cause of problems for the person with dementia stems from the person's neurological impairment

**EROTOMANIC:** Delusions that another person, usually of higher status, is in love with the individual

**ETHICS:** Collection of philosophical principles that examine the rightness and wrongness of decisions and conduct as human beings

**ETHNICITY:** Selected cultural characteristics used to classify people into groups or categories considered to be significantly different from others

**EXPLOITATION PHASE:** Phase of Peplau's nurse-patient relationship where the bulk of the work is accomplished with the patient taking full advantage of the nursing services offered. This phase encompasses all of the therapeutic activities that are initiated to reach the identified goal

**FAMILY THERAPY:** As insight oriented therapy with the goal of altering interactions between or among family members, thus improving the functioning of the family as a unit or any individual within the family

**FEAR:** Feelings consistent with panic and phobias

**FIDELITY:** Ethical principle focusing on acting as promised

**FLOODING:** Technique that exposes the patient to the anxiety-provoking or feared situation all at once

**FORENSIC NURSING:** Specialty practice that provides services to the legal and criminal system; forensic science is combined with the biopsychological education of registered nurses in scientific investigation, evidence collection, preservation, and analysis, and prevention and treatment of trauma- and/or death-related medical-legal issues

**GENOGRAM:** Tool developed to show a map of the multigenerational family structure and process, geography (urban or rural), gender, age, disability status, and risk status related to sex and gender

**GEROPSYCHIATRY:** The study of psychiatric and mental illness in the aging population

**GESTALT:** Human experience of being whole

**GRAND THEORIES:** Theories that are the most abstract and broad in scope

**GRANDIOSE:** Delusions of inflated worth, power, or knowledge; possibly involving special relationships with deity or famous person

**GROUP:** Any collection of two or more individuals who share at least one commonality or goal, such that the relationship is interdependent

**GROUP DYNAMICS:** Forces that produce patterns within the group as the group moves toward its goals

**GROUP PROCESS:** Interaction among group members

**GROUP THERAPY:** Process by which group leaders with advanced educational degrees and experience provide psychotherapy with members to improve their interpersonal functioning

**HALLUCINATION:** Most commonly auditory or visual but erroneous or false sensory perceptions

**HOMELESS PERSON:** One who lacks a fixed, regular, and adequate nighttime residence; this can be a supervised, publicly or privately operated shelter, a temporary residence for individuals intended to be institutionalized, or a public or private place not ordinarily used as a regular sleeping accommodation for human beings

**HONOR KILLINGS:** Killings based on the belief that women are the property of male relatives and embody the honor of the men to whom they "belong"

**HOPE:** A mental state characterized by the desire to gain an end or accomplish a goal combined with some degree of expectation that what is desired or sought is attainable

**HUMAN BEING:** Unique irreplaceable individual, a one-time being in this world, like yet unlike any person who has ever lived or ever will live

**HUMAN SEXUALITY:** Understanding how people experience themselves as sexual beings

**HUMANISTIC PSYCHOLOGY THEORY:** A group of psychologies that includes early and emerging orientations and perspectives, including Rogerian, existential, transpersonal, phenomenological, hermeneutic, feminist, and other psychologies

**HYPOMANIA:** A sublevel of mania

**HYSTERIA:** Greek for uterus; term used to describe anxiety and anxiety related disorders specifically in women in the 17th and 18th centuries

**IDENTIFICATION PHASE:** Second phase of Peplau's nurse-patient relationship in which the patient recognizes his or her needs for health care for which the nurse can provide assistance

**IMPULSE CONTROL DISORDERS:** Several psychiatric conditions characterized by behavior seeking a small, short-term gain at the expense of a large, long-term loss. Individuals are not able to resist the impetuous behavior

**IN-PATIENT PSYCHIATRIC CASE MANAGEMENT MODEL:** Case management model involving the use of a managed care agent to perform the initial assessment and develop an initial treatment plan

**INSOMNIA:** Difficulty initiating or maintaining sleep

**INTELLECTUAL DISABILITY:** Mental retardation; term used when a person's ability to learn at an expected level and function in daily life are limited

**INTERMITTENT EXPLOSIVE DISORDER:** Failure to resist aggressive impulses leading to serious property destruction or assaults

**INTERPERSONAL MODELS:** Models that focus on the interaction of the person with others)

**INTERPERSONAL RELATIONSHIP:** The connection that exists between two or more individuals with observation, assessment, communication, and evaluation skills serving as the foundation

**INTIMATE PARTNER VIOLENCE:** Violence among spouses or domestic partners

**INTOXICATION:** Reversible substance-specific syndrome with central nervous system response and related behavioral and psychological changes after exposure or ingestion of a substance

**INVOLUNTARY COMMITMENT:** Involuntary admission; the patient admitted against his or her wishes

**JUSTICE:** Ethical principle focusing on fair and equal treatment

**KANTIANISM:** Ethical theory focusing on performing one's duty rather than the "rightness" or "wrongness" of the outcome

**KLEPTOMANIA:** Recurrent failure to resist the impulse to steal

**LEAST RESTRICTIVE ENVIRONMENT:** The safest environment with the minimum restrictions on personal liberty necessary to maintain safety of the patient and the public, and to allow the patient to achieve independence in daily living as much as possible

**LIBIDO:** The driving force behind pleasure-seeking behavior

**LIMIT SETTING:** Specific parameters for what a person can and cannot do

**LINES OF RESISTANCE:** Internal factors that an individual uses to help defend against stressors

**LINGUISTIC COMPETENCE:** Capacity to communicate effectively and convey information in a manner that is easily understood by diverse audiences including persons with limited English proficiency, those who have low literacy skills or are not literate, and individuals with disabilities that impair communication and comprehension

**LOBBYING:** Any action undertaken by an individual or group to influence the thinking and decision making of an elected official at any level of government

**LONELINESS:** An unnoticed inability to do anything while alone

**MAGICAL THINKING:** Belief that thoughts are all-powerful

**MALIGNANT SOCIAL PSYCHOLOGY:** The damaging effects of the negative attitudes and prejudices of other people on someone's personhood

**MANAGED CARE AGENT:** Individual who performs an initial assessment and initiates a treatment plan

**MANAGED CARE ORGANIZATION:** Agencies providing case management, such as insurance companies

**MANIA:** Mental disturbances such as elevated mood, grandiosity, difficulty with attention span

**MATURATIONAL CRISIS:** Crisis that occurs during an individual's normal growth and development, at any point of change

**MELANCHOLIA:** Term (literal meaning, "black bile") used by Hippocrates to describe sad or dark moods noted in patients with depression

**MENTAL HEALTH RECOVERY:** View that encompasses the whole person

**MENTAL ILLNESS:** Mental disorders that are diagnosable conditions characterized by abnormalities in cognition, emotion, or mood, or the highest integrative aspects of behavior, such as social interactions or planning of future activities

**MICRO-LEVEL THEORIES:** Theories that are the least abstract and narrow in scope

**MIDDLE-RANGE THEORIES:** Theories that are less abstract than grand theories; more concrete

**MILIEU MANAGEMENT:** The provision and assurance of a therapeutic environment that promotes a healing experience for the patient

**MOOD:** A person's overall emotional status

**NEUROFIBRILLARY TANGLES:** Thick clots of protein that reside inside damaged neurons and are made from a protein called tau

**NEUROLEPTIC MALIGNANT SYNDROME:** A syndrome where the patient displays muscle rigidity, high fever, unstable blood pressure, diaphroesis, pallor, delirium, tachycardia, tachypnea, and rapid deterioration of mental status

**NONMALEFICENCE:** Ethical principle focusing on doing no harm

**NORMAL LINE OF DEFENSE:** Usual response to stressors, represents the individual's usual state of wellness

**NURSING PROCESS:** Systematic method of problem solving that provides the nurse with a logical, organized framework from which to deliver nursing care

**OBESITY:** A body mass index (BMI) greater than or equal to 30 (kg/m²). *See also* Overweight

**OBJECT PERMANENCE:** The ability of the child to realize that an object is no longer visible despite the fact that it still exists

**OBSESSIONS:** Recurrent and persistent thoughts, impulses, or images experienced at some time during the disturbance that are intrusive and inappropriate, causing marked anxiety or distress

**OPERANT CONDITIONING:** Also called instrumental conditioning; differs from Pavlov's classical conditioning in that it addresses consequences (or responses) and the modification of future behavior based upon the (positive or negative) reinforcement, punishment, or extinction associated with the consequence (response)

**ORIENTATION PHASE:** First phase of Peplau's nurse-patient relationship that includes the initial contact the nurse has with the patient

**ORIGINAL ENCOUNTER:** First phase of Travelbee's model characterized by first impressions by the nurse of the ill person and by the ill person of the nurse. Both the nurse and the ill person perceive each other in stereotypical or traditional roles

**OVERWEIGHT:** A body mass index (BMI) greater than or equal to 25 (kg/m²). *See also* Obesity

**PANIC DISORDER:** Sudden, intense, and unprovoked feelings of terror and dread

**PARAPHILIAS:** Sexual disorders involving recurrent, intense sexual urges, fantasies, or behaviors involving unusual objects, activities, or situations

**PATHOLOGICAL GAMBLING:** Persistent maladaptive gambling behavior

**PERSONALITY:** Who a person is and how that person behaves, which influences an individual's thoughts, feelings, attitudes, values, motivations, and behaviors

**PERSONALITY DISORDERS:** A long-term maladaptive way of thinking and behaving that is ingrained and inflexible

**PERSONALITY TRAITS:** Distinct set of qualities demonstrated over an extended period of time that characterize an individual

**PHOBIA:** Intense fear about certain objects or situations

**PICA:** Persistent eating of one or more nonnutritive substances for a period of at least one month

**PLAY THERAPY:** A method of psychotherapy that uses fantasy and symbolic meanings expressed during play as a medium for communicating and understanding a child's behavior

**POLICY:** In institutions, agencies and governments, policy is the sets of rules, guidelines, procedures, and processes that allow workers or officials to know how to go about conducting their daily tasks

**POLICY MAKING:** A broad term that embodies all the processes in political action. Policy making may also occur on a smaller level as within a family or a hospital unit

**POLITICAL ACTION:** Accomplished by people organizing themselves into a group to influence others to make changes

**POLITICS:** The process of influencing the allocation of resources, whether these are time, money, energy, services, and so on

**POLYPHARMACY:** Use of multiple medications beyond the clinically identified needs of the individual, including prescribed medications, over-the-counter medications, and herbal and homeopathic products

**POSITIVE PERSON WORK:** Means of how one could uphold the personhood of an individual with dementia

**PRIMARY PREVENTION:** Interventions that delay or avoid the onset of illness

**PROCESS GROUPS:** Traditional form of psychotherapy where deep feelings, reactions, and thoughts are explored and processed in a structured way

**PROCESS RECORDING:** The written report of an interaction between the patient and nurse, recorded verbatim to the extent possible and includes both verbal and nonverbal communication of both parties. The content of the interaction is analyzed for meaning and pattern of interaction

**PROGRESSIVELY LOWERED STRESS THRESHOLD:** Model that proposes that a person has a stress threshold firmly established by adulthood but which can be temporarily altered during times of illness, or permanently altered during episodes of brain damage such as in dementia

**PROTECTIVE FACTOR:** Characteristic, variable, or trait that guards against or buffers the effect of risk factors

**PSYCHODYNAMIC THEORIES:** Theories that focus on the unconscious and assert that underlying unconscious or repressed conflicts are responsible for conflicts, disruptions, and disturbances in behavior and personality

**PSYCHOEDUCATIONAL GROUPS:** Groups designed at imparting specific information about a select topic such as medication

**PSYCHOEDUCATIONAL INTERVENTION:** Interventions that include a significant educational component

**PSYCHOMIMETIC DISORDERS:** Medical disorders that mimic psychiatric disorders

**PSYCHONEUROIMMUNOLOGY:** Study of the connection among the immune, nervous, and endocrine systems

**PSYCHOPHARMACOLOGY:** Use of drugs to treat mental illness and its symptoms

**PSYCHOSIS:** Condition involving hallucinations, delusions, or disorganized thoughts, behaviors, or speech

**PYROMANIA:** Fire-setting for pleasure and gratification

**QUALITY OF LIFE:** A state of complete physical, mental, and social well-being and not the absence of disease or infirmity

**RACE:** Biological characteristics and variations within humans, originally consisting of a more or less distinct population with anatomical traits that distinguish that population clearly from others

**RAPPORT:** Nursing actions that alleviate an ill person's distress; a concern and an active interest in others; a belief in the worth, dignity, uniqueness, and irreplaceability of each individual human being; and an accepting, nonjudgmental approach

**REALITY ORIENTATION:** Technique used to improve the quality of life of confused older adults by assisting them to gain a more accurate understanding of their surroundings by regularly presenting confused persons with information about time, place, etc., in an effort to orient them to the here and now

**RELIGIOSITY:** Specific behavioral and social characteristics that reflect religious observance within an identified faith

**REMINISCENCE THERAPY:** The discussion of past activities, events, and experiences with another person or group of people

**RESILIENCE:** The process of adapting well in the face of adversity, trauma, tragedy, threats, or even significant sources of stress

**RESOLUTION PHASE:** Last phase of Peplau's nurse-patient relationship occurring when the patient's needs have been met through the collaborative work of nurse and patient

**REVERSIBILITY:** Concept in which a child realizes that certain things can turn into other things and then back again, such as water and ice

**RISK FACTORS:** Issues that increase an individual's chance for developing an illness

**SCHIZOPHRENIA:** Diagnostic category within the group of schizophrenia spectrum disorders

**SECLUSION:** Placement of the patient in a safe room alone

**SECONDARY PREVENTION:** Interventions focusing on treatment including identifying persons with disorders and standardizing treatment for disorders

**SELF:** The entire person of an individual; an individual's typical character and temporary behavior; the union of elements (body, emotions, thoughts, and sensations) that constitute the individuality and identity of a person

**SELF-AWARENESS:** The process of developing an understanding of one's own values, beliefs, thoughts, feelings, reactions, motivations, biases, strengths, and limitations and recognizing their effect on others

**SELF-DETERMINATION:** Freedom to make decisions without consulting others

**SELF-DISCLOSURE:** A nurse revealing genuine feelings or personal information about him- or herself

**SELF-EFFICACY:** The beliefs persons hold about their ability to accomplish something and about what the outcomes will be

**SELF-REFLECTION:** A process of becoming conscious of largely tacit or intuitive knowledge, motives, and attitudes that underlie a professional interpersonal interaction

**SENILE DEMENTIA:** Memory loss as part of normal aging

**SENSATE FOCUS:** Therapy involving a progression of sexual intimacy typically over the course of several weeks, eventually leading to penetration and orgasm

**SEROTONIN SYNDROME:** A life-threatening situation due to an overactivity of serotonin or disruption in the neurotransmitter's metabolism manifested by fever, sweating, agitation, tachycardia, hypotension, and hyperreflexia

**SEXUAL DISORDERS:** Also called paraphilias; recurrent, intense sexual urges, fantasies, or behaviors involving unusual objects, activities, or situations

**SEXUAL DYSFUNCTIONS:** Conditions characterized by a disturbance in the processes involved in the sexual response cycle

**SEXUAL FUNCTIONING:** The actual act of expressing yourself sexually either for pleasure or for reproductive purposes

**SEXUAL HEALTH PROMOTION:** The integration of the somatic, emotional, intellectual, and social aspects of sexual beings in ways that are positively enriching and that enhance personality, communication, and love

**SITUATIONAL CRISIS:** Crisis that stems from an unanticipated life event that threatens one's sense of self or security

**SOCIAL CRISIS:** Also called an adventitious crisis; crisis that results from an unexpected and unusual social or environmental catastrophe that can either be natural or man-made

**SOCIAL LONELINESS:** Loneliness due to loss of contact with peers, friends, or groups that have shared and supported the needs of the elderly individual

**SOCIAL PSYCHOLOGICAL THEORY:** The study of the effect of social variables on individual behavior, attitudes, perceptions, and motives

**SOMATIC:** Referring to the body

**SPECIFIC PHOBIA:** Marked and persistent fear and avoidance of a specific object or situation

**SPIRITUALITY:** Cognitions, values, and beliefs that address ultimate questions about the meaning of life, God, and transcendence, which may or may not be associated with formal religious observance

**SPLITTING:** Viewing reality in polarized categories

**STATUTORY RAPE:** Sexual intercourse with an adolescent between the ages of 13 and 18

**STRESS:** An increase in an individual's level of arousal created by a stimulus

**STRESS-VULNERABILITY-COPING MODEL:** One way of understanding how risk factors are involved with the development of psychiatric-mental health disorders; identification of risk factors according to three categories: biological, personal, and environmental

**SUBSTANCE ABUSE:** Recurrent substance use that leads to failure to meet obligations, puts the individual in hazardous situations, causes legal problems, or results in social, interpersonal, or professional problems

**SUBSTANCE DEPENDENCE:** Maladaptive pattern of behavior characterized by progression, tolerance, withdrawal, and preoccupation with the behavior regardless of any consequences, which has the potential to be fatal

**SUFFERING:** Feeling of displeasure that range from simple transitory mental, physical, or spiritual discomfort to extreme anguish, and to those phases beyond anguish, namely, the malignant phase of despairful not caring and the terminal phase of apathetic indifference

**SUICIDAL IDEATION:** Intruding thoughts of harming one's self

**SUICIDE:** Taking of one's own life; a behavior, not a disorder; an act of ambivalence often resulting from an affective disorder

**SYMBOLIC PLAY:** A child's ability to separate behaviors and objects from their actual use and instead use them for play

**SYMPATHY:** Phase of Travelbee's model occurring when the nurse desires to alleviate the cause of the patient's illness or suffering

**SYSTEM:** Any group of components sufficiently related to identify patterns of interaction

**SYSTEMATIC DESENSITIZATION:** Process in which a subject is gradually introduced to the source of a fear or anxiety, over the course of time and under controlled conditions

**TELEHEALTH:** Psyhciatric intervention via telecommunications such as phone or video conferencing

**TEMPERAMENT:** Innate aspects of personality that determine how a person tends to respond to the world; distinctive behavior involved with activity and adaptation

**TERTIARY PREVENTION:** Interventions focusing on maintenance including decreasing relapse or recurrence, and providing rehabilitation

**THEORY:** An organized set of concepts that explains a phenomenon or set of phenomena

**THERAPEUTIC:** Of or relating to the treatment of disease or disorders by remedial agents or methods

**THERAPEUTIC COMMUNICATION:** A patient-focused interactive process involving verbal and nonverbal behaviors

**THERAPEUTIC GROUPS:** Groups used to promote psychologic growth, development, and transformation

**THERAPEUTIC MILIEU:** A climate and environment that is therapeutic and conducive to psychiatric healing within a structured group setting; it encompasses the elements of trust, safety, peer support, and recovery psychoeducation to enable patients to work through psychological issues

**THERAPEUTIC USE OF SELF:** A process of self awareness through one's own growth and development and one's interaction with others

**THOUGHT DISORDER:** Broad term applying to illnesses involving disordered thinking and disturbances in reality orientation and social involvement

**TIME OUT:** A situation in which the nurse allows the patient to get away from the area and go to a safe, non-stimulating place to regain emotional control

**TOLERANCE:** Need for markedly increased amounts of a substance to achieve the desired effect; conversely, a markedly diminished effect with continued use of same amount of a substance

**TRANSFERENCE:** A psychodynamic term to describe the patient's emotional response to the health care provider

**TRANSINSTITUTIONALIZATION:** The transfer of mental health care from mental hospitals to jails and prisons where there are three times more mental health patients than in mental hospitals and where one in six detainees is diagnosed with a mental illness

**TRICHOTILLOMANIA:** Recurrent pulling out of one's hair for pleasure or tension relief

**UTILITARIANISM:** Ethical theory in which decisions should be based on producing the best outcome or the greatest happiness for the greatest number of people

**VALIDATION THERAPY:** A popular psychosocial intervention involving the affirmation of the person's feelings and the adoption of a non-judgmental approach on the part of the caregiver

**VALUES:** Abstract positive and negative concepts that represent ideal conduct and goals

**VERACITY:** Ethical principle focusing on honesty and truthfulness

**VOLUNTARY ADMISSION:** Patient agrees or consents to admission

**VULNERABLE POPULATIONS:** Groups of individuals typically defined by race/ethnicity, socio-economic status, geography (urban or rural), gender, age, disability status, and risk status related to sex and gender

**WITHDRAWAL:** Substance-specific syndrome with significant physical and psychological distress and impairment in areas of functioning that occur after reducing or stopping heavy and prolonged use of the substance

**WORRY:** A term indicative of symptoms such as anxious misery, apprehensive expectations, and obsessions

# ANSWERS to NCLEX PREP QUESTIONS

## Chapter 1
**1.** c; **2.** d; **3.** b; **4.** c; **5.** a

## Chapter 2
**1.** c; **2.** c; **3.** a; **4.** d; **5.** b; **6.** a

## Chapter 3
**1.** a; **2.** c; **3.** b; **4.** b; **5.** d

## Chapter 4
**1.** c; **2.** b; **3.** a; **4.** d; **5.** b

## Chapter 5
**1.** b; **2.** d; **3.** a; **4.** c; **5.** b

## Chapter 6
**1.** a; **2.** c; **3.** d; **4.** c; **5.** a

## Chapter 7
**1.** c; **2.** a; **3.** b; **4.** c; **5.** d

## Chapter 8
**1.** c; **2.** a, b, e; **3.** d; **4.** b; **5.** a

## Chapter 9
**1.** a; **2.** b; **3.** c; **4.** d; **5.** c; **6.** b; **7.** b

## Chapter 10
**1.** c; **2.** a; **3.** d; **4.** c; **5.** b

## Chapter 11
**1.** d; **2.** b; **3.** c; **4.** a, b, d; **5.** d; **6.** d; **7.** a

## Chapter 12
**1.** b; **2.** c; **3.** b; **4.** a; **5.** b; **6.** b; **7.** d; **8.** d; **9.** c

## Chapter 13
**1.** c; **2.** a; **3.** d; **4.** b; **5.** a; **6.** b

## Chapter 14
**1.** b, d; **2.** b; **3.** a; **4.** c; **5.** d; **6.** a

## Chapter 15
**1.** a; **2.** b; **3.** c; **4.** b; **5.** b, c, d; **6.** b; **7.** a; **8.** c

## Chapter 16
**1.** b; **2.** d; **3.** c; **4.** b; **5.** a; **6.** c, e, f

## Chapter 17
**1.** a; **2.** c; **3.** d; **4.** a, b, d, e; **5.** c

## Chapter 18
**1.** b; **2.** d; **3.** b, c; **4.** a; **5.** b, d, c, a

## Chapter 19
**1.** d; **2.** c; **3.** d; **4.** c; **5.** a

## Chapter 20
**1.** c; **2.** c, a, e, d, b; **3.** a; **4.** d; **5.** b

## Chapter 21
**1.** a; **2.** d, b, f, c, e, a; **3.** c; **4.** d; **5.** b; **6.** a

## Chapter 22
**1.** b; **2.** a; **3.** c; **4.** a, b, e; **5.** a, b, c, e

## Chapter 23
**1.** a; **2.** b; **3.** a; **4.** c; **5.** d; **6.** b

## Chapter 24
**1.** d; **2.** b; **3.** c; **4.** b, c, a, d, f, e, g; **5.** a; **6.** c

## Chapter 25
**1.** d; **2.** b; **3.** a; **4.** c; **5.** b

## Chapter 26
**1.** b; **2.** c; **3.** b, c, d, e; **4.** a; **5.** a, b, c, d, e

## Chapter 27
**1.** c; **2.** b; **3.** b; **4.** d; **5.** a

## Chapter 28
**1.** d; **2.** a; **3.** c; **4.** a, c, b, d; **5.** b; **6.** c

## Chapter 29
**1.** a; **2.** c; **3.** b; **4.** a; **5.** d

# NCLEX REVIEW QUESTIONS

1. The nurse is providing care to a patient with frontotemporal dementia. The nurse develops a plan of care for this patient, integrating knowledge about which of the following?

    a. The patient has a much shorter life expectancy.
    b. The patient has probably experienced multiple ministrokes.
    c. The patient's memory will remain intact.
    d. The patient is at risk for falls due to muscle rigidity.

2. A group of nursing students are reviewing information about systems theory. The students demonstrate the need for additional review when they identify which of the following?

    a. The interactions of a system are viewed in a linear fashion.
    b. The parts of a closed system are isolated from the environment.
    c. A change in one component affects other components.
    d. An open system is dynamic and constantly changing.

3. A nurse is providing an in-service presentation for staff members of a clinic about how the clinic is promoting culturally competent care. Which of the following would the nurse include?

    a. Emphasis on mental health as a separate entity from primary health care
    b. Services that are broad in scope, reflecting general cultural concepts
    c. Services that are focused primarily on the major cultural group
    d. Focus on the help-seeking behaviors of the unique populations being served

4. A nurse assesses a patient and determines that the patient is in the alarm stage of responding to stress. Which of the following would the nurse most likely assess?

    a. Pupil constriction
    b. Decrease in heart rate
    c. Rapid respirations
    d. Dry skin

5. A patient is being admitted to the inpatient unit with a diagnosis of borderline personality disorder. When preparing to assess this patient, which of the following would the nurse need to keep in mind?

    a. The patient is likely to demonstrate behaviors to get attention.
    b. The patient's behavior typically reflects a need to prevent abandonment.
    c. The patient most likely has a history of involvement with law enforcement.
    d. The patient will exhibit an extreme suspiciousness about others.

6. After reviewing information related to the symptoms of schizophrenia, a group of nursing students indicate the need for additional review when they identify which of the following as a positive symptom?

    a. Delusion
    b. Hallucination
    c. Affective flattening
    d. Echolalia

7. During an interpersonal relationship, a patient identifies that a nurse reminds him of his grandmother and begins to respond to the nurse as he would his grandmother. The nurse recognizes this as which of the following?

    a. Boundary testing
    b. Transference
    c. Boundary crossing
    d. Counter-transference

8. After teaching a group of students about housing services along the continuum of care, the instructor determines that the students need additional teaching when they identify which of the following as an example?

    a. Halfway house
    b. Psychiatric home care
    c. Supervised apartment
    d. Therapeutic foster care

9. A nurse is assessing a patient with an eating disorder for complications. Which of the following might the nurse assess?

    a. Hypertension
    b. Increased muscle strength
    c. Cold intolerance
    d. Tachycardia

10. A group of nursing students are reviewing information about Peplau's phases of the nurse-patient relationship and how they apply to the nursing process. The students demonstrate understanding of the information when they identify which of Peplau's phases as correlating to the implementation step of the nursing process?

    a. Orientation
    b. Identification
    c. Exploitation
    d. Resolution

11. A student nursing government organization (SNGO) has become aware of an important issue needing addressed at the college. The SNGO decides that they can address the issue through political action because:

    a. It is a group of people organizing themselves to influence others to make changes.
    b. They can threaten a lawsuit if their demands are not met.
    c. They want to proceed cautiously to avoid upsetting the administration.
    d. They don't want to damage their future careers as nurses.

12. A nursing instructor is creating a teaching plan for a class about critical thinking. Which of the following would the instructor be least likely to include as a necessary cognitive skill?

    a. Analysis
    b. Creativity
    c. Inference
    d. Self-regulation

13. The nurse is assessing a patient in whom pathological gambling is suspected. Which statement(s) would the nurse interpret as reflecting the diagnostic criteria for this condition? Select all that apply.

    a. "I find myself going back to the casino the next day to get even."
    b. "I started out with small amounts, but now I'm using half of my paycheck."
    c. "I might bet $5 on a football pool every so often."
    d. "I'm going to hit the jackpot again, like I did once before."
    e. "I went to the racetrack after I told my wife I had to work late."

14. While interacting with a patient, the patient says, "How about we meet later after you are done with work and go grab a cup of coffee and talk?" Which response by the nurse would be most appropriate?

    a. "That sounds like fun but I'm busy after work."
    b. "Remember, I'm here as a professional to help you."
    c. "Don't be silly. I can't meet you after work."
    d. "Okay, but this needs to be our secret."

15. A group of nursing students is reviewing information about the interpersonal theorists, Peplau and Travelbee. The students demonstrate understanding of the information when they identify which person as a key influence on Peplau?

    a. Harry Sullivan
    b. Victor Frankl
    c. Ida Orlando
    d. Sigmund Freud

16. A nurse is preparing a presentation about polypharmacy to a local church group of seniors. Which of the following would the nurse least likely include as a common unresolved issue contributing to this problem?

    a. Depression
    b. Fear
    c. Anxiety
    d. Pain

17. A nurse is preparing an in-service presentation about sexual dysfunction for a group of nurses involved in a continuing education course. As part of the presentation, the nurse is planning to describe the classic male sexual response cycle. Place the phases of the cycle in the order in which the nurse would present the information.

    a. Resolution
    b. Desire
    c. Orgasm
    d. Excitement

18. A nursing instructor is preparing a class discussion about the development of mental health care over time. Which of the following would the instructor include as occurring first?

    a. Development of psychoanalytic theory
    b. Establishment of the National Institute of Mental Health
    c. Use of medical treatments such as bloodletting and immobilization
    d. Emphasis on supportive, sympathetic care in a clean, quiet environment

19. A nurse is working with a patient diagnosed with dementia to foster the patient's personhood. Which of the following would be appropriate to use? Select all that apply.
    a. Intimidation
    b. Labeling
    c. Acceptance
    d. Objectification
    e. Collaboration
    f. Recognition

20. A patient is diagnosed with schizophrenia, catatonic type. Which of the following would the nurse expect to assess? Select all that apply.
    a. Stereotyped movements
    b. Mutism
    c. Absence of delusions
    d. Echopraxia
    e. Odd beliefs

21. A group of nurses in the emergency department (ED) are discussing a patient who has been admitted almost every holiday with suicide ideation. One of the nurses stated that the patient is not serious about hurting himself and should not be admitted the next time he comes in. Which response by the charge nurse would be most appropriate?
    a. "Telling him we cannot see him may be the answer to stop this behavior."
    b. "Each episode must be individually evaluated and all options explored."
    c. "He obviously needs support that he is not getting elsewhere."
    d. "We should avoid showing any emotion to him the next time he comes in."

22. A group of students are reviewing information about the classification of addictive disorders. The students demonstrate understanding of the information when they identify which of the following as a substance use disorder?
    a. Substance dependence
    b. Substance-induced disorder
    c. Susbstance intoxication
    d. Substance withdrawal

23. An elderly patient is experiencing social loneliness. Which of the following most likely would be involved?
    a. Loss of contact
    b. Loss of intimacy
    c. Loss of independence
    d. Loss of support

24. A patient with PTSD is exhibiting hypervigilence. Which statement would the nurse interpret as indicating this?
    a. "I'm having trouble sleeping at night."
    b. "I've been really irritable and angry."
    c. "I always have to watch my back."
    d. "I just can't seem to relax."

25. The following are phases identified by the model proposed by the anti-violence movement in Oregon. Place them in the proper sequence from beginning to end.
    a. Setup
    b. Fantasy
    c. Planning
    d. Abuse
    e. Rationalize
    f. Guilt
    g. Normal

26. Applying Freud's theory, which of the following stages would occur first in the development of personality?
    a. Oral
    b. Phallic
    c. Latency
    d. Anal

27. A group of students are reviewing information about the numerous issues that impact the mental health of physically ill patients. The students demonstrate a need for additional study when they identify which of the following?
    a. Unhealthy lifestyle practices as an adult can be traced to negative events in childhood.
    b. Grief is an abnormal response that interferes with a person's ability to heal.
    c. Neuropeptides and their actions are addressed with psychoneuroimmunology.
    d. Pain causes increased secretion of cortisol, which disrupts the immune system.

28. A patient with addiction is undergoing treatment that focuses on redirecting dysfunctional thought processes. The patient is involved in which of the following?
    a. Motivational enhancement therapy
    b. Cognitive behavioral therapy
    c. Mindfulnesss
    d. Community reinforcement

29. A group of nursing students are reviewing information on boundaries, boundary crossings, and boundary violations. The students demonstrate understanding of the information when they state which of the following?
    a. "Most times, a boundary crossing will lead to a boundary violation."
    b. "Boundary violations can be therapeutic in some instances."
    c. "Boundaries are unnecessary if the patient and nurse view each other as equals."
    d. "Boundary crossings can result in a return to established boundaries."

30. A nurse is interviewing a child diagnosed with a conduct disorder. Which of the following would the nurse expect to assess?
    a. Repetitive, stereotypical behaviors
    b. Difficulty organizing tasks
    c. Lack of follow-through with directions
    d. Bullying behaviors

31. While working with a patient diagnosed with an antisocial personality disorder, the nurse notes that the patient is beginning to exhibit signs that he is losing emotional control. The nurse assists the patient in moving to a safe, quiet area to regain his control. The nurse is using which of the following?
    a. Time out
    b. Limit setting
    c. Confrontation
    d. Cognitive restructuring

32. A woman is brought by her husband to the emergency department. The woman has significant swelling surrounding her right eye and bruising over the right side of her face. She is also holding her right upper arm that is covering a large bruised area. The nurse suspects intimate partner violence. When interviewing the woman, which statement would indicate that the woman is in the honeymoon phase of the cycle of violence?
    a. "I feel like I'm walking on eggshells."
    b. "He said he was sorry and wouldn't do it again."
    c. "I need to make sure I don't make him angry."
    d. "It was my fault because I didn't have dinner ready on time."

33. The following are the steps of Bailey's Journey of Grief Model. Place the steps in their proper sequence after the experience of loss.
    a. Searching
    b. Reinvestment
    c. Protest
    d. Reorganization
    e. Despair

34. When applying Maslow's hierarchy of needs, which needs category would be the highest level to be achieved?
    a. Safety
    b. Self-actualization
    c. Love
    d. Self-esteem

35. Travelbee identifies three major concepts for her theory. Which concept provides the nurse with the most powerful intervention?
    a. Hope
    b. Suffering
    c. Human being
    d. Empathy

36. The psychiatric-mental health nurse is using the CAGE assessment tool to screen for alcohol abuse. Which question would the nurse ask first?
    a. "Have you ever had a drink first thing in the morning to steady your nerves?"
    b. "Have people annoyed you by criticizing your drinking?"
    c. "Have you ever felt you should cut down on your drinking?"
    d. "Have you ever felt bad or guilty about your drinking?"

37. A nurse is interviewing an adolescent for indications of suicidal ideation. Which patient statement would be a cause for concern?
    a. "Don't worry, I'm not going to be bothering anyone anymore."
    b. "Sometimes I feel like my parents are dictators."
    c. "I used to like to draw, but I've found music is more relaxing."
    d. "School is okay but I'd much rather play sports."

38. A psychiatric-mental health nurse is a member of several groups. Which of the following would be considered an informal group?
    a. Treatment team
    b. Specialty nursing association
    c. Friends from work
    d. Nurses working on the unit

39. The following tasks reflect the stages of growth and development as identified by Sullivan. Place them in the order in which they would occur beginning with infancy.
    a. Self-identity development
    b. Delayed gratification
    c. Same-sex relationships
    d. Oral gratification
    e. Opposite-sex relationships
    f. Peer relationships

40. A situation with a patient is escalating and the staff determines that restraints are necessary. Which of the following would occur first?

    a. Explaining that the staff is there to help
    b. Approaching the patient slowly as a unit
    c. Taking down the patient to apply the restraints
    d. Obtaining an order for the restraints

41. When describing the results of integrating interpersonal models in psychiatric-mental health nursing, which of the following would be least appropriate to include?

    a. Therapeutic communication
    b. Milieu management
    c. Psychopharmacology
    d. Process groups

42. When describing physical boundaries to a group of nursing students, which of the following would the instructor use as an example of this type of boundary?

    a. Feelings
    b. Choices
    c. Touching
    d. Spirituality

43. A nurse is preparing a presentation for a local senior citizen group about dementia and delirium. When describing delirium, which of the following would the nurse include?

    a. It occurs gradually over a period of time.
    b. It is usually due to an underlying medical condition.
    c. It requires medication to slow its progression.
    d. It remains fairly constant throughout the day.

44. The nurse is assessing a female adolescent who engages in self-harming behavior. Which of the following would the nurse identify as a possible trigger? Select all that apply.

    a. Rejection by friends
    b. Substance misuse
    c. Feelings of power
    d. Worthlessness
    e. Parental divorce

45. A nurse is interviewing a patient who came to the area after she fled her home country, during a political revolution. When assessing the patient, the nurse notes that the patient has adopted several of the local customs of the area. The nurse identifies this as which of the following?

    a. Ethnicity
    b. Enculturation
    c. Spirituality
    d. Religiosity

46. The roots of theory building and policy generation are very similar because:

    a. Both can be a very politically influenced.
    b. There are multiple levels, each with a different implication.
    c. Neither can ever be proven as fact.
    d. Both start with observation of repeated instances of things that are puzzling or processes that seem to be wrong or in need of repair.

47. A nurse who will be providing care to a psychiatric-mental health patient is in the orientation phase of the relationship. The nurse would most likely assume which role?

    a. Counselor
    b. Teacher
    c. Stranger
    d. Surrogate

48. A psychiatric-mental health nurse is engaged in a therapeutic dialogue with a patient. The patient states, "I've been feeling so down lately." Which of the following would the nurse identify as being congruent with the patient's statement?

    a. Wide facial grin
    b. Low tone of voice
    c. Fidgeting
    d. Erect posture

49. When providing care to individuals involved in a community disaster, which of the following would be the priority?

    a. Food and water
    b. Safety
    c. Shelter
    d. Referrals

50. Which of the following best depicts a psychiatric-mental health nurse case manager acting in the role of a consultant?

    a. Instructing the patient about the need for adhering to his medication schedule.
    b. Promoting patient access to the least restrictive treatment method.
    c. Recommending possible vocational services that would be appropriate.
    d. Proactively identifying potential barriers that may affect the patient.

51. A nursing instructor is developing a class for a group of students about the theories of mental health and illness. When gathering information for a discussion on cognitive theories, which of the following would the instructor most likely include?

    a. Development of psychoanalytic theory
    b. Thorndike
    c. Seligman
    d. Beck
    e. Bandura

52. A group of nursing students are reviewing information about substance abuse in adolescence. The students demonstrate an understanding of the information when they identify which of the following as the most commonly abused substance in adolescence?

    a. Cocaine
    b. Cannabis
    c. Alcohol
    d. Amphetamines

53. A PMHN is engaged in advocacy for patients of a local clinic. The nurse is employing which ethical principle?

    a. Beneficence
    b. Fidelity
    c. Kantianism
    d. Veracity

54. The same SNGO meets to decide on its first approach to taking political action. They agree to lobby select administrators for the changes they feel are important. How would they initially be most effective?

    a. Buy radio time to get their message across.
    b. Put up flyers around the campus.
    c. Meet with the administrators individually.
    d. Send out college wide emails.

55. A psychiatric-mental health nurse (PMHN) is preparing a presentation for a group of student nurses about psychiatric-mental health nursing. Which statement would the nurse include in the presentation about this specialty?

    a. A PMHN needs to obtain a graduate level degree for practice.
    b. Advanced practice PMHNs can engage in psychotherapy.
    c. Basic level PMHNs mainly focus on the patient's ability to function.
    d. PMHNs primarily work in acute in-patient settings.

56. A psychiatric-mental health nurse is working as a case manager and has a caseload of 120 patients. The nurse is responsible for assessing the patients' needs and arranging for services. The nurse is functioning within which case management model?

    a. Broker case management
    b. Clinical case management
    c. Intensive case management
    d. Continuum of care

57. When describing the possibility of developing a psychiatric-mental health disorder related to a medical condition, which disorder would the nurse identify as most common and problematic?

    a. Schizophrenia
    b. Acute stress disorder
    c. Personality disorder
    d. Depression

58. In planning care for a patient newly admitted with severe major depressive disorder, the primary nursing intervention would be to:

    a. Avoid a stressful situation by asking for the patient's participation in the plan.
    b. Teach the patient about relapse and the signs and symptoms of mania.
    c. Assess if the patient has more than two weeks worth of medication.
    d. Evaluate the patient's cognitive functioning and ability to participate in planning care.

59. A group of nursing students is reviewing class information about the different types of personality disorders. The students demonstrate understanding of this information when they identify which of the following as a Cluster A personality disorder? Select all that apply.

    a. Borderline personality disorder
    b. Paranoid personality disorder
    c. Avoidant personality disorder
    d. Schizoid personality disorder
    e. Narcissistic personality disorder
    f. Antisocial personality disorder

60. A nurse is planning to implement complementary and alternative medicine therapies with a patient. In which of the following would the nurse include energy biofield therapies?

    a. Meditation
    b. Visualization
    c. Aromatherapy
    d. Acupuncture

61. A child is diagnosed with ADHD. When reviewing the child's history, which of the following would the nurse expect to find?

    a. Exposure to a traumatic event
    b. Difficulty engaging in quiet leisure activities
    c. Frequent losses of temper
    d. Previous diagnosis of oppositional defiant disorder

62. An older adult patient is admitted to the acute care facility for treatment of bacterial pneumonia for which the patient is receiving oxygen therapy and antibiotics. When assessing the patient, the nurse notes that the patient has suddenly become confused and agitated and is having increasing difficulty staying focused. The nurse suspects which of the following?

    a. Depression
    b. Dementia
    c. Delirium
    d. Generalized anxiety disorder

63. Which of the following patients would be least likely to require involuntary commitment?
    a. Patient convicted of substance abuse required to undergo treatment
    b. Patient who is actively experiencing suicidal ideation
    c. Patient with depression who is in need of treatment
    d. Patient deteriorating from a severe, persistent mental illness

64. The three primary concerns targeted by health care reform are:
    a. Source, prevention, and waste
    b. Quality, access, and value
    c. Limitation, categorization, and chronicity
    d. Ageism, comprehensiveness, and expense

65. While interviewing a middle-aged woman who has come to the mental health care facility, the woman states, "My oldest son just left for college last week. I'm so lost without him. The house seems so empty." The nurse would interpret the woman's statement as suggesting which type of crisis?
    a. Maturational
    b. Situational
    c. Social
    d. Adventitious

66. A nurse is establishing boundaries with a patient who is coming to a community mental health center for treatment. Which of the following would be least appropriate to do during the orientation phase?
    a. Give the patient some information about the nurse's personal life.
    b. Explain to the patient the reason for the nurse being there.
    c. Describe what it is that the nurse can provide for the patient.
    d. Discuss the time, place, and frequency for the meetings.

67. A group of nursing students are reviewing information related to the development of psychiatric-mental nursing. The students demonstrate understanding of the information when they identify which person as emphasizing the use of the interpersonal process?
    a. Florence Nightingale
    b. Linda Richards
    c. Dorothea Dix
    d. Hildegard Peplau

68. Which statement would the nurse expect a newly admitted married patient with mania to make? "I can:
    a. not do anything right anymore."
    b. manage our finances better than any accountant."
    c. understand why my spouse is so upset that I spend so much money."
    d. not understand where all our money goes."

69. The nurse is assessing a patient and determines that the patient is experiencing a normal grief response based on which of the following?
    a. Openly expresses anger
    b. Non-intact reality testing
    c. Persistent sleeping problems
    d. Consistently dysphoric

70. Influencing means using one's persuasive powers. Psychiatric nurses are well-equipped to participate in the political process because they are skilled at:
    a. Influencing people to change their views, consider new options, have new perspectives and open their minds to new ideas
    b. Developing treatment plans that affect change for the individual
    c. Understanding personalities and personality disorders
    d. Juggling multiple facets of a person's care and tend to think holistically

71. The nurse is working with group of patients who have immigrated to the United States from several Latin American and South American countries and is reviewing the situation for possible barriers to accessing mental health services. Which of the following would the nurse identify as an environmental barrier?
    a. No translator on staff at the facilities
    b. Knowledge about the mental health problems
    c. Availability of family support
    d. Beliefs of mental illness caused by demon

72. A group of students are reviewing information about the various types of sexual disorders and dysfunctions. The students demonstrate understanding of this topic when they identify which of the following as examples of sexual disorders? Select all that apply.
    a. Vaginismus
    b. Exhibitionism
    c. Pedophilia
    d. Premature ejaculation
    e. Male erectile disorder

73. A group of nursing students is reviewing information about anxiety disorders. The students demonstrate a need for additional study when they identify which of the following as a compulsion?
    a. Hearing voices that tell a person he is the king
    b. Repeatedly washing hands
    c. Touching the door knob three times before leaving
    d. Walking in a specific pattern when entering a room

74. When developing the plan of care for a patient who has attempted suicide, an understanding of which of the following would be most critical for the nurse to integrate into the plan?

    a. Patients who attempt suicide and fail will not try again.
    b. The more specific the plan, the greater the risk of suicide.
    c. People who talk about suicide rarely go ahead and attempt it.
    d. People who attempt suicide and fail do not really want to die.

75. A group of nursing students is reviewing the different types of drugs that may be used to treat dementia of the Alzheimer's type. The students demonstrate a need for additional study when they identify which of the following as an example of a cholinesterase inhibitor?

    a. Donepezil
    b. Rivastigmine
    c. Galantamine
    d. Atorvastatin

76. While performing a routine health check-up on a teenager who is 5 feet tall and 100 lbs, a nurse begins to suspect that a patient may be experiencing an eating disorder. Which statement by the patient would lead the nurse to suspect this?

    a. "Look at me, look at how fat I am."
    b. "My last period was about 6 weeks ago."
    c. "I just lost 5 pounds so I could fit into my prom dress."
    d. "I usually like to swim about 3 times a week."

77. When applying the Power and Control Wheel to evaluate a victimizer's behavior, which of the following would indicate intimidation?

    a. Calling the victim names
    b. Making the victim feel guilty
    c. Destroying property
    d. Controlling who the victim talks to

78. A nurse breaches a patient's confidentiality and shares this confidential information in writing. The nurse would most likely be charged with which of the following?

    a. Slander
    b. Medical battery
    c. Libel
    d. Assault

79. An elderly patient comes to the clinic complaining of difficulty sleeping, stating, "It just started about a week or so ago." When obtaining the patient's history, which of the following would the nurse identify as potentially contributing to the patient's complaint?

    a. Hypertensive agent added to his medications
    b. History of arthritis
    c. Dinner usually consumed at 5:30 p.m.
    d. Routine bedtime at 11:00 p.m.

80. A group of nursing students is reviewing information about adjustment disorders in children. The students demonstrate a need for additional study when they identify which of the following as a possible stressor?

    a. Witness to the death of a parent
    b. Moving away of a close friend
    c. Parental divorce
    d. Bullying by a classmate

81. When applying the therapeutic use of self during assessment, which of the following would be important for the nurse to demonstrate? Select all that apply.

    a. Genuineness
    b. Respect
    c. Empathy
    d. Adherence to rigid rules
    e. Honesty

82. A nurse is preparing a presentation for a local community group about adolescence and mental health problems. Which of the following would the nurse expect to include?

    a. Time typically heals any problems that adolescents experience.
    b. Problems in adolescence can continue into adulthood if not addressed.
    c. Adolescents primarily experience disorders that are uncommon in adults.
    d. The stigma associated with mental disorders is seen less frequently with adolescents.

83. A patient comes to the clinic for a routine check-up and is to have laboratory testing completed. During the assessment, the patient reveals that he is afraid of needles and begins to hyperventilate. The patient also becomes diaphoretic and complains of a lump in his throat. The nurse would suspect which of the following?

    a. Generalized anxiety disorder
    b. Posttraumatic stress disorder
    c. Acute stress disorder
    d. Specific phobia

84. The most important reason why a full physical health assessment is warranted for patients with depressive symptoms is that:
    a. they are less likely to complain about their physical health and may have an undiagnosed medical problem.
    b. physical health complications are likely to arise from antidepressant therapy.
    c. the attention afforded to the patient during the assessment is beneficial in decreasing social isolation.
    d. physiological changes may be the underlying cause of depression, and, if present, must be addressed.

85. A nurse is integrating Travelbee's theory of the nurse-patient relationship into the care being provided to a patient. Which of the following is demonstrated when the nurse implements actions to alleviate the ill person's distress?
    a. Emerging identities
    b. Empathy
    c. Sympathy
    d. Rapport

86. A patient states, "I get so anxious sometimes. I just don't know what to do." The nurse responds by saying, "You should try to do some exercise when you start to feel this way. I know it helps me when I get anxious." The nurse is using which of the following?
    a. Clarifying
    b. False reassurance
    c. Validating
    d. Giving advice

87. A group of psychiatric-mental health nurses are preparing an inservice presentation about stress and crisis. Which of the following would the group most likely include in the presentation?
    a. Crisis can be a chronic situation due to stress.
    b. An unknown stimulus is responsible for the crisis.
    c. The stress associated with crisis must be real.
    d. Crisis is not considered a mental illness.

88. When implementing secondary prevention strategies, which of the following would the psychiatric-mental health nurse do first?
    a. Conduct community screening
    b. Identify existence of risk factors
    c. Teach about coping skills
    d. Make referrals for immediate treatment

89. A patient is brought to the emergency department by an emergency medical team because the patient was behaving violently. When talking with the patient, the nurse notices that he suddenly shifts the conversation from one topic to another but the topics are completely unrelated. The nurse would document this finding as which of the following?
    a. Delusion
    b. Hallucination
    c. Neologism
    d. Loose association

90. The nurse is preparing to assess a patient with acute psychosis for the first time. Which of the following would be a priority?
    a. Providing a gentle touch to calm the patient
    b. Taking as long as necessary to gather all the information
    c. Focusing on the type of delusions the patient is experiencing
    d. Assessing for indications of suicidal ideation

91. A nursing instructor is preparing a class on anxiety disorders and the biological influences associated with this group of illnesses. Which of the following would the instructor include as a primary neurotransmitter involved in the anxiety response?
    a. Gamma-aminobutyric acid (GABA)
    b. Serotonin
    c. Dopamine
    d. Norepinephrine

92. A patient with alcohol intoxication and a blood alcohol level of 190 mg percent is exhibiting signs of withdrawal. Which of the following would the nurse expect to assess? Select all that apply.
    a. Restlessness
    b. Visible hand trembling
    c. Hypersensitivity to light
    d. Auditory hallucinations
    e. Pulse rate less than 89 beats per minute
    f. Seizures

93. A nurse is engaged in assessing a male patient and has determined that it is appropriate to move on to assessing the patient's sexual history. Which of the following would be most important for the nurse to do first?
    a. Make sure that the nurse and patient are alone
    b. Ask the patient about whether or not he is sexually active
    c. Question the patient about any history of sexual abuse
    d. Obtain the patient's permission to ask him questions about this area

94. The nurse is reviewing the medical record of a patient, that reveals that the patient experiences intense sexual arousal when being bound and humiliated. The nurse interprets this information as characteristic of which of the following?

    a. Sexual masochism
    b. Sexual sadism
    c. Frotteurism
    d. Fetishism

95. A nurse is observing the behavior of an 18-month-old child. The child is playing with a toy that involves placing different shaped blocks into the appropriately shaped opening. The child is attempting to place a round block into the round hole. The nurse interprets this as indicating which of the following?

    a. Circular reaction
    b. Object permanence
    c. Symbolic play
    d. Magical thinking

96. A nurse is preparing a presentation for a local community group about abuse and violence. Which of the following would the nurse most likely include?

    a. Abuse is primarily seen in lower socioeconomic areas where poverty is rampant.
    b. Children typically are around the ages of 8 to 10 when they suffer abuse.
    c. Abuse indicates an underlying mental health disorder that is out of control.
    d. An abuser frequently uses more than one method to achieve the goal.

97. A nurse is thinking about working in a correctional facility. Which characteristic would be important for the nurse to have?

    a. Self-awareness
    b. Prejudice
    c. Cultural bias
    d. Inflexibility

98. A nurse working at a homeless shelter in a large downtown area should be aware that there are many factors that contribute to homelessness of the mentally ill. Which of the following would the nurse identify as potentially contributing to homelessness? Select all that apply.

    a. Substance abuse
    b. Poverty
    c. Inadequate housing
    d. Low-paying jobs
    e. Rise in public assistance
    f. Affordable health care

99. When assessing an older adult for suspected abuse, the nurse interviews the victim together with the caregiver based on which rationale?

    a. To evaluate the patient and caregiver relationship
    b. To identify inconsistencies in their statements
    c. To confirm the patient's level of alertness
    d. To determine the need for adult protective services

100. A nurse is working in an area that has a high concentration of Asian immigrants and is developing a plan to minimize possible risk factors for poor mental health. Which of the following would the nurse least likely address?

    a. Social isolation
    b. Interaction with new culture
    c. Feelings of persecution
    d. Stress of acculturation

101. A group of students are reviewing information about the impact of culture, race, and ethnicity on mental health and mental health care delivery. The students demonstrate understanding when they identify which of the following as reflecting cognitive styles?

    a. Methods for processing information
    b. Information denoting evidence for change
    c. Primary locus of decision making
    d. Sources of anxiety and anxiety reduction

102. A nurse is preparing a presentation for a local community group about health care disparities and minorities. The nurse uses the African American population as an example. Which of the following would the nurse include in the presentation?

    a. They are more likely to receive a diagnosis for mental health conditions.
    b. The rates for suicide are lower in this population.
    c. They tend to report physical complaints related to mental illness.
    d. Lower doses of psychotropic medications are commonly prescribed.

103. A patient is being referred for a Level 2 ambulatory behavioral health care service. Which of the following might the nurse expect to be used?

    a. Partial hospitalization program
    b. Assertive community treatment
    c. Day treatment program
    d. Clubhouse program

104. A nurse is preparing a presentation for a senior citizen group about stresses that may affect their physical and mental health. Which of the following would the nurse least likely include as an effect of stress?

    a. Increased physiologic aging
    b. Enhanced immune function
    c. Slowing of normal mental changes
    d. Increased risk for depression

105. The nurse is working with the parents of a child with a mental health problem in developing a system of rewards and punishments for the child's behavior. The nurse is demonstrating integration of which theorist?

    a. Freud
    b. Pavlov
    c. Skinner
    d. Erikson

106. A patient with anorexia is admitted to the in-patient facility because of cardiovascular problems. The patient's minimal normal acceptable weight is 125 pounds. Which weight would the nurse interpret as indicative of anorexia?

    a. 118 pounds
    b. 112 pounds
    c. 107 pounds
    d. 100 pounds

107. A patient with dementia of the Alzheimer's type is demonstrating increasing problems with wandering. In addition, the patient's caregiver reports that the patient has wandered into the kitchen during the night and left the stove on several times over the past few weeks. Which of the following would be a priority nursing diagnosis for this patient?

    a. Chronic confusion related to effects of dementia
    b. Risk for injury related to increased wandering
    c. Deficient knowledge related to effects of illness
    d. Disturbed sleep pattern related to frequent nighttime awakenings

108. A patient is brought to the emergency department by a friend who states, "He's been in a lot of pain and has been using oxycodone quite a bit lately." Which of the following would lead the nurse to suspect that the patient is experiencing intoxication?

    a. Tachycardia
    b. Pinpoint pupils
    c. Rhinorrhea
    d. Gooseflesh

109. When assessing a patient with dyspareunia, which of the following would the nurse expect the patient to report?

    a. Inability to attain adequate lubrication in response to sexual excitement
    b. Recurrent pain in the genital area with sexual intercourse
    c. A deficient last of desire for sexual activity
    d. An avoidance for engaging in sexual activity

110. A group of students are reviewing medications used to treat depression in the older adult. The students demonstrate a need for additional study when they identify which agent as approved for use in the elderly?

    a. Escitalopram
    b. Paroxetine
    c. Duloxetine
    d. Aripiprazole

111. A group of students are reviewing information related to the variables associated with the levels of ambulatory behavioral care. The students demonstrate understanding when they identify which of the following as a service variable?

    a. Risk/dangerousness
    b. Social system support
    c. Level of functioning
    d. Milieu

112. The following are examples of therapy that may be used with a patient experiencing a psychiatric-mental health problem. Place the treatments in the proper order based on the concept of the least restrictive environment.

    a. Talk therapy
    b. Involuntary medication administration
    c. Behavioral therapy
    d. Seclusion

113. A nurse is working in the community and is preparing a presentation for a local group of parents about child abuse. Which of the following would the nurse most likely include in this presentation?

    a. Physicians are the individuals responsible for reporting suspected child abuse.
    b. Child abuse primarily involves emotional and sexual abuse.
    c. The perpetrator is commonly someone the child knows.
    d. When children do reveal abuse, they experience revictimization.

114. The nurse is implementing validation therapy with a patient diagnosed with dementia of the Alzheimer's type. Which of the following would the nurse do?

    a. Confirm the patient's version of reality
    b. Place cards on the bathroom and bedroom doors
    c. Repeatedly tell the patient what day it is
    d. Have the patient discuss past events

115. A group of students are reviewing information about eating disorders. The students demonstrate an understanding of the topic when they identify which of the following as being associated with bulimia nervosa?

    a. Greater occurrence in males
    b. Use of severe fasting rituals
    c. More common in women in their 20s and 30s
    d. High correlation with overweight and obesity

116. A patient is experiencing heroin withdrawal and develops hypertension. Which of the following would the nurse expect to administer?

    a. Phenobarbital
    b. Diazepam
    c. Clonidine
    d. Acamprosate

117. A patient with antisocial personality disorder is observed taking an other patient's belongings. Which initial nursing intervention would be most appropriate?

    a. Tell the patient's primary nurse what happened
    b. Obtain an order for an antipsychotic medication
    c. Confront the patient about his behavior
    d. Encourage the patient to discuss his angry feelings

118. The nurse is developing a plan of care for a patient diagnosed with a schizotypal personality disorder. Which of the following would be most appropriate to include in the plan?

    a. Setting specific boundaries for behavior
    b. Teaching problem-solving techniques
    c. Fostering decision-making skills
    d. Implementing social skills training

119. When engaging in therapeutic communication for the initial encounter with the patient, which of the following would be most appropriate for the nurse to use?

    a. Silence
    b. "What would you like to discuss?"
    c. "Are you having any problems with anxiety?"
    d. "Why do you think you came here today?"

120. Deinstitutionalization occurred as a result of which of the following?

    a. Mental Retardation Facilities and Community Mental Health Centers Act
    b. National Mental Health Act
    c. Omnibus Budget Reconciliation Act (OBRA)
    d. The Surgeon General's Report on Mental Health

121. A group of nursing students in a psychiatric-mental health rotation are reviewing information about various theorists associated with self, therapeutic use of self, and the therapeutic relationship. The students demonstrate understanding of the materal when they identify which theorist as having identified three core conditions for a therapeutic relationship?

    a. Hildegard Peplau
    b. Phil Barker
    c. Carl Rogers
    d. Joyce Travelbee

122. A nursing instructor is preparing a class for a group of students about case management in psychiatric-mental health nursing. Which of the following would the instructor most likely include about psychiatric-mental health case management?

    a. It is a method of care delivery that is unique to psychiatric-mental health nursing.
    b. It is a health care financing strategy aimed at reducing costs.
    c. It involves multi-disciplinary collaboration to achieve outcomes.
    d. It involves reducing fragmentation of care during illness episodes.

123. When integrating critical thinking, clinical decision making, the interpersonal relationship, and the nursing process, which of the following would be of primary importance?

    a. Nurse's self-awareness
    b. Setting for care
    c. Patient's needs
    d. Achievement of outcomes

124. A nurse is providing primary prevention to a local community group about psychiatric-mental health disorders. Which of the following would the nurse include as a protective factor? Select all that apply.

    a. Flexibility
    b. High intelligence
    c. Limited social relationships
    d. Absence of recreational activities
    e. Adequate economic resources

125. During a group session, the group leader notices that a member is boasting about his accomplishments in an effort to get the group to focus on him rather than focus on the task of the group. The leader would identify this behavior as reflecting which role?

    a. Encourager
    b. Energizer
    c. Recognition seeker
    d. Standard setter

126. A patient has been severely depressed and expressing suicidal thoughts. She was started on antidepressant medication four days ago. She is now more energized and communicative. Which of the following would be most important for the nurse to do?

    a. Allow the patient to have unsupervised passes to her home.
    b. Encourage the patient to participate in group activities.
    c. Increase vigilance with the patient's suicidal precautions.
    d. Recognize that the patient's suicidal potential has decreased.

127. The psychiatric nurse understands that dysthymia differs from a major depression episode in that dysthymia:
    a. Typically has an acute onset.
    b. Involves delusional thinking.
    c. Is a chronic low-level depression.
    d. Does not include suicidal ideation.

128. The psychiatric-mental health nurse is working with a patient diagnosed with alcohol abuse and is describing the 12-step program of Alcoholics Anonymous. Which of the following would the nurse include?
    a. Participants are selected based on their ability to attend meetings.
    b. The desire to quit drinking is the underlying concept.
    c. Sponsors are selected by the leader of the group meeting.
    d. Sobriety requires that the person focus on future events.

129. Which of the following would the nurse identify as a major issue involved with intermittent explosive disorder?
    a. Fear of discovery
    b. Ineffective health maintenance
    c. Injury
    d. Substance abuse

130. A group of nursing students are reviewing information related to impulse control disorders. The students demonstrate an understanding of the information when they identify which behavior as characteristic of trichotillomania?
    a. Fire setting
    b. Stealing
    c. Pulling out of hair
    d. Property destruction

131. A patient with anorexia nervosa disorder engages in binge eating and purging behaviors. Which of the following would the patient be least likely to use for purging?
    a. Diuretics
    b. Enemas
    c. Laxatives
    d. Antiemetics

132. The nurse is developing a teaching plan for a patient with an impulse control disorder. The nurse integrates knowledge of which of the following in this plan?
    a. An increase in tension leads to an increase in arousal.
    b. The act immediately leads to feelings of regret.
    c. A need for pleasure is the driving force for acting.
    d. Increased arousal leads to a rise in stress.

133. A PMHN is working with patients with psychiatric-mental health disorders who are incarcerated. The nurse is engaging in which of the following?
    a. Forensic nursing
    b. Disaster response
    c. Case management
    d. Telehealth

134. When describing vulnerable populations to a group of students, which of the following would the nursing instructor include?
    a. They typically experience increased risks for depression.
    b. Advocacy is a primary nursing role.
    c. The patient is usually completely dependent on the nurse.
    d. Children are more vulnerable than the elderly.

135. A group of nursing students are reviewing ethical principles and theories. They demonstrate understanding of the information when they identify utilitarianism as which of the following?
    a. Honesty
    b. Fair and equal treatment
    c. Doing no harm
    d. Greater good

136. A patient who is exhibiting acute psychotic symptoms is determined to be of threat to himself. Which level of care would be most appropriate for the patient to receive?
    a. Acute inpatient care
    b. Partial hospitalization
    c. Psychiatric emergency care
    d. Residential services

137. When describing Travelbee's view of suffering to a class, which of the following would the instructor include?
    a. It is confined to situations involving physical illness.
    b. It is easily controlled through communication.
    c. It can range from simple discomfort to extreme anguish.
    d. It determines how a person will survive.

138. A nursing instructor is preparing a class lecture about impulse control disorder. When describing kleptomania, which of the following would the instructor include?
    a. The patient needs the item for personal use.
    b. The item is too expensive for the patient to purchase.
    c. The object reflects an expression of anger.
    d. The person lacks a need for the object.

139. A psychiatric-mental health nurse identifies a nursing diagnosis of defensive coping for a patient being treated for alcohol intoxication. Which statement would support this diagnosis?
    a. "I really just drink when my life gets really stressful."
    b. "My employer said I might lose my job if things don't change."
    c. "I just can't do anything right, I'm such a failure."
    d. "My family just seems to be falling apart lately."

140. A patient with an anxiety disorder is asked to imagine specific aspects of the feared situation while engaged in relaxation. The nurse identifies this as which of the following?
    a. Flooding
    b. Systematic desensitization
    c. In vivo exposure
    d. Implosion therapy

141. A group of nursing students are reviewing the different classes of antidepressants. The students demonstrate understanding of the information when they identify sertraline as exerting its action on which neurotransmitter?
    a. Serotonin
    b. Dopamine
    c. Gamma-aminobutyric acid (GABA)
    d. Norepinephrine

142. Which statement by a patient with bipolar disorder would indicate the need for additional education about his prescribed lithium carbonate therapy? "I will:
    a. drink about 2 liters of liquids daily."
    b. restrict my intake of salt."
    c. take my medications with food."
    d. have my blood drawn like the doctor ordered."

143. During a group session, a member states that she feels embarrassed about being arrested for trying to steal clothing from a department store. Several other group members then share similar feelings about their involvement with law enforcement, which then leads to a discussion about thinking about consequences and learning from the experience.
    The leader interprets this interaction as reflecting which curative factor?
    a. Instillation of hope
    b. Universality
    c. Altruism
    d. Imitative behavior

144. A nursing instructor is preparing a teaching plan for a class about nursing theories. Which of the following would the instructor include when describing the Neuman Systems Model?
    a. The person is an energy field continually interacting with the environment.
    b. Each patient has a central core that includes survival factors common to all.
    c. A proper environment is necessary to promote the patient's reparative powers.
    d. The nurse and patient engage in an interpersonal process to reach a desired goal.

145. A group of nursing students are reviewing the various risk factors associated with psychiatric-mental health disorders. The students demonstrate understanding of the information when they identify which of the following as a family risk factor?
    a. Poverty
    b. High crime rate
    c. Placement in foster care
    d. Temperament

146. The following are phases associated with a crisis. Which of the following occurs first?
    a. Distress occurs as every method of coping fails.
    b. Anxiety increases as past coping methods are ineffective.
    c. Exposure to a stressor leads to use of past coping mechanisms.
    d. New and different coping strategies are tried.

147. When describing the concept of self, which of the following would be most appropriate to include?
    a. Discovery of personal identity throughout life
    b. A typically positive process of feedback
    c. The similarities shared with others in the environment
    d. An interaction among two or more individuals

148. During the orientation phase of the nurse-patient relationship, the nurse focuses communication on which of the following?
    a. Reason for the patient seeking help
    b. The patient as a whole
    c. Expected routines
    d. Time frame for interaction

149. After teaching a group of students about risk and protective factors, the nursing instructor determines that additional teaching is needed when the students state which of the following about resilience?
    a. "Everyone is born with resilience but not everybody uses it."
    b. "It is a protective factor that helps balance out the risk factors."
    c. "Individuals need time to develop resilience."
    d. "Resilience promotes better coping with trauma or stress."

150. When engaging in critical thinking, the psychiatric-mental health nurse draws a reasonable conclusion after looking at the evidence and proposing alternatives. The nurse is using which cognitive skill?
    a. Evaluation
    b. Explanation
    c. Interpretation
    d. Inference

151. A psychiatric-mental health patient requires level two case management services. Which of the following most likely would be involved?
    a. Crisis prevention
    b. Extensive services
    c. Crisis management
    d. Supportive services

152. After engaging in an argument with a friend at work, a person becomes angry. Moments later, upon returning to his/her office, he punches the wall. The person is demonstrating which defense mechanism?
    a. Suppression
    b. Rationalization
    c. Denial
    d. Displacement

153. A nurse is in the resolution phase of the interpersonal relationship with a patient. The nurse would also be engaged in which step of the nursing process?
    a. Assessment
    b. Planning
    c. Implementation
    d. Evaluation

154. A patient with schizophrenia is about to start medication therapy with clozapine. Which of the following would be most important for the nurse to do?
    a. Obtain a baseline white blood cell count
    b. Monitor the patient for high fever
    c. Suggest the use of hard candy to alleviate dry mouth
    d. Assess for cogwheel rigidity

155. Which of the following would the nurse expect to assess in a patient who is diagnosed with an obsessive-compulsive personality disorder?
    a. Preoccupation with details
    b. Suspiciousness of others
    c. Exaggerated sense of self-importance
    d. Unwillingness to get involved with others

156. A patient with panic disorder is prescribed venlafaxine. The nurse identifies this agent as which of the following?
    a. Selective serotonin reuptake inhibitor (SSRI)
    b. Serotonin/norepinephrine reuptake inhibitor (SNRI)
    c. Benzodiazepine
    d. Atypical antipsychotic

157. When engaging in critical thinking, which of the following would the nurse ask first?
    a. "What would be the best course of action?"
    b. "What is the issue at hand?"
    c. "What could have been missed?"
    d. "What factors might be affecting the patient?"

158. A psychiatric-mental health nurse case manager is reviewing a patient's assessment information and determines that more information is needed to determine why the patient stopped coming to the clinic for his medication prescription. The nurse is demonstrating which of the following?
    a. Communication
    b. Critical thinking
    c. Negotiation
    d. Collaboration

159. A mother and her adult daughter are experiencing a conflict. As a result, the mother turns to her sister and focuses her attention on her. The adult daughter then begins to focus on her work role. Applying the Bowen Family Systems Model, which of the following is present?
    a. Differentiation of self
    b. Emotional triangle
    c. Multigenerational transmission
    d. Corrective recapitulation of the primary family group

160. A group is in the orientation phase of development. The group facilitator would be involved with which of the following?
    a. Keeping the group on task
    b. Clarifying what is happening in the group
    c. Reviewing group accomplishments
    d. Describing group expectations

161. A patient is receiving a second-generation antipsychotic agent. Which of the following might this be?
    a. Chlorpromazine
    b. Haloperidol
    c. Fluphenazine
    d. Aripiprazole

162. The nurse is assessing an elderly patient. The nurse determines that the patient is at risk for suicide based on which of the following? Select all that apply.
    a. Female gender
    b. Living alone
    c. History of diabetes, arthritis, and stroke
    d. Polypharmacy
    e. Recent death of spouse

163. The nurse is conducting an interview with a patient diagnosed with schizophrenia. Throughout the conversation, the patient responds to questions and statements with, "okay." The nurse interprets this as reflecting which of the following?
    a. Affective flattening
    b. Alogia
    c. Avolition
    d. Anhedonia

164. A group of nursing students are reviewing information about theories of mental illness. The students demonstrate a need for additional review when they attribute which of the following as a concept identified by Albert Bandura?
    a. Reciprocal determination
    b. Behavior modeling
    c. Cognitive dissonance
    d. Self-efficacy

# ANSWERS to NCLEX REVIEW QUESTIONS

1. c
2. a
3. d
4. c
5. b
6. c
7. b
8. b
9. c
10. c
11. a
12. b
13. a, b, d, e
14. b
15. a
16. b
17. b, d, c, a
18. c
19. c, e, f
20. a, b, d
21. b
22. a
23. a
24. c
25. b, c, a, d, f, e, g
26. a
27. b
28. b

29. d
30. d
31. a
32. b
33. c, a, e, d, b
34. b
35. a
36. c
37. a
38. c
39. d, b, f, c, e, a
40. b
41. c
42. c
43. b
44. a, b, e
45. b
46. d
47. c
48. b
49. a
50. c
51. c
52. c
53. a
54. c
55. b
56. a

57. d
58. d
59. b, d
60. d
61. b
62. c
63. c
64. b
65. a
66. a
67. d
68. b
69. a
70. a
71. c
72. b, c
73. a
74. b
75. d
76. a
77. c
78. c
79. a
80. a
81. a, b, c, e
82. b
83. d
84. d

85. d
86. d
87. d
88. b
89. d
90. d
91. a
92. b, c, d
93. d
94. a
95. a
96. d
97. a
98. a, b, c, d, e
99. a
100. b
101. a
102. c
103. b
104. b
105. c
106. d
107. b
108. b
109. b
110. d
111. d
112. a, c, b, d

113. c
114. a
115. c
116. c
117. c
118. d
119. b
120. a
121. c
122. c
123. c
124. a, b, e
125. c
126. c
127. c
128. b
129. c
130. c
131. d
132. a
133. a
134. b
135. d
136. c
137. c
138. d
139. a
140. b

141. a
142. b
143. b
144. b
145. c
146. c
147. a
148. b
149. a
150. d
151. d
152. d
153. a
154. a
155. a
156. b
157. b
158. b
159. b
160. d
161. d
162. b, c, d, e
163. b
164. c